Traumatic Stress and Long-Term Recovery

Katie E. Cherry
Editor

Traumatic Stress and Long-Term Recovery

Coping with Disasters and Other Negative Life Events

Springer

Editor
Katie E. Cherry
Department of Psychology
Louisiana State University
Baton Rouge, LA
USA

ISBN 978-3-319-18865-2 ISBN 978-3-319-18866-9 (eBook)
DOI 10.1007/978-3-319-18866-9

Library of Congress Control Number: 2015945811

Springer Cham Heidelberg New York Dordrecht London

Printed on acid-free paper

Springer International Publishing AG Switzerland is part of Science+Business Media (www.springer.com)

Preface

Natural and technological disasters, acts of terrorism, wars, and interpersonal violence are frequent occurrences in the world today. When traumatic events happen, their impact may be felt personally and across many societal levels—locally, nationally, and globally. Given the ubiquity of such events, one possible response is to *look away*. Perhaps, we have become desensitized to traumatic happenings, where events that capture media attention briefly no longer invite our continued attention or concern. Another response is to *look at* catastrophic events, remember the survivors and their losses, and consider how these events may have changed peoples' lives and shaped history. For individuals who have been directly affected by disaster, the experience may be overwhelming, bringing stress and prolonged suffering that threatens health and well-being. Yet, resilience and recovery are also among the many psychological outcomes associated with traumatic event exposure. Years after the event, people remember what happened, revisiting disastrous events in memories driven by calendar–year anniversaries or perhaps brought to mind by commemorative activities that mark the passage of time.

The 10-year anniversary of the 2005 Atlantic Hurricanes, Katrina and Rita that dealt a catastrophic blow to the US Gulf Coast, is in the minds and hearts of many who experienced these two disasters either directly or indirectly. My earlier edited volume focused on the 2005 hurricanes, Katrina and Rita, from a lifespan developmental perspective (Cherry 2009). After completing this volume, I began to consider the long-term effects of natural disaster exposure and the consequences of catastrophically destructive events for peoples' daily lives. Finding an answer to the seemingly simple question, "How do post-disaster psychological reactions play out over time?" was important to me. I sought a research-based, scientifically valid answer to the question of how disasters affect people in the years after these events. Having an answer to this question would be gratifying and valuable for several reasons. Personally, I would have something useful to say about coping and recovery to hurricane survivors in south Louisiana. Professionally, as a social scientist, I know that empirical research and theory on disaster-related traumatic stress and the longevity of effects may provide direction for the development of evidence-based interventions to lessen suffering and mitigate adversity.

Promoting healing and recovery for those whose lives have been disrupted by disaster is a common rallying cry heard among a variety of health and wellness professionals, faith-based communities, clergy, and concerned citizens. In south Louisiana, I knew that 2015 would be a year set aside for observing the 10-year Katrina anniversary. However, anticipation of the year 2015 led to a deeper realization; 2015 also marks the 70-year anniversary of the liberation of Auschwitz, the deadly Nazi concentration camp in occupied Poland, and a dark reminder of the World War II Holocaust. The longevity of emotional pain and potential pathways to healing for hurricane survivors brought a gradual awareness that the platform of disaster exposure and long-term recovery is much wider and far more temporally expansive than I had initially thought. Consequently, this volume is written with the expressed intent of providing a broader context for understanding disaster effects, their consequences, and how suffering may (or may not) be resolved over time.

The present volume contains 23 chapters written by scholars from around the globe, many of whom are prolific leaders in their areas of expertise. These chapters provide the reader with a diverse array of research and theory, along with a unique glimpse into the experiences of many different populations whose lives have been altered by traumatic events. For convenience in exposition, this volume is organized into three main sections: (1) Traumatic Experiences: On Events that Change Lives, (2) Consequences of Trauma Exposure, and (3) Healing after Trauma: Resilience and Long-Term Recovery. This three-part presentation is intentionally linear, although most people will quickly realize that traumatic experiences may neither unfold so neatly nor necessarily run their course in such an orderly sequence. The reader will also detect a developmental perspective within these chapters, consistent with an urgent need to recognize that traumatic events not only disrupt lives, but also may alter the developmental context and trajectories of growth and change for individuals and families over time and across generations. A glimpse of the content of this volume follows.

Section I focuses on traumatic experiences. The opening chapter offers an elegant conceptual tour of traumatic stress (which differs from the stresses of ordinary life only by degree). The *Conservation of Resources* theory is highlighted, providing a useful conceptual framework for understanding the dynamic relationships among the loss of valued resources and post-disaster psychological reactions over time. The next four chapters bring an array of natural and technological disasters into sharp focus: wildfires, tornadoes, multiple hurricanes and the British Petroleum Deepwater Horizon oil spill as well as the Great East Japan earthquake and the resulting tsunami and nuclear disaster. The last three chapters in this section focus on traumatic events delivered by the hands of humanity: mass shootings in public places, soldiers' experience of war captivity and torture, and the potential transmission of extreme trauma across generations directly affected by the World War II Holocaust.

Section II casts a spotlight on the consequences of traumatic event exposure. This section opens with an ambitious and insightful chapter on early childhood adversity in relation to health outcomes across the lifespan. The next five chapters separately address a variety of psychosocial consequences following disaster: the long-term emotional consequences of severe stress exposure for adolescents; stress appraisal and coping self-efficacy; relocating permanently or rebuilding hurricane-damaged homes and communities; chaos, upheaval, and survival after disaster; and the successes (and failures) of faith-based communities after the 2005 hurricanes Katrina and Rita. This section closes with a cogent chapter on ambiguous loss—a unique type of loss experienced when an individual is presumed dead (e.g., the thousands washed away in the 2011 tsunami) although there is no body to bury, hence no opportunity for normal pathways of grief resolution to be realized.

Section III addresses healing after trauma, including discussions of resilience and long-term recovery. The lead chapter highlights the unique challenge for older persons exposed to trauma (either currently or earlier in their developmental history) and the dual realities of vulnerability and resilience experienced in later life. A conceptual model is presented, *The Pursuit of Happiness in a Hostile World*, which offers promising new directions for research on subjective well-being and lifetime adversities. The next five chapters address different but complementary facets of long-term recovery: ego development and lost possible selves; younger and older coastal fishers facing hurricane losses; trauma, religion, and spirituality as pathways to healing; faith and coping after disaster; and benefit finding and looking for potentially positive outcomes after disaster. The penultimate chapter covers the concept of complicated grief, along with an efficacious method of treatment. The final chapter with the last word on healing comes from a World War II Holocaust survivor whose perspective on forgiveness offers a uniquely liberating approach to releasing oneself from the pain of the past.

The present volume offers scholarly insights and a rich and diverse array of behavioral evidence concerning the experience of traumatic stress and long-term recovery. The intent of this volume has been to illuminate traumatic events that change lives, their consequences, and the process of healing after trauma based on theory and research and perhaps, most importantly through voices of people who have faced and survived catastrophic disasters and other forms of trauma. The scholarly pursuit of understanding traumatic events and their long-term effects by academicians and practitioners is not new (cf. Freedy and Hobfoll 1995). In the words of the late clinical psychologist Charles R. Snyder, an accomplished scholar in the field of stress and coping, "Undeniably, therefore, stressors keep rolling in like waves onto the psychological shores of humanity" (Snyder 2001, p. *x*). Indeed, the ongoing wave of present-day disasters interspersed among turbulent world events serves to remind us of the critical challenges that lie ahead for health and wellness professionals in the twenty-first century.

Louisiana State University Katie E. Cherry

References

Cherry, K. E. (Ed.) (2009). *Lifespan perspectives on natural disasters: Coping with Katrina, Rita and other storms*. New York: Springer.

Freedy, J., R., & Hobfoll, S. E. (1995). *Traumatic stress: From theory to practice.* New York: Plenum Press.

Snyder, C. R. (Ed.). (2001). *Coping with stress: Effective people and processes.* New York: Oxford University Press.

Contents

Contributors

Donice M. Banks Department of Psychology, University of New Orleans, New Orleans, LA, USA

Charles C. Benight Department of Psychology, Trauma Health & Hazards Center, University of Colorado at Colorado Springs, Colorado Springs, CO, USA

Pauline Boss Department of Family Social Science, College of Education and Human Development, University of Minnesota, St. Paul, MN, USA

Rachel Adamek Department of Psychology, Louisiana State University, Baton Rouge, LA, USA

Daphna Canetti School of Political Sciences, University of Haifa, Haifa, Israel

Katie E. Cherry Department of Psychology, Louisiana State University, Baton Rouge, LA, USA

Susan Delaney Irish Hospice Foundation, Dublin, Ireland

Sandro Galea School of Public Health, Boston University, Boston, MA, USA

James I. Gerhart Department of Behavioral Sciences, Rush University Medical Center, Chicago, IL, USA

Anna R. Harper Department of Psychology and Counseling, Southern Nazarene University, Bethany, OK, USA

Trevan G. Hatch School of Social Work, Louisiana State University, Baton Rouge, LA, USA

Stevan E. Hobfoll Department of Behavioral Sciences, Rush University Medical Center, Chicago, IL, USA

Chikako Ishii TELL Counseling, Tokyo, Japan

Laura A. King Department of Psychology, University of Missouri, Columbia, MO, USA

Eva Mozes Kor CANDLES Holocaust Museum and Education Center, Terre Haute, IN, USA

Keri L. Kytola Department of Psychology, Oklahoma State University, Stillwater, OK, USA

Sarah R. Lowe Department of Epidemiology, Mailman School of Public Health, Columbia University, New York, NY, USA

Yaxin Lu Louisiana Department of Education, Baton Rouge, LA, USA

Bethany A. Lyon Department of Psychology, Louisiana State University, Baton Rouge, LA, USA

Masaharu Maeda Department of Disaster Psychiatry, School of Medicine, Fukushima Medical University, Fukushima, Japan

Loren D. Marks School of Family Life, Brigham Young University, Provo, Utah, USA

Gerald L. Mitchell Department of Psychology, University of Missouri, Columbia, MO, USA

Jennifer N. Morey Department of Psychology, University of Kentucky, Lexington, KY, USA

Pamela F. Nezat Department of Psychology, Louisiana State University, Baton Rouge, LA, USA

Misari Oe Department of Neuropsychiatry, Kurume University, School of Medicine, Kurume, Japan

Yuval Palgi Department of Gerontology and the Center for Research and Study of Aging, University of Haifa, Haifa, Israel

Kenneth I. Pargament Department of Psychology and Counseling, Southern Nazarene University, Bethany, OK, USA

Judith R. Phillips Department of Psychology, California State University San Marcos, San Marcos, CA, USA

Abraham Sagi-Schwartz Center for the Study of Child Development, University of Haifa, Haifa, Israel

Suzanne C. Segerstrom Department of Psychology, University of Kentucky, Lexington, KY, USA

M. Katherine Shear School of Social Work, Columbia University, New York, NY, USA

Dov Shmotkin School of Psychological Sciences and the Herczeg Institute on Aging, Tel Aviv University, Tel Aviv, Israel

Amit Shrira Interdisciplinary Department of Social Sciences, Bar-Ilan University, Ramat Gan, Israel

Jennifer Silva Brown Department of Behavioral Sciences, Drury University, Springfield, MO, USA

Avigal Snir Mass Trauma Research Lab, Bob Shapell School of Social Work, Tel Aviv University, Tel Aviv, Israel

Zahava Solomon Mass Trauma Research Lab, Bob Shapell School of Social Work, Tel Aviv University, Tel Aviv, Israel

Jacob Y. Stein Mass Trauma Research Lab, Bob Shapell School of Social Work, Tel Aviv University, Tel Aviv, Israel

Edward E. Waldrep Department of Psychology, Kent State University, Kent, OH, USA

Carl F. Weems Department of Human Development and Family Studies, Iowa State University, Ames, IA, USA

Part I
Traumatic Experiences: On Events that Change Lives

Chapter 1
Traumatic Stress in Overview: Definition, Context, Scope, and Long-Term Outcomes

James I. Gerhart, Daphna Canetti and Stevan E. Hobfoll

Introduction

Traumatic events that threaten life, health, body integrity, and the lives of others are ubiquitous and have life-altering impacts for a substantial portion of individuals. This chapter introduces the topic of traumatic stress with special emphasis on long-term effects of trauma exposure and extreme adversity. Common traumatic events are reviewed, and the nature of traumatic stress, acute stress disorder (ASD), and post-traumatic stress disorder (PTSD) is discussed within the frameworks of conservation of resources (COR) theory (Hobfoll, 2004) and ecological and contextual psychology (Benight & Bandura, 2004; Bronfenbrenner, 1997; Hayes, Barnes-Holmes, Wilson, 2012; Smith & Thelen, 1996) with an emphasis on understanding how constellations of environmental stressors shape traumatic stress reactions over the course of development.

The *Diagnostic and Statistical Manual of Mental Disorders,* 5th edition (DSM-V) defines trauma as, "Exposure to actual or threatened death, serious injury, or sexual violence …" (American Psychiatric Association, 2013). Trauma may be directly experienced or witnessed, or it may be indirectly experienced via trauma to loved ones or as part of one's work with trauma survivors (American Psychiatric Association, 2013). In today's world, the horrors of war, terrorism, abuse, natural disasters, and other catastrophic events have the potential to elicit powerful emotions of

J. I. Gerhart (✉)
Department of Behavioral Sciences, Rush University Medical Center, 1725 W. Harrison, St 950, Chicago, IL 60612, USA
e-mail: james_gerhart@rush.edu

S. E. Hobfoll
Department of Behavioral Sciences, Rush University Medical Center, 1645 W. Jackson Blvd, Suite 400. Chicago, IL 60612, USA
e-mail: stevan_hobfoll@rush.edu

D. Canetti
School of Political Sciences, University of Haifa, Room 4021Terrace Bldg, Haifa 31905, Israel
e-mail: dcanetti@poli.haifa.ac.il

K. E. Cherry (ed.), *Traumatic Stress and Long-Term Recovery,*
DOI 10.1007/978-3-319-18866-9_1

terror, fear, and rage and set in motion cycles of loss that cascade across multiple domains of living (Hobfoll, 1989, 2004).

Although trauma is ubiquitous, the long-term response to trauma is complex and ideographic, with individuals showing unique reactions to the traumatic event based on the unique ecology in which they live. Equifinality is evident in the fact that individuals may develop similar symptoms in response to vastly different losses. Individuals have developed symptoms of PTSD in response to war and mass destruction (Cicchetti & Rogosch, 1996), agricultural crises (Olff, Koeter, Van Haaften, Kersten, & Gersons, 2005), and other non-life-threatening stressors (Bodkin, Pope, Detke, & Hudson, 2007; Scott & Stradling, 1994). Multifinality is evident in the fact that individuals exposed to the exact same event may differ drastically in their response and symptomatology (Cicchetti & Rogosch, 1996). Based on current DSM-V criteria, there are over 600,000 possible PTSD presentations (Galatzer-Levy & Bryant, 2013). Some individuals show considerable resilience in the face of trauma (Bonanno, 2004) and even report positive benefit in the face of adversity (Tedeschi & Calhoun, 1996). Yet for many others, trauma and loss may be overwhelming with long-term effects that persist throughout an individual's lifetime and impact later generations (Polusny & Follette, 1995). Given the vast heterogeneity in the etiology of traumatic stress and its outcomes, there is a need to analyze the individuals in their ecological context (see Chaps. 10 and 12, this volume).

COR theory is an ecological theory of stress (Hobfoll, 1989). It begins with the assumptions that humans continually strive to obtain and preserve valued resources, and that much of human behavior is organized around the collection and preservation of valued resources. Although what is valued is somewhat ideographic, evolutionary and cultural processes have led to common cross-cultural themes. Across individuals and groups, survival resources (e.g., food, water, shelter, safety), intrapersonal resources (e.g., hope, engagement, vigor), and interpersonal resources (e.g., attachments, relationships, social roles; Hobfoll & Lilly, 1993) tend to be highly valued.

Resource caravans refer the positive associations between resources or the tendency for resources to co-occur together and to "follow" the individual or system over time. For instance, access to stable work may also entail access to safer housing, beneficial relationships with peers, and a generally positive self-regard (Hobfoll, 2011). Wealth, social supports, and other resources are often accumulated within the family unit and transferred through inheritances, gifts, and favors and provide an example of *resource caravan passageways,* the psychosocial processes that favor the codevelopment of resources within individuals and groups (Hobfoll, 2011). The local community and neighborhood are other examples of *resource caravan passageways* to the extent that they can provide safe housing, clean environments, social capital, entertainment, effective policing, and access to adequate health care.

The origins of traumatic stress begin with loss or threatened loss of these objectively valued resources (Hobfoll, 1989, 2004), and in the case of traumatic stress, these loss cycles are typically rapid, momentous, and involve key personal, social, and material resources. Moreover, traumatic stress often places a heavy tax on energy resources, including stamina and finances. PTSD and related disorders occur in response to the loss or threatened loss of valued resources that are central to survival, social life, and the sense of self, and they are often characterized by a rapid speed of loss. COR provides a broader perspective to organismic and cognitive theories of stress that have emphasized the mediating roles of subjective and private mental processes (e.g., Folkman & Lazarus, 1988). The primacy of resource loss also provides a parsimonious explanation for how non-life-threatening events such as the loss of cattle, housing, and divorce may evoke PTSD and related distress. This perspective is also consistent with other environmental approaches to psychopathology that posit distress emerges in aversive environmental contexts where reinforcement schedules are inadequate to maintain effective behavior (Ferster, 1973). Key corollaries of the COR theory are that loss is developmental and tends to occur in negative spirals, the impact of loss outweighs the positive impact of gain, and individuals with fewer reserves of resources are more sensitive to loss and gain (Hobfoll, 2004).

Risk factor caravans refer the positive correlations between trauma risk factors such that exposure to trauma increases the likelihood of reexposure and greater sensitivity to stress (Layne et al., 2014; McFarlane, 2010). For instance, exposure to childhood abuse is associated with reexposure to violence in adulthood, limited social support, difficulty regulating emotion, and negative health behaviors (Layne et al., 2014; Stevens et al., 2013; see also Chap. 9, this volume, for related discussion). The associations among resources and risk factors are explained by the presence of *resource and risk factor passageways* that emerge out of social and cultural structures (Hobfoll, 2011). These concepts highlight that the process of trauma involves multiple transactions across levels of trauma exposure.

This ecological and developmental perspective of COR theory highlights that psychological trauma is inherently multileveled: Biological and psychological reactions to trauma are nested within individuals over time and may shape development (see Chap. 10, this volume). Moreover, these trauma-exposed individuals are nested within families, communities, and cultures that reciprocally shape and are shaped by these life-threatening events (Hobfoll, 2004).

Traumatic Stress: A Historical Synopsis

Although the contemporary nosological models of traumatic stress in the form of ASD and PTSD are by definition relatively young, fear, anger, avoidance, and other reactions to traumatic events have likely served important survival functions prior to recorded human history (Hobfoll, 2004). Resource caravan passageways emerged as individuals, families, and tribes collaborated extensively to pool and preserve survival resources. However, threats ranging from volatile geological and meteorological catastrophes to infectious biological agents and intergroup conflict have repeatedly threatened our evolutionary ancestors and selected individuals populations, and cultural practices that were able to survive. Biologically, vigilance to threat, fear reactions, and related avoidance behavior enabled our ancestors to allocate physiological resources to escape from threatening predators and competitors and prevented additional loss of health, life, and other valued resources (McNally, 2003). Likewise, anger in the presence of trauma likely motivated individuals to persist in the face of extreme adversity and to eliminate threats posed by predators and conflicting tribes. To the extent that individuals exhibited these reactions in early human history, they were more likely to survive, reproduce, and foster the reproduction of related kin who might carry similar traits (Hobfoll, 2004).

The development of language-based learning played a significant role in the elaboration and coordination of resource caravan passageways. In particular, the sharing of information about trauma enabled individuals to avoid trauma without having directly encountered life-threatening events in the past (Hayes & Long, 2013; Hayes, Wilson, Gifford, Follette, & Strosahl, 1996). With the development of language, stories of trauma were folded into and relayed in our most important tales, myths, and legends. Thus, evidence of PTSD symptoms can be found throughout the earliest works of documented human history. Ancient literary works such as Gilgamesh and ancient religious texts including the book of Genesis, the first book of the Holy Bible, provide numerous examples of individuals who have struggled to comprehend and move forward in the face of trauma (Kienzler, 2008; Luger, 2010). In the Epic of Gilgamesh, the ancient king is torn with profound grief and guilt at the death of his friend and spends the remainder of his life battling against fate in a search of immortality (Birmes, Hatton, Brunet, & Schmitt, 2003; Kienzler, 2008). These early examples highlight the profound and life-altering effects of trauma and loss that have repeatedly occurred throughout history in the aftermath of war and terror, epidemic disease, natural disasters, and other large-scale traumas.

The twentieth century brought additional refinements to theory as important advancements in the philosophy and science of human behavior were made, and th Wilson e world was witness to two major world wars (Wilson, 1995). Formal diagnostic criteria for traumatic stress reactions were first introduced by the American Psychiatric Association's DSM in 1952 as transient situation personality disorder—gross stress reactions and were reintroduced as adjustment reaction of adult life in DSM-II. Following the Vietnam War, there was increased pressure on the American Psychiatric Association to fully acknowledge and codify the extreme stress of war veterans following the onslaught of the Vietnam War. PTSD was first introduced in DSM-III in 1980 and has been retained with revisions until the current DSM-V (American Psychiatric Association, 2013; Wilson, 1995).

The Initial Impact: Acute Physiological and Psychological Response to Trauma

Exposure to life-threatening traumatic events is inherently distressing and has the ability or power to elicit instinctive psychophysiological "flight-or-fight" reactions (McNally, 2003). These initial behavioral responses to threat are mediated by the sympathetic nervous system and include instinctive freezing and hypervigilance followed by attempts to flee the situation or attack and overcome the threat (Bracha, Ralston, Matsukawa, Williams, & Bracha, 2004). These responses are accompanied by a range of physiological alterations including release of catecholamines such as norepinephrine and epinephrine along with vasoconstriction, tachycardia, increased respiration, muscle tension, and suppression of digestive functions. As metabolic resources are diverted to enhance physical performance in the face of threat, additional physiological changes occur to prepare the body for potential physical trauma. Clotting is increased to prevent potential blood loss in the event of tissue damage. An upsurge of inflammatory processes occurs in preparation for exposure to infectious agents following bodily harm.

The initial freezing and hypervigilance may have helped our evolutionary ancestors avoid detection by potential predators, while flight reactions facilitated rapid escape from the situation and fight responding prepared the organism to overcome the threat through aggressive measures (Bracha et al., 2004; Cannon, 1929). In some cases, humans may respond to traumatic threats by fainting. The fainting response tends to occur following a rapid increase and then abrupt decrease in blood pressure. The potential evolutionary function of fainting is speculative, but in early human close quarters combat, an individual who had fainted would be more likely to be ignored by opposing groups and therefore survive the skirmish, reproduce, and support the survival of genetic relatives (Bracha et al., 2004).

Psychologically, at the time of exposure, individuals may experience intense fear, horror, or rage, and they may have a subjective sense of helplessness (American Psychiatric Association, 2013). Attention to threat is magnified as sense experience is altered such that hearing may become dulled, and vision becomes tunneled. In some cases, the individual may experience a sense of dissociation and feel as if the event is surreal or not actually happening.

The Dust Settles: The Individual Aftermath of Trauma

In the time following the onset of trauma, the individual transitions from a stage of alarm and anxiety and attempts to adapt or cope with the stressor and preserve resources. Eventually, coping resources are overwhelmed, the individual is exhausted, and the potential for physical and psychological impairment is increased (Selye, 1946). Following acute reactions to trauma just described individuals may relive trauma through unwanted thoughts, nightmares, and flashbacks; feel emotionally numbed or flat; avoid internal and external reminders of the trauma; experience intense physiological reactions; and have difficulty sleeping. The DSM-V organizes these reactions to trauma under the diagnostic criteria for the diagnoses of ASD and PTSD (American Psychiatric Association, 2013). The disorders are similar with regard to symptoms of psychological reexperiencing of trauma, avoidance, negative cognition and mood, and hyperarousal. Timing is the primary distinction between ASD and PTSD. Traumatic stress symptoms occurring within the first 3 days to month after trauma fall under the umbrella of ASD symptoms. Traumatic stress symptoms occurring after 1 month fall under the umbrella of PTSD symptoms. The prevalence of both disorders varies across the nature of trauma and other risk factors. It is estimated that approximately 8 % of individuals will experience PTSD at some point in their lives (Kessler, Sonnega, Bromet, Hughes, & Nelson, 1995).

PTSD symptoms are aggregated into five symptoms clusters. Current PTSD criterion A pertains to exposure to trauma in the form of death, death threats, actual or threatened physical or sexual harm to oneself or another (American Psychiatric Association, 2013). Trauma may be directly witnessed or may occur when one learns that a close relative or friend was exposed to actual or threatened violent or accidental death. Individuals may also be traumatized by repeated exposure to trauma via professional duties. The current criteria rule out indirect media exposure as an indirect source of posttraumatic stress.

PTSD criterion B or reexperiencing symptoms pertains to the presence of reexperiencing symptoms or intrusion symptoms. Individuals exposed to trauma experience upsetting memories of the traumatic event and trauma-related nightmares. Individuals may also experience flashbacks in which they vividly relive the trauma as if it were occurring again. Related symptoms within this cluster include repeated intense distress and physiological reactivity that may mimic the initial reaction to trauma.

PTSD criterion C or avoidance symptoms pertains to attempts to avoid and escape trauma-related cognitions and stimuli. The sources of trauma-related stimuli may be internal to the individual in the form of memories, cognitions, and physical sensations. Trauma-related stimuli may also be found in the individuals' external environment and serve as reminders of the traumatic event.

PTSD criterion D symptoms pertain to negative alterations in mood and cognition related to the traumatic event. Individuals may report an impaired memory of the traumatic event. Individuals may also develop negative expectations of self and others and experience an increase in negative trauma-related emotions and mood states.

PTSD criterion E or hyperarousal symptoms pertains to alterations in arousal and reactivity including irritability, aggression, exaggerated startle responses, hypervigilance, and disturbed sleep. Symptoms must persist for 1 month and produce significant distress or impairment (American Psychiatric Association, 2013).

Spiraling Distress: Related Disorders and Expressions of Trauma

The risk factor caravans specified by COR theory are particularly salient among the highly comorbid and correlated conditions that occur in the aftermath of trauma (Bremner, 1999; Kessler et al., 1995). PTSD is also associated with other anxiety disorders (Bremner, 1999), substance abuse, and antisocial and borderline personality disorder (Keane & Kaloupek, 1997). More than 79 % of individuals with PTSD are expected to present with some comorbid psychiatric diagnosis (Keane &

Kaloupek, 1997). Further, 30–50% of patients with PTSD qualify for a comorbid diagnosis of major depressive disorder (Campbell et al., 2007). Conversely, in some settings, over one third of patients with major depressive disorder qualify for a comorbid diagnosis of PTSD (Campbell et al., 2007). Factor analytic work has suggested that trauma-related PTSD and depressive symptoms may fall along a single dimension of severity with depression symptoms and suicidal ideation constituting the most severe symptoms (Elhai et al., 2011).

Exposure to traumatic stress and PTSD is also associated with anger and hostility (Orth & Wieland, 2006). Intense anger and aggression may occur in relation to the elicitation of fight-or-flight responding as aggression may function to eliminate perceived threats in the environment (Novaco & Chemtob, 1998). Anger and aggression may also serve avoidant functions to the extent that these reactions provide distraction from anxiety and fear (Feeny, Zoellner, & Foa, 2000; Gardner & Moore, 2008). PTSD may also increase the frequency and severity of hostile cognitions so that individuals are attuned to the presence of annoyance and threat from other individuals. Although PTSD and anger often occur among individuals with military war experiences that could have shaped their fight reactions in the face of trauma, individuals exposed to health trauma, disasters, criminal victimization, and other traumas also demonstrate significant associations between PTSD and anger (Orth & Wieland, 2006).

Sleep disturbances are also common in the context of traumatic stress. Insomnia is a common comorbid condition among individuals with PTSD (Maher, Rego, & Asnis, 2006). Difficulty sleeping may contribute to the perpetuation of PTSD and related symptoms over time, because individuals have difficulty regulating their coping resources when tired and exhausted (Gerhart, Hall, Russ, Canetti, & Hobfoll, 2014).

Patterns of Posttraumatic Adjustment over Time

Across DSM-V trauma categories, the prevalence of PTSD diagnosis is approximately 29% (range: 3.1–87.5%) and decreases to 17% (range: 0.6–43.8%) at 1 year following the trauma (Santiago et al., 2013). This overall pattern is suggestive of both resilience and recovery in the face of trauma. Resilience is demonstrated in that the vast majority of individuals do not develop diagnosable PTSD in response to trauma exposure. Recovery is demonstrated by the overall reduction in diagnosable PTSD and presumed ongoing adjustment. Despite this overall pattern, there is considerable variability observed in the course of PTSD prevalence and symptom severity over time (Bonanno & Mancini, 2012; Santiago et al., 2013).

Although measures of central tendency are informative for characterizing general responses to stress, these measures may also mask the significant individual variability in PTSD symptoms over time (Bonanno & Mancini, 2012). Multilevel and latent growth modeling techniques have been especially helpful for characterizing overall slopes of PTSD symptom severity and indentifying factors that are associated with change in PTSD over time (Murphy, Johnson, Chung, & Beaton, 2003). For example, PTSD symptoms among bereaved parents have been shown to decrease significantly over time, but individual characteristics such as gender and social support are associated with differences in rate of change. Latent growth class analysis and latent growth mixture modeling assume that reactions to traumatic events may be heterogeneous, and analysis reveals there are approximately four typical trajectories of posttrauma adjustment: resilience, recovery, chronic stress, and delayed onset reactions (Bonanno & Mancini, 2012; see Fig. 1.1).

Resilience tends to be the most frequent response to trauma exposure. Individuals in the resilient category may experience some transient stress reactions in the form of anxiety or sleep disturbance but experience little to no disruption in day-to-day function (Bonanno, 2004). Recovery pertains to moderate-to-severe symptoms of posttraumatic stress that gradually decrease over the course of time. This is evidenced by the finding that nearly half of all cases of PTSD resolve in approximately 3 months following diagnosis (American Psychiatric Association, 2013). Chronic stress is marked by severe levels of PTSD symptoms that remain high and cause significant disruption in function and quality of life. Delayed onset of PTSD is marked by moderate symptoms that increase over time. With regard to total prevalence, delayed onset PTSD is relatively uncommon with few meeting criteria beginning 6 months post trauma, and even fewer reporting an onset 1 year following the trauma.

Although resilience often emerges as a common response to trauma, evidence suggests that patterns of distress vary across context. Patterns of chronic distress are particularly common in the presence of risk factor caravan passageways. In the case of citizens of the Palestinian Authority where repeated exposure to political violence is high, and access to valued resources is more limited, the modal response to trauma is trajectory of moderate distress that recovers over time (Hobfoll, Man-

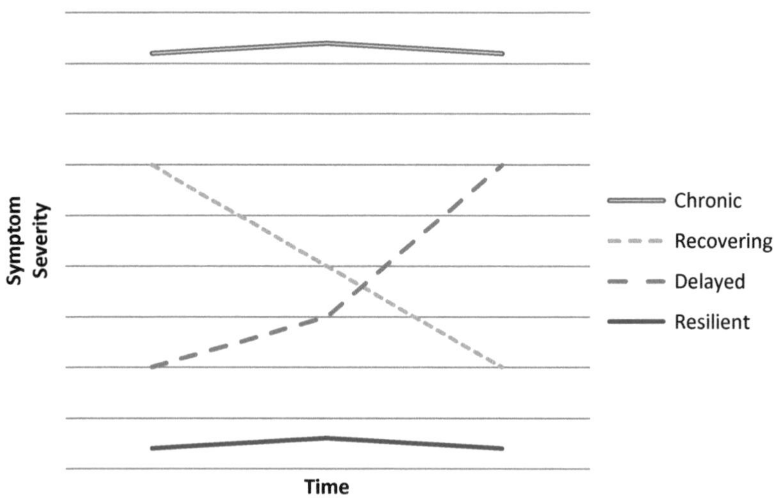

Fig. 1.1 Prototypical trajectories of distress

cini, Hall, Canetti, & Bonnano, 2011). In this context, individuals who fared better tended to have less exposure to political violence and loss.

Long-Term Correlates of Trauma

Although the general trajectory of trauma is that of recovery, evidence suggests that the impacts of varied traumas may persist throughout the lifetime (Layne et al., 2014; Polusny & Follette, 1995), particularly when losses are not recoupable as in the case of physical disability, geographical displacement, and the death of loved ones. Survivors of the Jewish Holocaust following exposure to torture, death of immediate family, isolation, and other traumatic loss experienced high rates of PTSD and had continued heightened sensitivity to loss and trauma 58 years following the end of World War II (Dekel & Hobfoll, 2007; see also Chap. 23, this volume). The long-term impacts of trauma have also been demonstrated in World War II and Korean War veterans. Approximately 50 years post war, over one third reported significant war-related stress (Hunt & Robbins, 2001). These symptoms are explained in part by the long-term impacts of war-related injury (i.e., a risk factor caravan of disability and daily trauma reminders) and illness along with ongoing intrusion and avoidance symptoms.

The long-term impacts of trauma are also evident among survivors of childhood sexual abuse who experience increased risk of anxiety, borderline personality disorder, and other negative psychological outcomes in adulthood (Hillberg, Hamilton-Giachritsis, & Dixon, 2011). Risk factor caravans are especially salient in the co-occurrence of childhood abuse, as sexual and physical abuses are frequently accompanied by psychological maltreatment that further impacts adjustment and well-being (Spinazzola et al., 2014). The detrimental effects of childhood abuse are multiplicative such that psychological maltreatment may amplify the effects of co-occurring abuse and trauma.

Less is known about the long-term impacts of isolated mass trauma. Consistent with the resilience literature, many acute psychological symptoms resolve for many individuals in the aftermath of mass trauma, but risk for substance abuse, physical distress, and greater medical utilization may remain elevated (Galea, 2007).

Impact on Physical Health and Morbidity

Whereas the presentation of traumatic stress in the form of PTSD and related symptoms is salient, research conducted in the field of health psychology continues to reveal the insidious impacts of trauma on long-term physical health and functional status (see Chap. 9, this volume). PTSD is significantly associated with an array of debilitating physical conditions such as pain and cardiovascular disease (Galea, 2007; McFarlane, 2010; Taylor-Clift et al. 2015). Moreover, PTSD is associated with cardiovascular-related mortality and all-cause mortality (Boscarino, 2006, 2008).

There are a number of biobehavioral mechanisms that may explain the associations between trauma, PTSD, and physical morbidity. Chronic inflammation and risky health behaviors are two particularly plausible passageways that may explain the associations between trauma and disease. Inflammatory markers including C-reactive protein (CRP) are elevated among individuals exposed to a host of traumatic stressors including interpersonal violence (Heath et al., 2013) and terrorism (Canetti, Russ, Luborsky, Gerhart, & Hobfoll, 2014). Trauma and PTSD may also indirectly impact health status through behavioral mechanisms such as smoking, overeating, sedentary behavior, and poor medical compliance (see Chap. 9, this volume, for related discussion). To some extent, these behaviors may function to assuage psychological distress at the cost of long-term health (Weiss, Tull, Viana, Anestis, & Gratz, 2012).

Untangling the Web: Trauma Types, Risk Factors, and Mechanisms

The heterogeneity in reactions to trauma begs the question of why some individuals decompensate in the face of traumatic stress, when many remain resilient. From the perspective of COR theory, these differences can be explained by the complete field of resource and risk factor caravan passageways (Hobfoll, 2004; Hobfoll et al., 2009; Layne et al., 2014). Figure 1.2 depicts the multilevel model of trauma and resource loss. As can be seen, trauma impacts intrapersonal, interpersonal, and community resources (one-way arrows), and the negative impacts of trauma may

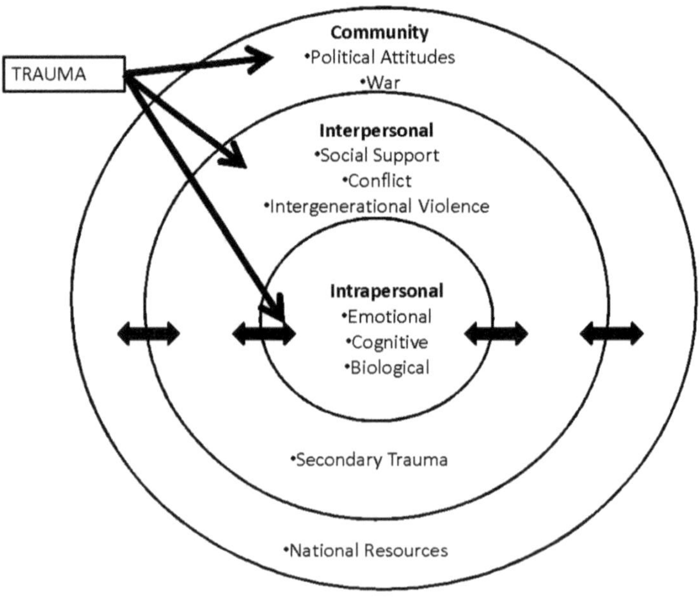

Fig. 1.2 Multilevel model of trauma and resource loss

spiral across levels (two-way arrows). Although individuals and social structures are highly motivated to preserve and enhance resources through resource caravan passageways of education, financial planning, and social engagement, traumatic stress may engender multiple cycles of resource loss. Thus, some of what is called resilience is actually a reflection of the fact that the degree of personal, social, and material loss is different for different people experiencing a trauma, and what is misconstrued as more "resilient" in many cases may rather be a reflection of experience less of the trauma burden. Further, the available of external resources is not uniform. Some have more family and availability of government and emergency aid. Some circumstances may limit access to that external aid, and some environments are themselves too resource poor to provide more than a minimum of aid.

The Nature of the Trauma

Adverse reactions to trauma are linked to the type, severity and chronicity of the initiating traumatic events (Brewin, Andrews, & Valentine, 2000). In the aftermath of trauma, individuals who reported higher levels of PTSD symptoms tend to have experienced more severe and chronic trauma exposure (Brewin et al., 2000; Hobfoll et al., 2009). Individuals directly exposed versus witness to trauma and individuals closer in proximity to the trauma may be at increased risk for PTSD and related symptoms, because the level of objective threat is higher. Individuals exposed to the repetitive nature of combat trauma tend to report more adverse outcomes compared to individuals exposed to more isolated incidents of civilian terrorism and work-related accidents (Amir, Kaplan, & Kotler, 1996). Ongoing warfare and natural disasters have the potential to initiate larger cycles of loss, because individuals and communities may be directly traumatized and also experience ongoing losses of key resources (Hobfoll, 2011; see Chap. 12, this volume).

The timing and frequency of trauma are also linked to the development of PTSD symptoms. Individuals exposed to interpersonal trauma early in life tend to experience greater difficulty with emotion regulation and PTSD symptoms compared to those with trauma that occurs less frequently and later in life (Ehring & Quack, 2010). In addition to adding to the total number of traumas likely to accumulate over the lifetime, trauma has been shown to have compounding effects with regard to sensitization and kindling (McFarlane, 2010). With repeated exposure, individuals may become primed to be increasingly psychologically and physiologically reactive to stressful and traumatic events in the environment so that each additional trauma magnifies the risk of adverse psychological and physical reactions (McFarlane, 2010).

The Intrapersonal Context of Trauma

Individuals' personal characteristics may afford important coping resources for facing adversity and trauma and remaining engaged in their environment (Hobfoll & Lilly, 1993). Engagement refers to the individual's personal affective-motivational reserves of energy (vigor), commitment (dedication), and excitement (absorption) needed to maintain activities of living (Hobfoll, 2011; Schaufeli, Salanova, González-Romá, & Bakker, 2002). The physical, cognitive, and emotional energy underlying engagement is often inherently valued in its own right and facilitates the ongoing development of resources in occupation and social settings (Armon, Melamed, & Shirom, 2012; Hobfoll, 2011). Traumatic contexts tend to have punishing effects that drain engagement reserves, and other individual characteristics may potentiate this drain.

Neuroticism is a stable personality trait that refers to an individual's overall proclivity to experience negative mood and affect in the form of anxiety, worry, anger, and sadness and lends increased sensitivity to trauma (Costa & McCrae, 2008). To the extent that neurotic individuals are prone to the view the world as threatening, they may also experience greater draining of their vigor and engagement (Armon et al., 2012) and experience vulnerability for emotional disorders in general (Barlow, Sauer-Zavala, Carl, Bullis, & Ellard 2014). Individuals also differ with regard to the strategies that they utilize to regulate affective distress. Emotion regulation strategies pertain to the efforts to modify or maintain the form, frequency, and impact of emotion (Gross & Thompson, 2007). Difficulties in emotion regulation may arise when individuals are unable or unwilling to identify, accept, and acknowledge negative emotional states and when individuals behave in an impulsive manner to escape uncomfortable emotions (Bond et al., 2011; Gratz & Roemer, 2004). Experiential avoidance, the tendency to negatively evaluate, suppress, and avoid uncomfortable thought and emotion, has been shown to be a significant mediator in the relationship between neuroticism and PTSD (Goldsmith, Gerhart, Chesney, et al., 2014; Maack, Tull, & Gratz, 2012; Shenk, Putnam, Rausch, Peugh, & Noll, 2014) and may lead to generalized vulnerability to psychopathology and interpersonal problems (Gerhart, Baker, Hoerger, & Ronan, 2014; Goldsmith, Gerhart, Chesney, et al., 2014; Levin et al., 2014; Shenk, Putnam, & Noll, 2014). Avoidance of trauma reminders may trigger social withdrawal and reduce contact with rewarding events in the external environment which trigger ongoing loss spirals (Carvalho & Hopko, 2011) to the extent that individuals ruminate with peers, and permit smaller problems to escalate (Holahan, Moos, Holahan, Brennan, & Schutte, 2005).

Other personal characteristics including female gender, lower socioeconomic status, education, age, and intelligence have been linked to higher levels of PTSD following traumatization (Brewin et al., 2000). To a great extent, factors such as socioeconomic status, education, and intelligence provide pathways to greater access to resources (Hobfoll et al., 2011). As such, these individuals are less affected by stress and trauma, because they have greater reserves to fall back on. Gender differences may be explained in part by physiological differences, including hypothalamic–pituitary–adrenal (HPA) axis response to trauma (DeSantis et al., 2011), but these associations may also be mediated by gender norm differences in cognitive appraisal such that females may be more likely to adopt self-blame and develop world views that are more threatening (Tolin & Foa, 2006). From a life span perspective age and prior development are important for understanding reactions and recovery from trauma. Older adults may be more physically vulnerable to trauma and have fewer instrumental resources needed to recuperate from loss (Sharkey, 2007).

The Interpersonal Context

Although constructs such as neuroticism, emotion regulation, and trauma cognitions are situated within the individual, they occur in response to a much broader ecological context. Exposure to childhood trauma is significantly associated with neuroticism assessed in adulthood (Roy, 2002). Self-efficacy tends to be positively associated with social support (Hobfoll, 2011; Karademas, 2006), children's self-talk increasingly tracks family, and peer assessments of their competence over the course of development (Cole, Jacquez, & Maschman, 2001), and caregivers play important roles in shaping emotion regulation and social skills (Eisenberg, Fabes, & Murphy, 1996). These deficits in cognitive and emotion regulation are often part of a larger constellation of risk factors that include abuse and a lack of nurturing interactions (Fruzzetti, Shenk, & Hoffman, 2005; Stevens et al., 2013). As such, subjective psychological events within the individual are often reciprocally intertwined with their social ecology.

The social context of trauma plays a crucial role in adjustment in the aftermath of trauma as the family system or local community is often the primary vehicle for the consolidation and protection of resources through the provision of emotional support, love, and validation needed to process difficult emotion, along with instrumental and financial supports needed to navigate the world (Hobfoll, 2011; Hobfoll & Vaux, 1993). Inversely, problems and deficits in these areas can lead to significant distress and maladjustment (Brewin et al., 2000; Hobfoll, 1989; Layne et al., 2014; Stevens et al., 2013). These social resources are complex, dynamic, and impact posttrauma adjustment through multiple social-cognitive mechanisms (Benight & Bandura, 2004; see Chap. 11, this volume). As noted earlier, even subjective reactions to trauma and stress may have been directly and indirectly shaped within the family system (Hobfoll, 2011).

The ability to form secure and stable attachments affords a sense of stability and safety in the face of environmental adversity (Bowlby, 1969). The tendency to identify with and attach to others in early life has played a crucial role in survival throughout much of human history. Secure attachments enable the developing individual to acquire strategies for seeking and providing help, internalize adaptive coping strategies, and develop realistic expectations about supportive relationships (Mikulincer, Shaver, & Pereg, 2003). Whereas caregivers may share a proclivity to positive cognitions through their communication (Donnelly, Renk, Sims, & Mcquire, 2011), they may also pass on a proclivity to shame and negative self-evaluation through negativistic parenting styles (Alessandri & Lewis, 1993; Mills et al. 2007). When exposed to trauma, individuals with less secure attachment styles (i.e., anxiety and avoidance) tend to report higher levels of perceived stress, and in turn experience higher levels of PTSD symptoms (Besser, Neria, & Haynes, 2009). Attachment anxiety is also linked to poorer perceived social support in the aftermath of trauma (Besser & Neria, 2010).

The concept of social support is broadly defined as relationships and other interpersonal interchanges that provide a sense of connection to others and provide help and assistance to the individual (Hobfoll & Stokes, 1988). Thus, social support includes close attachments and other helpful relationships. Poor positive social support is consistently linked with poor adjustment in the aftermath of trauma (Brewin et al., 2000). This may be so as the traumatized individual has less access to emotional support in the form of validation and encouragement, less instrumental support in the form of physical assistance, and less access to models of positive coping strategies (Benight & Bandura, 2004; Hobfoll, 2004). Although the previous examples are of positive social support, negative social support in the form of criticism, hostility, and judgment may provoke additional distress that outweighs the benefit of positive support (Hobfoll, 2004). Whereas social resources are sometimes mistakenly conceptualized as a static buffer against PTSD and related distress, social support interacts dynamically with symptoms and other resources, such that support may be eroded over time (Hobfoll & Stokes, 1988). In some instances, PTSD symptoms, depression, and poorly regulated anger may overwhelm supportive others and reduce the likelihood of helpful interactions (Gerhart, Sanchez Varela, Burns, Hobfoll, & Fung, 2014; Gerhart et al., 2014; Lane & Hobfoll, 1992). Risk factor caravans are exemplified among individuals who are exposed to ongoing trauma, have limited social and financial resources, lack the ability to permanently escape the threatening family, home, or neighborhood environment, and as a result remain at high risk for ongoing interpersonal violence (Fleury, Sullivan, & Bybee, 2000; Stevens et al., 2013). These escalating cycles of violence and re-traumatization may reinforce and lead to trajectories of chronic posttraumatic stress and contribute to health disparities (Layne et al., 2014; Taylor-Clift et al. 2015).

Aftershocks: Shared Trauma, Intergenerational Violence, and War

Given that trauma occurs within dynamic social systems, there is a potential for consequences of trauma to apply at the group level. These patterns highlight that resources, losses, and PTSD cluster within social systems, and that many traumas may impact the individual and the social system through direct and indirect effects. In these cases, trauma becomes a shared experience that may limit coping resources across the group level (Tosone et al., 2003). These events highlight the occurrence of trauma as inherently multileveled with the potential for transactions between the individual and group context (Kawachi, Subramanian, & Kim, 2008).

Shared and Secondary Trauma

Trauma experienced at the group level can produce emergent processes. Shared trauma is a concept from the psychotherapy literature that refers to situations in which the common experience of a trauma (e.g., terrorism, war, natural disaster) among patient and therapist who reside in the same community may alter the work of therapy, as the provider may be more acutely vulnerable to stress and therefore more emotionally reactive to the content and process of psychotherapy (Baum, 2010; Saakvitne, 2002; Tosone, Nuttman-Shwartz, & Stephens, 2012). In order to provide effective services, the clinician must monitor and address their personal reactions to trauma (Tosone et al., 2012).

Individuals often turn first to emotional support from friends and family before larger community supports and psychotherapy (Elliott & Pais, 2006). Although professional training, role boundaries, and support may help offset potential resource losses in the context of therapy (Tosone et al., 2012), loss spirals may persist in less structured social roles and relationships. Coping and adjustment are highly nested within a couple such that an individual's traumatic stress is positively associated with the traumatic stress of the spouse, and patterns of reciprocal hostility, criticism, and withdrawal may emerge within couples (Dekel & Monson, 2010). Emotion-focused coping within the dyad may be especially detrimental for both members as it is associated with distress within the individual (Gilbar, Weinberg, & Gil, 2011). Trauma may also affect group-level processes more indirectly through secondary or vicarious traumatization. In these instances, the trauma is not necessarily shared among individuals, but one may develop posttraumatic reactions through hearing and empathizing with stories of trauma.

Intergenerational violence may also contribute to the spiraling effects of trauma throughout social systems. Growing up in abusive and traumatic environments does not entail a future trajectory of imitating abusive behavior, but there are some small-to-moderate links between witnessing and experiencing violence and abuse and later perpetration of abuse in the family system (Stith et al. 2000). From a social learning perspective, trauma-exposed individuals may learn abusive behaviors from caregivers and other role models in childhood, and mimic these learned behaviors as adults with their spouses and children (Bandura, 1977). In the case of borderline personality disorder, risk factor caravan passageways may occur through inconsistent parenting practices that vacillate widely between hostility and disengagement (Stepp, Whalen, Pilkonis, Hipwell, & Levine, 2012).

Impact on Political Attitudes and War

Spirals of resource loss may also occur at the national or cultural level, through cycles of retaliatory violence. In the face of trauma and particularly threat to one's life, individuals often attempt to manage terror and threat perceptions by strengthening attitudes of support for their own cultural or national group and also becoming more committed to attitudes against their cultural out-groups (Greenberg et al. 1990). In the areas of chronic conflict (e.g., Israel and the Palestinian Authority; Northern Ireland), direct and indirect exposure to war-related trauma is significantly associated with support for more military action and war (Hayes & McAllister, 2001). Just as the nature of the trauma has important impacts on traumatic stress reactions, the type of trauma also impacts political attitudes. Chronic war entails repeated traumatization that may shape increasingly hostile political attitudes over time (Hobfoll, Canetti-Nisim, & Johnson, 2006).

The mechanisms of war and terror-related trauma's impact on political attitudes are complex, but evidence suggests that these relationships are explained in part by a desire for defensive political measures to escape existential insecurity (Canetti, Halperin, Hobfoll, Shapira, & Hirsch-Hoefler, 2009). In the face of war and trauma, core beliefs about safety and security may be drastically altered (Janoff-Bulman, 1992; Magwaza, 1999). As a result, individuals are primed to be vigilant for ongoing threats and increasing their support for violent military action (Bonanno & Jost, 2006). Conflict may escalate rapidly as opposing groups and nations participate in cycles of retaliation (Haushofer, Biletzki, & Kanwisher, 2010). Addressing the impact of chronic war and terror-related trauma on political process may be crucial for healing long-standing conflict (Canetti, Hall, Greene, Kane, & Hobfoll, 2014).

Summary

This chapter introduced the topic of traumatic stress and its long-term impacts within the context of COR theory (Hobfoll, 1989, 2004). This ecological and developmental perspective of trauma highlights that traumatic stress from the initial horror to its long-term fallouts is dynamic and multileveled. The concept of risk factor caravans is introduced to highlight the nesting and statistical covariation of risk factors and trauma sequelae within individuals and social groups. Although individuals demonstrate considerable resilience in the face of adversity, traumatic stress has the power to disrupt emotional and social lives through ongoing spirals of loss. Paradoxically, individuals in an effort to avoid and compensate for traumatic losses may inadvertently contribute to ongoing cycles of traumatization.

References

Alessandri, S. M., & Lewis, M. (1993). Parental evaluation and its relation to shame and pride in young children. *Sex Roles, 29*(5–6), 335–343.

American Psychiatric Association. (2013). *Diagnostic and statistical manual of mental disorders* (5th ed.). Washington: American Psychiatric Association.

Amir, M., Kaplan, Z., & Kotler, M. (1996). Type of trauma, severity of posttraumatic stress disorder core symptoms, and associated features. *The Journal of General Psychology, 123*(4), 341–351.

Armon, G., Melamed, S., & Shirom, A. (2012). The relationship of the job demands-control-support model with vigor across time: Testing for reciprocality. *Applied Psychology: Health and Well-Being, 4*(3), 276–298.

Bandura, A. (1977). Self-efficacy: Toward a unifying theory of behavioral change. *Psychological Review, 84*(2), 191–215.

Barlow, D. H., Sauer-Zavala, S., Carl, J. R., Bullis, J. R., & Ellard, K. K. (2014). The nature, diagnosis, and treatment of neuroticism back to the future. *Clinical Psychological Science, 2*(3), 344–365.

Baum, N. (2010). Shared traumatic reality in communal disasters: Toward a conceptualization. *Psychotherapy: Theory, Research, Practice, Training, 47*(2), 249.

Benight, C. C., & Bandura, A. (2004). Social cognitive theory of posttraumatic recovery: The role of perceived self-efficacy. *Behaviour Research and Therapy, 42*(10), 1129–1148.

Besser, A., & Neria, Y. (2010). The effects of insecure attachment orientations and perceived social support on posttraumatic stress and depressive symptoms among civilians exposed to the 2009 Israel–Gaza war: A follow-up cross-lagged panel design study. *Journal of Research in Personality, 44*(3), 335–341.

Besser, A., Neria, Y., & Haynes, M. (2009). Adult attachment, perceived stress, and PTSD among civilians exposed to ongoing terrorist attacks in Southern Israel. *Personality and Individual Differences, 47*(8), 851–857.

Birmes, P., Hatton, L., Brunet, A., & Schmitt, L. (2003). Early historical literature for post-traumatic symptomatology. *Stress and Health, 19*(1), 17–26.

Bodkin, J. A., Pope, H. G., Detke, M. J., & Hudson, J. I. (2007). Is PTSD caused by traumatic stress? *Journal of Anxiety Disorders, 21*(2), 176–182.

Bonanno, G. A. (2004). Loss, trauma, and human resilience: Have we underestimated the human capacity to thrive after extremely aversive events? *American Psychologist, 59*(1), 20.

Bonanno, G. A., & Jost, J. T. (2006). Conservative shift among high-exposure survivors of the september 11th terrorist attacks. *Basic and Applied Social Psychology, 28*(4), 311–323.

Bonanno, G. A., & Mancini, A. D. (2012). Beyond resilience and PTSD: Mapping the heterogeneity of responses to potential trauma. *Psychological Trauma: Theory, Research, Practice, and Policy, 4*(1), 74–83.

Bond, F. W., Hayes, S. C., Baer, R. A., Carpenter, K. M., Guenole, N., Orcutt, H. K., et al. (2011). Preliminary psychometric properties of the acceptance and action questionnaire–II: A revised measure of psychological inflexibility and experiential avoidance. *Behavior Therapy, 42*(4), 676–688.

Boscarino, J. A. (2006). Posttraumatic stress disorder and mortality among US army veterans 30 years after military service. *Annals of Epidemiology, 16*(4), 248–256.

Boscarino, J. A. (2008). A prospective study of PTSD and early-age heart disease mortality among Vietnam veterans: Implications for surveillance and prevention. *Psychosomatic Medicine, 70*(6), 668–676.

Bowlby, J. (1969). *Attachment and loss, volume i: Attachment*. New York: Basic Books.

Bracha, H., Ralston, T. C., Matsukawa, J. M., Williams, A. E., & Bracha, A. S. (2004). Does "fight or flight" need updating? *Psychosomatics, 45*(5), 448–449.

Bremner, J. D. (1999). Acute and chronic responses to psychological trauma: where do we go from here? *American Journal of Psychiatry, 156*(3), 349–351.

Brewin, C. R., Andrews, B., & Valentine, J. D. (2000). Meta-analysis of risk factors for posttraumatic stress disorder in trauma-exposed adults. *Journal of Consulting and Clinical Psychology, 68*(5), 748–766.

Bronfenbrenner, U. (1977). Toward an experimental ecology of human development. *American Psychologist, 32*(7), 513.

Campbell, D. G., Felker, B. L., Liu, C. F., Yano, E. M., Kirchner, J. E., Chan, D., et al. (2007). Prevalence of depression–PTSD comorbidity: Implications for clinical practice guidelines and primary care-based interventions. *Journal of General Internal Medicine, 22*(6), 711–718.

Canetti, D., Halperin, E., Hobfoll, E. S., Shapira, O., & Hirsch-Hoefler, S. (2009). Authoritarianism, perceived threat and exclusionism on the eve of the Disengagement: Evidence from Gaza. *International Journal of Intercultural Relations, 33*, 463–474.

Canetti, D., Hall, B. J., Greene, T., Kane, J. C., & Hobfoll, S. E. (2014). Improving mental health is key to reduce violence in Israel and Gaza. *The Lancet, 384*(9942), 493–494.

Canetti, D., Russ, E., Luborsky, J., Gerhart, J. I., & Hobfoll, S. E. (2014). Inflamed by the flames? The impact of terrorism and war on immunity. *Journal of Traumatic Stress, 27*(3), 345–352.

Cannon, W. B. (1929). Vob. IX JULY, 1929 No. 3 Organization for physiological homeostatis. *Physiological Reviews, 9*(3), 399–431.

Carvalho, J. P., & Hopko, D. R. (2011). Behavioral theory of depression: Reinforcement as a mediating variable between avoidance and depression. *Journal of Behavior Therapy and Experimental Psychiatry, 42*(2), 154–162.
Cicchetti, D., & Rogosch, F. A. (1996). Equifinality and multifinality in developmental psychopathology. *Development and Psychopathology, 8*(04), 597–600.
Cole, D. A., Jacquez, F. M., & Maschman, T. L. (2001). Social origins of depressive cognitions: A longitudinal study of self-perceived competence in children. *Cognitive Therapy and Research, 25*(4), 377–395.
Costa, P. T., & McCrae, R. R. (2008). The revised neo personality inventory (NEO-PI-R). *The SAGE Handbook of Personality Theory and Assessment, 2,* 179–198.
Dekel, R., & Hobfoll, S. E. (2007). The impact of resource loss on holocaust survivors facing war and terrorism in Israel. *Aging and Mental Health, 11*(2), 159–167.
Dekel, R., & Monson, C. M. (2010). Military-related post-traumatic stress disorder and family relations: Current knowledge and future directions. *Aggression and Violent Behavior, 15*(4), 303–309.
DeSantis, S. M., Baker, N. L., Back, S. E., Spratt, E., Ciolino, J. D., Maria, M. S., et al. (2011). Gender differences in the effect of early life trauma on hypothalamic–pituitary–adrenal axis functioning. *Depression and Anxiety, 28*(5), 383–392.
Donnelly, R., Renk, K., Sims, V. K., & McGuire, J. (2011). The relationship between parents' and children's automatic thoughts in a college student sample. *Child Psychiatry and Human Development, 42*(2), 197–218.
Ehring, T., & Quack, D. (2010). Emotion regulation difficulties in trauma survivors: The role of trauma type and PTSD symptom severity. *Behavior Therapy, 41*(4), 587–598.
Eisenberg, N., Fabes, R. A., & Murphy, B. C. (1996). Parents' reactions to children's negative emotions: Relations to children's social competence and comforting behavior. *Child Development, 67*(5), 2227–2247.
Elhai, J. D., de Francisco Carvalho, L., Miguel, F. K., Palmieri, P. A., Primi, R., & Frueh, B. C. (2011). Testing whether posttraumatic stress disorder and major depressive disorder are similar or unique constructs. *Journal of Anxiety Disorders, 25*(3), 404–410.
Elliott, J. R., & Pais, J. (2006). Race, class, and Hurricane Katrina: Social differences in human responses to disaster. *Social Science Research, 35*(2), 295–321.
Feeny, N. C., Zoellner, L. A., & Foa, E. B. (2000). Anger, dissociation, and posttraumatic stress disorder among female assault victims. *Journal of Traumatic Stress, 13*(1), 89–100.
Ferster, C. B. (1973). A functional analysis of depression. *American Psychologist, 28*(10), 857–870.
Fleury, R. E., Sullivan, C. M., & Bybee, D. I. (2000). When ending the relationship does not end the violence: Women's experiences of violence by former partners. *Violence Against Women, 6*(12), 1363–1383.
Folkman, S., & Lazarus, R. S. (1988). The relationship between coping and emotion: Implications for theory and research. *Social Science and Medicine, 26*(3), 309–317.
Fruzzetti, A. E., Shenk, C., & Hoffman, P. D. (2005). Family interaction and the development of borderline personality disorder: A transactional model. *Development and Psychopathology, 17*(04), 1007–1030.
Galatzer-Levy, I. R., & Bryant, R. A. (2013). 636,120 ways to have posttraumatic stress disorder. *Perspectives on Psychological Science, 8*(6), 651–662.
Galea, S. (2007). The long-term health consequences of disasters and mass traumas. *Canadian Medical Association Journal, 176*(9), 1293–1294.
Gardner, F. L., & Moore, Z. E. (2008). Understanding clinical anger and violence: The anger avoidance model. *Behavior Modification, 32,* 897–912.
Gerhart, J. I., Sanchez Varela, V., Burns, J. W., Hobfoll, S. E., & Fung, H. C. (2014). Anger, provider responses, and pain: Prospective analysis of stem cell transplant patients. *Healthy Psychology, 33*(4), 197–206.

Gerhart, J. I., Baker, C. N., Hoerger, M., & Ronan, G. F. (2014). Experiential avoidance and interpersonal problems: A moderated mediation model. *Journal of Contextual Behavioral Science, 3*(4), 291–298.

Gerhart, J. I., Hall, B. J., Russ, E. U., Canetti, D., & Hobfoll, S. E. (2014). Sleep disturbances predict later trauma-related distress: Cross-panel investigation amidst violent turmoil. *Health Psychology, 33*(4), 365–372.

Gilbar, O., Weinberg, M., & Gil, S. (2011). The effects of coping strategies on PTSD in victims of a terror attack and their spouses: Testing dyadic dynamics using an actor-partner interdependence model. *Journal of evidence-based complementary & alternative medicine, 19*, 0265407511426939.

Goldsmith, R. E., Gerhart, J. I., Chesney, S. A., Burns, J. W., Kleinman, B., & Hood, M. M. (2014). Mindfulness-Based Stress Reduction for Posttraumatic Stress Symptoms Building Acceptance and Decreasing Shame. *Journal of evidence-based complementary & alternative medicine, 19* (4), 227–234.

Gratz, K. L., & Roemer, L. (2004). Multidimensional assessment of emotion regulation and dysregulation: Development, factor structure, and initial validation of the difficulties in emotion regulation scale. *Journal of Psychopathology and Behavioral Assessment, 26*(1), 41–54.

Greenberg, J., Pyszczynski, T., Solomon, S., Rosenblatt, A., Veeder, M., Kirkland, S., et al. (1990). Evidence for terror management theory II: The effects of mortality salience on reactions to those who threaten or bolster the cultural worldview. *Journal of Personality and Social Psychology, 58*(2), 308.

Gross, J. J., & Thompson, R. A. (2007). Emotion regulation: Conceptual foundations. In J.J. Gross (Ed.), *Handbook of emotion regulation,* (pp. 3–24). New York: Guilford Press.

Hankin, B. L., & Abela, J. R. (Eds.). (2005). *Development of psychopathology: A vulnerability-stress perspective*. Thousand Oaks: Sage.

Haushofer, J., Biletzki, A., & Kanwisher, N. (2010). Both sides retaliate in the Israeli–Palestinian conflict. *Proceedings of the National Academy of Sciences, 107*(42), 17927–17932.

Hayes, S. C., & Long, D. (2013). Contextual behavioral science, evolution, and scientific epistemology. In S. C. Hayes & D. Long (Eds.), *Advances in Relational Frame Theory: Research and application*, (pp. 5–26). Oakland: New Harbinger.

Hayes, B. C., & McAllister, I. (2001). Sowing dragon's teeth: Public support for political violence and paramilitarism in Northern Ireland. *Political Studies, 49*(5), 901–922.

Hayes, S. C., Wilson, K. G., Gifford, E. V., Follette, V. M., & Strosahl, K. (1996). Experiential avoidance and behavioral disorders: A functional dimensional approach to diagnosis and treatment. *Journal of Consulting and Clinical Psychology, 64*(6), 1152.

Heath, N. M., Chesney, S. A., Gerhart, J. I., Goldsmith, R. E., Luborsky, J. L., Stevens, N. R., et al. (2013). Interpersonal violence, PTSD, and inflammation: Potential psychogenic pathways to higher C-reactive protein levels. *Cytokine, 63*(2), 172–178.

Hillberg, T., Hamilton-Giachritsis, C., & Dixon, L. (2011). Review of meta-analyses on the association between child sexual abuse and adult mental health difficulties: A systematic approach. *Trauma, Violence, and Abuse, 12*(1), 38–49.

Hobfoll, S. E. (1989). Conservation of resources: A new attempt at conceptualizing stress. *American Psychologist, 44*(3), 513.

Hobfoll, S. E. (2004). *Stress, culture, and community: The psychology and philosophy of stress*. New York: Springer.

Hobfoll, S. E. (2011). Conservation of resources theory: Its implication for stress, health, and resilience. In S. Folkman (Ed.), *The oxford handbook of stress, health, and coping* (pp. 127–147). New York: Oxford University Press.

Hobfoll, S. E., & Lilly, R. S. (1993). Resource conservation as a strategy for community psychology. *Journal of Community Psychology, 21*(2), 128–148.

Hobfoll, S. E., & Stokes, J. P. (1988). The process and mechanics of social support. In S. Duck, D. F. Hay, S. E. Hobfoll, B. Ickes, & B. Montgomery (Eds.), *The handbook of research in personal relationships*. London, New York: Wiley.

Hobfoll, S. E., & Vaux, A. (1993). Social support: Social resources and social context. In L. Goldberger & S. Breznitz (Eds.), *Handbook of stress: Theoretical and clinical aspects* (2nd ed., pp. 685–705). New York: Free Press.
Hobfoll, S. E., Canetti-Nisim, D., & Johnson, R. J. (2006). Exposure to terrorism, stress-related mental health symptoms, and defensive coping among Jews and Arabs in Israel. *Journal of Consulting and Clinical Psychology, 74*(2), 207–218.
Hobfoll, S. E., Palmieri, P. A., Johnson, R. J., Canetti-Nisim, D., Hall, B. J., & Galea, S. (2009). Trajectories of resilience, resistance, and distress during ongoing terrorism: The case of Jews and Arabs in Israel. *Journal of Consulting and Clinical Psychology, 77*(1), 138–148.
Hobfoll, S. E., Mancini, A. D., Hall, B. J., Canetti, D., & Bonanno, G. A. (2011). The limits of resilience: Distress following chronic political violence among Palestinians. *Social Science and Medicine, 72*(8), 1400–1408.
Holahan, C. J., Moos, R. H., Holahan, C. K., Brennan, P. L., & Schutte, K. K. (2005). Stress generation, avoidance coping, and depressive symptoms: A 10-year model. *Journal of Consulting and Clinical Psychology, 73*(4), 658.
Hunt, N., & Robbins, I. (2001). The long-term consequences of war: The experience of world war II. *Aging and Mental Health, 5*(2), 183–190.
Janoff-Bulman, R. (1992). *Shattered assumptions*. New York: The Free Press.
Karademas, E. C. (2006). Self-efficacy, social support and well-being: The mediating role of optimism. *Personality and Individual Differences, 40*(6), 1281–1290.
Kawachi, I., Subramanian, S. V., & Kim, D. (2008). *Social capital and health* (pp. 1–26). New York: Springer.
Keane, T. M., & Kaloupek, D. G. (1997). Comorbid psychiatric disorders in PTSD. *Annals of the New York Academy of Sciences, 821*(1), 24–34.
Kessler, R. C., Sonnega, A., Bromet, E., Hughes, M., & Nelson, C. B. (1995). Posttraumatic stress disorder in the national comorbidity survey. *Social Science & Medicine, 67(2), 218–227.*
Kienzler, H. (2008). Debating war-trauma and post-traumatic stress disorder (PTSD) in an interdisciplinary arena. *Archives of General Psychiatry, 52*(12), 1048–1060.
Lane, C., & Hobfoll, S. E. (1992). How loss affects anger and alienates potential supporters. *Journal of Consulting and Clinical Psychology, 60*(6), 935.
Layne, C. M., Briggs, E. C., & Courtois, C. A. (2014). Introduction to the special section: Using the Trauma History Profile to unpack risk factor caravans and their consequences. *Psychological Trauma: Theory, Research, Practice, and Policy, 6*(S1), S1–S8.
Levin, M. E., MacLane, C., Daflos, S., Seeley, J. R., Hayes, S. C., Biglan, A., & Pistorello, J. (2014). Examining psychological inflexibility as a transdiagnostic process across psychological disorders. *Journal of Contextual Behavioral Science, 3*(3), 155–163.
Luger, S. (2010). Flood, salt, and sacrifice: Post traumatic stress disorders in genesis. *Jewish Bible Quarterly, 38,* 124–126.
Maack, D. J., Tull, M. T., & Gratz, K. L. (2012). Experiential avoidance mediates the association between behavioral inhibition and posttraumatic stress disorder. *Cognitive therapy and research, 36*(4), 407–416.
Magwaza, A. S. (1999). Assumptive world of traumatized South African adults. *The Journal of social psychology, 139*(5), 622–630.
Maher, M. J., Rego, S. A., & Asnis, G. M. (2006). Sleep disturbances in patients with post-traumatic stress disorder: Epidemiology, impact and approaches to management. *CNS Drugs, 20,* 567–690.
McFarlane, A. C. (2010). The long-term costs of traumatic stress: Intertwined physical and psychological consequences. *World Psychiatry, 9*(1), 3–10.
McNally, R. J. (2003). Psychological mechanisms in acute response to trauma. *Biological Psychiatry, 53*(9), 779–788.
Mikulincer, M., Shaver, P. R., & Pereg, D. (2003). Attachment theory and affect regulation: The dynamics, development, and cognitive consequences of attachment-related strategies. *Motivation and Emotion, 27*(2), 77–102.

Mills, R. S., Freeman, W. S., Clara, I. P., Elgar, F. J., Walling, B. R., & Mak, L. (2007). Parent proneness to shame and the use of psychological control. *Journal of Child and Family Studies, 16*(3), 359–374.

Murphy, S. A., Johnson, L. C., Chung, I. J., & Beaton, R. D. (2003). The prevalence of PTSD following the violent death of a child and predictors of change 5 years later. *Journal of Traumatic Stress, 16*(1), 17–25.

Novaco, R. W., & Chemtob, C. M. (1998). Anger and trauma: Conceptualization, assessment, and treatment. In V. M. Follette, J. I. Ruzek, & F. R. Abueg (Eds.), *Cognitive-behavioral therapies for trauma* (pp. 162–190). New York: Guilford.

Olff, M., Koeter, M. W., Van Haaften, E. H., Kersten, P. H., & Gersons, B. P. (2005). Impact of a foot and mouth disease crisis on post-traumatic stress symptoms in farmers. *The British Journal of Psychiatry, 186*(2), 165–166.

Orth, U., & Wieland, E. (2006). Anger, hostility, and posttraumatic stress disorder in trauma-exposed adults: A meta-analysis. *Journal of Consulting and Clinical Psychology, 74*(4), 698.

Polusny, M. A., & Follette, V. M. (1995). Long-term correlates of child sexual abuse: Theory and review of the empirical literature. *Applied and Preventive Psychology, 4*(3), 143–166.

Roy, A. (2002). Childhood trauma and neuroticism as an adult: Possible implication for the development of the common psychiatric disorders and suicidal behaviour. *Psychological Medicine, 32*(08), 1471–1474.

Saakvitne, K. W. (2002). Shared trauma: The therapist's increased vulnerability. *Psychoanalytic Dialogues, 12*(3), 443–449.

Santiago, P. N., Ursano, R. J., Gray, C. L., Pynoos, R. S., Spiegel, D., Lewis-Fernandez, R., et al. (2013). A systematic review of PTSD prevalence and trajectories in DSM-5 defined trauma exposed populations: Intentional and non-intentional traumatic events. *PLoS ONE, 8*(4), e59236.

Schaufeli, W. B., Salanova, M., González-Romá, V., & Bakker, A. B. (2002). The measurement of engagement and burnout: A two sample confirmatory factor analytic approach. *Journal of Happiness Studies, 3*(1), 71–92.

Scott, M. J., & Stradling, S. G. (1994). Post-traumatic stress disorder without the trauma. *British Journal of Clinical Psychology, 33*(1), 71–74.

Shenk, C. E., Putnam, F. W., Rausch, J. R., Peugh, J. L., & Noll, J. G. (2014). A longitudinal study of several potential mediators of the relationship between child maltreatment and posttraumatic stress disorder symptoms. *Development and psychopathology, 26*(01), 81–91.

Selye, H. (1946). The gerneral adaptation syndrome and the diseases of adaptation 1. *The Journal of Clinical Endocrinology and Metabolism, 6*(2), 117–230.

Sharkey, P. (2007). Survival and death in New Orleans: An empirical look at the human impact of Katrina *Journal of Black Studies, 37*(4), 482–501.

Spinazzola, J., Hodgdon, H., Liang, L. J., Ford, J. D., Layne, C. M., Pynoos, R., et al. (2014). Unseen wounds: The contribution of psychological maltreatment to child and adolescent mental health and risk outcomes. *Psychological Trauma: Theory, Research, Practice, and Policy, 6*(S1), S18.

Stepp, S. D., Whalen, D. J., Pilkonis, P. A., Hipwell, A. E., & Levine, M. D. (2012). Parenting behaviors of mothers with borderline personality disorder: A call to action. *Personality Disorders: Theory, Research, and Treatment,* 3(1), 104–106.

Stevens, N. R., Gerhart, J., Goldsmith, R. E., Heath, N. M., Chesney, S. A., & Hobfoll, S. E. (2013). Emotion regulation difficulties, low social support, and interpersonal violence mediate the link between childhood abuse and posttraumatic stress symptoms. *Behavior Therapy, 44*(1), 152–161.

Stith, S. M., Rosen, K. H., Middleton, K. A., Busch, A. L., Lundeberg, K., & Carlton, R. P. (2000). The Intergenerational Transmission of Spouse Abuse: A Meta-Analysis. *Journal of Marriage and Family, 62*(3), 640–654

Taylor-Clift, A., Hobfoll, S. E., Gerhart, J. I., Richardson, D., Calvin, J. E., & Powell, L. H. (2015). Posttraumatic stress and depression: potential pathways to disease burden among heart failure patients. *Anxiety, Stress, & Coping*, (ahead-of-print), 1–14.

Tedeschi, R. G., & Calhoun, L. G. (1996). The posttraumatic growth inventory: Measuring the positive legacy of trauma. *Journal of Traumatic Stress, 9*(3), 455–471.
Thelen, E., & Smith, L. B. (1996). A dynamic systems approach to the development of cognition and action. Cambridge, MA: MIT press.
Tosone, C., Lee, M., Bialkin, L., Martinez, A., Campbell, M., Martinez, M. M., et al. (2003). Shared trauma: Group reflections on the September 11th disaster. *Psychoanalytic Social Work, 10*(1), 57–77.
Tosone, C., Nuttman-Shwartz, O., & Stephens, T. (2012). Shared trauma: When the professional is personal. *Clinical Social Work Journal, 40*(2), 231–239.
Weiss, N. H., Tull, M. T., Viana, A. G., Anestis, M. D., & Gratz, K. L. (2012). Impulsive behaviors as an emotion regulation strategy: Examining associations between PTSD, emotion dysregulation, and impulsive behaviors among substance dependent inpatients. *Journal of Anxiety Disorders, 26*(3), 453–458.
Wilson, J. P. (1995). The historical evolution of PTSD diagnostic criteria. In G. S. Everly & J. M. Lating (Eds.), *Psychotraumatology: Key papers and core concepts in post-traumatic stress* (pp. 9–26). New York: Plenum.

Chapter 2
Natural Disasters: On Wildfires and Long-Term Recovery of Community-Residing Adults

Judith R. Phillips

Introduction

A wildfire is defined as a large, uncontrolled, fast-moving, and destructive fire. Various names are used to describe it such as bushfire, wildland fire, brushfire, grass fire, and forest fire. They occur throughout the world (Brotak, 2012). Examples of this can be seen recently from February 2014 through September 2014: California's King wildfire, Washington State's Carlton Complex wildfire, Spain's Costa del Sol wildfire, the Valparaiso Chile wildfire, and South Australia's Victoria wildfire.

Wildfires appear to be occurring more frequently due to a combination of factors including global climate changes (Brotak, 2012). Not only do wildfires damage or destroy structures, plants, and animals but they may also kill or injure firefighters and community residents. Economic losses can range in the billions of dollars (Brotak, 2012). Adverse health effects can also be seen, as a community's air quality is poorer after a wildfire, resulting in respiratory system problems for those residing in the area (Caamano-Isorna et al., 2011; Finlay, Moffat, Gazzard, Baker, & Murray, 2012). Psychiatric and psychological consequences of wildfire destruction have also been found (Finlay et al., 2012).

In this chapter, I examine the impact of wildfires on the long-term mental health of community-residing adults. This chapter is organized as follows. I begin with an overview of past research on short-term and long-term psychological well-being after a wildfire event. In the next section, I present select data from the 2007 northern San Diego County wildfire study. Specifically, I describe this study's assessment of the impact of demographic and psychosocial predictors on the mental well-being of community-residing adults aged 30–94 years of age. I conclude by reflecting on the implications of these findings for disaster planning and preparation for community-residing adults.

J. R. Phillips (✉)
Department of Psychology, California State University San Marcos, 3226 Social & Behavioral Sciences Building, San Marcos, CA 92096, USA
e-mail: jphillip@csusm.edu

K. E. Cherry (ed.), *Traumatic Stress and Long-Term Recovery*,
DOI 10.1007/978-3-319-18866-9_2

Literature Review

The literature on short-term and long-term effects on the mental health outcomes of community-residing adults after a wildfire is limited. A review of research investigating the short-term effects of a wildfire on mental well-being includes studies on wildfires in California, one occurred in 2003 (Marshall, Schell, Elliott, Rayburn, & Jaycox, 2007) and others occurred in 2008–2009 (Afifi, Felix & Afifi, 2012), and a wildfire in Greece in 2007 (Mellon, Papanikolau, & Prodromitis, 2009).

Mental health outcomes for community-residing adult participants were comparable for Marshall et al. (2007) who surveyed at 3 months after the wildfire and Mellon et al. (2009) who surveyed at 6 months. Both of these researchers found poorer mental health and evidence of psychopathology for those directly affected by the wildfires. On the other hand, Afifi et al. (2012), who surveyed at approximately 5 months after the wildfire with the largest number of evacuees, did not find the mental health of community-residing adults who evacuated to be significantly different from those adults who did not evacuate, although differences approached significance. One of the better predictors of psychopathology in the short term after a wildfire was damage to property or home (Marshall et al., 2007). Afifi et al. (2012) found that older adults and women reported better mental health than younger adults and men.

Although there was not a consensus in these studies, many adults, especially those who had the greatest exposure to the wildfire, exhibited poor psychological health (Afifi et al., 2012; Marshall et al., 2007; Mellon et al., 2009). Does this trend continue throughout the long term or does it increase or decrease? A review of five studies that have explored the mental health of community-residing adults for at least 1 year after a wildfire disaster provides some answers.

Three studies were conducted on the long-term effects of wildfires on the mental health of community-residing adults after various Australian bushfires. McFarlane, Clayer, and Bookless (1997) surveyed 20 months after the 1983 Ash Wednesday bushfire; Camilleri et al. (2010) investigated 3 years after the 2003 Canberra bushfires, and Bryant et al. (2014) probed 3–4 years after the 2009 Victorian Black Saturday bushfires. A fourth study by Papanikolaou, Adamis, and Kyriopoulos (2012) continued to investigate the effects of the 2007 wildfires in Greece 3 years after the wildfire. Caamano-Isorna et al. (2011) assessed respondents 1 year after the 2006 Galician Spain wildfires for the use of anxiolytic–hypnotic drugs (anxiety drugs).

In three studies, the majority of respondents reported good mental health or low levels of psychological distress at the time of assessment (Bryant et al., 2014; Camilleri et al., 2010; McFarlane et al., 1997). When examining for the effect of exposure to the wildfire, Bryant et al. (2014), Caamano-Isorna et al. (2011) and Papanikolaou et al. (2012) found a trend of those respondents in the more directly affected communities to report higher levels of depression, higher levels of post-traumatic stress disorder, or poorer psychological health than those respondents in the medium or low affected areas or unaffected areas. Papanikolaou et al. (2012) found that older adults and women exhibited poorer psychological health, while

Caamano-Isorna et al. (2011) discovered that men used more anxiolytics–hypnotic drugs than women in the affected area.

Camilleri et al. (2010) also assessed the sources and types of support that those impacted by the wildfire perceived to be helpful in their recovery. These participants indicated that family, friends, and neighbors who provided emotional support such as kindness, listening, understanding, and tangible support such as offering housing, clothing, and financial aid facilitated their recovery. They also mentioned that aid from governmental and community services was important to their recovery.

From this review of short- and long-term effects of a wildfire on mental health, the reader can see that the psychological well-being of most community-residing adults appears to return after a period of time (Afifi et al., 2012; Bryant et al., 2014; Caamano-Isorna et al., 2011; Camilleri et al., 2010; Marshall et al., 2007; McFarlane et al., 1997; Mellon et al., 2009; Papanikolaou et al., 2012). There was a trend which showed that those who were most directly exposed to the wildfire in the short- and long-term period had poorer psychological health than those outside of the direct line of the wildfire (Bryant et al., 2014; Caamano-Isorna et al., 2011; Marshall et al., 2007; Papanikolaou et al., 2012). There were mixed findings for age and gender on psychological health in the short- and long-term time frame after a wildfire (Afifi et al., 2012; Caamano-Isorna et al., 2011; Papanikolaou et al., 2012).

San Diego County Wildfires

Four undergraduate research assistants and I explored similar variables in our study assessing community-residing adults 4.5 years after the 2007 northern San Diego County wildfires. Specifically, we investigated the severity of wildfire exposure, age, and gender on the mental well-being of community residents (Phillips, Cruz, Cuadra, Martinez, & Perdomo, 2013a, b).

We also examined the influence of sources of and types of social support on long-term recovery as did Camilleri et al. (2010). Past research has found that receiving social support is important for those recovering from the effects of a disaster and lessens psychological vulnerability (Acierno, Ruggiero, Kilpatrick, Resnick, & Galea, 2006; Camilleri et al., 2010).

The Disaster

On Sunday, October 21, 2007, multiple wildfires began in San Diego County during a major Santa Ana wind event. During the following days, the fires burned over 300,000 acres and destroyed or damaged approximately 1350 homes. Ten people were killed. Half a million residents were evacuated from their homes.

The targeted fire in this study, the Witch Creek fire, was the primary wildfire in northern San Diego County. This was the largest of these October wildfires and is considered the fourth largest fire in California's history. It started to the east in the foothills and moved west towards the coast. It burned approximately 200,000 acres, destroyed 1125 residences, damaged 77 residences, and caused the deaths of two community residents. Raging uncontrolled for 10 days, this fire was finally 100% contained on October 31. Yet as widespread as this wildfire was, there were areas in northern San Diego County where community residents did not sustain loss of property or have to be evacuated.

Participants

One hundred and ninety-one community residents of northern San Diego County who ranged in age from 30 to 94 years in 2012 (M=63.25 years, SD=14.59) responded to the questionnaire. They were mostly Caucasian, non-Hispanic (88.00%), married at the time of the wildfire (77.00%) and at the time of data collection (75.40%). The majority of these adults had an annual income of $75,001 to $100,000+(58.70%) and had insurance on their property and valuables (91.60%). One hundred and ten were female (57.60%). All participants were residents of northern San Diego County at the time of the 2007 wildfire and in 2012 as well. All were at least 25 years of age at the time of the wildfire.

The severity of exposure to the wildfire differed for the community participants. For this study, primary victim status was assigned to those participants who had responded to a survey question that they had experienced structural damage (total or partial) to their residence as a result of the wildfires. They may or may not have been evacuated, depending on whether they were at home or were away from home when the wildfire occurred. Thirty-six respondents were determined to be primary victims (18.85%) with 27 reporting total loss of their home or apartment and nine reporting partial loss of their residence.

Secondary victim status was assigned to those who reported that they had evacuated from their homes, but they did not experience any structural damage to their residence. Because they were evacuated from their residence, they lived in close proximity to the path of the wildfire. There were 100 participants in this category (52.36%).

Non-victim status was assigned to those community residents who responded that they did not have to evacuate and that they had no property damage. These 54 participants (28.27%) lived in northern San Diego County but not in or near the path of the wildfire. These three categories were based on work by Bolin (1985) and Norris and Murrell (1988).

Community residents were classified into five age groups: those in their 30s (M=5, F=6), those in their 40s (M=5, F=16), those in their 50s (M=25, F=26), those in their 60s (M=16, F=26), those in their 70s (M=15, F=22), those in their 80s (M=12, F=11), and those in their 90s (M=3, F=3). Table 2.1 presents details of respondents' severity of exposure and age in decades.

Table 2.1 Age and victim status

Age in decades	Victim status		
	Primary	Secondary	Non-victim
30–39	2	4	5
40–49	3	10	8
50–59	16	19	16
60–69	7	19	16
70–79	3	26	8
80–89	5	13	4
90–94	0	6	0

Materials and Procedure

The questionnaire was composed of mostly closed-ended questions. Demographic questions pertained to age, gender, and marital status at two points in time; racial background; total household income for 2011; home or rental insurance; and property damage information and evacuation experience during the wildfire.

Received social support was measured by the *Inventory of Postdisaster Social Support* scale (Kaniasty & Norris, 2000; Norris, Murphy, Kaniasty, Perilla, & Ortis, 2001). Participants were asked to estimate how often they received different types of social support within a clearly established time frame anchored between the October wildfires (Oct 21, 2007) and around New Year's Day 2008. This support was related to the wildfires. It was modified to include 30 items to measure three types of support: emotional (three questions), informational (three questions), and tangible (four questions). Emotional social support assessed actions such as being comforted or shown signs of affection, someone expressing concern about your well-being, and knowing that others would be around if they were needed. Informational social support measured someone suggesting some action to take, understanding a situation you were in, and being given information on how to do something. Tangible social support referred to being given/loaned/offered money, furniture tools, food, and a place to stay. Three distinct sources of support were measured: family (ten items), friends, including neighbors and coworkers (ten items), outsiders, including people outside respondent's immediate support circle such as community leaders, voluntary organizations, and professional service providers (ten items). These questions were scored on a four-option response set ((0) = never to (3) = many times). In the current study, there was very good total internal consistency with a Cronbach alpha coefficient of 0.95. Others have found internal consistency coefficient of 0.93 with 36 total items (Kaniasty & Norris, 2000).

The *Center for Epidemiologic Studies Depression Scale* (CES-D; Radloff, 1977) was used to assess nonclinical depressive mood and symptoms and is intended for the general population. A 20-item scale was used and scored on a four-option response set ((0) = rarely or none of the time to (3) = most or all of the time). In the general population, a score of 16 or greater suggests a high level of depressive symptoms, and a score lower than 16 reflects lower levels of symptoms (Myers & Weissman, 1980). In the current study, the Cronbach's alpha coefficient was 0.85.

Researchers included a prompt at the end of the questionnaire asking for additional comments related to participants' experiences after the wildfires. Narrative data were collected from 46 participants.

The snowball sampling technique was used to disperse the seven-page questionnaire during the months of May through July 2012. Undergraduate research assistants and I distributed the questionnaire to adult community residents who then distributed it to other community-residing adults and so forth. An information sheet was attached to each questionnaire. This information sheet invited community-residing adults to participate in the study if they lived in the area that was involved in the 2007 northern San Diego County wildfires and if they were at least 25 years old in October 2007. These adults were told that every resident's experiences were wanted whether they experienced damage to their homes or apartments or had no damage and whether they had to evacuate or did not have to evacuate. They were told that the survey would take about 30 min to fill out and asked questions about social support encountered during and after the wildfires and about their experiences during the wildfires and in 2012.

Participants were not compensated for their time. They completed the questionnaire in their place of their choice and mailed it back to the main researcher in an attached addressed and stamped envelope. There was a response rate of 45.7 %.

Results

Mental Health

The mean for all respondents for CES-D score was 8.88 (standard deviation (*SD*) = 7.86, range = 0–46) at 4.5 years after the wildfire. This mean is below the cutoff for depressive symptomology and indicates that most participants were below the clinical indicator for depressive symptoms. Demographic comparisons revealed that there was a significant effect for age in decades, $F(6, 163) = 2.91$, $p = 0.10$. Post hoc comparisons using the Tukey honest significant difference (HSD) test indicated that the mean CES-D score for those in their 60s ($M = 10.97$, $SD = 10.37$, range = 0–46) was significantly different from those in their 70s ($M = 5.26$, $SD = 4.4$, range = 0–15), $p = 0.03$. No significant differences were found between the other decades, although mean CES-D scores did approach significance between those in their 70s ($M = 5.26$, $SD = 4.4$, range = 0–15) and those in their 90s ($M = 15.33$, $SD = 10.29$, range = 3–30), $p = 0.051$. Table 2.2 provides CES-D mean and *SD* and age in decade data.

When victim status groups and participants' gender were compared with CES-D scores, no main effects were found, but there was an interaction, $F(2, 176) = 3.93$, $p = 0.02$. Specifically, women respondents' CES-D scores declined as their exposure to the wildfire declined; men's CES-D scores in-

Table 2.2 Mean CES-D and standard deviation scores and age in decades

Age in decades	Mean CES-D scores (*SD*)
30	10.64 (7.32)
40	7.40 (6.79)
50	9.37 (7.46)
60	10.97 (10.37)
70	5.27 (4.47)
80	8.32 (6.20)
90	15.33 (10.29)

CES-D center for epidemiologic studies depression scale

Table 2.3 Mean CES-D and standard deviation scores, victim status, and gender

Victim status/gender	CES-D Mean (*SD*)
Primary	
Male	5.55 (5.05)
Female	12.83 (11.81)
Secondary	
Male	6.95 (5.22)
Female	8.79 (7.77)
Non-victim	
Male	11.09 (7.58)
Female	8.48 (7.57)

CES-D center for epidemiologic studies depression scale

creased as their exposure to the wildfires declined. Table 2.3 presents CES-D mean and *SD*, gender, and victim status data.

Women ($M=9.58$, $SD=8.83$; range = 0–46) of all ages showed more depressive symptomology than the men ($M=7.92$, $SD=6.21$; range = 0–37); however, there was no significant effect between females and male participants, $t(181)=-1.49$, $p=0.14$ (two-tailed).

Although primary victims ($M=10.11$, $SD=10.42$, range = 0–46) reported more depressive symptomology during a week in 2012 than secondary victims ($M=8.01$, $SD=6.79$, range = 0–30) and non-victims ($M=9.65$, $SD=7.66$, range = 0–37), analysis of the three victim status groups and their mental health at 4.5 years after the wildfire yielded no significant effect, $F(2, 163)=1.51$, $p=0.22$. After looking at these data, the large *SD* for the primary victim status group showed scores ranging from 0 to 46 with six participants' scores being 16 and above and eight participants' scores being 3 and below; therefore, it confirmed a wide range of values indicative of a large *SD*.

Received Social Support

Overall, the mean total social support given to these respondents between the 2007 wildfire and New Year's Day 2008 was 24.26 ($SD=19.87$). No significant differences were found between depressive symptomology and total social support, but the total social support given to primary victims ($M=49.9$, $SD=19.22$) was significantly different from that given to secondary victims ($M=19.68$, $SD=15.45$) and non-victims ($M=15.87$, $SD=12.94$),

$F(2,168) = 54.17$, $p = .00$. The total social support given to secondary victims did not differ significantly from that given to non-victims.

Types of received social support. There were three different types of received social support: informational, emotional, and tangible, and each was analyzed with the three-victim statuses—primary, secondary and non-victim.

Informational social support. The effect of victim status and received informational social support was significant, $F(2, 85.44) = 37.65$, $p = 0.00$; range = 0–27 with primary victims ($M = 14.87$, $SD = 7.25$) receiving informational social support significantly more than secondary victims ($M = 4.93$, $SD = 5.69$) and non-victims ($M = 4.18$, $SD = 4.85$). One primary victim mentioned in the narrative data that United Policyholders, a nonprofit organization, gave invaluable information on filing insurance claims.

Emotional social support. There was a significant effect of victim status on received emotional social support, $F(2, 152.3) = 29.95$, $p = 0.00$; range = 0–27. Primary victims ($M = 20.28$, $SD = 5.31$) received more emotional social support than secondary victims ($M = 11.04$, $SD = 8.12$) and non-victims ($M = 8.85$, $SD = 7.50$). One primary victim mentioned in the narrative data that it took a lot of work to "suck it up" and keep going, but her strong marriage and deep faith definitely helped in recovering from the fire.

Secondary victims did not receive significantly more emotional social support than non-victims did, but respondents from both groups reported in the narrative data that they did receive emotional support. A secondary victim wrote that supportive family and friends were important, and a non-victim wrote that many people called to ask about them.

Tangible social support. The effect of victim status and received tangible social support was significant, $F(2, 46.3) = 65.63$, $p = 0.00$, range = 0–36. Primary victims ($M = 16.81$, $SD = 8.6$) received more tangible social support than secondary victims ($M = 4.10$, $SD = 4.47$) and non-victims ($M = 1.98$, $SD = 2.52$). In the narrative data, one non-victim respondent wrote that because he did not experience any personal property loss, he donated furniture and money to those who had lost their homes. Another non-victim respondent stated that he took a truckload of replacement items such as clothing and a TV to a friend who lost a home.

A secondary victim who had lost her home in the 2003 Cedar Fire in San Diego wrote of providing tangible social support by working at the donation center as a "personal shopper" where she was matched with an individual/family to assess their needs and to help gather necessary goods. She also helped give out a Fire Survivors Handbook, "a how-to and what-to-do guide that was assembled from our collective experiences from 2003 and the months that followed."

In this analysis, secondary victims received significantly more tangible social support than non-victims did. One secondary victim wrote in the narrative data that as she was evacuated she fell and hurt her back. A neighbor took her to the hospital.

Sources of social support. There were three types of sources of social support in this study: family, friends, and others. Each was analyzed with the three-victim statuses—primary, secondary, and non-victim. Scores ranged from 0 to 30.

Social support from family. A significant effect of victim status was found for family social support, $F(2, 80.2)=20.91$, $p=0.00$ with primary victims ($M=16.75$, $SD=8.56$) receiving more social support from family members than secondary victims ($M=8.00$, $SD=6.44$) and non-victims ($M=7.26$, $SD=5.66$). One primary victim mentioned in the narrative data that without the support of family, recovery would have been more difficult.

Secondary victims did not receive significantly more support from family members than did non-victims, but through the narrative data, secondary victims and non-victims wrote of the support that family provided. For example, one secondary victim mentioned "supportive family."

Social support from friends. The effect of victim status and friends' social support was significant, $F(2, 178)=56.78$, $p=0.00$. Primary victims ($M=18.75$, $SD=6.90$) received social support from friends, neighbors, and coworkers more often than did secondary victims ($M=7.69$, $SD=5.95$) and non-victims ($M=5.25$, $SD=4.97$). There were many comments in the narrative data from primary victims related to received social support from friends, neighbors, and coworkers. For example, one primary victim wrote that she and her husband were blessed to have had great friends to help them. She went on to say that this "taught my husband and me what matters" (see Chap. 21, this volume, for related discussion).

Secondary victims received significantly more social support from friends, work colleagues, and neighbors than non-victims did. One secondary victim wrote that her neighbors helped to take care of her for three weeks as she had hurt her back when evacuating and was unable to stand and walk for those weeks.

Social support from others. A significant effect of victim status was found for others' social support, $F(2, 58.76)=59.21$, $p=0.00$ with primary victims ($M=16.53$, $SD=7.92$) receiving more social support from outsiders such as community leaders, voluntary organizations, and professional service providers than secondary victims ($M=4.36$, $SD=4.8$) and non-victims ($M=2.94$, $SD=3.73$). Another primary victim stated that there was a group called Fired Up Sisters (FUS) that was created to support women whose homes were destroyed or damaged and that this support system helped her tremendously. She stated, "we cried, we solved problems, we moved forward. After a couple of months, friends and families didn't want to hear about our constant problems so with our FUS group, we found a 'new' normal" (see Chap. 12, this volume, for a related discussion). Another primary victim mentioned the biggest encouragement was the outpouring of concerns and help from those outside her immediate circle.

Secondary victims did not receive significantly more social support from outsiders such as community leaders, voluntary organizations, and professional service providers than did non-victims. A secondary victim mentioned in the narrative data "the kindness of strangers was completely overwhelming."

Conclusions

In summary, these community-residing adults who responded to the questionnaire in 2012 on the 2007 northern San Diego County wildfire showed good psychological health. Our findings were similar to those of Bryant et al. (2014), Camilleri et al. (2010), and McFarlane et al. (1997). While Bryant et al. (2014), Caamano-Isorna et al. (2011), and Papanikolaou et al. (2012) found that respondents in the more directly affected communities or primary victims showed poorer psychological health than those adults in the medium or low affected areas or unaffected areas, this result was not replicated in our study (Phillips et al., 2013a, b). Although the mean score for depressive symptoms was higher in the primary victim group, there were no significant differences among the scores of the three exposure groups on the depressive symptomology measure.

There was agreement between our study and Papanikolaou et al.'s (2012) which showed that older adults exhibited poorer psychological health; specifically, though it was those in their 60s who showed more depressive symptoms than those in their seventies in our study. This exception noted that there were no other differences among the seven age groups here. Unlike Caamano-Isorna et al. (2011) or Papanikolaos et al. (2012), we did not find any gender differences. We did find an interaction between gender and victim status. Women in the primary victim group had higher mean depressive symptoms than those women in the secondary and non-victim groups, but men showed the opposite pattern.

Although there was no significance in total social support and depressive symptomology, our findings agreed in kind with Camilleri et al. (2010). Primary victims were helped significantly more than the other two victim groups by family, friends, and outside sources, and they were provided three types of social support: informational, emotional, and tangible social support.

Camilleri et al. (2010) mentioned that after the wildfire in Canberra, Australia, residents formed new groups to help with recovery. This was seen in this study with the formation of the Fired Up Sisters (FUS) organization. This support group began in November 2007 for those women who were primary victims of the 2007 northern San Diego County wildfire. It was foremost an emotional support group for these women, but it also provided discounts from local merchants and solicited donations of tangible goods and services to help primary victim families (Rossi, 2010). In the narrative data, this organization was mentioned several times, including a primary victim who wrote that she had amazing friendship and support from all "my Fired Up Sisters."

Implications

While wildfires, as do all natural disasters, have an immediate impact on the mental health of those affected individuals, the findings from the 2007 northern San Diego wildfire study continue to provide promise for long-term recovery and good psychological health of those community-residing adults affected by wildfires in the years after this event, particularly those hardest impacted residents whose homes were destroyed or damaged. One participant in the 2007 wildfire study stated in the narrative data that she, as a primary victim of an earlier San Diego wildfire, "provided proof that life surely can return to normal."

Found in both qualitative and quantitative research, key factors in the recovery process appear to include social support from three sources (Camilleri et al., 2010; Phillips et al., 2013a). Family, friends, neighbors, and coworkers should reach out to aid victims in the direct path of the wildfire, those in medium affected areas, and those in low affected areas. Those outside the immediate circle, including community leaders, professional service providers, and voluntary organizations, are excellent sources of additional social support. Organizations such as FUS should be encouraged and supported by community funds and community backing. A community effort is needed not only to physically rebuild an area devastated by wildfire but also to psychologically rebuild its residents (see Chap. 12, this volume).

The three types of social support are needed, but no one needs to provide all three. Some sources can provide emotional support, while others can provide informational or tangible support. Not all residents will need all three types of support; individual differences will appear based on victim status, age, and gender. Therefore, it is important for communities to put considerable effort into establishing a system of support built to provide multiple options and selections of service based on an individual's needs.

In conclusion, it is essential for researchers to continue to study the effects of wildfires on the psychological health of adult community residents for many years after the wildfire event. It is also crucial for community leaders to heed researchers' findings to aid in the psychological recovery of community-residing adults. Such alliances will offer hope for those affected by wildfires.

Acknowledgments The author would like to thank former students Moe Perdomo, David Martinez, Sean Cuadra, and Araceli Cruz for their help in the development of this study and entering and checking data. The author is also grateful to these students, Joe Phillips, and all individuals who distributed the questionnaire. A California State University San Marcos CHABSS Lecturer Professional Development Grant supported this research.

References

Acierno, R., Ruggiero, K. J., Kilpatrick, D. G., Resnick, H. S., & Galea, S. (2006). Risk and protective factors for psychopathology among older versus younger adults after the 2004 Florida hurricanes. *The American Journal of Geriatric Psychiatry, 14*, 1051–1059. doi:10.1097/01.JGP.0000221327.97904.b0.

Afifi, W. A., Felix, E. D., & Afifi, T. D. (2012). The impact of uncertainty and communal coping on mental health following natural disasters. *Anxiety, Stress & Coping, 25*, 329–347. doi:10.1080/10615806.2011.603048.

Bolin, R. (1985) Disaster characteristics and psychosocial impacts. In B. J. Soder (Ed.), *Disasters and mental health: Selected contemporary perspectives* (pp. 3–28). Rockville: National Institute of Mental Health.

Brotak, E. (2012, March 14). Wildfires getting worse around the world. *Earth Island Journal.* http://www.earthisland.org/journal/index.php/elist/eListRead/wildfires_getting_worse_around_the_world. Accessed 22 July 2014.

Bryant, R. A, Waters, E., Gibbs, L., Gallagher, H. C., Pattison, P., Lusher, D., et al. (2014, May 22). Psychological outcomes following the Victorian Black Saturday bushfires. Retrieved from http://anp.sagepub.com/content/48/7/634. Accessed 25 June 2014.

Caamano-Isorna, F., Figueiras, A., Sastre, I., Montes-Martinez, A., Taracido, M., & Pineiro-Larnas, M. (2011). Respiratory and mental health effects of wildfires: An ecological study in Galician municipalities (North-West Spain). *Environmental Health, 10*, 48–56. doi:10.1186/1476-069X-10-48.

Camilleri, P., Healy, C., Macdonald, E. M., Nicholls, S., Sykes, J., Winkworth, G., et al. (2010). Recovery from bushfires: The experience of the 2003 Canberra bushfires three years after. *Journal of Emergency Primary Heath Care, 8*, 1–15.

Finlay, S. E., Moffat, A., Gazzard, R., Baker, D., & Murray, V. (2012, November 2). Health impacts of wildfires. *PLOS Currents Disasters, 1*, 1–27. doi:10.1371/4f959951cce2c. http://currents.plos.org/disasters/article/health-impacts-of-wildfires/. Accessed 13 June 2014.

Kaniasty, K., & Norris, F. H. (2000). Help-seeking comfort and receiving social support: The role of ethnicity and context of need. *American Journal of Community Psychology, 28*, 545–581. doi:10.1023/A:1005192616058.

Marshall, G. N., Schell, T. E., Elliott, M. N., Rayburn, N. R., & Jaycox, L. H. (2007). Psychiatric disorders among adults seeking emergency disaster assistance after a wildland-urban interface fire. *Psychiatric Services, 58*, 509–514. doi:10.1176/appi.ps.58.4.509.

McFarlane, A. C., Clayer, J. R., & Bookless, C. L. (1997). Psychiatric morbidity following a natural disaster: An Australian bushfire. *Social Psychiatry and Psychiatric Epidemiology, 32*, 261–268. doi:10.1007/BF00789038.

Mellon, R. C., Papanikolau, V., & Prodromitis, G. (2009). Locus of control and psychopathology in relation to levels of trauma and loss: Self-reports of Peloponnesian wildfire survivors. *Journal of Traumatic Stress, 22*, 189–196. doi:10.1002/jts.

Myers, J. K., & Weissman, M. M. (1980). Use of a self-report symptom scale to detect depression in a community sample. *The American Journal of Psychiatry, 137*, 1081–1084.

Norris, F. H., & Murrell, S. A. (1988). Prior experience as a moderator of disaster impact on anxiety symptoms in older adults. *American Journal of Community Psychology, 16*, 665–683. doi:10.1007/BF00930020.

Norris, F. H., Murphy, A. D., Kaniasty, K., Perilla, J. L., & Ortis, D. C. (2001). Postdisaster social support in the United States and Mexico: Conceptual and contextual considerations. *Hispanic Journal Of Behavior Sciences, 23*, 469–496. doi:10.1177/0739986301234008.

Papanikolaou, V., Adamis, D., & Kyriopoulos, J. (2012). Long term quality of life after a wildfire disaster in a rural part of Greece. *Open Journal of Psychiatry, 2*, 164–170. doi:10.4236/ojpsych.2012.22022.

Phillips, J. R., Cruz, A., Cuadra, S., Martinez, D., & Perdomo, M. (2013a). Predictors of mental health after a disaster: A study of older adults four years after the 2007 San Diego County wildfires. *The Gerontologist, 53*(S1), 109.

Phillips, J. R., Cruz, A., Cuadra, S., Martinez, D., & Perdomo, M. (2013b). Middle-aged and older adults' long-term responses to the 2007 Southern California wildfires. *The Gerontologist, 53*(S1), 158.

Radloff, L. S. (1977). The CES-D scale: A self-report depression scale for research in the general population. *Applied Psychological Measurement, 1*(3), 385–401. doi:10.1177/014662167700100306.

Rossi, N. (2010, May 15). Fired Up Sisters was born out of tragedy: Wildfire support becomes relief group. *San Diego Union Tribune*. http://www.utsandiego.com/. Accessed 05 Oct 2014.

Chapter 3
On Tornados: Storm Exposure, Coping Styles, and Resilience

Jennifer Silva Brown

Introduction

The psychosocial consequences of natural disaster exposure, which include threats to psychological health, physical well-being, social networks, are all well documented in the existing literature (Bonanno, Galea, Bucciarelli, & Vlahov, 2007; Logue, Melick, & Stuening, 1981b; Polusny et al., 2008). These disasters not only bring about damage to ones' possessions, home, and/or community but they simultaneously create a long-term stressor that challenges psychological resiliency. While exposure to an earthquake, hurricane, wildfire, tornado, or other disaster may be viewed as an isolated event, subsequent individual role changes have the potential to chronically tax physical and mental health. Ongoing challenges surrounding housing, employment, and health status, all have the potential to prolong post-disaster recovery.

While disaster exposure may consist of similar levels of widespread damage and health consequences, it should be noted that not all natural disasters are equal. Earthquakes commonly happen with no little to warning, tornados frequently materialize within minutes, and others, such as hurricanes and possibly wildfires, have the potential to provide residents with days of advance notice. Affording persons in the affected areas with warning that a disaster is imminent may produce differing individual and community post-storm outcomes. Furthermore, there are various demographic distinctions among those populations affected. Some disaster survivors may reside within an area that is statistically more likely to experience one disaster type over another (i.e., Gulf Coast/hurricanes; West Coast/earthquakes; Midwest/tornados). These storm and population differences warrant continued investigation into the factors that promote post-disaster resilience, which is essential for individual and community recovery.

J. Silva Brown (✉)
Department of Behavioral Sciences, Drury University, 900 N. Benton Avenue, Springfield, MO 65802, USA
e-mail: jsilvabrown@drury.edu

K. E. Cherry (ed.), *Traumatic Stress and Long-Term Recovery*,
DOI 10.1007/978-3-319-18866-9_3

Overall, there are two primary objectives of the current chapter. The first is to provide a summary of the literature pertaining to coping and resilience following disaster exposure within adult survivor populations. The second objective pertains to the presentation of data from the Joplin Impact Project (JIP), a research initiative designed to identify factors which contribute to the health and well-being of persons exposed to the 2011 Joplin tornado. The JIP data are utilized in a discussion regarding the predictive significance of post-disaster coping methods to psychological resilience.

Resilience

Resilience is generally referred to as the successful adaptation to an adversity that would most likely lead to a negative outcome (Bonanno, 2004; Masten, 2001). The lack of psychopathology development after a traumatic event has been regarded as necessary but not sufficient to infer resilience within an individual. The construct has been largely viewed at as a measurement outcome post trauma, a psychological aftermath which becomes evident over time. Regarding a uniform operational definition of resilience, it is generally agreed upon that an individual must be exposed to negative events/experiences; however, the specifics continue to be debated (Luthar & Cicchetti, 2000). Furthermore, a contemporary debate exists as to whether resilience should be assessed as a static trait or as a fluid process (DeHaan, Hawley, & Deal, 2002; Rutter, 2012).

Pioneer resilience theorists focused on outcomes of "at-risk" youth who had grown up in impoverished homes and/or violent communities (Benard, 1991; Rutter, 1985). Early theory posited that these risks or "vulnerabilities" consisted of personal characteristics or experiential deficits, which would make one more likely to succumb to adverse psychological sequelae. Risks consisted of such factors as low socioeconomic status, trauma exposure, lack of social support, and/or unemployment (Benard, 1991). The early goal was simply to identify all of the qualities associated with deleterious outcomes such as psychopathology or distress. It was presumed that if one could pre-identify potential risk factors and subsequently intervene to reduce such risk, then there would be a corresponding reduction in negative outcomes. However, during this *deficit-focused* approach to research, it was noted that about half to two thirds of the persons who were exposed to these risk factors were thriving and developed positive outcomes (Benard & Slade, 2009; Masten, 2001; Rutter, 2006). Consequently, these findings gave rise to the shift from "historical" risk to "modern" protective factors.

Research investigating protective factors is regarded to be *strengths-based,* recognizing strengths that one may possess which would allow him/her to thrive in the face of adversity. Protective factors refer to either internal or external influences with the potential to modify, improve, or alter a one's response to a hazard that is linked to a maladaptive outcome (Rutter, 1985;Werner & Smith, 1992). Initially, protective factors were regarded as positive experiences that might simply outweigh the negative experiences and events. This presumption was deemed inaccurate, and consequently modern theory recognizes that protective factors may be associated with a wide variety of personal characteristics and situational variables.

When investigating the concurrent contribution of risk and protective factors on resilience outcomes, several conceptualizations emerge. The main effects hypothesis presumes an additive effect of an individual's risk and protective factors, where the positive would outweigh the vulnerabilities in order to increase the probability of a good or "resilient" outcome (Luthar, Ciccetti, & Becker, 2000). This view is most consistent with the compensatory model of resilience, which assumes that protective factors directly counteracts or opposes the risk (Fraser, Richman, & Galinsky, 1999).

Resilience has also been regarded as an interactive process, where different persons may possess the same risk and protective factors, but yet have very diverse outcomes (Greene & Greene, 2009), results of which are not consistent with the "additive" formulation. Other resilience theorists have examined various resilience outcome trajectories in order to explain the method by which risk and protection factors interact among one another (Fraser et al., 1999). The *cumulative* view assumes that protective factors are primarily internal characteristics (e.g., gender, IQ) that directly impact the level of risk to which one may be exposed. The *buffering* view suggests that protective factors directly modify the level of risk so that one still experiences that particular risk, but exposure is less severe with these "protections" in place.

The concept of resilience, while complex in scope, is a still a relatively novel area of study; the results of which can conceivably impact post-trauma/disaster recovery processes. It is well documented that personal (intrinsic) characteristics are highly important to positive adaptation following risk exposure, however, continued resilience research will pinpoint those societal (extrinsic) factors that promote recovery within the affected community (see Chap. 2, this volume, for related discussion). Specifically, investigations focused on post-storm resilience, and adaptability will identify areas lacking in post-disaster supportive action. Lastly, continued resilience investigations will contribute to the development of evidence-based interventions that are designed to reduce suffering and promote effective preparation and post-disaster management.

Coping Styles

Resilience is commonly investigated, and incorrectly defined synonymously, with the presence of coping during stress. Modern theorists regard resilience as a related yet distinct concept; the presence of which is observed post stress and is the product of adaptive coping. As coping is to be investigated during stress, resilience is most appropriately assessed as a post-stress and coping outcome measure. Therefore, while resilience may be highly correlated with coping, it should not be inferred without incorporation of an operationalized measure (Fletcher & Sarkar, 2013).

It has been well documented that the use of adaptive coping strategies can mitigate the deleterious effects of stress. (Eisenbarth, 2012). Early theoretical work depicted coping as a survival response, where an organism would react to any threatening situation in order to maintain life (see Lazarus & Folkman, 1984 for review). This view posited that the relationship between emotion and coping was unidirectional and static, where coping was necessary to alleviate feelings of distress. Most interpretations regarded coping as a simple and direct response to a situation that an individual perceived as threatening, harmful, or challenging (Folkman & Lazarus, 1988; Lazarus & Folkman, 1984). As the body of literature expanded, focus was directed toward examining coping as a cognitive and behavioral process with ability to influence well-being, social functioning, and overall health.

Lazarus and Folkman (1984, 1987) were among the first to view coping not simply as a responsive action but instead as a bidirectional or transactional process. Their transactional theory holds that emotion can influence selected coping style, but that subsequent coping could mediate the emotional response. Lazarus and Folkman suggested that coping responses are mediated by a variety of preexisting individual difference factors, which consist of available resources, personality traits, self-perceived competences, and past experiences. These authors suggested that the context of the situation, as appraised by the person, was significantly important in shaping the coping process. They also assumed that coping decisions were determined after a two-component *appraisal* of the situation. During *primary appraisal,* one must define an event as being irrelevant, benign positive, or stressful. This initial appraisal classifies an event as harmful (damage has already occurred), threatening (potential for damage), and/or challenging (potential for gain or mastery). The *secondary appraisal* process concerns a decision on what can be done about the event. It seeks to answer the question "*What can be done about this?*" During this process, individuals take stock of their resources (e.g., social support, material, psychological) and evaluate their coping options.

Lazarus and Folkman (1984) present two distinct forms of coping and make note that individuals select a style based on "goodness of fit." The purpose of the first form is to alter the troubled person–environment relationship *(problem-focused coping),* while the second is aimed at relieving emotional distress *(emotion-focused coping)*. Zakowski, Hall, Klein, and Baum (2001) found that if one deems the situation controllable, a *problem-focused coping* strategy was usually employed. This form of coping consists of approaches that directly target the situation and source of stress (i.e., confrontational or interpersonal strategies). Alternatively, *emotion-focused coping* frequently usually occurs when one perceives the problem to be unchangeable, and a determination that little (or nothing) can be done is made. Persons who use this strategy may employ acceptance, positivity (find a silver lining), denial, or attempt to limit negative thinking. It is important to note that selection of coping style is not a static trait, as it can vary both across and between stressful encounters (Krohne, 1996).

Resilience and Coping After Disaster

Early disaster research has generated a wealth of descriptive data on disasters, including information such as type/duration of storm, number of injuries/casualties, rates of physical health consequences, and psychopathology rates (Green, 1982; Logue, Melick, & Hansen, 1981a). In recent years, however, increased attention has been directed to the impact of natural disaster exposure on collective psychosocial well-being, coping responses, and resilience among survivors(Bonanno et al., 2007; Cherry, Silva, & Galea, 2009; Cherry et al., 2011; Galea et al., 2002; Silva, Marks, & Cherry, 2009; Silva Brown et al., 2010). This body of literature includes a variety of analytical techniques to describe the psychological sequelae following disaster. Findings have yielded mixed results, with some authors reporting relatively minor rates of psychological distress following exposure and others revealing severe mental health impact (Norris et al., 2002a; Norris, Friedman, & Watson 2002b).

Lack of methodological consistency may be in part to blame for the lack of reliable results from these investigations. Norris et al. (2002a) and (2002b) compiled research from 160 samples of 102 disasters worldwide and subsequently noted that many investigators utilize differing research protocols (e.g., measurement tools, time frames for assessment, and sampling techniques). Furthermore, the type of disaster investigated strongly varied across studies, with natural disasters being the most common form examined, followed by man-made disasters (oil spills) and man-neglect/harm disasters (mass shootings/bombings). Despite these inconsistencies, Norris and colleagues were able to identify a "dose-dependent" relation within numerous publications, where disaster severity was a reliable predictor of psychosocial response within an extensive proportion of studies. In sum, research has consistently shown the consequences of disaster exposure but has yet to examine how to resolve or prevent survivors from succumbing to negative outcomes. These authors fittingly argue that disaster researchers should move forward to examine how risk and protective factors foster resilience within those who reside in disaster-affected communities.

What is the post-disaster trajectory of a resilient individual? Bonanno (2004) has argued there is a distinction between *resilience* and *recovery* following exposure to disaster (see Chaps. 1 and 10, this volume, for related discussion). Resilience, he theorizes, reflects an ability to maintain a stable equilibrium, where individuals do not succumb, but continually uphold their level of current functioning. On the other hand, Bonanno links recovery with a downward trajectory to where dysfunction in time eventually returns to pre-disaster levels. He also argues that resilience has been underestimated in the current literature. In contrast, others presume *adaptability* or the ability to "bounce back" as a hallmark component of individual (and community) resilience post disaster (Norris, Stevens, Pfefferbaum, Wyche, & Pfefferbaum, 2008; Sherrieb, Norris, & Galea, 2010).

Regardless of the debated resilience trajectory, recent research has begun to document the predictors of psychological resilience post disaster. Investigations of post-disaster resilience have inferred the presence of resilience from established correlates. Lee, Shen, and Tran (2009) assessed the predictors of resilience among a sample of 363 African American evacuees from Hurricane Katrina. This study employed structural equation modeling to explain the variance of post-disaster resilience and psychological distress. Resilience was defined as self-reported ability to recover from the disaster at some future point. Distress was measured based upon self-reports of depression, anger, and fear. The results demonstrated that human loss and income were significantly related to the author's concept of resilience.

The presence of long-term resilience among 3812 individuals following the 2004 Indian Ocean tsunami has also been investigated (Frankenberg, Sikoki, Sumantri, Suriastini, & Thomas, 2013). These authors utilized preexisting baseline data and conducted a follow-up nearly 5 years post tsunami. Measurements included demographic data, storm impact assessment (e.g., displacement, need for government assistance), post-traumatic stress reactivity (via post-traumatic stress disorder (PTSD) measures), and level of household economic resources. Regression analyses examined levels of change, and subsequent results revealed education to be predictive of greater resilience, as defined by psychosocial health and household economic resources. These authors also did not incorporate an operationalized measure of resilience, but rather inferred post-disaster resilience from the presence of these positive outcome variables.

Rodriguez-Llanes, Vos, and Guha-Sapir (2013) highlight the importance of creating evidence-based measures of resilience for post-disaster investigations. This work reemphasizes the lack of a clear and consistent definition of resilience across studies, which in conjunction with heterogeneous protocols hampers the assessment of those factors that promote post-disaster adaptation. Adequate measurement tools, such as the Connor–Davidson Resilience Scale (CD-RISC; Connor & Davidson, 2003), the Ego Resilience Scale (Block & Kremen, 1996), and the Brief Resilience Scale (Smith et al., 2008), all provide scale-based scores and have been well validated within the existing literature. Subsequent post-disaster studies should utilize an operationalized resilience measurement.

There is also an even smaller but still growing body of literature that surveys the impact of coping behaviors on post-disaster outcomes (Grattan et al., 2011; McFarlane & Spurrell, 1993; Oni, Harville, Xiong, & Buekens, 2012; Silver, Homlan, McIntosh, Poulin, & Gil-Rivas, 2002). The results from these investigations, while limited, suggest that coping behaviors are potential mediators of mental health. Similar to the science of resilience, the conceptualization of coping varies within the literature; however, many investigations employ the Brief COPE (Carver, 1997) as their primary measurement tool.

Oni, Harville, Xiong, and Buekens (2012) recruited 192 women following Hurricane Katrina. Coping styles of these women were assessed using the Brief COPE (Carver, 1997), in addition to PTSD and depression symptoms. Results reported that denial, behavioral disengagement, venting were related to greater levels of PTSD, while lessened levels were linked with positive reframing and use of humor. Silver et al. (2002) examined coping strategies (measured via Brief COPE) following the September 11th terrorist attacks among 2729 residents of New York City approximately 2 weeks, 2 months, and 6 months after the attacks. Results showed that behavioral disengagement, denial, and self-distraction to be predictive of post-event PTSD scores, while active coping was linked with decreased levels of global distress. Silver et al. concluded that the utilization of disengagement coping strategies increased the odds of psychological distress post disaster. Lastly, Grattan et al. (2011) also utilized the Brief COPE as a measurement indicator of coping response following the British Petroleum Deepwater Horizon Oil Spill (see Chap. 4, this volume). The authors assessed fishing communities that were either directly ($N=23$) or indirectly ($N=71$) economically impacted by the disaster. Income loss was significantly linked with behavioral disengagement strategies and lower resilience levels, measure via the CD-RISC (Connor & Davidson, 2003). Resilience scores did not differ between the two groups.

To summarize, the concepts of coping and resilience, albeit distinct, are related and predictive of one another. The aforementioned review of literature has firmly established the need for post-disaster research that incorporates operationalized measurements of both constructs, as the protective factors contributing post-disaster adaptation remain ambiguous. The successful identification and incorporation of effective coping strategies have the potential to improve post-disaster resilience outcomes. The limited literature warrants the continued investigation of these concepts within post-disaster survivors.

The current study utilized the Brief COPE inventory (Carver, 1997) to evaluate the relationship between coping styles and post-disaster resilience scores, measured via the CD-RISC (Connor & Davidson, 2003), among survivors of the May 22, 2011, Joplin, MO, tornado. The main objective of this study was to isolate characteristics linked with adaptive coping and greater post-tornado resilience among survivors. It was hypothesized that adaptive and maladaptive coping styles would predict post-storm resilience. It was also expected that prior storm exposure would predict resilience scores. This prediction is consistent with the stress inoculation hypothesis, which posits that prior stress exposure fosters resilience to future stress or trauma (Eysenck, 1983; see also Chap. 16, this volume).

Joplin Impact Project

On the early evening of May 22, 2011, disaster struck Joplin, MO, in the form of an EF-5 tornado. The multiple-vortex tornado had a reported width varying between three-quarters and one mile, internal winds over 200 miles per hour, and a destruction path over 22 miles (the US Department of Commerce, National Oceanic and Atmospheric Administration, National Weather Service Central Region Headquarters 2011). Warning sirens were activated 24 min before the storm touched down at 5:34 p.m. When the storm dissipated at 6:12 p.m., only 38 min after arrival, over three quarters of the city had suffered extensive damage. One quarter of Joplin was completely destroyed, taking the lives of 158 people and injuring over 1000 individuals. In the days and weeks following the storm, the Joplin community rallied together to begin the rebuilding of their ravaged community.

The JIP at Drury University was developed during the summer immediately following the tornado. This research initiative examined the psychological and physical health consequences of the tornado in an adult community sample. Data for the JIP came from 87 residents of Joplin, MO. Participants ranged in age from 19 to 86 years (M=37.58; SD=15.61), with 57.5% of the sample being female and 88.5% Caucasian. The majority of participants were recruited from a disaster relief supply bank, where tornado survivors could receive tangible assistance upon providing the necessary documentation from the Federal Emergency Management Agency (FEMA). The remaining participants were recruited via word-of-mouth. Informed consent was obtained, and participants were asked to complete a series of survey instruments (described below). These measures were designed to evaluate storm impact, levels of physical and mental health, coping behaviors, and post-storm resilience. Survey administration occurred in a single session at either the supply bank or a public location (e.g., coffee shop, restaurant) of the participants' choosing. Completion time took approximately 20–25 min, and all participants were compensated with a $25 gift card for their time. Participants were subsequently debriefed and provided with information regarding no-cost counseling resources. Data collection occurred between September 22 and October 7, 2011 (4 months post storm). The protocol and all survey materials were reviewed and approved by the Institutional Review Board at Drury University.

Overview of Dependent Measures

The measures described here are a subset of a larger battery of instruments that were administered to all participants.

Demographic Information Participants completed a series of self-reported demographic items designed to assess their current age, gender, marital status, annual household income, and highest level of education.

Tornado Impact This questionnaire was modeled after an instrument designed to investigate the psychological consequences of 2005 Hurricanes Katrina and Rita (Cherry et al., 2010). The questionnaire contained four separate modules; each intended to address specific elements of the tornado. The *storm exposure and threat to self and family/property* module included questions that assessed storm-related damage, fear for safety, storm impact on self/family/friends. The *storm-related disruption and stressors* module included questions about environmental/property issues (i.e., experienced power loss and/or property damage) and the types of disruption created by the storms. The *social support* module assessed the availability of help if needed before and after the storms, charitable giving, volunteer work done for others, and other psychosocial issues (housed displaced family members or other evacuees; helped evacuees in other ways, such as volunteering or assisting with relief efforts). The *lifetime exposure to potentially traumatic events* module documented participants' exposure to other stressful or disturbing events, such as previous disaster experience(s), serious accidents, physical attacks, and/or military combat.

Data for this report stem primarily from the *storm exposure and threat to self and family/property* module. This study utilized the impact questionnaire to examine four exposure factors: *presence of tornado damage* (0=no, 1=yes), *displacement due to tornado* (0=no, 1=yes), *exposure to another natural disaster exposure* (0=no, 1=yes), and *level of fear during the tornado* (0=not afraid, 1=a little afraid, 2=fairly afraid, 3=moderately afraid, and 4=extremely afraid).

Objective Health Status Health status was based on a cumulative index reflecting the self-reported presence of six chronic conditions (i.e., hypertension, cardiovascular disease, diabetes, asthma, cancer, and self-reported physical disability). These conditions were selected in order to provide a broad assessment of health in an adult population. Conditions range in severity from mild/moderate (e.g., hypertension) to more severe (e.g., cardiovascular disease). Prior research has shown that the number of chronic conditions systematically increases with age (Administration on Aging, 2013), and consequently, this is seen as an adequate index of health. For each participant, scores of 0 (absence) and 1 (presence) were assigned for each health condition. These individual condition scores were then added to create a cumulative, composite index of health, ranging from 0 to 6 points. This version of the Chronic 6 Index was adapted from Cherry et al. (2013).

Psychological Functioning Current level of anxiety, depression, and PTSD was assessed for each participant. Anxiety and depression were measured using Public Health Questionnaires 7 (PHQ-7) and 9 (PHQ-9), respectively. These diagnostic tools incorporate a series questions and assign scores based on responses of *not at all* (0), *several days* (1), *more than half the days* (2), and *nearly every day* (3). Total anxiety scores can range from 0 to 21, with cutoff scores of 5 (mild), 10 (moderate), and 15 (severe). Total depression scores can range from 0 to 27, with cutoff scores of 5 (mild), 10 (moderate), 15 (moderately severe), and 20 (severe). Both the PHQ-7 and PHQ-9 are well-validated measures that have been deemed appropriate for use in a general adult population (Dear et al., 2011; Kroenke, Spitzer, & Williams, 2001).

PTSD scores were assessed using the PTSD checklist—Civilian Version (Weathers, Litz, Herman, Huska, & Keane, 1993). This self-report measurement scale uses a series of 17 items designed to reflect current diagnostic criteria. Individual response items are scored from 1 to 5 with 1=*not at all,* 2=*a little bit,* 3=*moderately,* 4=*quite a bit,* and 5=*extremely*. Total PSTD checklist scores range from 17 to 85, and summing of the *moderately, quite a bit,* and *extremely* reported items can be associated with the number of symptoms and severity of the disorder. Scores ranging from 17 to 33 indicate low PTSD, from 34 to 43 indicate moderate PTSD, and scores above 44 indicate high PTSD. The psychometric properties of the PTSD checklist are well documented in the literature (Ruggiero, Del Ben, Scotti, & Rabalais, 2003).

Coping Style The Brief COPE (Carver, 1997) was administered to examine the presence of unique styles of coping among tornado survivors. Participants were instructed to reflect upon the tornado and choose the frequency of their post-disaster coping behaviors. The 28 individual response items were coded on a Likert scale ranging from 1 to 4, with 1=*I have not been doing this at all,* 2=*I have been doing this a little bit,* 3=*I have been doing this a medium amount,* and 4=*I have been doing this a lot*. Response items were combined and summed to produce scores for 14 subscales, where higher scores reflecting greater frequency.

Scores for the 14 distinct coping styles were subsequently clustered and summed together to create three broad coping categories: Problem-focused (active coping, planning, religion, and instrumental support subscales), active emotional (venting, positive reframing, acceptance, humor, and emotional support subscales), and avoidant emotional (denial, behavioral disengagement, and self-distraction, substance abuse, and self-blame subscales), after Schneider, Elhai, and Gray (2007). Favorable psychometric properties are well documented in the current literature, and the Brief COPE has been deemed appropriate for use within the general adult population (Windle, Bennert, & Noyes, 2011).

Resilience Post-disaster resilience scores were obtained from the CD-RISC (Connor & Davidson, 2003). This 25-item scale was scored on a 5-point scale from 0=*not true at all,* 1=*rarely true,* 2=*sometimes true,* 3=*often true,* and 4=*nearly true all the time*. Individual CD-RISC items are summed together to create a composite score ranging from 0 to 100, where a higher score reflects a greater level of post-storm resilience. The CD-RISC has shown sound psychometric properties among nonclinical and clinical populations in recent years (Ahern, Kiehl, Sole, & Byers, 2006).

Results

Descriptive Statistics Sample characteristics, demographic, and mental and physical health scores appear in Table 3.1. Participants ranged in age between 19 and 86 years ($M=37.58$; $SD=15.61$). The sample was distributed relatively well between male (42.5 %) and female (57.5 %) participants, with the majority of persons identifying as Caucasian (88.5 %). Most of the individuals identified as married (42.5 %), followed by single (36.8 %), divorced (19.5 %), and then widowed (1.1 %). Regarding educational status, over one quarter of persons reported having less than a high school diploma (27.6 %), with 26.4 % having a high school diploma, and the remaining identified as either having some college training (34.5 %) or bachelors/masters degree (10.3 %). The breakdown of annual income was as follows: $10,000 or under (21.8%), $10,001–$20,000 (25.3%), $20,001–$30,000 (24.1%), $30,001–$40,000 (12.6%), $40,001–$50,000 (2.3%), US$ 50,0001 or more (6.9 %), and a subset reported, “Don’t know/decline” (6.9 %).

Table 3.1 Participant characteristics (N=87)

	N		%	
Sex				
Male	37		42.5	
Female	50		57.5	
Race/ethnicity				
African American	4		4.6	
Asian American	2		2.3	
Caucasian	77		88.5	
Native American	1		1.1	
Multiracial	2		2.3	
Other	1		1.1	
Education[a]				
Less than high school	24		27.6	
High school	23		26.4	
Some college	30		34.5	
Bachelors	6		6.9	
Masters	3		3.4	
Doctorate	0		0	
Marital status				
Single	32		36.8	
Married	37		42.5	
Divorced	17		19.5	
Widowed	1		1.1	
Annual household income				
$0–$10,000	19		21.8	
$10,0001–$20,000	22		25.3	
$20,001–$30,000	21		24.1	
$30,001–$40,000	11		12.6	
$40,000–$50,000	2		2.3	
$50,001+	6		6.9	
Decline/do not know	6		6.9	
	Mean	SD	Minimum	Maximum
Age[a]	37.58	15.61	19	86
Chronic 6	0.63	0.88	0	3
Anxiety (PHQ-7)	7.43	5.78	0	21
Depression (PHQ-9)	7.95	6.72	0	26
PTSD checklist	35.83	16.13	17	85
Resilience (CD-RISC)	70.70	20.27	1	100

PHQ Public Health Questionnaire, *PTSD* post-traumatic stress disorder, *CD-RISC* Connor–Davidson Resilience Scale

[a]Indicates missing data

Tornado Exposure Table 3.2 presents the results of the storm impact questionnaire. Out of the 87 persons who completed the inventory, 82.8% (N=72) reported being present in Joplin when the tornado touched down. Nearly all (93.1%) of the

Table 3.2 Storm impact questionnaire ($N=87$)

	N	%
Were you in Joplin when the tornado occurred?		
Yes	72	82.8
No	15	17.2
Were family/friends in Joplin when the tornado occurred?		
Yes	81	93.1
No	3	3.4
Don't know	3	3.4
Did the tornado damage your property?		
Yes	60	69.0
No	27	31.0
Did the tornado damage family/friends' property?		
Yes	80	92.0
No	5	5.7
N/A	2	2.3
Were you displaced as a result of the tornado?		
Yes	39	44.8
No	48	55.2
Were family/friends displaced as a result of the tornado?		
Yes	63	72.4
No	22	25.3
N/A	2	2.3
How afraid were you that you may be seriously killed or injured?[a]		
Not afraid at all	17	19.8
A little afraid	14	16.3
Moderately afraid	19	22.1
Extremely afraid	36	41.9
How afraid were you that your family/friends may be seriously killed or injured?		
Not afraid at all	2	2.3
A little afraid	12	13.8
Moderately afraid	17	19.5
Extremely afraid	54	62.1
N/A	2	2.3
Looking back, how safe do you really think you were?		
Not safe at all	26	30.2
Not too safe	24	27.9
Fairly safe	26	30.2
Very Safe	10	11.6
Looking back, how safe do you really think your family/friends were?		
Not safe at all	39	44.8
Not too safe	32	36.8
Fairly safe	12	13.8
Very Safe	2	2.3
N/A	2	2.3

[a]Indicates missing data

participants reported having family or friends in the Joplin area. For those persons who reported having no family or friends in the Joplin area, a "*non-applicable*" option was available on subsequent questions. A large portion (69 %) of the sampled population suffered personal property damage, with 44.8 % reporting being displaced from their residence. In accordance with the level of reported damage, over half of all participants (63.7 %) stated that they were either extremely (41.6 %) or moderately afraid (22.1 %) during the tornado. Additionally, the majority of participants had family or friends who suffered property damage (92 %) and/or were displaced (72 %) from their homes.

Mental and Physical Health The PHQ-9 depression total scores ranged from 0 to 26 ($M=7.95$; $SD=6.72$). Regarding depression severity, 39.01 % ($N=34$) of the sample was considered minimal/not depressed, 27.59 % ($N=24$) was mildly depressed, 14.94 % ($N=13$) was moderately depressed, 10.34 % ($N=9$) was moderately severe depressed, and 8.46 % ($N=7$) was severely depressed. The PHQ-7 generalized anxiety total scores ranged from 0 to 21 ($M=7.43$; $SD=5.78$). Regarding anxiety severity, 36.78 % ($N=32$) of the sample was considered minimal/not anxious, 31.03 % ($N=27$) was mildly anxious, 18.39 % ($N=16$) was moderately anxious, and 13.79 % ($N=12$) was severely anxious. The PTSD checklist total scores ranged from 17 to 85 ($M=35.83$; $SD=16.13$). Regarding PTSD severity, 32.18 % ($N=28$) of the sample was considered to exhibit high levels of post-traumatic stress. Resilience (CD-RISC) scores ranged from 1 to 100 with an average sample score of 70.70 ($SD=20.27$). The Chronic 6 Index scores ranged from 0 to 3 ($M=0.63$; $SD=0.88$).

Correlational analyses (Table 3.3) were conducted among PHQ-7, PHQ-9, PTSD checklist, Chronic 6 Index, and CD-RISC measures. Correlation results revealed significant negative relationships of PHQ-7 anxiety ($r=-.475$, $p<.001$), PHQ-9 depression ($r=-.815$, $p<.001$), and PTSD checklist ($r=-.366$, $p<.001$), with CD-RISC resilience. The PHQ-7 anxiety, PHQ-9 depression, and PTSD checklist all showed significant positive correlations with one another. The Chronic 6 Index did not significantly correlate with any variables.

Regression Analysis A two-stage hierarchical regression analysis was conducted to determine the predictive impact of age, gender, marital status (entered as yes/no), income (enter as greater/less than $20,000 per year), prior storm exposure (entered as yes/no), and three coping styles (problem-focused, active emotional, and avoidant emotional) on resilience among adult survivors. Listwise deletion was selected to address missing data, which resulted in a total of 77 participants for this analysis. Demographic factors (age, gender, marital status, income, prior storm exposure) were entered on the first step, while the three distinct coping styles were entered on the second step. Results are shown in Table 3.4. The overall model predicting resilience from demographic factors was not significant (F (5, 71)$=.92$, $p=.473$) and accounted for only 6 % of the variance. Introducing the three coping style variables was significant and explained an additional 50 % of the variance in resilience (F (3, 68)$=10.87$ $p<.001$). The avoidant emotional coping style was the greatest predictor of resilience and uniquely accounted for 31 % of the variance ($B=-2.48$, $p<.001$,

Table 3.3 Spearman correlations among anxiety (PHQ-7), depression (PHQ-9), PTSD (PCL checklist), resilience (CD-RISC), and physical health (Chronic 6 Index)

	1	2	3	4
Anxiety (1)	–	–	–	–
Depression (2)	*0.876**	–	–	–
N	87	–	–	–
PTSD(3)	*0.816**	*0.818**	–	–
N	87	–	–	–
Resilience (4)	*–.475**	*–.518**	*–.366**	–
N	87	87	87	–
Chronic 6 (5)	.139	.104	.144	.016
	87	87	87	87

**p* <.01

Table 3.4 Regression analysis predicting resilience from demographic measures and coping styles

	R^2	ΔR^2	B	β	sr^2	F
Step 1 (demographics)	.06	.06	–	–	–	$F(5, 71)=0.92$
Age	–	–	.05	.04	.001	–
Gender	–	–	−1.37	–.03	–.001	–
Marital status (Y/N)	–	–	7.40	.18	.03	–
Household Income (</>US$ 20,000)	–	–	–3.27	–.08	–.005	–
Prior storm exposure (Y/N)	–	–	2.91	.07	.005	–
Step 2 (coping styles)	.56	.50	–	–	–	$F(8, 68)=10.87$**
Problem-focused	–	–	*1.64***	.43	.12	–
Active emotional	–	–	*1.09**	.23	.03	–
Avoidant emotional	–	–	*–2.48***	–.59	–.31	–

*Significant at the .05 level
**Significant at the .01 level

$sr^2=-.31$). Problem-focused coping was the second greatest predictor of resilience ($B=1.64$, $p=.001$, $sr^2=.12$), accounting for 12 % of the variance. Lastly, active emotional coping was also a significant predictor of resilience ($B=1.09$, $p<.05$, $sr^2=.03$), accounting for 3 % of the variance.

Conclusion and Future Directions

This chapter provides new evidence concerning storm exposure, coping style, and resilience among residents of Joplin, MO, following the 2011 tornado. Two primary findings emerged from the analyses. First, the storm impact data reveal substantial destruction and devastation due the Joplin tornado. A majority (69 %) of participants reported damage to their personal property, and nearly half (44.8 %) had been displaced. The strong sense of fear during the tornado was also documented, as nearly two thirds (64 %) of the sample stated they were moderately to extremely afraid that they might be killed or seriously injured. While cross-disaster comparisons are limited due to distinctions in terms of disaster severity and type, one can reasonably argue that the severity of the Joplin tornado could relate to greater psychosocial sequelae among survivors. This is consistent with Norris and colleagues (see Norris et al., 2002a, b), who identified a dose-dependent relationship between disaster severity and psychosocial outcomes. Also, JIP data did not support the notion that an "inoculation" effect occurred (Eysenck, 1983), as prior storm exposure did not relate to increased levels of resilience among JIP participants. Consequently, it is recommended that post-storm "on-the-ground" interventions be based in part on self-reported fear of survivors, as well disaster type and destruction levels.

The second finding revealed that the mental health measures and coping styles were significantly related to post-storm resilience levels within this Joplin sample. These data provide a novel contribution to the existing literature on coping and resilience among disaster survivors. Specifically, all three mental health measures negatively correlated ($p<.001$) with psychological resilience as measured by the CD-RISC. Outcomes from the two-tier regression analysis revealed that the three coping styles, problem-focused ($p<.001$), active emotional ($p=.030$), and avoidant emotional ($p<.001$), were all significant predictors of CD-RISC scores. Age, gender, marital status, income, and prior storm exposure were not significant predictors of CD-RISC scores. This study indicates that Joplin residents who engaged in problem-focused (e.g., active coping, planning) or active emotional (e.g., positive reframing, humor, acceptance) coping strategies reported greater levels of resilience, while those who engaged in avoidant emotional (e.g., denial, behavioral disengagement) coping reported lower levels of resilience.

These results are consistent with other disaster-based literature that was previously discussed. Oni et al. (2012) found that the use of behavioral disengagement coping styles was predictive of lessened PTSD symptoms among survivors of Hurricanes Katrina. Silver et al. (2002) found behavioral disengagement, denial, and self-distraction to be predictive of PTSD scores, while active coping was linked with decreased levels of global distress among survivors of the September 11, 2001, terrorist attacks. Lastly, Grattan et al. (2011) also reported a negative relationship between behavioral disengagement coping strategies and resilience scores (measure via the CD-RISC) among residents impacted by the BP Deepwater Horizon Oil Spill. The collective inspection of these findings uncovers similar post-disaster trends, all of which speak to the hypothesis that an overreliance on avoidant emotional coping styles may lead to adverse psychological outcomes post disaster. Consequently, the pre-identification of persons who utilize avoidant strategies, in addition to the fostering of active coping methods, may be effective methods for clinicians and health professionals to employ during post-disaster assessments.

Three primary methodological limitations of the current study should be addressed. First, the lack of pre-storm baseline data does not permit inferences regarding changes in mental health and resilience scores due to the tornado. While the literature may suggest that anxiety, depression, and PTSD scores increase post disaster, without the availability of baseline data, these conclusions are not warranted. Second, data for the JIP were collected approximately 4-months post storm in order to assess immediate impact. Prior disaster literature has shown that psychological responses change with time (Silver et al., 2002); therefore, additional follow-up studies would be necessary to infer mental health change or infer community "recovery" with time. Lastly, the JIP sample size (N=87) was relatively small, and consequently, one may contend that this sample is not generalizable to the larger Joplin (or another tornado impacted) community. Yet notwithstanding the smaller sample size, the participant and diversity characteristics closely resemble the population demographics of Joplin (The Heller School, 2012). To speak to this concern, subsequent investigations may want to increase external validity through the use of an increased sample size.

In closing, the present results provide a novel contribution to the small but growing body of literature on psychosocial functioning and well-being post disaster. Results demonstrate the importance of acknowledging that disasters, while destructive in nature, do not produce equivalent psychological aftermaths. Preparatory experiences, as well as personal experiences amid the storm, may lead to differing levels of distress across individuals and communities. Furthermore, the dependence on avoidant coping strategies may be associated with elevated PSTD scores, while consequently lowering psychological resilience. In light of these findings, further research into evidence-based interventions that increase storm preparation and promote post-disaster adaptational coping skills should be conducted.

Acknowledgments I would like to thank Alexandra Duello, Bailey Greene, Blake Herd, Spencer Prevalett, Morgan Merrell, Melanie Messick, and Paige Nichols for their assistance with data collection for the JIP. This research was supported by the Office of the Vice President for Academic Affairs, the Department of Behavioral Sciences, and the Hammons School of Architecture at Drury University. This support is gratefully acknowledged.

References

Administration on Aging, U.S. Department of Health and Human Services. (2013). *A profile of older Americans:* 2013. http://www.aoa.gov/Aging_Statistics/Profile/2013/14.aspx. Accessed August 2014.

Ahern, N. R., Kiehl, E. M., Sole, M. L., & Byers, J. (2006). A review of instruments measuring resilience. *Issues in Comprehensive Pediatric Nursing, 29,* 103–125.

Benard, B. (1991). *Fostering resiliency in kids: Protective factors in the family, school and community*. Portland: Northwest Regional Educational Laboratory.

Benard, B., & Slade, S. (2009). Listening to students: Moving from resilience research to youth development practice and school connectedness. In R. Gilman, E. S. Huebner, & M. J. Furlong (Eds.) *Handbook of positive psychology in schools* (pp. 353–370). New York: Routledge.

Block, J., & Kremen, A. M. (1996). IQ and ego-resiliency: Conceptual and empirical connections and separateness. *Journal of Personality and Social Psychology, 70,* 349–361.

Bonanno, G. A. (2004) Loss, trauma, and human resilience: Have we underestimated the human capacity to thrive after extremelyaversive events? *American Psychologist, 59,* 20–28.

Bonanno, G. A., Galea, S., Bucciarelli, A., & Vlahov, D. (2007). What predicts psychological resilience after disaster? The role of demographics, resources, and life stress. *Journal of Consulting and Clinical Psychology, 75,* 671–682.

Carver, C. S. (1997). You want to measure coping but your protocol's too long: Consider the Brief COPE. *International Journal of Behavioral Medicine, 4,* 92–100.

Cherry, K. E., Silva, J., & Galea, S. (2009). Natural disasters and the oldest-old: A psychological perspective on coping and health in late life. In K. E. Cherry (Ed.), *Lifespan perspectives on natural disasters: Coping with Katrina, Rita and other storms* (pp. 171–193). New York: Springer.

Cherry, K. E., Galea, S., Su, J. L., Welsh, D. A., Jazwinski, S. M., Silva, J. L., & Erwin, M. J. (2010). Cognitive and psychosocial consequences of Hurricanes Katrina and Rita among middle aged, older and oldest-old adults in the Louisiana Healthy Aging Study (LHAS). *Journal of Applied Social Psychology, 40,* 2463–2487.

Cherry, K. E., Silva Brown, J., Marks, L. D., Galea, S., Volaufova, J., Lefante, C., et al. (2011). Longitudinal assessment of cognitive and psychosocial functioning after hurricanes Katrina and Rita: Exploring disaster impact on middle-aged, older, and oldest-old adults. *Journal of Applied Biobehavioral Research, 16,* 187–211.

Cherry, K. E., Jackson Walker, E. M., Silva Brown, J. L., Volaufova, J., LaMotte, L. R., Su, L. J., et al. (2013). Social engagement and health in younger, older, and oldest-old adults in the Louisiana Healthy Aging Study (LHAS). *Journal of Applied Gerontology, 32,* 51–75.

Connor K. M., & Davidson, J. R. T. (2003). Development of a new resilience scale: The Connor–Davidson Resilience Scale (CD-RISC). *Depression and Anxiety, 18,* 76–82.

Dear, B. F., Titov, N., Sunderland, M., McMillan, D., Anderson, T., Lorian, C. & Robinson, E. (2011). Psychometric comparison of the GAD-7 and the PSWQ for measuring response during treatment of generalized anxiety disorder. *Cognitive Behavior Therapy, 40,* 216–227.

DeHaan, L., Hawley, D., & Deal, J.E. (2002). Operationalizing family resilience: A methodological strategy. *American Journal of Family Therapy, 30,* 275–291

Eisenbarth, C. (2012). Coping profiles and psychological distress: A cluster analysis. *North American Journal of Psychology, 14,* 485–496.

Eysenck, H. (1983). Stress, disease, and personality: The inoculation effect. In C. L. Cooper (Ed.), *Stress research* (pp. 121–146). New York: Wiley.

Fletcher, D., & Sarkar, M. (2013). Psychological resilience: A review and critique of definitions, concepts and theory. *European Psychologist, 18,* 12–23.

Folkman, S., & Lazarus, R. S. (1988). Coping as a mediator of emotion. *Journal of Personality and Social Psychology, 54,* 466–475.

Frankenberg, E., Sikoki, B., Sumantri, C., Suriastini, W., & Thomas, D. (2013). Education, vulnerability, and resilience after a natural disaster. *Ecology and Society, 18,* 16.

Fraser, M, Richman, J, & Galinsky, M. (1999). Risk, protection, and resilience: Towards a conceptual framework for social work practice. *Social Work Research, 23,* 131–144.

Galea, S., Ahern, J., Resnick, H., Kilpatrick, D., Bucuvalas, M., Gold, J., & Vlahov, D. (2002). Psychological sequelae of the September 11 terrorist attacks in New York City. *New England Journal of Medicine, 346*(13), 982–987.

Grattan, L., Roberts, S., Mahan, W., McLaughlin, P., Otwell, W. S., & Morris J. G. J. (2011). The early psychological impacts of the Deepwater Horizon oil spill on Florida and Alabama communities. *Environmental Health Perspectives, 119,* 838–843.

Green, B. L. (1982). Assessing level of psychological impairment following disaster. *Journal of Nervous & Mental Disease, 170,* 544–552.

Greene, R. R., & Greene, D. G. (2009). Resilience in the face of disasters: Bridging micro- and macro-perspectives. *Journal of Human Behavior in the Social Environment, 19,* 1010–1024.

The Heller School for Social Policy and Management (2012). *Population demographics and diversity for Joplin, Missouri.* http://diversitydata.sph.harvard.edu/Data/Profiles/Show.aspx?loc!!/span>=716. Accessed August 2014.

Krohne, H. W. (1996). Individual differences in coping. In M. Zeidner & N. S. Endler (Eds.), *Handbook of coping: Theory, research, applications* (pp. 381–409). New York: Wiley.

Kroenke, K., Spitzer, R. L., & Williams, J. B. W (2001). The PHQ-9: Validity of a brief depression severity measure. *Journal of General Internal Medicine, 16,* 606–613.

Lazarus, R. S., & Folkman, S. (1984). *Stress, appraisal, and coping.* New York: Springer.

Lazarus, R. S., & Folkman, S. (1987). Transactional theory and research on emotions and coping. *European Journal of Personality, 1,* 141–169.
Lee, E. O., Shen, C., & Tran, T. (2009). Coping with Hurricane Katrina: Learning from African American survivors. *Journal of Black Psychology, 35,* 1–23
Logue, J. N., Melick, M. E., & Hansen, H. (1981a). Research issues and directions in the epidemiology of health effects of disasters. *Epidemiologic Reviews, 3,* 140–162.
Logue, J. N., Melick, M. E, & Stuening, E. L. (1981b). A study of health and mental health status following a major natural disaster. In R. Simons (Ed.), *Research in community health* (pp. 217–274). Greenwich: JAI.
Luthar, S. S., & Cicchetti, D. (2000). The construct of resilience: Implications for intervention and social policy. *Development and Psychopathology, 12,* 857–885.
Luthar, S.S., & Cicchetti, D., & Becker, B. (2000). The construct of resilience: A critical evaluation and guidelines for future work. *Child Development, 71,* 543–562.
Masten, A. S. (2001). Ordinary magic: Resilience processes in development. *American Psychologist, 56,* 227–238.
McFarlane, A. C., & Spurrell, M. (1993). Posttraumatic stress disorder and coping after a natural disaster. *Social Psychiatry and Psychiatric Epidemiology, 28,* 194–200.
Norris F. H., Friedman M. J., Watson P. J., Byrne, C. M., Diaz, E., & Kaniasty, K. (2002a). 60,000 disaster victims speak: Part I. An empirical review of the empirical literature, 1981–2001. *Psychiatry, 65,* 207–239.
Norris F. H, Friedman M. J., & Watson P. J. (2002b). 60,000 disaster victims speak: Part II. Summary and implications of the disaster mental health research. *Psychiatry, 65,* 240–260.
Norris, F. H., Stevens, S. P., Pfefferbaum, B., Wyche, K. F., & Pfefferbaum, R. L. (2008). Community resilience as a metaphor, theory, set of capacities, and strategies for disaster readiness. *American Journal of Community Psychology, 41,* 127–150.
Oni, O., Harville, E. W., Xiong, X., & Buekens, P. (2012). Impact of coping styles on post-traumatic stress disorder and depressive symptoms among pregnant women exposed to Hurricane Katrina. *American Journal of Disaster Medicine, 7,* 199–209.
Polusny, M., Ries, B. J., Schultz, J. R., Calhoun, P., Clemensen, L., & Johnsen, I. (2008). PTSD symptom clusters associated with physical health and health care utilization in rural primary care patients exposed to natural disaster. *Journal of Traumatic Stress, 21,* 75–82.
Rodriguez-Llanes, J. M., Vos, F., & Guha-Sapir, D. (2013). Measuring psychological resilience to disasters: Are evidence-based indicators an achievable goal? *Environmental Health, 12,* 115–136.
Ruggiero, K. J., Del Ben, K., Scotti, J. R., & Rabalais, A. E. (2003). Psychometric properties of the PTSD Checklist—civilian version. *Journal of Traumatic Stress, 16,* 495–502.
Rutter, M. (1985). Resilience in the face of adversity: Protective factors and resistance to psychiatric disorder. *British Journal of Psychiatry, 147,* 598–611.
Rutter, M. (2006). Implications of resilience concepts for scientific understanding. *Annals of the New York Academy of Science, 1094,* 1–12.
Rutter, M. (2012). Resilience as a dynamic process. *Developmental Psychopathology, 24,* 335–344.
Schneider, K. R., Elhai, J. D., & Gray, M. J. (2007). Coping style predicts posttraumatic stress and complicated grief symptom severity among college students reporting traumatic loss. *Journal of Counseling Psychology, 54,* 344–350.
Sherrieb, K., Norris, F. H., & Galea, S. (2010). Measuring capacities for community resilience. *Social Indicators Research, 99,* 227–247.
Silva, J. L., Marks, L. D., & Cherry, K. E. (2009). The psychology behind helping and prosocial behaviors: An examination from intention to action. In K. E. Cherry (Ed.), *Lifespan perspectives on natural disasters: Coping with Katrina, Rita and other Storms* (pp. 219–240). New York: Springer.
Silva Brown, J., Cherry, K. E., Marks, L. D., Jackson, E. M., Volaufova, J., Lefante, C., & Jazwinski, S. M. (2010). After Hurricanes Katrina and Rita: Gender differences in health and religiosity in middle-aged and older adults. *Health Care for Women International, 31,* 997–1012.

Silver, R. C., Holman, E. A., McIntosh, D. N., Poulin, M., & Gil-Rivas, V. (2002). Nationwide longitudinal study of psychological responses to September 11. *Journal of the American Medical Association, 288,* 1235–1244.

Smith, B. W., Dalen, J., Wiggins, K., Tooley, E., Christopher, P., & Bernard, J. (2008). The brief resilience scale: Assessing the ability to bounce back. *International Journal of Behavioral Medicine, 15,* 194–200.

U.S. Department of Commerce, National Oceanic and Atmospheric Administration, National Weather Service Central Region Headquarters (July 2011). *NWS Central Region Service Assessment: Joplin, Missouri, Tornado – May 22, 2011*. Kansas City, Missouri. http://www.nws.noaa.gov/om/assessments/pdfs/Joplin_tornado.pdf. Accessed December 2014.

Werner, E., & Smith, R. (1992). *Overcoming the odds: High risk children from birth to adulthood.* Ithaca: Cornell University Press.

Weathers, F. W., Litz, B. T., Herman, D. S., Huska, J. A., & Keane, T. M. (1993). The PTSD checklist: Reliability, validity, and diagnostic utility. Presented at the Annual Meeting of the International Society for Traumatic Stress Studies. San Antonio, TX, October 1993.

Windle, G., Bennett, K., & Noyes, J. (2011). A methodological review of resilience measurement scales. *Health and Quality of Life Outcomes, 9,* 8.

Zakowski, G. S., Hall, M. H., Klein, L. C., & Baum, A. (2001). Appraised control, coping, and stress in a community sample: A test of the goodness-of-fit hypothesis. *Annals of Behavioral Medicine, 23,* 158–165.

Chapter 4
When Multiple Disasters Strike: Louisiana Fishers in the Aftermath of Hurricanes and the British Petroleum Deepwater Horizon Oil Spill

Bethany A. Lyon, Pamela F. Nezat, Katie E. Cherry and Loren D. Marks

Introduction

The 2010 Deepwater Horizon oil spill devastated the US Gulf Coast, particularly Louisiana, Mississippi, Alabama, and Florida. Many coastal residents, especially commercial fishers, were directly impacted by the approximately 200 million gallons[1] of oil that spilled into the Gulf Coast. Years after the spill, lasting effects to the coastal communities can still be seen. Louisiana Gulf Coast fishers and their families offer a prototypical example of cumulative adversity, given that Hurricanes Katrina and Rita ravaged this same region in 2005, followed by severe Hurricanes Gustav and Ike in 2008. Given the paucity of research on both natural and technological disaster exposure, individuals and families who have weathered storms and are striving to endure the uncertainties of the BP oil spill have unique insights to offer on cumulative adversity during a historically difficult period of time and circumstance. Our objective in this chapter is to capture and express the fears and

[1] There are 42 gallons in a barrel of oil, placing the British Petroleum (BP) oil spill at roughly 5 million barrels. Spill estimates range from 185 to 205 million gallons of oil.

B. A. Lyon (✉) · P. F. Nezat · K. E. Cherry
Department of Psychology, Louisiana State University, 236 Audubon Hall,
Baton Rouge, LA 70803-5501, USA
e-mail: blyon2@tigers.lsu.edu

P. F. Nezat
e-mail: pamela.nezat@gmail.com

K. E. Cherry
e-mail: pskatie@lsu.edu

L. D. Marks
School of Family Life, Brigham Young University, 2092C Joseph F. Smith Building,
Provo, Utah 84602, USA
e-mail: loren_marks@byu.edu

K. E. Cherry (ed.), *Traumatic Stress and Long-Term Recovery*,
DOI 10.1007/978-3-319-18866-9_4

concerns faced by commercial fishers and to convey the resilience exemplified by many of the individuals and families who shared their experience with us during structured interviews conducted at least 12 months after the BP oil spill.

Overview of Literature

In the paragraphs that follow, we briefly review previous studies that span three catastrophic oil spills: the North Sea oil rig disaster, the *Exxon Valdez* oil spill, and early findings from the BP Deepwater Horizon oil spill. We then turn our attention to the concept of cumulative adversity and a closely related notion, the *pileup* of demands that impact family stress and adaptation in the wake of multiple stressors.

The 1980 North Sea Oil Rig Disaster

The 1980 North Sea oil rig disaster occurred between the United Kingdom and Norway. One of the rig legs broke and the entire oil rig capsized due to poor weather conditions. Of the 212 men on board, only 89 survived the disaster (Holgersen, Klöckner, Boe, Weisæth & Holen, 2011). Holgersen et al. (2011) carried out a longitudinal study focused on long-term mental health after the oil rig disaster, testing participants in 1980, 1981, 1985, and 2007. Based on analyses of participants' symptoms of post-traumatic stress disorder (PTSD), four symptom trajectories were revealed: resilient, recovery, chronic, or relapse. The largest group was the resilient group ($n=43$), which had diminishing PTSD scores after the disaster—and in many cases reduced to a score of zero after just a few years. The recovery group ($n=10$) showed a gradual decline in PTSD symptoms across the 27-year span. The chronic group ($n=8$) showed essentially no reduction in symptoms across time, and the relapse group ($n=9$) followed the initial gradual reduction of symptoms in the first few months post disaster, but then experienced a gradual increase in symptoms over the course of the next 27 years. These trajectories and typologies convey widely differential adjustment patterns across individuals experiencing the same disaster. Additional research is needed to help determine (and perhaps predict) which people impacted by a disaster are most at risk for falling into one of the latter, more negatively impacted and less resilient groups.

The 1989 Exxon Valdez Oil Spill

The Exxon Valdez supertanker disaster on March 24, 1989, on Bligh Reef in Prince William Sound, Alaska was (at the time) the worst oil spill in the US history. Many studies document long-term threats to mental health in commercial fishers affected by the *Exxon Valdez* oil spill. For instance, Palinkas, Petterson, Russell, and Downs

(1993) tested participants in 13 Alaskan communities affected by the *Exxon Valdez* oil spill 1 year after the disaster occurred. The researchers determined that participants who were highly exposed to the oil spill (those who resided in coastal areas) had higher rates of mental health problems than those from a community further from the disaster area. Arata, Picou, Johnson, and McNally (2000) also studied commercial fishers 6 years after the *Exxon Valdez* oil spill. Their findings indicated that those who suffered economic loss after the spill showed higher levels of depression, PTSD, and anxiety than those who did not experience economic losses.

Comparisons Between the Exxon Valdez and BP Deepwater Horizon Oil Spills

The *Exxon Valdez* findings,which document profound and lasting harm for those whose livelihood depends on natural resources, provide historical precedent for understanding the current circumstances of the US Gulf Coast fishers (including shrimpers and oystermen) affected by the BP Deepwater Horizon spill. Gill, Picou, and Ritchie (2012) reported a direct comparison between the *Exxon Valdez* disaster and the BP Deepwater Horizon oil spill for the mental and social health of people directly affected by the spills 5 months after these events. High stress levels were found in both groups of participants, with the strongest predictors of high stress levels being family health concerns, commercial ties to the renewable resources, [uncertain] economic future, economic loss, and exposure to the oil.

The 2010 BP Deepwater Horizon Oil Spill

The 2010 BP Deepwater Horizon oil spill was reported to be the worst spill this continent has ever seen, with estimates of 200 million gallons of oil that poured into the Gulf of Mexico (Gill et al., 2012). The spill has been devastating to the commercial fishing and seafood industries. The long-term impacts of an oil spill of this magnitude on the environment and the industries tied to the environment are still undetermined. When an event of an unprecedented scale occurs, experts have no direct point of reference. Some researchers have looked to previous oil spills in order to extrapolate and to establish some hypothetical expectations to relieve the uncertainty felt by coastal residents, as well as anticipating the environmental implications, but this is not an easy charge. It is, of course, a more attainable goal to estimate damage done versus predicting future effects.

Indeed, there is evidence pertaining to the immediate psychosocial impacts of the 2010 BP Deepwater Horizon oil spill. For instance, Grattan et al. (2011) compared coastal community residents directly impacted by the oil to those who were indirectly impacted but found no differences in psychological distress between the two groups. Differences in mental health were found, however, between those who faced economic loss and those that did not, with those experiencing economic loss also experiencing psychological impacts after the disaster, consistent with the Arata et al. (2000) findings from the *Exxon Valdez* spill.

Lee and Blanchard (2012) surveyed coastal residents to assess community attachment, negative affective states, including anxiety and fear, and other sociodemographic characteristics while the oil from the BP spill was still flowing (June 2010). Analyses of the full sample (935 households) and subsequent analyses aggregated by household type (family member employed in the oil industry; fishing/seafood industry; no involvement in either industry) indicated that greater attachment to their community of residence was associated with higher levels of psychological distress. This finding was surprising in that community attachment has been widely recognized as having a beneficial effect on community resilience and well-being. Lee and Blanchard's (2012) findings imply that the salutary effects of community attachment may not hold in crisis conditions immediately after a technological disaster. The authors also suggested that a high level of community attachment may have made residents less likely to leave even though they were living in a social atmosphere full of stress, worry, and negative affect. In a follow-up investigation, Cope, Slack, Blanchard, and Lee (2013) reported additional survey data collected in the same geographic region using different household samples tested at two later intervals: wave 2 (4 months out from baseline, October 2010) and wave 3 (1 year from the explosion date, April 2011). Cope et al. found that physical and mental health effects were worse at wave 1 baseline assessment when the spill was still flowing compared to waves 2 and 3, implying that uncertainty is a major factor in post-disaster distress. They also found that stronger community attachment was associated with *reduced* psychological distress in the later waves of testing overall. For fishing households, however, significant interaction effects with the time of testing variable indicated that the negative mental health impacts at wave 1 remained evident at waves 2 and 3, suggesting that fishers may be uniquely vulnerable to distress associated with the BP oil spill 1 year later (see Cherry et al., 2015, for related discussion). Interpretative caution is warranted, because different household samples were compared across the three waves of testing. Nonetheless, Cope et al.'s results highlight the complex relationship one's stress level has with the community they are surrounded by, which also appear to vary over time for coastal community residents directly impacted by technological disaster.

Cumulative Adversity and the "Pileup" of Demands

As documented in the existing literature, dealing with traumatic life events can be difficult and trying: but *multiple* traumas, especially within a narrow time frame, can have devastating effects, particularly if a second trauma occurs before the victim has recovered from the first one (Marks, Nesteruk, Hopkins-Williams, Swanson, & Davis, 2006). In the 5 years preceding the BP Deepwater Horizon oil spill, Gulf Coast residents had been forced to navigate their way through the aftermath of four major Hurricanes (Katrina, Rita, Gustav, and Ike). Mental health becomes a prevalent concern when individuals, families, and communities face so much adversity, particularly in such a compressed period of time. Mong, Niguchi, and Ladner (2012) tested Gulf Coast residents for PTSD and their use of coping strategies, 1–2 months after the BP spill was stopped. Mong and colleagues found that 28% of their sample showed significant levels of PTSD symptoms. Further, negative coping strategies were positively correlated with PTSD symptoms for the participants directly affected by the oil spill. These results could be due in part to the immediate time frame of the study, in which the participants are still in a type of aftershock. Positive coping strategies, however, were negatively correlated with PTSD symptoms. Mong and colleagues stressed the importance of studying potential long-term impacts of the oil spill to learn more (regarding both positive and negative coping).

Keinan, Shrira, and Shmotkin (2012) examined lifetime cumulative adversity faced by middle-age Israelis. Their findings suggest the more trauma an individual faces, the higher the level of distress. However, those who experienced two or less adverse life events also reported lower well-being (as gauged by quality of life and optimism/hope) than those who experienced three adverse life events. The authors suggested that cumulative adversity may activate both positive and negative effect, in distress and well-being. The authors also note that their index of cumulative adversity does not gauge duration or severity of the traumatic event, which are likely critical variables to consider.

Seery et al. (2010) have also studied cumulative adversity through the course of one's life and resilience against the negative outcomes associated with those events. Their findings show that mental health and well-being were the highest for those that reported some adversity, compared to those that report none as well as those that report the higher levels of adversity. The average number of adverse life events (i.e., bereavement, loved one's illness, relationship stress, violent events, social stress, personal illness, and disasters) experienced by participants was 7.69 events. Participants who had lived through a small number of traumatic life experiences exhibited lower scores of distress, less functional impairment, fewer symptoms of PTSD, and higher life satisfaction. Those who have been through more than the average number of traumatic experiences showed a reversal of these findings, with higher marks on the negative outcomes and lower satisfaction with life, revealing a U-shaped curved function with relation to the number of adverse events.

As implicitly noted in our brief overview of research related to catastrophic oil spills, psychological trauma, and cumulative adversity, the extant literature primarily contains findings based on psychometrically sound measures yielding strictly quantitative data. The current chapter's findings are based on qualitative data derived from in-depth interviews and participants' responses to open-ended questions. Qualitative research allows for a unique opportunity to highlight what the participants consider important and can allow them to elaborate their thoughts, feelings, and concerns in a much more detailed manner than a closed response paper and pencil measure (Marks & Dollahite, 2011).

Method

Participants

In all, 64 commercial fishers and their family members were tested (*M* age = 54.7 years, *SD* = 15.7; age range = 21–90 years; 34 men and 30 women). They were enrolled in a research program on post-Katrina resilience described more fully elsewhere (see Cherry et al., 2015). All had experienced catastrophic losses in the 2005 Hurricanes Katrina and Rita and were directly affected by the 2010 BP oil spill. They were recruited from multiple sources in St. Bernard and Plaquemines parishes (counties) and through a mailing to the United Commercial Fishermen's Association (UCFA).

Procedure, Coding, and Analyses

Participants were interviewed in their homes or in a community location across two (or more) sessions, separated by at least a week. The procedures used in this study were reviewed and approved by the Institutional Review Board of Louisiana State University in Baton Rouge, LA. All participants were assigned a three-digit number (301–364) to preserve anonymity, as referenced throughout this chapter. A more complete description of the method is provided in Chap. 12 (this volume). In this chapter, we focus on participants' responses to one multifaceted, open-ended question:

> Have you been directly affected by the recent oil spill in the Gulf Coast? If so, in what way? Please tell us how the oil spill has affected you, your family and your community.

Of the 64 participants, four couples responded to this question jointly and one participant declined for a total of 59 completed open-ended responses (digitally recorded and transcribed verbatim). Narrative data were then content analyzed in a manner consistent with grounded theory methodology (Strauss & Corbin, 1998). One coding team of four members (one graduate student, three undergraduate students) met weekly during the fall semester of 2013 to carry out the open coding process (see Chap. 12, this volume, for description). Each week the coders discussed the prevalent ideas and themes covered in the 10–12 interviews coded that week, until all 61 interviews had been coded.

Findings

In all, seven core themes were identified in these data. Given the richness of these data, many of the salient issues and themes evident in our participants' narratives will require additional attention in future work. In this chapter, we have limited ourselves to three of the most central and pervasive themes that emerged from our interviews with Louisiana Gulf Coast fishers, shrimpers, and oystermen. These themes work together to present a textured picture of the lived experience of the participants' over the past decade.

Theme 1: Troubled Present, Uncertain Future conveys the uncertainty fishers felt regarding how the spill would play out over time, and what would become of their fishing careers and lifestyles. The water provides a way of life for these fishers, and those interviewed expressed belief that the BP oil spill threatened to strip them of their livelihood. *Theme 2: Environmental Devastation* reflects the fishers' profound concerns with changes that have already occurred in the environment. *Theme 3: The "Pileup" Effect after a Decade of Disasters* captures the fishers' reports regarding recent catastrophic hurricanes as sources of accumulated anguish over the past decade. To the degree possible, we provide firsthand accounts and primary data from the participants themselves. Direct quotations and narratives are offered to support and illustrate each of the themes, respectively.

Theme 1: Troubled Present, Uncertain Future

Uncertainty of the extent of damage and how the Deepwater Horizon oil spill would impact the lifestyle of commercial fishers was a major theme addressed in many of the interviews. Not knowing how and when the effects of the oil spill would be resolved was a serious source of stress and worry for those interviewed. The fishers' almost haunting reality is that no one knows exactly how much damage the oil spill has caused or what the long-term fallout will be. This was, and is, very unsettling for the fishers and their families—as well as for other Gulf Coast residents who fish and enjoy the water recreationally. A 52-year-old male explained that:

> 326: [The Deepwater Horizon oil spill] could possibly be more devastating than what Katrina was to us. I knew after Katrina that one day, as far as…the fishing industry…that everything would be fine. But as I told you the first day, that nobody knows what the effects of this is.

For many of the participants, fishing was their sole source of income, and the oil spill threatened to take that away from them. The uncertainty fishers and their families face was captured by a 50-year-old woman:

> 318: It is unnerving. It is stressful because this is what [my husband] has done all his life, and it is uncertain. *There is uncertainty of the future*.

As the following participants note, fishing means far more to them than an occupation, or even a career; it is a way of life. The catching and harvesting of fish, shrimp, and oysters are not only an economic base, they are also part of the cultural heritage of lifelong coastal residents in south Louisiana. The more mature generation of fishers feel responsible for this heritage—and for the next generation (see Chap. 18, this volume, for related discussion). The thought of this heritage, livelihood, and life fading is devastating to some, as illustrated by the following interview excerpts.

> 313: It is more than just a job. You feel like if we are the generation that loses this, then we are responsible for losing our heritage (47-year-old male).

> 301: At my age it isn't going to affect me that bad, but the younger people who want to be fishermen, who are fishermen, it's going to affect them for years and years and years to come. It may even be the end of their way of life (77-year old male).

> 330: It is definitely going to be a thing of the past. After this generation, I do not think they will have any more commercial fishermen. I think it will just be in history books after this (43-year old female).

Not everyone felt pessimism weighing them down, however. One wife of a coastal fisherman said,

> 316: I guess I wasn't afraid of the outcome [or worried about] if we could survive it. I knew we could. Maybe not doing what he was going to—you know, fishing, but we would survive and I was confident that…that the Gulf would take care of it. I mean I prayed, I prayed about it. And everybody else prayed about it. It was just the uncertainty (51-year old female).

Even for the more optimistic, like 316, the uncertainty of how bad this disaster will be for them in both loss of their heritage and livelihood seemed uncomfortable at best and terrifying at worst.

> 320: I'm not sure what to do right now…I see it coming to an end really, really fast here. And…I'm just…really kind of scared. I mean, it costs a lot of money to live…(48-year-old male).

However, uncertain the fishers and their spouses were about their own livelihood, every related report indicated that this man-made disaster was going to be hard on the environment. As one participant summarized:

> 325: Mother Nature can destroy something and build it back, but like with the oil spill, we never had an oil spill before and we do not know what is going to [happen. It could] be a long, long-term [disaster] (60-year old male).

The environmental effects noted by the commercial fishermen interviewed are covered in the second major theme, which we turn to next.

Theme 2: Environmental Devastation

The second theme addresses the environmental effects of the oil spill. After five million barrels (about 200 million gallons) of oil gushed into the Gulf of Mexico, the ecosystems of the sea and coastline took a catastrophic hit. Fishermen witnessed and continue to see these devastations first hand. And while the full extent of the damage remains unknown, some environmental effects witnessed by the participants were heartbreaking to them, as described in the next excerpts:

> 302: I have seen dead pelicans out there. I have seen dead turtles. I have seen all, all the catfish especially. And these catfish, I mean, big hearty catfish…this huge [shows size with hands], the whole bank for miles and miles and miles full of dead catfish (59-year old male).

> 352: Our fish died, our oysters died, our crabs are deformed, our shrimp are deformed. They are born with no eyes. We have shrimp with no eyes. Yes, we have crabs with holes in the shells. We have oysters with pits in them from bacteria. It has never been seen before. We have things that we see that have never been seen before. We have shrimp that are growing [in deformed ways]…. When you do this type of work and you sell bait, shrimp mainly… you got a product that cannot be sold. You are out of business (46-year old male).

A great number of the fishers spoke of a chemical agent used in the clean-up efforts called the dispersant. Dispersant changes the properties of the oil, both chemically and physically, in order to change the potentially hazardous effects of surface oil slicks (National Research Council, 2005, p. 10). The dispersant was developed to bind with the oil on the surface moving the dispersed oil droplets into the water column thus reducing the surface oil that would threaten the coastal wetlands. Dispersants ideally balance the risks and dangers of oil between the surface and shoreline and the underwater ecosystems in the water column and on the seafloor (National Research Council, 2005, p. 2; see National Commission on the BP Deepwater Horizon Oil Spill and Offshore Drilling, 2011 for a more detailed description of the BP Deepwater Horizon oil spill clean-up efforts). Unfortunately, the dispersant reportedly had some unforeseen complications as noted by the following participants:

> 310: That dispersant that they actually used all over here was not supposed to be used in sixty feet of water or less. We do not have many places in Louisiana that have sixty feet of water, so [virtually] every place it was used was illegal. And EPA told them not to, but they [did] (55-year-old male).

> 358: When they shoved that dispersant in there and made the oil sink, we still got oil coming up. Today. That dispersant, first good storm you get out in the Gulf's going to roll that bottom up, and that dispersant's going to wash free, and that stuff's going to come up again. You have oil all over the place again (71-year old male).

The dispersant caused problems in particular for oyster production because it killed the spat, which is essentially the juvenile stage in oyster development. Eastern oyster *(Crassostrea virginica)* is the most prevalent species of oyster harvested in the US Gulf Coast (Oyster Technical Task Force, 2012). The term spat is used to describe any small or immature oyster with shell length ranging from 0.3 up to 25.0 mm, where the adult oyster shell length is classified as longer than 75 mm (Oyster Technical Task Force, 2012, p. 37). Oysters in the Gulf of Mexico typically reach adult size in 18–24 months, after 5–6 years oyster size could grow to 150 mm (Oyster Technical Task Force, 2012, p. 44). In the mobile larval stage, oysters' movement is determined primarily by water currents and salinity (Oyster Technical Task Force, 2012, p. 44). This delicate life cycle of oysters worried many of the fishers. One participant reported that the damage seemed to be:

> 358: From the pollution…not so much from the oil, as from the dispersant they [used]. The dispersant not only screwed up the oyster beds, but it killed all the reproduction. So there's no spats. So that means we don't know how many years that'll be before they [the oysters] start reproducing on their own (71-year old male).

Oyster fishermen also had to deal with freshwater diversions. The diversions were used to stop the Gulf water from making landfall, but these diversions threw off the delicate balance between salt water and freshwater that oysters need to thrive.

As a result, the oyster fishing suffered great losses. The following two reports from oystermen are reflective:

> 347: Oysters are something…it ain't like your other seafood. It takes a long time to grow. They ran a lot of fresh water for that BP spill to try to push the oil out. And when they did that, it made the mussels grow on the oysters that were back alive (60-year old male).

> 360: [The oyster] resource has been severely impacted…the serious thing that we are waiting to see whether it comes back…[is] the production of oysters that we see, the resource rebound. We have not seen it yet, and that is disturbing us—disturbing the people with the state, the oystermen, the Wildlife and Fisheries, the biologists (55-year old male).

A comparatively younger participant still saw a "silver lining" to all the environmental damage caused by the oil spill (see Chap. 21, this volume, for a related discussion). He spoke of coastal erosion being a serious and long-standing issue for the Louisiana coastline, and now from his perspective, people are finally paying attention to this issue due to the attention drawn by the BP oil spill:

> 349: Actually it's improving it now because they are actually doing something to try to prevent coastal erosion. Since the oil spill there's been more people looking at [coastal erosion], and it's more concentrated, so it might actually help more than it does harm, in my opinion (28-year old male).

Such optimism, however, was the exception not the rule in the participants' interviews. The combination of haunting uncertainty regarding the future (Theme 1) and serious concerns about the delicate environmental balance in the Gulf and surrounding waterways seemed to be perennial stressors for many that we interviewed. The economic, psychological, and emotional blow dealt by Deepwater Horizon was not only severe—in the eyes of many, it remains a long-term if not permanent one. The blow leveled by Deepwater Horizon was not, however, the first or even the second that these hardy individuals and families have weathered. We now turn to the third and final theme, *The "Pileup" Effect after a Decade of Disasters*.

Theme 3: The "Pileup" Effect after a Decade of Disasters

As discussed at the outset of this chapter, the Louisiana Gulf Coast fishers and their families provide a unique and prototypical opportunity to learn about severe, cumulative adversity. The Deepwater Horizon oil spill is the newest stressor added to a long list of adversities that these individuals have faced over the last decade. These fishermen have experienced back-to-back Hurricanes Katrina and Rita in August and September of 2005, were then slammed by another set of back-to-back hurricanes (Gustav and Ike) in 2008, and were then dealt a third blow of the Deepwater Horizon oil spill in 2010.

The third theme established by the fishers' narrative text is consistent with what family stress scholars refer to as the "pileup" of demands associated with normative events and nonnormative crises that impact families over time. The "pileup" of pre- and post-crisis demands figures prominently in the double ABC-X model of family stress and adaptation (cf. Lavee, McCubbin, & Patterson, 1985; see also

Chap. 21, this volume). Here, we borrow the concept of "pileup" to broadly characterize post-disaster stressors such as catastrophic losses of homes and property. In addition to disaster-related material losses, we interpret "pileup" to include possibly diminished resources to cope with prior and current environmental stressors. Several of these fishers have survived hurricanes where they lost many of their material possessions, including boats, docks, and marinas. After regrouping from the catastrophic combinations of Katrina/Rita and Gustav/Ike, the respondents were faced with the adversity of the oil spill, pushing many perilously close to a breaking point. Several respondents addressed their sense of pileup or "exacerbated" cumulative stress, including the following:

> 310: So financially, [the oil spill] is a big deal financially and then emotionally, because you were pulling yourself out of the Katrina/Rita/Gustav era. You were digging your way out once again. And now you come up with a manmade disaster and that is what exacerbates this whole situation (55-year old male).

> 313: We lost our quality of life. And so soon after Katrina and Rita. It is like the double whammy (47-year old male).

> 340: It ruined my lifestyle. Getting compensated is not the same as not having it happen to you at all. Katrina made everybody move and now the storm's finishing us off (51-year old male).

Not only have these participants faced financial hardships, they also referenced an impact on their quality of life, now diminished relative to earlier times. Fishing used to be a comfortable life doing what they love, but for some it has turned into a source for worry and fear.

The natural and man-made disasters striking the same region in such a short window of time reportedly impacted many aspects of participants' lives. For some, everything seemed to be piling up. For one woman, when the shrimping disappeared, her household lost:

> 363: …our income coming in. We could not go shrimping. I lost my job. What more could happen? Then they had the hurricane, then this [oil spill]. It kills you. Then my Momma dies and my boyfriend dies, back-to-back (51-year old female).

Another participant said of her husband:

> 311: … when the kids needed him the most, he was dealing with Katrina stuff, and now [he's] dealing with the oil spill stuff (54-year old female).

One man (321) seemed to succinctly capture the sentiment of many, "Every time we started doing good, something happens" (67-year-old male). Another woman commented that is getting harder for her to stay positive about her families' career in the oyster business and explained that, for her:

> 324: The oil spill, just made it that much tougher to be optimistic about being an oyster fisherman or any kind of fisherman (55-year old female).

In general the fishermen of Louisiana's Gulf Coast are tough; they are a hardy and resilient crowd. Even though they have been on the receiving end of at least three major blows that can objectively be considered catastrophic, some appear to have hope that things will get better one day, and that they will be able to see themselves through all of the hardships. The following excerpts reflect this optimistic view:

> 313: You know, I still have hope that somewhere along the line things will straighten out (47-year old male).
>
> 332: Yeah, well…it's okay…what doesn't kill you makes you stronger. God doesn't give you anything you can't handle. You know, I just wish he didn't think my shoulders were as broad as they are (52-year old female).
>
> 319: Bae[2], things always work out all the time, in some fashion (44-year-old female).

Time will reveal whether the fishermen of Louisiana's Gulf Coast can absorb this "third blow" of Deepwater Horizon and find their way back to their feet. This blow will likely be the final one for some, but given our firsthand opportunity to witness the remarkable resilience of many of these individuals and families, we expect that many will not only find their feet, they will once again find their sea legs.

Conclusion

The commercial fishers of south Louisiana have been hit hard by both natural and man-made disasters. The uncertainty of what will become of their future, their finances, and their lifestyle weighs heavily, causing stress years after the spill had been capped. The uncertainty spreads into the environment, as both the oil and the dispersant used have caused horrible death and detriment to the seafood crops and industry. The uncertainty and worry of those employed by the seafood industry is extremely clear in the devastating footage of Hurricane Katrina aftermath (United Commercial Fishermen's Association & Barisich 2011), as well as the aftershock of the BP Deepwater Horizon oil spill (Stencel & Hopkins, 2013). Each film was made shortly after the disasters wreaked havoc on the Gulf Coast. The film *Dirty Energy* (Stencel & Hopkins, 2013) especially highlights the region as a unique culture in danger of losing their fishing lifestyle, potentially making commercial fishing just a cherished memory.

The present research dives firsthand into how the fishers are faring in the years after the 2005 Hurricanes Katrina and Rita, after the 2008 Hurricanes Gustav and Ike, and the 2010 BP Deepwater Horizon oil spill. The worry and fear are ever present, as well as the financial and emotional drains. The results of our study indicate that fishers are working to keep their lifestyles, family, environment, and community afloat years after the spill. The Gulf Coast has been battered with adversity. At the same time, the coast features a community of tough, hardworking individuals that have made it through turbulent and disaster-riddled times. Further research to address the long-term impacts of these disasters and the development of interventions tailored specifically toward mitigating cumulative adversity are warranted.

[2] "Bae," is a slang expression similar to "Baby." (Definition of Bae, 2010)

Acknowledgments We thank George Barisich, President of the United Commercial Fishermen's Association, for his help with recruitment and Frank Campo of Campo's Marina in Yscloskey (southeastern St. Bernard) for providing space for interviews. We also thank Ashley Cacamo, Annie Crapanzano, and Benjamin Staab for assistance with data collection and Rachel Adamek, Devon Welsch, Kristina Fitzgerald, Claire Bernacchio, and Dina Anbinder for help with data scoring. We are grateful to Sr. Mary Keefe, Huey Gonzales, Charlie Robin, Lauren Denley, John Tesvich, and Eva Vujnovich for their contribution to the research effort, and Matthew Lee, Vijay John, and John E. Supan for their assistance in exposition concerning spat and dispersants.

This research was supported by grants from the Louisiana Board of Regents and the BP Gulf of Mexico Research Initiative, Office of Research and Economic Development, Louisiana State University. This support is gratefully acknowledged.

Correspondence concerning this chapter should be addressed to Katie E. Cherry, Department of Psychology, Louisiana State University, Baton Rouge, LA 70803-5501 (e-mail: pskatie@lsu.edu).

References

Arata, C. M., Picou, J. S., Johnson, G. D., & McNally, T. S. (2000). Coping with technological disaster: An application of the conservation of resources model to the *Exxon Valdez* oil spill. *Journal of Traumatic Stress, 13*(1), 23–39.

Cherry, K. E., Sampson, L., Nezat, P. F., Cacamo, A., Marks, L. D., & Galea, S. (2015). Long-term psychological outcomes in older adults after disaster: relationships to religiosity and social support. *Aging & Mental Health, 19*(5), 430–443.

Cope, M. R., Slack, T., Blanchard, T. C., & Lee, M. R. (2013). Does time heal all wounds? Community attachment, natural resource employment, and health impacts in the wake of the BP Deepwater Horizon disaster. *Social Science Research, 42*, 872–881.

Definition of Bae. (2010). http://onlineslangdictionary.com/meaning-definition-of/bae. Accessed 23 June 2014.

Gill, D. A., Picou, J. S., & Ritchie, L. A. (2012). The *Exxon Valdez* and BP oil spills: A comparison of initial social and psychological impacts. *American Behavioral Scientist, 56*(1), 3–23.

Grattan, L. M., Roberts, S., Mahan, W. T., Jr., McLaughlin, P. K., Otwell, S., & Morris, J. G., Jr. (2011). The early psychological impacts of the Deepwater Horizon oil spill on Florida and Alabama communities. *Environmental Health Perspectives, 119*(6), 838–843.

Holgersen, K. H., Klöckner, C. A., Boe, H. J., Weisæth, L., & Holen, A. (2011). Disaster survivors in their third decade: Trajectories of initial stress responses and long-term course of mental health. *Journal of Traumatic Stress, 24*(3), 334–341.

Keinan, G., Shrira, A., & Shmotkin, D. (2012). The association between cumulative adversity and mental health: Considering dose and primary focus of adversity. *Quality of Life Research, 21*, 1149–1158.

Lavee, Y., McCubbin, H. I., & Patterson, J. M. (1985). The double ABCX model of family stress and adaptation: An empirical test by analysis of structural equations with latent variables. *Journal of Marriage and the Family*, 47, 811–825.

Lee, M. R., & Blanchard, T. C. (2012). Community attachment and negative affective states in the context of the BP Deepwater Horizon disaster. *American Behavioral Scientist, 56*(1), 24–47.

Marks, L. D., & Dollahite, D. C. (2011). Mining the meanings from psychology of religion's correlation mountain. *Journal of Psychology of Religion and Spirituality, 3*, 181–193.

Marks, L. D., Swanson, M., Nesteruk, O., & Hopkins-Williams, K. (2006). Stressors in African American marriages and families: A qualitative study. *Stress, Trauma, and Crisis: An International Journal, 9*, 203–225.

Mong, M. D., Noguchi, K., & Ladner, B. (2012). Immediate psychological impact of the Deepwater Horizon oil spill: Symptoms of PTSD and coping skills. *Journal of Aggression, Maltreatment, and Trauma, 21*, 691–704.

National Research Council of the National Academies. (2005). *Oil spill dispersants: Efficacy and effects*. Washington, D.C.: National Academies Press.
National Commission on the BP Deepwater Horizon Oil Spill and Offshore Drilling. (2011). The use of surface and subsea dispersants during the BP Deepwater Horizon oil spill. In C. A. Farrugia (Ed.), *Dispersant and oil monitoring in the Deepwater Horizon spill* (pp. 1–28). New York: Nova Science Publishers, Inc.
Oyster Technical Task Force. (2012). *The oyster fishery of the Gulf of Mexico, United States: A fisheries management plan, 2012 revision* (pp. 31–45). Ocean Springs, MS: Gulf States Marine Fisheries Commission.
Palinkas, L. A., Petterson, J. S., Russell, J., & Downs, M. A. (1993). Community patterns of psychiatric disorders after the *Exxon Valdez* Oil Spill. *American Journal of Psychiatry, 150*(10), 1517–1523.
Seery, M. D., Holman, E. A., & Silver, R. C. (2010). Whatever does not kill us: Cumulative lifetime adversity, vulnerability, and resilience. *Journal of Personality and Social Psychology, 99*(6), 1025–1041.
Stencel, E., Hopkins B. D. (Producers), & Hopkins, B. D. (Director). (2013). *Dirty energy* [Motion picture]. United States: Cinema Libre Studio.
Strauss, A., & Corbin, J. (1998). *Basics of qualitative research: Techniques and procedures for developing grounded theory*. Thousand Oaks: Sage.
United Commercial Fishermen's Association (Producers), & Barisich, G. (Producer). (2011). *Post Katrina: The plight of the Gulf Coast fishermen* [Motion picture]. Available from George Barisich, 3413 Don Redden Court, Baton Rouge, LA, 70802.

Chapter 5
The Great East Japan Earthquake: Tsunami and Nuclear Disaster

Masaharu Maeda and Misari Oe

Introduction

On March 11, 2011, a huge earthquake with a magnitude of 9.0, which was later named as the Great East Japan Earthquake, struck the Tohoku region in the northern part of the main island of Japan. A tsunami following the earthquake caused serious damages especially in three prefectures, Iwate, Miyagi, and Fukushima, and created over 300,000 refugees in Tohoku region. Subsequently, the tsunami totally damaged all of the cooling system at the Fukushima Daiichi Nuclear Power Plant and led to several explosions of the plant buildings and widespread diffusion of radioactive materials. The whole of Japan fell into a severe nuclear crisis during the several weeks after the accident. A nuclear emergency was declared for the first time in Japan, and 140,000 residents within 20 km of the plant were evacuated.

The tsunami and the nuclear accident eventually resulted in terrible effects across widespread domains in Japan as well as the Tohoku region: Lives of numerous residents were disrupted, as were communities, economy, and policy. Especially, there have been various types of psychosocial influence on the residents and their communities: Not only psychiatric problems such as post-traumatic stress disorder (PTSD), grief reaction, or depression but also more complicated psychosocial issues such as prejudice, discrimination, disparities, and fragmentation were seen in communities. In other words, the tsunami and nuclear disaster affected all dimensions

M. Maeda (✉)
Department of Disaster Psychiatry, School of Medicine, Fukushima Medical University,
1 Hikarigaoka, Fukushima, 960-1295, Japan
e-mail: masagen@fmu.ac.jp

M. Oe
Department of Neuropsychiatry, Kurume University, School of Medicine,
67 Asahimachi, Kurume, 830-0011, Japan
e-mail: oe_misari@kurume-u.ac.jp

K. E. Cherry (ed.), *Traumatic Stress and Long-Term Recovery*,
DOI 10.1007/978-3-319-18866-9_5

and levels of society, from psychiatric disorders at the individual and family level to prejudice and fragmentation of small communities and the extended population.

In this chapter, we described the multiple psychosocial effects caused by both the tsunami and the Fukushima nuclear power plant accident. More emphasis, however, was put on the adverse effects from the nuclear disaster because of long-term and serious consequences for people living in or out of Fukushima Prefecture and the worldwide concern it caused. Also, in order to more deeply understand the current complicated situation in Fukushima, we reviewed three major nuclear accidents, including one that occurred in Japan.

Mental Health Effects After the Great East Japan Earthquake and Tsunami

The earthquake and the tsunami that followed it devastated the coastal areas, and as of July 2014, 15,887 people have been confirmed dead and 2,612 are still missing (Japanese National Police Agency, JNPA, 2012). Almost all of the victims died not by the earthquake but by the tsunami. People living along the coast have been well trained for tsunami-evacuation procedures, according to the past tsunami experiences; namely, the Meiji Sanriku Tsunami in 1896 which killed about 20,000 people and the 1933 Showa Sanriku Tsunami which killed about 3,000 people (Ishigaki, Higashi, Sakamoto & Shibahara, 2013). However, the 2011 tsunami was much greater than expected. The tsunami also impacted the seacoast areas of the Soma plain in the Fukushima Prefecture, including the Fukushima Daiichi Nuclear Power Plant. According to the Japan Meteorological Agency, the height of the tsunami was 9.3 m in Soma.

One of the most systematic surveys on mental health effects was conducted 6–11 months after the disaster (Yokoyama et al., 2014). The Kessler 6-item scale (K6; Kessler et al., 2003) was used to measure the mental health problems of 10,025 study participants in three municipalities in Iwate Prefecture (3,934 male and 6,091 female, mean age 61.0 years). The respondents were classified into moderate (5–12 of K6) and serious mental health problems (13+). A total of 42.6% of the respondents had moderate or serious mental health problems. They revealed that female gender, health complaints, severe economic status, relocations, and lack of a social network were associated with mental health problems.

The psychological consequences caused by the earthquake and the tsunami in Fukushima posed serious problems. However, in reality, the mental or psychosomatic health effects caused by the nuclear plant disaster were more extensive by comparison and should be considered with greater urgency. In actuality, over 120,000 people were evacuated mainly due to the radioactive contamination. In the next section, we reviewed previous major nuclear plant disasters to broaden the context for discussion of the Fukushima Daiichi Nuclear Power Plant disaster.

Review of Three Major Nuclear Plant Accidents

To illustrate the psychological consequences of prior radiation disasters, we chose three nuclear plant accidents (Chernobyl accident, Three Mile Island (TMI) accident, and Tokaimura accident) and the descriptive review of the long-term effects was conducted with PubMed. Additionally, we also referred to the grant database of the Health, Labour and Welfare Ministry, Japan, for the review of Tokaimura accident. Chernobyl and TMI disasters were chosen because of the severity and the abundance of the literature; Tokaimura accident was chosen because it was the first fatal nuclear accident in Japan.

Chernobyl Accident

Brief Summary of the Accident The Chernobyl accident occurred on April 26, 1986, at the Chernobyl Nuclear Power Plant in the former Ukrainian Republic of the Soviet Union. This was the most severe in the history of the nuclear power industry and caused a huge release of radionuclides over large areas of Belarus, Ukraine, and the Russian Federation. More than 600,000 people were registered as emergency and recovery workers ("liquidators") and some 300,000 residents were relocated (International Atomic Energy Agency, IAEA, 2006). It was registered as level 7 on the International Nuclear and Radiological Event Scale by the IAEA, 2008.

After 20 years, the Chernobyl Forum report summarized that there is no clearly demonstrated increase in the incidence of solid cancers or leukemia due to radiation, apart from the dramatic increase in incidents of thyroid cancer among those exposed at a young age (IAEA, 2006). Nevertheless, the mental health effects were regarded as the most significant public health consequence of the accident (Bromet, Havenaar, Guey, 2011).The summary of key findings of the Chernobyl disaster in the long term is seen in Table 5.1.

Mental Health Effects in the Long Term Three groups have been the target of research on the mental health consequences of Chernobyl (Bromet et al. 2011). The group of cleanup workers is focused upon because they worked near the damaged reactor. The second group consists of children exposed in utero or as young infants and their parents because of an elevated rate of thyroid cancer in children. The adult population with varying levels of exposure is the third group.

For cleanup workers, higher suicide risk (Rahu et al., 2006) and higher prevalence of depression and PTSD (Loganovsky et al., 2008) were observed. A research group in Latvia assessed the associations of various exposure variables with mental and psychosomatic distress in a sample of 1412 Latvian liquidators drawn from the State Latvian Chernobyl Clean-up Workers Registry (Viel et al., 1997). They revealed that length of work (>28 days) in a 10-km radius from the reactor, work (>1 time) on the damaged reactor roof, forest work, and fresh fruit consumption were risk factors for mixed mental-psychosomatic disorder, which consisted of

Table 5.1 Summary of key findings of the Chernobyl accident

Outcomes	Sample	Results	Method	References
Mental and psychosomatic effects in the long term				
Psychological well-being	Adolescents who exposed in utero to radiation from the Chernobyl accident and their mothers, in the affected area in Norway	Adolescents themselves reported few problems; the level of problems reported by the mothers was generally lower than that reported by the adolescents	The Child Behavior Checklist (CBCL), the Youth Self-Report (YSR)	Heiervang, Mednick, Sundet, & Rund, 2011
Depression, anxiety, somatization	General population adults from two geographic areas of differing radiation contamination within Belarus	Degree of chronic daily stressors showed a significant positive relationship with psychological distress, whereas mastery/controllability showed a significant inverse relationship with distress	Brief Symptom Inventory depression, anxiety, and somatization subscale	Beehler et al., 2008
Depression, PTSD, Headaches	Cleanup workers	More frequent than controls	WHO Composite International Diagnostic Interview	Loganovsky et al., 2008
Depression, Anxiety Spectrum Complaints, PTSD	General population adults, immigrants to the USA from the former Soviet Union, within 50 km from Chernobyl	More frequent than 50–150 km or over 150 km	Beck Depression Inventory, Beck Anxiety Inventory, Revised Civilian Mississippi PTSD Scale	Foster & Goldstein, 2007
Suicide risk	Cleanup workers	Higher than controls	Standard mortality rate	Rahu, Rahu, Tekkel, & Bromet, 2006
Anxiety, depression, fear, somatization, mother's report of psychological well-being	11-year-old children who were exposed in utero to age 15 months when the accident occurred and their mothers	No statistically significant differences on the self-report; the evacuee mothers rated their children's well-being as significantly worse, especially with respect to somatic symptoms	The Children's Manifest Anxiety Scale, the Depression Self-Rating Scale, the Fear Inventory, the Children's Somatization Inventory, CBCL	Bromet et al., 2000
Anxiety	Mothers and fathers of the children who had been exposed in the prenatal period at the time of the accident in Belarus	An increased prevalence of high personal anxiety compared to the control group	The State-Trait Anxiety Inventory	Igumnov & Drozdovitch, 2000

Table 5.1 (continued)

Outcomes	Sample	Results	Method	References
Mood Disorders, depression symptoms, Anxiety Disorders, psychosomatic distress, psychological well-being	General population adults in the affected area in Belarus	No statistically significant differences in DSM diagnosis for mood disorders and anxiety disorders; more frequent than controls in self-rating scale	DSM-III-R, Brief Scales for Anxiety and Depression, depression subscale, Bradford Somatic Inventory score, 12-item General Health Questionnaire	Havenaar et al., 1997
Psychosomatic distress	Cleanup workers	Length of work (>28 days) in a 10-km radius from the reactor, work (>1 time) on the damaged reactor roof, forest work, and fresh fruit consumption were risk factors	Depression, cardiovascular physiologic malfunction arising from mental factors and unspecified disorders of the autonomic nervous system by ICD-9	Viel et al., 1997
Neurocognitive effects in the long term				
IQ	Adolescents who were exposed in utero to radiation from the most contaminated areas in Norway	Scored significantly lower in full-scale IQ than unexposed adolescents; the difference was restricted to verbal IQ	Two subtests from the Wechsler Abbreviated Scale of Intelligence	Heiervang, Mednick, Sundet, & Rund, 2010
IQ, school performance, attention, memory, subjective appraisals of memory problems	Children who were in utero to age 15 months, evacuated to Kyiv from the 30 km zone and their mothers	No statistically significant differences (vs. classmates) in IQ, school performance, attention and memory; more evacuee mothers subjectively reported memory problems in their children than classmates' mothers, but these reports were not correlated with performance on the neuropsychological tests or grades in school	The symbolic relations subtest of the Detroit Tests of Learning Aptitude, GPA, two forms of the VSAT, The Benton Visual Retention Test A	Litcher et al., 2000; Taormina et al., 2008
Accuracy and efficiency of cognitive performance	Cleanup workers, foresters and agricultural workers	Averaged levels of performance of the exposure groups were significantly lower than those of the controls	The ANAMUKR battery	Gamache, Levinson, Reeves, Bidyuk, & Brantley, 2005

Table 5.1 (continued)

Outcomes	Sample	Results	Method	References
IQ	Children who had been exposed in the prenatal period at the time of the accident in Belarus	At the age of 6–7: lower mean full-scale IQ compared to the control group; by the age of 10–12: no statistically significant differences	The Wechsler Intelligence Scale for Children	Igumnov & Drozdovitch, 2000

DSM Diagnostic and Statistical Manual of Mental Disorders, *ICD* International Classification of Diseases, *GPA* Graded Prognostic Assessment, *VSAT* Verbal Scholastic Aptitude Test, *ANAM-KUKR* Ukrainian Subset of Automated Neuropsychological Assessment Metrics, *PTSD* post-traumatic stress disorder

depression, cardiovascular physiologic malfunction arising from mental factors, and unspecified disorders of the autonomic nervous system, according to International Classification of Diseases (ICD)-9 coding system.

In the second group, an increased prevalence of high personal anxiety of the parents in Belarus was reported (Igumnov & Drozdovitch, 2000). In this article, a moderate correlation between high personal anxiety in parents and emotional disorders in children was also reported. In another study (Bromet et al., 2000), although there were no statistical differences in the self-reports of psychological well-being between the adolescents who were exposed in utero to age 15 months and controls, the evacuee mothers rated their children's well-being as significantly worse, especially with respect to somatic symptoms. Interestingly, it seems that the geographical closeness is related to the anxiety level of the parents in the long term. A study in Norway showed that adolescents themselves reported few problems, and the level of problems reported by the mothers was generally lower than that reported by the adolescents (Heiervang et al., 2011). A possible explanation for this discrepancy between investigations is that the mothers of the Norwegian participants experienced less Chernobyl-related anxiety, due to fortunate circumstances in Norway and perceived physical and psychological distance from the disaster (Heiervang et al., 2011).

For general population adults in the affected area, the long-term effects might be at a moderate or subclinical level (Havenaar et al., 1997; Foster & Goldstein, 2007; Beehler et al. 2008). Compared to the residents who had lived over 50 km from the plant, depression, anxiety, and PTSD symptoms were greater for those living within 50 km of the accident site at 15 years post Chernobyl (Foster & Goldstein, 2007). Beehler et al. (2008) conducted a multilevel analysis and revealed that female gender, greater number of chronic stressors, and the perception of family problems were associated with psychological distress. By contrast, higher mastery/controllability was significantly predictive of lower depression, lower anxiety, and lower somatization scores, 20 years after the accident.

Neurocognitive Effects in the Long Term Most of the studies have been focused on the exposed children who were in utero in April, 1986. The results concerning intellectual development are conflicting. The evacuee children in Ukraine who were in utero to age 15 months, evacuated to Kyiv from the 30-km zone, showed no statistically significant differences compared to their classmates, 11 and 19 years after the accident (Litcher et al., 2000; Taormina et al., 2008). In a Belarusian study, 250 exposed in utero children at the age of 6–7 and 10–12 years were compared to a control group of 250 children of the same age from non- and slightly contaminated areas of Belarus (Igumnov & Drozdovitch, 2000). It was a noteworthy feature that despite the lower mean full-scale IQ at 6–7 years compared to the control group (the Wechsler Intelligence Scale for Children; 89.6 ± 10.2 vs. 92.1 ± 10.5, $p = 0.007$), there were no statistically significant differences (94.3 ± 10.4 vs. 95.8 ± 10.9, $p = 0.117$) by the age of 10–12. These results suggest that the intellectual development might reduce the gap between the exposed children and the non-exposed children. However, another study conducted in Norway (Heiervang, et al., 2010) showed that the mean IQ of exposed group (84 adolescents who were exposed in utero to radiation from the most contaminated areas at 19 years) was 100.4 ± 13.1, and the mean IQ of the control group was 105.4 ± 12.1 by two subtests from the Wechsler Abbreviated Scale of Intelligence.

Another study focused on parents of the exposed children. The subjective appraisals about the memory problems of their children were examined (Litcher et al., 2000). More evacuee mothers subjectively reported memory problems in their children than classmates' mothers, but these reports were not correlated with performance on the neuropsychological tests or grades in school. This result is consistent with a study of Igumnov and Drozdovitch (2000), which showed an increased prevalence of high personal anxiety in mothers and fathers.

A 4-year longitudinal study of the cognitive effects of exposure (Gamache, et al., 2005) showed that the average levels of the exposed groups, including eliminators (who are assigned "cleanup"duties at or very near the accident site), forestry workers, and agricultural workers, were significantly lower than those of the controls on most measures. They also reported the significant declines in accuracy and efficiency, as well as psychomotor slowing, for all exposed groups over the 4-year period.

Three Mile Island Accident

Brief Summary of the Accident The accident at TMI nuclear facility on March 28, 1979 in Pennsylvania was registered as a level 5 on the International Nuclear and Radiological Event Scale by the International Atomic Energy Agency (IAEA). After the accident, there was no increase in cancer morbidity or mortality. Moreover, the evacuation was voluntary and temporary, and almost all the families returned within 2 weeks (Bromet, 2012).

In a report of the President's Commission on the accident at TMI, it is clearly stated that the major health effect of the accident appears to have been on the mental health of the people living in the region of TMI and of the workers (President's Commission on the accident at TMI, 1979). The reactor restarted in October 1985, after the extended legal conflict (Dew, Bromet, Schulberg, Dunn, & Parkinson, 1987). It should be considered that this restart also influenced the psychological consequences of the people, as discussed more fully next.

Mental Health Effects in the Long Term Here, we reviewed the mental or psychosomatic health effects in the long term (Table 5.2). A series of longitudinal epidemiologic studies was designed to focus on the mental health of the mothers of young children living within ten miles of the plant (Dew et al., 1987; Dew & Bromet 1993). It is noteworthy that symptom levels after restart were elevated over previous levels (Dew et al., 1987). The results from cluster analysis of this cohort 10 years following the accident showed two major subgroups of women: those whose temporal profiles were either (a) stable and at a low, clinically nonsignificant psychiatric symptom level across all measurements points (65 % of the sample), or (b) at consistently elevated levels of distress (35 % of the sample; Dew & Bromet, 1993). Multivariate analyses indicated that pre-accident characteristics as well as parameters reflecting respondents' initial involvement with and reactions to the accident were important for distinguishing between women within the two temporal profile groups. Meanwhile, Prince-Embury and Rooney (1995) revealed that an increased lack of control, a lack of faith in the radiation experts, and an increased fear of developing cancer were observed among the residents following the restart of the nuclear-powered generator.

Five years after the accident, another follow-up study (Houts, et al., 1991) was conducted for 1,880 mothers who gave birth within 12 months of the accident and lived in communities within 10 miles of the nuclear facility. Although the anxiety and depression symptoms had no statistically significant differences, the mothers rated their 5-year-old children's health as poorer than the mothers who gave birth from 13 to 24 months after the accident. The lowered subjective appraisals of their children are consistent with the studies after the Chernobyl accident (Litcher et al., 2000; Igumnov & Drozdovitch, 2000).

The mental health of 104 nuclear workers at the TMI plant was compared 2.5 years after the accident with that of 122 workers from another nuclear plant and 151 workers from two coal-fired generating plants (Parkinson & Bromet, 1983). This was the follow-up study of a telephone survey, which showed more hostility and psychophysiological symptoms at the time of the accident (Kasl, Chisholm, & Eskenazi, 1981a; b). Surprisingly, the coal-fired plant workers were somewhat more symptomatic than the nuclear plant workers, probably because of the workplace exposure problems. The research group suggested that the impact of the accident on workers at the plant was unremarkable in the long term.

Tokaimura Accident

Brief Summary of the Accident On September 30, 1999, a critical accident occurred in the conversion building at the uranium conversion facility of JCO Company Limited in Tokaimura, Ibaraki Prefecture, Japan (IAEA, 1999). It resulted in three JCO workers suffering acute radiation syndrome, and a number of workers and members of the public receiving radiation doses. Some 161 people were evacuated from within about 350 m of the facility, and some 310,000 people were advised

Table 5.2 Summary of key findings of the TMI accident

Outcomes	Sample	Results	Method	References
Mental and psychosomatic effects in the long term				
Psychological symptoms	Adult residents near TMI	A lowering of psychological symptoms between 1985 and 1989 in spite of increased lack of control, less faith in experts and increased fear of developing cancer	The Revised Symptom Checklist (SCL-90-R)	Prince-Embury & Rooney, 1995
Psychological symptoms, including depression, anxiety, and hostility	Mothers living within 10 miles of TMI	Pre-accident characteristics, as well as parameters reflecting respondents' initial involvement with, and reactions to the accident, were important for distinguishing between high and low level of distress	The depression, anxiety, and hostility subscales of the Symptom Checklist-90 (SCL-90)	Dew & Bromet, 1993
Anxiety and depression, subjective rating of their children's health	Pairs of mothers and children lived in communities within 10 miles of the nuclear facility	No statistically significant differences (vs. controls); mothers rated poorer mean ratings of their children than controls	The Hopkins Symptoms Checklist (HSCL)	Houts, Tokuhata, Bratz, Bartholomew, & Sheffer, 1991
Psychological symptoms, including depression, anxiety, and hostility	Mothers living within 10 miles of TMI	Symptom levels after restart were elevated over previous levels; history of diagnosable major depression and generalized anxiety following the accident, plus symptoms and beliefs about personal risk prior to the restart, best predicted post-restart symptoms	The depression, anxiety, and hostility subscales of the Symptom Checklist-90 (SCL-90)	Dew et al., 1987
Psychological symptoms	Nuclear plant workers	No statistically significant differences than another nuclear plant workers	The Symptom Checklist (SCL-90)	Parkinson & Bromet, 1983

TMI Three Mile Island

to stay indoors for about 18 h as a precautionary measure. This accident, which was ranked a level 4 on the IAEA Scale, was considered the worst civilian nuclear radiation accident in Japan prior to the Fukushima Daiichi Nuclear Power Plant accident.

Mental Health Effects Following the Tokaimura accident, Japanese psychiatrists began performing consultations of the 59 residents 2–4 weeks after the disaster and found that residents complained about concerns of their physical health, anxiety, insomnia, and irritability (Tomita & Nakajima, 1999). Furthermore, they also found that pregnant mothers were concerned about future risks to their pregnancy and the possible adverse effects on their child, including those who were exposed in utero.

Surveys on the symptoms of PTSD were also conducted after the interventional seminars for the residents around the site. The topics of the lectures were on PTSD symptoms and related psychological issues, titled "Care of Child (after the accident)". Surveys were also conducted at the consultation center (Konishi & Inamoto, 1999), and a screening questionnaire of PTSD symptoms (the Impact of Events Scale - Revised, IES-R) was also performed (Asukai, et al., 2002). Among the 424 event participants, 31 residents (7.2 %) were considered part of the high-risk group. Meanwhile, 47.5 % ($n=19$) of the consultation center visitors ($n=40$) were placed in the high-risk group. They also revealed that the close proximity and the subjective threat of death had also influenced the IES-R score.

Psychosocial Consequences of Fukushima Disaster

There were very complicated psychological impacts on the Fukushima people after the nuclear crisis. The variety of psychosocial reactions among those directly affected by this event can be summarized within five main issues: posttraumatic stress response, chronic anxiety and guilt, ambiguous loss, separated families and communities, and stigma (see Table 5.3). With the exception of posttraumatic stress responses, four of the five main issues are very unique in Fukushima and have never been seen in other Tohoku areas affected by the tsunami (Maeda and Oe, 2014). Figure 5.1 also shows these multidimensional psychosocial reactions and those relationships.

Three experiences (close experience of the explosion of the power plant, fear for the fall out and worries about labeling as being exposed to radiation) were considered to be key to understand the complex emotional responses. These three led various reactions among people living in/out of Fukushima. Also, the unique and specific reactions in the nuclear disaster were shown on the right side of the fig. 5.1.

Posttraumatic Stress Responses When the first explosion of the plant occurred following the disaster, most people, even those who lived near the plant, did not expect such a serious nuclear crisis to happen. They were so poorly prepared for such a crisis that they fell into a panic. The lack of the information from the government about the accident spurred the people further. Amid the confusion, most of the residents living within 30 km from the plant were trying to escape from their hometown. Although some people initially had been optimistic and refused to leave,

Table 5.3 Features of psychological impact on the Fukushima people after the accident

Psychological impact	Features
Posttraumatic stress responses	Traumatic memories of plant explosion and evacuation Hyper arousal Reexperiencing symptoms
Chronic anxiety and guilt	Fear of radioactive exposure, especially in the case of parents with young children Negative influence on children's development Guilt about abandoning friends and neighbors
Ambiguous loss experience	Loss of home through evacuation rather than damage Uncertainty of nuclear accident evacuees about returning home Depressive symptoms
Separated families/communities	Weakened resilience within community Increased conflicts within and between families Frustration of neighboring cities that take in evacuees
Self-stigma	Discrimination against workers and young women Concealment of history in Fukushima Righteous anger Loss of self-esteem

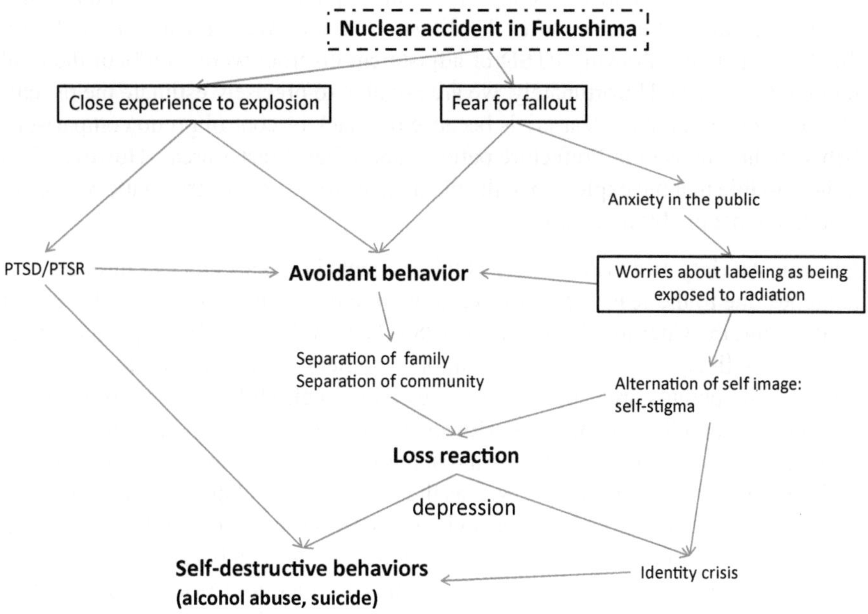

Fig. 5.1 Multidimensional psychosocial reactions in/out of Fukushima

most of them were eventually evacuated in fear of the meltdown and radioactive exposure.

Afterwards, the government gradually lifted the residential restriction and some of the evacuees returned to their hometown. However, even until today, they still have traumatic memories about the explosions and their evacuation, which have yielded various symptoms of PTSD, such as hyperarousal and reexperiencing symptoms (Maeda, 2012). The people returning to their hometown are still worried that another explosion at the plant might occur again in the near future. Their worries and anxieties are likely to make them emotionally unstable and may disturb return of the evacuees. Even in the coastal areas that contain low air levels of cesium (e.g., Minami-Soma city), many evacuees still hesitate to return to their hometown due to their close proximity to the plant. Their hesitation may indicate that the posttraumatic responses and the worries of another explosion among the evacuees continue to exist. Supporting this notion, a major cohort survey for approximately 210,000 people in the evacuation zone performed by the Fukushima Medical University about 1 year after the accident revealed that 21.6% of the total responders were estimated to be at risk of PTSD based on the result of PTSD Checklist (Weathers, Litz, Herman, Huska, Keane, 1993; Yabe et al., 2014).

Three months after the accident, Kyutoku et al. (2012) performed an online survey for the people in the Tohoku disaster area, and also revealed that the level of PTSD symptoms for the earthquake and tsunami were significantly higher than that of the nuclear accident. However, considering that the people living near the plant also lived in the coastal area affected by the disaster, both the tsunami and the nuclear crisis may have given them more fearful experiences than the people solely living far from the plant. In a study of the initial patients visiting psychiatric clinics in Fukushima Prefecture after the disaster (Miura, Wada, Itagaki, Yabe, Niwa, 2012), the patients showing PTSD or adjustment disorder were 13.9% of the total number (n=1321). Unfortunately, we are not able to precisely estimate the psychiatric influence of the nuclear crisis because of a lack of control group comparisons between the Fukushima Prefecture patients and other disaster areas. However, it is quite possible that the explosion at the plant gave rise to serious traumatic responses among the people living near the plant.

Chronic Anxiety and Guilt Many of the residents in Fukushima still have chronic anxieties due to the fear of radioactive contamination. Similar to the TMI accident in 1979 and the Chernobyl accident in 1986 (Dew & Bromet, 1993; Bromet et al., 2011), it is likely that the anxieties among mothers with young children are the highest. The parents are especially nervous about their children possibly touching or handling something dangerous. However, their concerns and the restrictions on their children's outdoor activities could actually have a negative influence on their children's psychological state, as well as their physical development (Save the Children, 2012). In a survey of 97 parents visiting a pediatric clinic in Fukushima city 5 months after the disaster, 77.2% answered that their children became more stressed due to the restrictions on their outdoor activities. Further, 85.1% also answered that they, if possible, hoped to move a less-affected area (Kitajo, 2011).

In addition, many of the parents who stayed behind in Fukushima have experienced guilt for their children and have expressed their fear of being accused of allowing their children to continue to be exposed to radiation by staying in Fukushima (Save the Children, 2012). Conversely, the parents who managed to relocate to other areas also felt guilty for escaping their hometown and abandoning their friends and neighbors (see Chap. 12, this volume, for related discussion).

It is important to note that the anxieties and guilt from the parents, especially the mothers, are likely to lead to their children's instability. The survey of the pediatric clinic described earlier (Kitajo, 2011) also showed that compared with those before the disaster, the children in Fukushima city tended to be more irritable, more easily offended, more apathetic, and more obsessive. Furthermore, the study using Strength and Difficulty Questionnaire (SDQ; which is completed by parents) revealed that the rate of children with some behavioral problems in Fukushima was considerably higher than that in the other areas in Japan (Yabe et al., 2014).

While interacting with their children having such problematic behavior, their mothers also tended to become more anxious. Furthermore, the mothers' anxieties might elicit negative reactions in their children again, creating a vicious circle. As Raphael (1986) described in her book, these strong interactions between parents and their children are quite common in disasters. Unfortunately, many of the parents and their children in Fukushima are facing these negative intrafamilial interactions, such as distress towards other family members.

Ambiguous Loss Experiences In Fukushima, there are still vast areas where people are in danger of radioactive contamination as well as in danger from the effects of the tsunami. Over 100,000 people have been evacuated, and many have lost their homes, their jobs, family members, or their sense of community. The elderly people are especially likely to have many difficulties in their readjustment, due to the difficulty in changing their jobs and adapting themselves to new circumstances.

Given these losses, we should note that the difference in the losses brought by the nuclear crisis are very ambiguous compared with those by tsunami. Though many houses where the evacuees lived before the disaster are not damaged in appearance, the evacuees were not allowed to stay or live there by the government's order. Even after the government lifted the restrictions, many evacuees are still hesitant about returning to their homes for several reasons, such as the fear of insufficient decontamination, difficulty in finding employment, or simply due to uncertainty. On the other hand, the tsunami survivors, despite their great and apparent loss, seemed to have overcome their traumatic experiences faster than the people affected by the nuclear accident.

The Fukushima evacuees continue to face a dilemma; they can continue waiting for their hometown to become habitable again someday, but it is unknown when such a situation will occur. Also, this uncertainty has led to difficulties in both compensations and the welfare service. Similar to having a missing loved one (Boss, 1999; see also Chap. 15, this volume), such ambiguous loss delays the recovery process of the evacuees and may lead to continuing psychiatric problems for the Fukushima people. In particular, we should pay attention to occurrence of depression or suicide. For example, in Fukushima Prefecture, 32.4% of the new outpatients having depression or PTSD answered that their symptoms are related to the nuclear accident (Miura et al., 2012). The major psychiatric survey using K6 questionnaire which was performed by the Fukushima Medical University about 1 year after the accident shows 14.6% of all responders were estimated to be at risk of depression (Yabe et al., 2014). This result shows that the prevalence rate of people at risk of depression in Fukushima was considerably higher than that of general population in Japan (Kawakami, 2007). Moreover, in regards to suicide, the Reconstruction Agency certified that 57 cases of suicide in Fukushima by September, 2014 were closely related to the disaster (The Reconstruction Agency, 2014). The certified number of suicides in Fukushima is much higher than those in other prefectures affected mainly by tsunami, such as Iwate and Miyagi. In Fukushima, the rehabilitation process was considerably delayed compared to other prefectures, and approximately 120,000 evacuees still exist (as of September, 2014). Considering the fact that the suicide rate in Kobe city started increasing dramatically 3 years after the Great Hanshin Awaji earthquake occurred in 1995 (Nishio et al., 2009), we should pay great attention to the further increase of suicide in Fukushima.

Separated Families and Communities In Fukushima, many people were relocated from the affected area both voluntarily and involuntarily. Multiple factors, such as the fear of radioactive exposure, along with residential restrictions, compensations, employment, and/or other personal reasons, divided the residents into two groups: those who decided to relocate and those who did not. Unfortunately, the dissonance between these two groups often arose, which broke the bonds between the original residents (see Chap. 12, this volume, for related discussion).

Generally, if a natural disaster strikes, the bonds and cohesiveness among residents tend to become stronger, and moreover, may enhance the resilience of communities and reduce mental health problems (see Chap. 4, this volume). The past epidemiological study (Kessler, Borges, Walters, 1999) also revealed that the prevalence of PTSD among the people who experienced natural disasters was considerably lower than that among those who experienced other man-made incidents (e.g., motor vehicle accidents, physical assaults, rapes, etc.). Japan is known for being affected by a large number of natural disasters, such as earthquakes, tsunamis, or typhoons, and the communities in Japan have developed a sense of resilience from such incidents. However, since the Fukushima disaster was essentially a man-made disaster rather than a natural one, the resilience of the communities and the families has weakened.

In Fukushima, there have been three types of discordance, each of which has led to dissonance within both families and the community, as follows:

- Family members having different opinions on the physical risk induced by radioactive exposure.
- Interfamilial conflicts caused by differences in residential restrictions or compensations.
- Frustrations between evacuees and neighboring members taking in large numbers of evacuees (e.g., Iwaki city).

As time passed since the disaster, the souring relationships among the community members and the evacuees has worsened due to several reasons: the delinquency of taxes, the unclear period of the evacuees' stay, an increase in population, and the rise in land cost. These three types of discordance have created tension within the population of Fukushima.

Stigma and Self-Stigma. Although the authorities such as the World Health Organization (2013) recommended that the people in Fukushima should not be fearful of the radiation risks in regards to their physical condition, many people are still skeptical. Taking into account the psychosocial burden of the evacuees, it is problematic that there is a public stigma forming through ignorance about the radiation. For example, Shigemura, Tanigawa, Saito, and Nomura (2012) showed that discrimination was associated with both general psychological distress and posttraumatic responses among the workers engaging in the repair of the destroyed plant. Furthermore, many young women in Fukushima are afraid of how people may look down on them due to assumptions regarding the influence of radiation on pregnancy or on genetic inheritance (Glionna, 2012). Some also believe that the women exposed to radiation should not be allowed to marry or reproduce. Unfortunately, due to these misconceptions, many evacuees are hiding the fact that they lived in Fukushima after moving to other prefectures (Save the Children, 2012).

This phenomenon reminds us of the atomic bomb survivors of Hiroshima and Nagasaki. They also tried to hide their life history and refused to discuss their experiences of the atomic bombing. In particular, the young female survivors also showed the same strong tendency of concealing their experience as those of Fukushima and showed worse psychological symptoms than those of the male survivors (Yamada & Izumi, 2002).

The self-awareness of both of the atomic bomb survivors and the Fukushima people can be regarded as a "self-stigma" induced by the public stigma related to radioactive contamination. According to the idea of Corrigan, Watson, & Barr, (2006), who studied the traits of self-stigma among people with mental disorders, the self-stigma would cause either righteous anger or a loss of self-esteem within the stigmatized people. Also, in the case of Fukushima, such self-stigmas are likely to cause emotional distress within the victims. Given the considerable psychological effects from the self-stigma, dispelling public stigma should be highly prioritized in order to prevent the Fukushima people of stigmatizing themselves further.

Conclusion and Future Directions

The Great East Japan Earthquake was the most severe complex disaster in recorded history. The psychosocial influence of this event was seen broadly and multidimensionally on people living in or out of Fukushima. We have endeavored to comprehensively demonstrate them in this chapter, yet it is difficult for us to describe the whole of the unique features brought by the disaster because of the variety, confusion, and ambiguity at the present time. Specifically, the findings or data concerning the psychosocial states of the Fukushima people are not sufficient to know the real extent of the traumatic stress experienced so far. Although, in reality, many researchers have tried to conduct various types of studies in Fukushima since the disaster occurred, targeted people often felt uncomfortable participating in research because of the feeling of being "an experimental animal" and declined to participate as a result. It is, therefore, still difficult to get reliable and useful data obtained from controlled and/or longitudinal studies. Considering the Fukushima people's distrust for researchers, we should spend more time to make better relationships with them and provide useful information and adequate care for them.

Given the complicated problems, as described earlier, regarding mental health among the Fukushima people, we recommend the following three approaches. First, we should focus on high-risk groups, such as mothers with young children, and provide effective psychological interventions for them. Second, we should provide adequate risk communication and programs involving the media to dispel the stigma towards the Fukushima people. Lastly, we should provide active support for the medical and welfare workers or public servants working in Fukushima to prevent their burnout or exhaustion. Various types of workers engaging in the rehabilitation of Fukushima for a long time were especially more likely to have serious psychiatric problems such as depression, alcohol abuse, or suicidal ideation. They should be regarded as one of the highest risk groups and need to receive more intensive care or treatment.

Considering the multiple and widespread psychosocial problems, establishing a community-based care network with various types of resources in Fukushima is key to success rather than finding one specific approach to resolve them. Although many facilities such as hospitals, clinics, health centers, schools, or nonprofit organizations are concerned with the rehabilitation of Fukushima, these facilities tend to provide interventions independently of each other. Therefore, a facility with a collaborative mission, functionally linking independent institutions and programs together as a center, is important to improve the current situation. A new facility, the Fukushima Center for Disaster Mental Health (FCDMH), has been in operation since about 10 months after the disaster. It has 50–60 staff members including psychiatrists, clinical psychologists, social workers, nurses, and occupational therapists and has been positively providing outreach service and psychoeducational programs for the evacuees, residents, or various stakeholders based on the transdisciplinary model. The FCDMH is expected to cooperate with other existing facilities and meet needs of evacuees, residents or communities with flexibility.

An important direction for further research concerns the continued assessment of mental health needs of those directly affected by the nuclear disaster. For example, the Mental Health and Lifestyle Survey (MHLS) performed by Fukushima Medical University is considered to be the most important longitudinal survey in order to obtain useful data concerning the mental health conditions of the 210,000 people who have once lived in the evacuation area (Yasumura et al., 2012). In this chapter, we have introduced several results of the MHLS concerning the prevalence of PTSD or depression. The MHLS was planned to do screening for the residents to identify people at risk for some psychiatric or lifestyle-related problems using several questionnaires (K-6, PCL, and SDQ). According to the results, interventions using telephone or through the mail have been provided for the responders by the support team belonging to the Fukushima Medical University (Yabe et al., 2014). If other mental health care providers use the data more effectively, more seamless care or treatment plan should be able to be provided for people who need help.

References

Asukai, N., Kato, H., Kawamura, N., Kim, Y., Yamamoto, K., Kishimoto, J., et al. (2002). Reliability and validity of the Japanese-language version of the Impact of Event Scale-Revised (IES-R-J): Four studies of different traumatic events. *The Journal of Nervous and Mental Disease, 190*(3), 175–182.

Beehler, G. P., Baker, J. A., Falkner, K., Chegerova, T., Pryshchepava, A., Chegerov, V., et al. (2008). A multilevel analysis of long-term psychological distress among Belarusians affected by the Chernobyl disaster. *Public Health, 122*(11), 1239–1249. doi:10.1016/j.puhe.2008.04.017.

Boss, P. (1999). *Ambiguous loss: Learning to live with unresolved grief.* Cambridge: Harvard University Press.

Bromet, E. J.(2012). Reflections on the mental health consequences of nuclear power plant disasters and implications for epidemiologic research in northeast Japan. *Japanese Bulletin of Social Psychiatry, 21,* 222–234.

Bromet, E. J., Goldgaber, D., Carlson, G., Panina, N., Golovakha, E., Gluzman, S. F., et al. (2000). Children's well-being 11 years after the Chornobyl catastrophe. *Archives of General Psychiatry, 57*(6), 563–571.

Bromet, E. J., Havenaar, J. M., & Guey, L. T. (2011). A 25 year retrospective review of the psychological consequences of the Chernobyl accident. *Clinical Oncology (Royal College of Radiologists (Great Britain)), 23*(4), 297–305. doi:10.1016/j.clon.2011.01.501; 10.1016/j.clon.2011.01.501.

Corrigan, P. W., Watson, A. C., & Barr, L (2006). The self–stigma of mental illness: Implications for self-esteem and self-efficacy. *Journal of Social and Clinical Psychology, 25*(8), 875–884.

Dew, M. A., & Bromet, E. J. (1993). Predictors of temporal patterns of psychiatric distress during 10 years following the nuclear accident at Three Mile Island. *Social Psychiatry and Psychiatric Epidemiology, 28*(2), 49–55.

Dew, M. A., Bromet, E. J., Schulberg, H. C., Dunn, L. O., & Parkinson, D. K. (1987). Mental health effects of the Three Mile Island nuclear reactor restart. *American Journal of Psychiatry, 144*(8), 1074–1077.

Foster, R. P., & Goldstein, M. F. (2007). Chernobyl disaster sequelae in recent immigrants to the United States from the former Soviet Union (FSU). *Journal of Immigrant Minority Health, 9*(2), 115–124. doi:10.1007/s10903-006-9024-8.

Gamache, G. L., Levinson, D. M., Reeves, D. L., Bidyuk, P. I., & Brantley, K. K. (2005). Longitudinal neurocognitive assessments of Ukrainians exposed to ionizing radiation after the Chernobyl nuclear accident. *Archives of Clinical Neuropsychology, 20*(1), 81–93. doi:10.1016/j.acn.2004.03.005.

Glionna, J. M. (2012). A year after tsunami, a cloud of distrust hangs over Japan: The Fukushima nuclear disaster has left residents doubting their government, their source of energy, even the food they eat. Los Angeles Times, 11 March, http://articles.latimes.com/2012/mar/11/world/la-fg-japan-quake-trust-20120311. Accessed 20 Jun 2013.

Havenaar, J. M., Rumyantzeva, G. M., van den Brink, W., Poelijoe, N. W., van den Bout, J., van Engeland, H., et al. (1997). Long-term mental health effects of the Chernobyl disaster: an epidemiologic survey in two former Soviet Regions. *American Journal of Psychiatry, 154*(11), 1605–1607.

Heiervang, K. S., Mednick, S., Sundet, K., & Rund, B. R. (2010). Effect of low dose ionizing radiation exposure in utero on cognitive function in adolescence. *Scandinavian Journal of Psychology, 51*(3), 210–215. doi:10.1111/j.1467-9450.2010.00814.x.
Heiervang, K. S., Mednick, S., Sundet, K., & Rund, B. R. (2011). The psychological well-being of Norwegian adolescents exposed in utero to radiation from the Chernobyl accident. *Child & Adolescent Psychiatry & Mental Health, 5*, 12. doi: 10.1186/1753-2000-5-12.
Houts, P. S., Tokuhata, G. K., Bratz, J., Bartholomew, M. J., & Sheffer, K. W. (1991). Effect of pregnancy during TMI crisis on mothers' mental health and their child's development. *American Journal of Public Health, 81*(3), 384–386.
Igumnov, S., & Drozdovitch, V. (2000). The intellectual development, mental and behavioural disorders in children from Belarus exposed in utero following the Chernobyl accident. *European Psychiatry, 15*(4), 244–253.
IAEA (International Atomic Energy Agency). (1999). *Report on the preliminary fact finding mission following the accident at the nuclear fuel processing facility in Tokaimura, Japan.* International Atomic Energy Agency, Vienna. http://www-pub.iaea.org/MTCD/publications/PDF/TOAC_web.pdf. Accessed 14 Nov 2014.
IAEA (International Atomic Energy Agency). (2006). *Chernobyl's legacy: Health, environmental and socio-economic impacts and recommendations to the governments of Belarus, the Russian federation and Ukraine, 2003–2005.* International Atomic Energy Agency, Vienna. http://www.iaea.org/Publications/Booklets/Chernobyl/chernobyl.pdf. Accessed 7 Aug 2014.
International Atomic Energy Agency (2008). The International Nuclear and Radiological Event Scale. Retrieved from http://www-ns.iaea.org/tech-areas/emergency/ines.asp. Accessed 24 June 2015.
Ishigaki, A., Higashi, H., Sakamoto, T., & Shibahara, S. (2013). The Great East Japan Earthquake and devastating tsunami: An update and lessons from the past great earthquakes in Japan since 1923. *The Tohoku Journal of Experimental Medicine, 229*(4), 287–299.
JNPA (Japanese National Police Agency). (2012). Damage situation and police countermeasures associated with 2011 Tohoku district—off the Pacific Ocean Earthquake. Retrieved from http://www.npa.go.jp/archive/keibi/biki/higaijokyo_e.pdf. Accessed 24 June 2015.
Kasl, S. V., Chisholm, R. F., & Eskenazi, B. (1981a). The impact of the accident at the Three Mile Island on the behavior and well-being of nuclear workers: Part II: Job tension, psychophysiological symptoms, and indices of distress. *American Journal of Public Health, 71*(5), 484–495.
Kasl, S. V., Chisholm, R. F., & Eskenazi, B. (1981b). The impact of the accident at the Three Mile Island on the behavior and well-being of nuclear workers; Part I: Perceptions and evaluations, behavioral responses, and work-related attitudes and feelings. *American Journal of Public Health, 71*(5), 472–483.
Kawakami, N. (2007). National Survey of Mental Health measured by K6 and factors affecting mental health status (in Japanese) in research on applied use of statistics and information. *Health Labour Sciences Research Grant Report 2006/2007.*
Kessler, R. C., Borges, G., & Walters, E. E. (1999). Prevalence of and risk factors for lifetime suicide attempts in the national comorbidity survey. *Archives of General Psychiatry, 56*(7), 617–626.
Kessler, R. C., Barker, P. R., Colpe, L. J., Epstein, J. F., Gfroerer, J. C., Hiripi, E., et al. (2003). Screening for serious mental illness in the general population. *Archives of General Psychiatry, 60*(2), 184–189.
Kitajo, T. (2011). Effects of Fukushima nuclear accident on children in Fukushima. *Nishoikaiho,* 42, 119–121.
Konishi, T., & Inamoto, E. (1999). The impacts of the residents near Tokaimura on the mental health consultations after the nuclear accident. In T. Yoshikawa (Ed.), *Health and Labour Sciences Research Grant report: PTSD research of residents after the disasters* (pp. 10–18). (Japanese). https://mhlw-grants.niph.go.jp/niph/search/NIDD00.do?resrchNum=199900066A#selectHokoku. Accessed 24 June 2015.
Kyutoku, Y., Tada, R., Umeyama, T., Harada, K., Kikuchi, S., Watanabe, E., Liegey-Dougall, A., Dan, I. (2012) Cognitive and psychological reactions of the general population three months

after the 2011, Tohoku earthquake and tsunami. *PLos One, 7*(2),:e31014. doi: 10.1371/journal.pone.0031014.

Litcher, L., Bromet, E. J., Carlson, G., Squires, N., Goldgaber, D., Panina, N., et al. (2000). School and neuropsychological performance of evacuated children in Kyiv 11 years after the Chornobyl disaster. *Journal Child Psychology Psychiatry, 41*(3), 291–299.

Loganovsky, K., Havenaar, J. M., Tintle, N. L., Guey, L. T., Kotov, R., & Bromet, E. J. (2008). The mental health of clean-up workers 18 years after the Chernobyl accident. *Psychological Medicine, 38*(4), 481–488. doi:10.1017/S0033291707002371.

Maeda, M. (2012) Difficulties of the staff working at Hibarigaoka Psychiatric Hospital in Minami-Soma. *Rishoseisinigaku, 41*(9), 1183–1191. (Japanese)

Maeda, M., & Oe, M. (2014). Disaster behavioral health: Psychological effects of the Fukushima Nuclear Power Plant accident. In K. Tanigawa and R. K. Chhem (Eds.), *Radiation disaster medicine* (pp. 79–88). Springer International Publishing.

Miura, I., Wada, A., Itagaki, S., Yabe, H., & Niwa, S. (2012). Relationship between psychological distress and anxiety/depression following Great East Japan Earthquake in Fukushima Prefecture. *Rinsho-seishinigaku, 41,* 1137–1142.

Nishio, A., Akazawa, K., Shibuya, F., Abe, R., Nushida, H., Ueno, Y., et al. (2009). Influence on the suicide rate two years after a devastating disaster: A report from the 1995 Great Hanshin-Awaji Earthquake. *Psychiatry and Clinical Neurosciences, 63,* 247–250.

Parkinson, D. K., & Bromet, E. J. (1983). Correlates of mental health in nuclear and coal-fired power plant workers. *Scand J Work Environ Health, 9*(4), 341–345.

President's Commission on the accident at Three Mile Island. (1979). *The need for change, the legacy of TMI: Report of the President's Commission on the accident at Three Mile Island.* Washington, D.C.: U.S. Government Printing Office.

Prince-Embury, S., & Rooney, J. F. (1995). Psychological adaptation among residents following restart of Three Mile Island. *Journal of Traumatic Stress, 8*(1), 47–59.

Rahu, K., Rahu, M., Tekkel, M., & Bromet, E. (2006). Suicide risk among Chernobyl cleanup workers in Estonia still increased: An updated cohort study. *Annals of Epidemiology, 16*(12), 917–919. doi:10.1016/j.annepidem.2006.07.006.

Raphael, B. (1986). *When disaster strikes: How individuals and communities cope with catastrophe*. New York: Basic Books.

Save the Children. (2012). Fukushima families: Children and families affected by Fukushima's nuclear crisis share their concerns one year on. http://www.savethechildren.org/atf/cf/%7B9def2ebe-10ae-432c-9bd0-df91d2eba74a%7D/JAPAN_FUKUSHIMA_FAMILIES_REPORT.PDF. Accessed 25 Jun 2013.

Shigemura, J., Tanigawa, T., Saito, I., & Nomura, S. (2012). Psychological distress in workers at the Fukushima Nuclear Power Plants. *JAMA, 308*(7), 667–669.

Taormina, D. P., Rozenblatt, S., Guey, L. T., Gluzman, S. F., Carlson, G. A., Havenaar, J. M., et al. (2008). The Chornobyl accident and cognitive functioning: A follow-up study of infant evacuees at age 19 years. *Psychological Medicine, 38*(4), 489–497. doi:10.1017/S0033291707002462; 10.1017/S0033291707002462.

The Reconstruction Agency Report. (2014). http://www.reconstruction.go.jp/topics/main-cat2/sub-cat2-1/20131224_kanrenshi.pdf. (Japanese)

Tomita, N., & Nakajima, S. (1999). Mental health of the affected residents. In T. Yoshikawa (Ed.), *Health and labour sciences research grant report: PTSD research of residents after the disasters*. (Japanese). https://mhlw-grants.niph.go.jp/niph/search/NIDD00.do?resrchNum=199900066A#selectHokoku. Accessed 24 June 2015.

Viel, J. F., Curbakova, E., Dzerve, B., Eglite, M., Zvagule, T., & Vincent, C. (1997). Risk factors for long-term mental and psychosomatic distress in Latvian Chernobyl liquidators. *Environmental Health Perspectives, 105*(Suppl 6), 1539–1544.

Weathers, F. W., Litz, B. T., Herman, D. S., Huska, J. A., & Keane, T. M. (1993, October). The PTSD checklist (PCL): Reliability, validity, and diagnostic utility. In International Society for Traumatic Stress Studies (Ed.), *Annual convention of the international society for traumatic stress studies*. San Antonio: International Society for Traumatic Stress Studies.

World Health Organization Report. (2013). Health risk assessment from the nuclear accident after the 2011 Great East Japan Earthquake and Tsunami based on a preliminary dose estimation.

Yabe, H., Suzuki, Y., Mashiko, H., Nakayama, Y., Hisata, M., Niwa, S. I., et al. (2014). Psychological distress after the Great East Japan Earthquake and Fukushima Daiichi Nuclear Power Plant accident: Results of a mental health and lifestyle survey through the Fukushima Health Management Survey in FY2011 and FY2012. *Fukushima Journal of Medical Science, 60*(1), 57–67.

Yamada, M., & Izumi. S. (2002) Psychiatric sequelae in atomic bomb survivors in Hiroshima and Nagasaki two decades after the explosions. *Social Psychiatry and Psychiatric Epidemiology,* 37(9):409–415.

Yasumura, S., Hosoya, M., Yamashita, S., Kamiya, K., Abe, M., Akashi, M., et al. (2012). Study protocol for the Fukushima Health Management Survey. *Journal of Epidemiology, 22*(5), 375–383.

Yokoyama, Y., Otsuka, K., Kawakami, N., Kobayashi, S., Ogawa, A., Tannno, K., et al. (2014). Mental health and related factors after the Great East Japan Earthquake and Tsunami. *PLoS One, 9*(7), e102497. doi:10.1371/journal.pone.0102497.

Chapter 6
Posttraumatic Stress in the Aftermath of Mass Shootings

Sarah R. Lowe and Sandro Galea

Introduction

Over the past few decades, mass shooting episodes in the USA have shocked the nation. Names like Columbine, Sandy Hook, and Aurora have become part of our national lexicon, and they bring to mind images of the horrors that took place during these tragic events. Although mass shootings capture public attention, they remain extremely rare events. For example, between 1990 and 2012, there were 25 mass shootings at secondary schools and college campuses that resulted in 135 deaths, accounting for only 0.4 % of national firearm homicides, with the average number of episodes remaining within the range of 0–3 per year (Shultz, Cohen, Muschert, & Flores de Apodaca, 2013).

Despite the continued rarity of mass shootings, key events over the past decade have led to an unusually large number of fatalities and injuries—for example, 33 fatalities and 23 injuries in the 2007 Virginia Tech massacre, 12 fatalities and 58 injuries in the 2012 Aurora, Colorado theatre shooting, and 28 fatalities and 2 injuries in the Sandy Hook elementary school shooting in Newtown, Connecticut (Follman, Aronsen, & Pan, 2014). These high-impact episodes in particular are likely to exert a psychological toll on their direct victims and members of the communities in which they took place. Yet, surprisingly little empirical research evaluates the mental health effects of mass shootings, and no efforts to our knowledge have been made to synthesize the extant literature.

S. R. Lowe (✉)
Department of Epidemiology, Mailman School of Public Health, Columbia University, Room 720-F, 722 West 168th Street, New York, NY 10032, USA
e-mail: srl2143@columbia.edu

S. Galea
School of Public Health, Boston University,
715 Albany Street, Talbot 301, Boston, MA 02118, USA
e-mail: sgalea@bu.edu

K. E. Cherry (ed.), *Traumatic Stress and Long-Term Recovery*,
DOI 10.1007/978-3-319-18866-9_6

In this chapter, we therefore aim to conduct a comprehensive review of empirical investigations on the mental health effects of mass shootings. We focus specifically on post-traumatic stress disorder (PTSD) diagnoses and severity of posttraumatic stress symptoms (PTSS), the most common outcomes assessed in the aftermath of traumatic events. We provide an overview of this body of research, including the prevalence of PTSD across different studies, and predictors associated with higher odds of PTSD or higher PTSS. Based on this review, we make recommendations for future research and post-incident interventions.

Overview of Studies

We conducted a comprehensive literature search in PsycInfo and PubMed databases, using both general terms (e.g., "shooting," "tragedy") and names of specific events (e.g., "Columbine," "Sandy Hook"). We limited our search to articles in peer-reviewed, English-language journals that included quantitative indices of PTSD and PTSS among the dependent variables. We therefore excluded qualitative studies and quantitative studies that focused on other outcomes (e.g., other psychiatric disorders, perceptions of social solidarity, coping strategies).

We identified a total of 35 studies on 14 different mass shooting incidents that took place from 1984 to 2008. One study focused on two different events combined. Table 6.1 provides basic information on each event (e.g., location, number of injuries and fatalities) in chronological order. Twelve events took place in the USA, and two took place in Finland. The majority of events ($n=8$) were in a secondary school or university context, whereas the remainder took place in other locations (e.g., local businesses). In organizing the results of the literature search, we noted instances in which data from the same sample were used across different analyses. In total, there were 19 independent samples (1 from the study focusing on 2 different events combined).

Posttraumatic Stress Disorder

Table 6.2 denotes the prevalences of PTSD across the studies, as well as the measures and classification systems used to determine them, if this information was available. The lowest PTSD prevalence reported was 3 % among parents of children exposed to an elementary school shooting 6–14 months post incident, determined using conservative diagnostic and statistical manual (DSM)-III-R criteria with the PTSD Reaction Index (PTSD-RI; Schwarz & Kowalski, 1991a). The highest prevalence reported was 91 % among children in the same study, using liberal (proposed) DSM-IV criteria and the children's version of the PTSD-RI (Schwarz & Kowalski, 1991b).

Table 6.1 Summary of mass shooting incidents and characteristics of peer-reviewed studies

Year	Location	Context	Perpetrator	Fatalities	Injuries	Peer-reviewed articles	Samples
1984	Los Angeles, CA	Elementary school	Adult African American male	3	14	2	1
1984	San Ysidro, CA	Fast-food restaurant	Adult white male	21	15	1	1
1987	Russellville, AR	Four local businesses	Adult white male	2	4	1	1
1988	Winnetka, IL	Elementary school	Adult white female	2	5	6	3
1991	Killeen, TX	Cafeteria-style restaurant	Adult white male	24	20	5	2
1992	St. Louis, MO	Courthouse	Adult white male	1	5	1	1
1993	San Francisco, CA	Office building	Adult white male	6	14	1	1
1994	Brooklyn, NY	Brooklyn Bridge	Adult Lebanese-born immigrant male	1	3	1	1
2006	Montreal, Quebec, Canada	University (Dawson College)	Adult Indo-Canadian male	2	17	1	1
2007	Tuusula, Finland	High school (Jokela High School)	Adolescent white male	9	19	2	1
2007	Blacksburg, VA	University (Virginia Polytechnic Institute and State University)	Adult South Korean male	33	25	4	2
2008	DeKalb, IL	University (Northern Illinois University)	Adult white male	6	18	7	1
2008	Conway, AR	University (University of Central Arkansas)	Four adult African American males	2	1	1	1
2008	Kauhajoki, Finland	University (Seinäjoki University of Applied Sciences)	Adult white male	11	1	1	1

Table does not include one study that focused on two different events (Vicary & Fraley, 2010)

Table 6.2 Summary of the findings from peer-reviewed studies on the psychological effects of mass shooting incidents

Author, year	*N*	Sample	Timing	PTSD assessment: measure; classification system	Prevalence	Predictors
1984: Elementary school in Los Angeles, CA						
(1a) Pynoos et al. (1987)	159	Elementary school students	1 month	PTSD-RI; DSM-III	60.4%	PTSS, 1 month: proximity to attack, greater acquaintance with the deceased victim
(1b) Nader, Pynoos, Fairbanks, and Frederick (1990)	100	[a]	1 month, 14 months	[a]	–	PTSS, 14 months: proximity to attack, greater acquaintance with the deceased victim; grief: greater acquaintance with the deceased
1984: Fast-food restaurant in San Ysidro, CA						
(1) Hough et al. (1990)	303	Middle-aged Mexican-American women from the community, but who were not directly involved in the incident	6–9 months	Scale derived for the study, based on the DIS, DSM-III	Post-incident, 12.6%; past month, 6.8%	Severe PTSD (significance of trends not tested): widowed, separated or divorced status, older age, no children at home, lower income, unemployment, having friends/relatives involved in event, fair–poor physical health, higher depression. Mild PTSD (significance of trends not tested): middle age, having three or more children at home, middle income, having friends/relatives involved in the event, fair–poor physical health
1987: Four local businesses in Russellville, AR						
(1) North, Smith, McCool, and Shea (1989)	18	Employees at two of the four local businesses who were either at work during the shooting ($n=15$) or absent ($n=11$)	4–6 weeks	DIS/disaster supplement; DSM-III	5.6%	–
1988: Elementary school in Winnetka, IL						

Table 6.2 (continued)

Author, year	*N*	Sample	Timing	PTSD assessment: measure; classification system	Prevalence	Predictors
(1a) Schwarz and Kowalski (1991a)	130	Elementary school students (n=64) and their parents (n=66)	6–14 months	PTSD-RI; DSM-III-R, liberal moderate and conservative criteria	Children, DSM-III-R: 50 % (liberal), 41 % (moderate), 8 % (conservative); parents, DSM-III-R, proposed: 39 % (liberal), 24 % (moderate), 3 % (conservative)	PTSD, children (predictors of diagnosis based on liberal, moderate, or conservative criteria): perception that he/she would get shot or was in danger during event, increased physical symptoms, increased visits to school nurse, increased or new fears, guilt. PTSD, parents (predictors of diagnosis based on liberal, moderate, or conservative criteria): felt numb, scared, or fearful that the alleged perpetrator was still on the loose
(1b) Schwarz and Kowalski (1991b)	130	[a]	6–14 months	PTSD-RI; DSM-III, DSM-III-R (same prevalences as Schwarz & Kowalski, 1991a), proposed DSM-IV: liberal, moderate, and conservative criteria	PTSD, children, DSM-III, proposed DSM-IV: 91 %, 41 % (liberal), 61 %, 41 % (moderate), 16 %, 9 % (conservative); PTSD, parents, DSM-III, proposed DSM-IV: 52 %, 54 % (liberal), 16 %, 24 % (moderate), 4 %, 6 % (conservative)	–
(2a) Schwarz and Kowalski (1992a)	24	School personnel	6 months	PTSD-RI; DSM-III	–	PTSS: personality traits—guilt and resentment, insecurity, psychasthenia
(2b) Schwarz and Kowalski (1992b)	24	[a]; subsample completed two waves (n=13)	6 months, 18 months	[a]	–	PTSS, 6 months: loss to follow-up

Table 6.2 (continued)

Author, year	*N*	Sample	Timing	PTSD assessment: measure; classification system	Prevalence	Predictors
(2c) Schwarz, Kowalski, and McNaly (1993)	24	[a]; subsample completed two waves (n=12)	6 months, 18 months	[a]	–	PTSS, 6 months: enlargement of recall of emotional experiences (hyperarousal), life-threat experiences (hyperarousal), and sensory experiences (avoidance, hyperarousal, total PTSS), lack of diminishment in recall of emotional experiences (intrusion); PTSS, 18 months: enlargement in recall of sensory experiences (hyperarousal)
(3) Sloan, Rozensky, Kaplan, and Saunders (1994)	140	Emergency responders	6 months	IES intrusion, and avoidance; unspecified	–	PTSS: five indicators of job stress during the event—exposure to traumatic stimuli, adverse work environment, time pressure, quantitative workload, qualitative workload (intrusion and avoidance)
1991: Cafeteria-style restaurant in Killeen, TX						
(1a) North, Smith, & Spitznagel (1994)	136	Survivors (e.g., restaurant patrons and employees, emergency responders)	1–2 months	DIS, DSM-III-R	28.6 %	PTSD: female gender, pre-incident Major Depression (MD) (among female participants only), any pre-incident psychiatric diagnosis (among female participants only), post-incident MD, any post-incident psychiatric disorder (among female participants only), seeing a doctor or counselor, taking medication
(1b) North, Smith, and Spitznagel (1997)	124	[a]	1–2 months, 1 year	[a]	At 1 year: 17.7 %	PTSD, either/both 1–2 months and 1 year: female gender, any pre-incident psychiatric diagnosis (among female participants only), any other post-incident psychiatric disorder, any other lifetime psychiatric disorder, pre-incident MD, MD at 1–2 months, lifetime MD

Table 6.2 (continued)

Author, year	*N*	Sample	Timing	PTSD assessment: measure; classification system	Prevalence	Predictors
(1c) North, Spitznagel, and Smith (2001)	136	[a]	1–2 months, 1 year, 3 years	[a]	–	PTSD, 1–2 months: lower active outreach and informed pragmatism coping at 1–2 months; PTSD, 1 year: lower informed pragmatism coping at 1–2 months; PTSD, 3 years: lower informed pragmatism coping at 1–2 months
(1d) North, McCutcheon, Spitznagel, and Smith (2002)	116	[a]	[a]	[a]	At 3 years: 18 %	Non-recovery from PTSD, 3 years: functional interference due to symptoms, having seen a mental health professional at 1–2 months
(2) Sewell (1996)	92	Persons either directly exposed (e.g., restaurant patrons) or indirectly exposed (e.g., relatives of directly exposed)	1 week, 3 months	Module from the PDI; DSM-IV	At 1 week: 38.7 %	PTSD, 1 week: pre-incident PTSD; PTSD non-recovery, 3 months: lower trauma-related construct elaboration
1992: Courthouse in St. Louis, MO						
(1) Johnson, North, and Smith (2002)	80	Employees at courthouse and offices of involved individuals; subsample completed two waves (*n*=77)	6–8 weeks, 1 year, 3 years	DIS/disaster supplement; unspecified	At 6–8 weeks: 5 %; at either 6–8 weeks, 1 year, or 3 years: 10 %	PTSS, 6–8 weeks: younger age, being married, lower education, feeling like the incident had caused them a great deal of harm (total PTSS, reexperiencing), reporting that the incident was very upsetting (avoidance), perceived lack of recovery (avoidance), mental health service utilization (reexperiencing, avoidance, and hyperarousal)
1993: Office building in San Francisco, CA						

Table 6.2 (continued)

Author, year	*N*	Sample	Timing	PTSD assessment: measure; classification system	Prevalence	Predictors
(1) Classen, Koopman, Hales, and Spiegel (1998)	36	Office employees; subsample completed two waves ($n=32$)	1 week, 7–10 months	IES, DTS; DSM-III-R	–	PTSD, 7–10 months: ASD symptoms (DTS total, IES-R intrusion, IES-R avoidance)
1994: Brooklyn Bridge in Brooklyn, NY						
(1) Trappler and Friedman (1996)	22	Youth who were in the van that was target of shooting (survivors); 11 students, age-matched and from the same community (comparison)	8 weeks	PTSD symptom scale, IES-R, clinical information; DSM-IV	Among survivors: 36.4 %	PTSS: being a survivor (vs. member of comparison group, intrusion and avoidance)
2006: Dawson College (DC) in Montreal, Quebec						
(1) Séguin et al. (2013)	948	DC students and employees	18 months	Measure adapted from the 2002 Canadian Community Health Survey; unspecified	Post-incident incidence rate: 1.8 %	–
2007: High school in Jokela, Finland						
(1a) Suomalainen, Haravuarti, Berg, Kiviruusu, and Marttunen (2011)	231	Jokela High School students. Unexposed comparison group of students from a different high school in Finland ($n=526$)	4 months	IES; unspecified	Among exposed: 19.2 %	PTSD: female gender, exposed (vs. unexposed), severe or extreme exposure (vs. mild to significant exposure), lower perceived support from family and friends
(1b) Murtonen, Suomalainen, Haravuori, and Marttunen (2012)	–	Jokela High School students	[a]	[a]	–	PTSD: not perceiving crisis support as helpful

Table 6.2 (continued)

Author, year	*N*	Sample	Timing	PTSD assessment: measure; classification system	Prevalence	Predictors
2007: Virginia Tech (VT) in Blacksburg, VA						
(1a) Littleton, Grills-Taquechel, and Axsom (2009)	293	Female VT students	Pre-incident, 2 months, 6 months	PSS-SR; DSM-IV	At 2 months: 30 %; at 6 months: 23 %	PTSS, 2 months: higher resource loss at 2 months post-incident. PTSS, 6 months: higher resource loss at 2 and 6 months
(1b) Littleton, Axsom, and Grills-Taquechel (2011a)	368	[a]	Pre-incident, 2 months, 6 months, 1 year	[a]	At 1 year: 27 %	PTSS, 6 months: PTSS at 2 months, maladaptive coping at 2 months; PTSS, 1 year: PTSS and maladaptive coping at 6 months
(1c) Littleton, Grills-Taquechel, Axsom, Bye, and Buck (2012)	215	[a]	Pre-incident, 2 months, 6 months, 1 year	[a]	–	PTSD, 1 year: pre-incident sexual victimization, lower benevolence beliefs at 2 months, lower family support at 2 months
(2a) Hughes et al., 2011	4639	VT students	3–4 months	TSQ; DSM-IV	15.4 %	PTSD: female gender, higher exposure to first incident of attack, inability to contact close friends during incident, death of a close friend, death of a friend of acquaintance
2008: Northern Illinois University (NIU) in Dekalb, IL						
(1a) Stephenson, Valentiner, Kumpula, and Orcutt (2009)	691	Female NIU students	Pre-incident, 2–4 weeks	DEQ; DSM-IV	–	PTSS, 2–4 weeks: higher anxiety sensitivity (physical and cognitive concerns), higher exposure

Table 6.2 (continued)

Author, year	*N*	Sample	Timing	PTSD assessment: measure; classification system	Prevalence	Predictors
(1b) Fergus, Rabenhorst, Orcutt, and Valentiner (2011)	58	[a]; subsample of participants with highest and lowest levels of exposure participated in a laboratory experiment	6 weeks	[a]	–	PTSS, 6 weeks: higher negative affect while writing and reading about event
(1c) Kumpula, Orcutt, Bardeen, and Varkovitsky (2011)	532	[a]	Pre-incident, 2–4 weeks, 8 months	[a]	Pre-incident—significant PTSS: 20.8%; at 2–4 weeks—significant PTSS: 49.4%; at 8 months—significant PTSS: 11.4%	PTSS, 2–4 weeks: non-White race/ethnicity (avoidance and hyperarousal), higher pre-incident trauma exposure, higher pre-incident experiential avoidance, higher peritraumatic dissociation; PTSS, 8 months: higher exposure, higher PTSS at 2–4 weeks, higher experiential avoidance at 2–4 weeks
(1d) Littleton, Kumpula, and Orcutt (2011b)	691	[a]	Pre-incident, 2–4 weeks, 8 months	[a]	–	PTSS, 2–4 weeks: non-African-American race/ethnicity, higher pre-incident trauma exposure, higher pre-incident stress, higher exposure; PTSS, 8 months: Asian-American race/ethnicity, higher pre-incident trauma exposure, higher pre-incident anxiety, higher exposure, higher PTSS at 2–4 weeks, higher resource loss
(1e) Mercer et al. (2012)	235	[a]; Subsample of participants who provided DNA samples	Pre-incident, 2–4 weeks	[a]	–	PTSS, change in symptoms from pre-incident to 2–4 weeks: rs25531 A/A genotype, 5-HTTLPR multimarker low-expressing genotypes

Table 6.2 (continued)

Author, year	N	Sample	Timing	PTSD assessment: measure; classification system	Prevalence	Predictors
(1f) Bardeen, Kumpula, and Ocrutt (2013)	691	[a]	Pre-incident, 2–4 weeks, 8 months	[a]	–	PTSS, 2–4 weeks: higher pre-incident posttraumatic stress, higher exposure, higher emotion regulation difficulties at pre-incident and 2–4 weeks; PTSS, higher emotion regulation difficulties at 2–4 weeks and 8 months
(1g) Orcutt, Bonanno, Hannon, and Miron (2014)	660	[a]	Pre-incident, 2–4 weeks, 8 months, 14 months, 20 months, 26 months, 32 months	[a]	–	Posttraumatic stress, chronic dysfunction trajectory: pre-incident trauma exposure, higher pre-incident experiential avoidance, higher exposure, higher emotion regulation difficulties (limited access to strategies, lack of emotional clarity) at 8 months
2008: Seinäjoki University of Applied Sciences (SUAS) in Kauhajoki, Finland						
(1) Turunen, Haravuori, Punamäki, Suomalainen, and Marttunen (2014)	137	SUAS students	4 months, 16 months, 28 months	IES, unspecified	–	PTSS, 4 months: preoccupied attachment style (total PTSS, avoidance subscale)
2007 and 2008: VT and NIU (combined)						
(1) Vicary and Fraley (2010)	284	VT (n=124) and NIU (n=160)	2 weeks, 8 weeks	PSS-SR, unspecified	At 2 weeks: 64 %; at 8 weeks: 22 %	PTSD, 2 weeks: female gender, knowing one of the victims

Under each event, numbering is used to denote when studies used data from the same sample, with studies presented in chronological order by publication date. For example, for the 1984 elementary school shooting in Los Angeles, CA, two studies from the same sample are listed and labeled accordingly: (1a) Pynoos et al., 1987 and (1b) Nader, Pynoos, Fairbanks, & Frederick, 1990. Bivariate associations were included only if multivariate results were unavailable If prevalence was reported in multiple publications for the same sample, then it went with one that included a higher # of participants.

DEQ distressing events questionnaire, *DIS* diagnostic interview schedule, *DTS* Davidson trauma scale, *IES* impact of events scale, *IES-R* impact of events scale-revised, *PSS-SR* PTSD symptom scale-self report, *PTSD* posttraumatic stress disorder, *PTSD-RI* post-traumatic stress disorder—reaction index, PTSS posttraumatic stress symptoms/severity, TSQ trauma screening questionnaire, *ASD* acute stress disorder, *DC* Dawson College

[a] Same description as the preceding study

Issues in Interpretation

There are several issues to consider when comparing the prevalence of PTSD across studies. First, variation in sample characteristics, as discussed in more detail later, could influence risk for PTSD, including variation in demographic characteristics and exposure to the incident. Second, there is wide variation in the timing of assessments, spanning from approximately 1 week to 32 months post incident. As shown in studies with multiple waves (e.g., Nader, Pynoos, Fairbanks, & Frederick, 1990; North, Smith, & Spitznagel, 1997) , the prevalence of psychiatric disorders tends to decrease over time, limiting the extent to which prevalences at varying time points after different events can be compared. Third, different measures and diagnostic criteria were used across the studies, which could certainly affect prevalence rates. The influence of diagnostic criteria on prevalence rates was most clearly demonstrated in the aftermath of the 1988 Illinois elementary school shooting, wherein the prevalence of PTSD among child survivors at 6–14 months post incident ranged from 8 to 91 % and among their parents from 3 to 54 % using conservative DSM-III-R criteria and liberal (proposed) DSM-IV criteria, respectively (Schwarz & Kowalski, 1991a, b).

An additional issue in interpretation is whether the prevalence of PTSD was due to direct exposure to the event or whether indirect exposure (e.g., hearing about the event through conversations or the media) could have led to similar figures. Two studies addressed this issue by comparing directly and indirectly exposed samples, with the results in each case indicating that exposure was associated with higher risk for adverse outcomes. First, students at Jokela High School in Finland, where a shooting took place in 2007, had significantly higher odds of PTSD than students in another city in Finland (Suomalainen et al., 2011). Second, in the aftermath of the 1994 Brooklyn Bridge shooting, levels of PTSS were higher in youth who directly experienced the attack than an age-matched comparison group of youth in the same community who were not directly exposed (Trappler & Friedman, 1996).

Predictors of Adverse Mental Health Outcomes

Table 6.2 also includes significant predictors of increased risk for PTSD or higher PTSS in each of the studies. These predictors can be divided roughly into three categories: (1) demographics and pre-incident characteristics, (2) incident exposure, and (3) post-incident functioning and psychosocial resources.

Demographic and Pre-incident Characteristics Demographic characteristics have frequently been included as predictors of PTSD and PTSS. Most consistently, female gender has been shown to be a predictor of adverse outcomes (e.g., North, Smith & Spitznagel, 1994; Suomalainen et al., 2011). One proposed explanation for this difference is that women are more likely to employ a ruminative coping style, increasing the severity and chronicity of their symptoms (e.g., McIntyre, Spence, & Lachlan, 2011; Palus, Fang, & Prawitz, 2012; see also Chap. 1 for related discussion).

Indicators of socioeconomic disadvantage, although less often included in post-incident studies, have also been consistently associated with poor outcomes. For example, in the aftermath of the 1984 shooting at a fast-food restaurant in California, higher prevalences of severe PTSD were documented among community members with lower income or who were unemployed, relative to their counterparts (Hough et al., 1990). Lower education was also associated with higher PTSS among survivors of the 1992 St. Louis courthouse shooting (Johnson, North, & Smith, 2002).

Other demographic characteristics have been less consistently associated with adverse outcomes. For example, older age was associated with increased risk for severe PTSD after the 1984 California fast-food restaurant attack (Hough et al., 1990), whereas younger age was associated with higher PTSS after the 1992 St. Louis courthouse shooting (Johnson et al., 2002). Racial/ethnic minority status has also been inconsistently associated with outcomes. For example, among female Northern Illinois University (NIU) students, African American ethnicity was associated with lower PTSS at 2–4 weeks post incident, whereas Asian ethnicity was associated with higher PTSS at 8 months post incident (Littleton, Kumpula, & Orcutt, 2011b).

Few studies have investigated whether marital and parent status affects risk for post-incident adversity. Hough et al. (1990) found higher prevalences of severe PTSD among widowed, divorced, or separated persons (relative to married and single persons) and among adults with no children at home (relative to those with one to two and three or more children); however, the statistical significance of these trends was not assessed. In contrast, Johnson et al. (2002) found that being married, relative to single or divorced, widowed, or separated, was associated with higher PTSS.

Only one study to our knowledge has investigated the role of genetic risk variants in predicting post-incident outcomes. Among a subsample of NIU female students who provided DNA samples, variants within the serotonin transporter gene were associated with significantly greater increases in PTSS from pre-incident to 2–4 weeks post incident (Mercer et al., 2012).

The results of several investigations have shown that pre-incident psychological functioning is a strong predictor of post-incident outcomes. A retrospective assessment of PTSD was found to predict post-incident PTSD among survivors of the 1991 Texas restaurant shooting (Sewell, 1996). In the aftermath of the same incident, reports of pre-incident psychiatric diagnosis were also associated with increased risk for PTSD among female survivors (North et al., 1994, 1997).

A related set of findings indicate that prior trauma exposure increases risk for psychological adversity in the aftermath of shooting incidents. For example, in the study of female Virginia Tech survivors, those who had experienced sexual victimization prior to the event were at increased risk of PTSS 1 year after the shooting (Littleton, Grills-Taquechel, Axsom, Bye, & Buck, 2012). Among the NIU student sample, higher pre-incident trauma exposure was predictive of higher PTSS at two post-incident time points (Littleton et al. 2011b), as well as increased odds of a non-resilient trajectory of PTSS over time (Orcutt, Bonanno, Hanna, & Miron, 2014). One possibility is that prior trauma exposure increases risk for post-incident psychological adversity through its association with pre-incident psychological symptoms; however, this pathway has not yet been explored empirically.

Incident Exposure Indices of greater incident exposure, including proximity to an attack, acquaintance with the deceased, and exposure inventories (with items assessing, for example, seeing or hearing the events and physical injuries), have consistently been associated with adverse outcomes (e.g., Littleton et al., 2011b; Pynoos et al., 1987). There is some evidence that the impact of milder forms of exposure on mental health decreases over time. For example, in the aftermath of the NIU shooting, moderate, severe, and extreme exposures (relative to no direct exposure) were associated with higher PTSS 2–4 weeks post incident, whereas only extreme exposure was associated with higher PTSS at 8 months post incident (Littleton et al., 2011b).

In addition, emotional reactions during and after the incident have been found to predict later psychological responses. For example, students' perceptions that they would be shot or were in danger during the 1988 Illinois elementary school shooting increased risk for PTSD (Schwarz & Kowalski, 1991a). Kumpula et al. (2011) assessed NIU students' experiences of *peritraumatic dissociation*—altered awareness and depersonalization or derealization—during the event and found them to be predictive of higher PTSS 2–4 weeks post incident. Other investigators have drawn on longitudinal data to show that earlier post-incident symptoms are positively associated with PTSS and risk for PTSD at later time points (e.g., Bardeen, Kumpula, & Orcutt, 2013; Littleton, Axsom, & Grills-Taquechel, 2011a). For example, acute stress disorder symptoms 1 week after the 1993 San Francisco office building shooting were associated with increased odds for PTSD 7–10 months post incident. Interestingly, Murtonen et al. (2012) found that students' perceptions that early crisis support was unhelpful were also associated with increased risk for PTSD, suggesting that survivors who do not benefit from early interventions might be at particular risk of adverse longer-term outcomes.

How events are perceived and remembered have also been found to predict outcomes. For example, after the 1992 St. Louis courthouse shooting, survivors' perception that the incident had caused them a great deal of harm, that it was very upsetting, and that they had not recovered were each associated with higher PTSS (Johnson et al., 2002). A small study of school personnel in the aftermath of the 1988 Illinois elementary school shooting assessed participants' changes in reports of emotional, life threat, and sensory experiences during the attack and found that those whose reports became more intense over time (*enlargement* of recall) or did not become less intense over time (lack of *diminishment* of recall) tended to have more severe PTSS (Schwarz, Kowalski, & McNaly, 1993).

Post-Incident Functioning and Psychosocial Resources As noted previously, early post-incident mental health responses have been found to prospectively predict later outcomes (e.g., Bardeen et al., 2013). In a similar vein, other classes of psychiatric symptoms have been positively associated with increased risk for PTSD and higher PTSS in cross-sectional assessments. For example, among female survivors of the 1991 Texas restaurant shooting, a diagnosis of any other psychiatric disorder was associated with increased odds of PTSD (North et al., 1994); among the full sample, there was also significant concordance between post-incident major depression and PTSD. A positive association between post-incident fears and PTSS has also been documented (Schwarz & Kowalski, 1991a).

Hough et al. (1990) have further suggested interrelations between PTSD and physical health problems. Specifically, the researchers found that higher prevalences of both mild and severe PTSD were observed in affected community members with fair or poor physical health versus those with good or excellent physical health, in the aftermath of the 1984 California fast-food restaurant shooting. Among children directly exposed to the 1988 Illinois elementary school shooting, increased physical symptoms and visits to the school nurse were associated with increased risk of PTSD (Schwarz & Kowalski, 1991a). In the absence of longitudinal research, the direction of the relationship between PTSD and physical health remains unclear.

In terms of psychosocial resources, researchers have focused on personality characteristics, beliefs and attitudes, coping styles, and social relationships as predictors of PTSD (see Chaps. 11 and 17, this volume, for related discussion). Personality characteristics that have been associated with higher PTSS include guilt and resentment, insecurity, and anxiety sensitivity (Schwarz & Kowalski, 1992a; Stephenson, Valentiner, Kumpula, & Orcutt, 2009). In contrast, perceived benevolence of others has been associated with decreased risk for PTSD (Littleton et al., 2012).

Coping styles have been differentially associated with outcomes. Forms of coping that involve taking action, cognitive processing of the incident, and acceptance have been associated with lower PTSS (e.g., North, Spitznagel, & Smith, 2001; Sewell, 1996), whereas ruminative and avoidant coping styles have been found to increase risk (e.g., Littleton et al., 2012). To some extent, means of coping in the aftermath of an incident could represent more pervasive difficulties and ways of approaching one's experiences. In this vein, studies drawing on pre-incident data have found that emotion regulation difficulties and *experiential avoidance,* or the tendency to disengage from difficult emotions, sensations, thoughts, and memories, to be prospective predictors of higher PTSS (e.g., Bardeen et al., 2013; Kumpula, Orcutt, Bardeen, & Varkovitzky, 2011).

Similarly, indicators of fewer social resources (e.g., lower perceived social support) have been consistently associated with adverse outcomes (e.g., Littleton et al., 2012; Suomalainen et al., 2011). These differences could be driven in part by stable personality characteristics. For example, nonsecure attachment styles were significantly associated with higher PTSS among students after a college campus shooting in Finland (Turunen, Haravuori, Punamäki, Suomalainen, & Marttunen, 2014).

On the other hand, researchers have been informed by conservation of resources (COR) theory (Hobfoll, 1989); see also Chap. 1, this volume), which suggests that *change* in psychosocial resources, rather than stability, increases risk for adverse psychological outcomes. Supporting COR theory, Littleton and colleagues found that survivors' reports of loss of life direction and pride, optimism, and interpersonal resources (e.g., companionship) were associated with higher PTSS (Littleton, Grills-Taquechel, & Axsom, 2009; Littleton et al., 2011b).

Only recently have investigators sought to explore the processes through which different predictors relate to each other in shaping mental health outcomes. For example, in the aftermath of the NIU shooting, Kumpula et al. (2011) found that students' pre-incident experiential avoidance was positively associated with their post-incident reports of peritraumatic dissociative experiences, which in turn were positively associated with PTSS. Similarly, among student survivors of the Virginia Tech attack, prior sexual victimization was found to be indirectly associated with PTSS through lower benevolence beliefs and social support (Littleton et al., 2012). Other studies have employed cross-lagged modeling and have found positive bi-directional relationships between PTSS and maladaptive coping (Littleton et al., 2011a), and PTSS and emotion regulation difficulties (Bardeen et al., 2013), suggesting that symptoms can perpetuate themselves over time by undermining psychological resources.

Discussion

Recent mass shooting incidents with unusually high numbers of injuries and fatalities have led to substantial concerns about these episodes and their long-term psychological effects on victims, communities, and the nation as a whole. Each event is unique, occurring in a particular time and place, committed by perpetrators who vary in their clinical and personal histories, and claiming different numbers of victims who themselves vary in age, gender, occupation, and so on. These sources of variation are likely to influence the psychological effects of any incident on affected communities. Despite this variation, our review of the research to date provides evidence that exposure to these events increases risk for PTSD. Risk is not distributed equally, however, and research has identified several risk factors for adverse outcomes, including demographic characteristics (e.g., female gender, lower socioeconomic status), higher pre-event trauma exposure and psychological symptoms, greater event exposure, and lack of psychosocial resources (e.g., emotional regulation difficulties, experiential avoidance, low social support).

Although the extant body of research offers some conclusions about posttraumatic stress in the aftermath mass shootings, more research is needed to better understand the mechanisms through which risk and protective factors contribute to longer-term outcomes. There is a particular need for studies in the aftermath of high-impact events. For example, we identified no studies of affected samples in two recent events with unusually high numbers of casualties—the 2012 shootings at the Aurora movie theatre and Sandy Hook elementary school. Researchers and institutional review boards might be hesitant to conduct studies in the aftermath of such events due to concerns about retraumatizing or otherwise taking advantage of victims. Notably, however, the majority (85 %) of NIU students who completed a post-incident experimental study reported that they would participate in the study again (Fergus, Rabenhorst, Orcutt, & Valentiner, 2011). Although replication is needed, these results imply that study participation might not have adverse effects.

Research in the aftermath of other traumatic events suggests that some persons who have experienced trauma may actually derive benefits from research participation (e.g., Griffin, Resick, Waldrop, & Mechanic, 2003).

Further studies that draw on pre-incident data from ongoing projects would provide greater insight into the role of pre-event functioning and trauma exposure on psychological responses. In a similar vein, studies that include multiple waves of follow-up data would allow for an enhanced understanding of longitudinal patterns of responses and the processes that lead to chronic symptoms. The research could also be enriched by further studies that incorporate additional sources of data, including genetic variants and information on community characteristics and resources.

In addition to further research on affected samples, more investigations are needed to understand the broader impact of mass shootings on unaffected communities. Although two studies in this review showed that indirectly exposed subsamples were at lower risk of PTSD or elevated PTSS than their exposed counterparts (Suomalainen et al., 2011; Trappler & Friedman, 1996) , the findings suggest that they experienced at least some degree of psychological adversity. Along these lines, research in the aftermath of the September 11th terrorist attacks suggested that indirect exposure could increase risk for PTSD far beyond the affected communities. For example, in the National Epidemiologic Survey of Alcohol and Related Conditions, indirect exposure to 9/11 through the media was associated with increased risk for PTSD, relative to no reported 9/11 exposure (Henricksen, Bolton, & Sareen, 2010). Further research could assess indirect exposure to mass shooting episodes in national samples, or follow-up on samples previously assessed for PTSS to determine whether intervening indirect exposure to a mass shooting episode was associated with symptom elevations.

Additional research would also inform interventions to prevent and treat post-incident PTSS among the directly and indirectly exposed. Of course, the first step in prevention would be to decrease the likelihood that mass shooting events occur in the first place. The rarity of these events precludes the use of statistical modeling to predict their occurrence (Swanson, 2011). Researchers have accordingly advised against the use of risk profiles, which have the potential for false positives bias, and stigmatization (Reddy et al., 2001). Instead, a deductive threat assessment approach, in which a team of professionals gathers information about a particular case to assess the likelihood that a violent episode will occur, and formulates a response based on that assessment, has been proposed (e.g., (Cornell & Allen, 2011; Reddy et al., 2001). Others have suggested the need for promoting positive school climates in which there is open dialogue between students, teachers, and administrators to reduce the likelihood of school shootings (Mulvey & Cauffman, 2001), and they also suggest efforts to improve access to and continuity of high-quality mental health services for people with serious mental illness to prevent violent behaviors among this group (Swanson, 2011).

Unfortunately, not all mass shooting incidents can be prevented, and it is therefore important to develop interventions to address mental health problems in their wake. Trained crisis response teams that establish safety, evaluate the psychological needs of victims, connect survivors with a range of services to meet their needs, and evaluate response efforts have been proposed to mitigate the effects of school violence (Crepeau-Hobson, Sievering, Armstong, & Stonis, 2012). Hobfoll et al. (2007) have also identified five empirically supported principles for mental health responses to mass trauma—promoting a sense of safety, calming, a sense of self-efficacy and community efficacy, connectedness, and hope.

The empirical research also lends support for approaches that identify survivors most at risk of adverse outcomes, including women, persons of lower socioeconomic status, those who faced higher levels of exposure, and persons lacking strong social support networks (see Chap. 5, for related discussion). Furthermore, they suggest interventions that enhance emotion regulation and active coping skills and that encourage engagement with and acceptance of emotions, thoughts, memories, and sensory experiences (e.g., Metz et al., 2013). These skill-building interventions could be part of the standard curriculum and could promote resilience after a range of traumatic events and stressors.

In summary, mass shooting incidents are extremely rare but highly publicized events, and limited research suggests that exposure to such episodes can increase risk for PTSD. A variety of risk and protective factors have been identified, including demographic characteristics, pre-event trauma exposure and functioning, event exposure, and psychosocial resources. Further research that explores the processes contributing to long-term outcomes will yield important implications for post-incident interventions to reduce mental health impacts.

References

Bardeen, J. R., Kumpula, M. J., & Orcutt, H. K. (2013). Emotion regulation difficulties as a prospective predictor of posttraumatic stress symptoms following a mass shooting. *Journal of Anxiety Disorders, 27,* 188–196. doi:10.1016/j.janxdis.2013.01.003.

Classen, C., Coopman, C., Hales, R., & Spiegel, D. (1998). Acute stress disorder as a predictor of posttraumatic stress symptoms. *American Journal of Psychiatry, 155,* 620–624.

Cornell, D., & Allen, K. (2011).Development, evaluation, and future directions of the Virginia Student Threat Assessment Guidelines. *Journal of School Violence, 10,* 88–106. doi:10.1080/15388220.2010.519432.

Crepeau-Hobson, F., Sievering, K. S., Armstrong, C., & Stonis, J. (2012). A coordinated mental health crisis response: Lessons learned from three Colorado school shootings. *Journal of School Violence, 11,* 207–225. doi:10.1080/15388220.2012.682002.

Fergus, T. A., Rabenhorst, M. M., Orcutt, H. K., & Valentiner, D. P. (2011). Reactions to trauma research among women recently exposed to a campus shooting. *Journal of Traumatic Stress, 24,* 596–600. doi:10.1002/jts.20682.

Follman, M., Aronsen, G., & Pan, D. (2014). *A guide to mass shootings in America*. http://www.motherjones.com/politics/2012/07/mass-shootings-map. Accessed 23 Aug 2014.

Griffin, M. G., Resick, P. A., Waldorp, A. E., & Mechanic, M. B. (2003). Participation in trauma research: Is there evidence of harm? *Journal of Traumatic Stress, 16,* 221–227. doi:10.1023/A:1023735821900.

Henricksen, C. A., Bolton, J. M., & Sareen, J. (2010). The psychological impact of terrorist attacks: Examining a dose-response relationship between exposure to 9/11 and Axis I mental disorders. *Depression & Anxiety, 27,* 993–1000. doi:10.1002/da.20742.
Hobfoll, S. E. (1989). Conservation of resources: A new attempt at conceptualizing stress. *American Psychologist, 44,* 513–524. doi:10.1037//0003-066X.44.3.513.
Hobfoll, S. E., Watson, P., Bell, C. C., Bryan, R. A., Brymer, M. J., Friedman, M. J., et al. (2007). Five essential elements of immediate and mid-term mass trauma intervention: Empirical evidence. *Psychiatry, 70,* 283–315. doi:10.1521/psyc.2007.70.4.283.
Hough, R. L., Vega, W., Valle, R., Kolody, B., Griswalddel Castillo, R., & Tarke, H. (1990). Mental health consequences of the San Ysidro McDonald's massacre: A community study. *Journal of Traumatic Stress, 3,* 71–92. doi:10.1007/BF00975136.
Hughes, M., Brymer, M., Chiu, W. T., Fairbank, J. A., Jones, R. T., Pynoos, R. S., et al. (2011). Posttraumatic stress among students after the shootings at Virginia Tech. *Psychological Trauma: Theory, Research, Practice, and Policy, 3,* 403–411. doi:10.1037/a0024565.
Johnson, S. D., North, C. S., & Smith, E. M. (2002). Psychiatric disorders among victims of a courthouse shooting spree: A three-year follow-up study. *Community Mental Health, 38,* 181–194.
Kumpula, M. J., Orcutt, H. K., Bardeen, J. R., & Varkovitzky, R. L. (2011). Peritraumatic dissociation and experiential avoidance as prospective predictors of posttraumatic stress symptoms. *Journal of Abnormal Psychology, 120,* 617–627. doi:10.1037/a0023927.
Littleton, H., Grills-Taquechel, A., & Axsom, D. (2009). Resource loss as a predictor of posttrauma symptoms among college women following the mass shooting at Virginia Tech. *Violence and Victims, 24,* 669–686. doi:10.1891/0886-6708.24.5.669.
Littleton, H., Axsom, D., & Grills-Taquechel, A. E. (2011a). Longitudinal evaluation of the relationship between maladaptive trauma coping and distress: Examination following the mass shooting at Virginia Tech. *Anxiety, Stress, and Coping, 3,* 273–290. doi:10.1080/10615806.2010.500722.
Littleton, H., Kumpula, M., & Orcutt, H. (2011b). Posttraumatic symptoms following a campus shooting: The role of psychosocial resource loss. *Violence and Victims, 26,* 461–476. doi:10.1891/0886-6708.26.4.461.
Littleton, H., Grills-Taquechel, A. E., Axsom, D., Bye, K., & Buck, K. S. (2012). Prior sexual trauma and adjustment following the Virginia Tech campus shootings: Examination of the mediating role of schemas and social support. *Psychological Trauma: Theory, Research, Practice, and Policy, 4,* 578–586. doi:10.1037/a0025270.
McIntyre, J. J., Spence, P. R., & Lachlan, K. A. (2011). Media use and gender differences in negative psychological responses to a shooting on a university campus. *Journal of School Violence, 10,* 299–313. doi:10.1080/15388220.2011.578555.
Mercer, K. B., Orcutt, H. K., Quinn, J. F., Fitzgerald, C. A., Conneely, K. N., Barfield, R. T., et al. (2012). Acute and posttraumatic stress symptoms in a prospective gene x environment study of a university campus shooting. *Archives of General Psychiatry, 69,* 89–97. doi:10.1001/archgenpsychiatry.2011.109.
Metz, S. M., Frank, J. L., Reibel, D., Cantrell, T., Sanders, R., & Broderick, P. C. (2013).The effectiveness of the Learning to BREATHE program on adolescent emotion regulation. *Research in Human Development, 10,* 252–272. doi:10.1080/15427609.2013.818488.
Mulvey, E. P., & Cauffman, E. (2001). The inherent limits of predicting school violence. *American Psychologist, 56,* 797–802. doi:10.IO.17//0O03-066X.56.10.797.
Murtonen, K., Suomalainen, L., Haravuori, H., & Marttunen, M. (2012). Adolescents' experiences of psychosocial support after traumatisation in a school shooting. *Child and Adolescent Mental Health, 17,* 23–30. doi:10.1111/j.1475–3588.2011.00612.x.
Nader, K., Pynoos, R., Fairbanks, L., & Frederick, C. (1990). Children's PTSD reactions one year after a sniper attack at their school. *American Journal of Psychiatry, 147,* 1526–1530.
North, C. S., Smith, E. M., McCool, R. E, & McShea, J. M. (1989). Short-term psychopathology in eyewitnesses to mass murder. *Hospital & Community Psychiatry, 40,* 1293–1295.

North, C. S., Smith, E. M., & Spitznagel, E. L. (1994). Posttraumatic stress disorder in survivors of a mass shooting. *American Journal of Psychiatry, 151,* 82–88.
North, C. S., Smith, E. M., & Spitznagel, E. L. (1997). One-year follow-up of survivors of a mass shooting. *American Journal of Psychiatry, 154,* 1696–1702.
North, C. S., Spitznagel, E. L., & Smith, E. M. (2001).A prospective study of coping after exposure to a mass murder episode. *Annals of Clinical Psychiatry, 13,* 81–86. doi:10.3109/10401230109148952.
North, C. S., McCutcheon, V., Spitznagel, E. L., & Smith, E. (2002). Three-year follow-up of survivors of a mass shooting episode. *Journal of Urban Health, 79,* 383–391. doi:10.1093/jurban/79.3.383.
Orcutt, H. K., Bonanno, G. A., Hanna, S. M., & Miron, L. R. (2014). Prospective trajectories of posttraumatic stress in college women following a campus mass shooting. *Journal of Traumatic Stress, 27,* 1–8. doi:10.1002/jts.21914.
Palus, S. R., Fang, S. S., & Prawitz, A. D. (2012). Forward, together forward: Coping strategies of students following the 2008 mass shootings at Northern Illinois University. *Traumatology, 18,* 13–26. doi:10.1177/1534765612437381.
Pynoos, R. S., Frederick, C., Nader, K., Arroyo, W., Steinberg, A., Eth, S., et al. (1987). Life threat and posttraumatic stress in school-age children. *Archives of General Psychiatry, 44,* 1057–1063. doi:10.1001/archpsyc.1987.01800240031005.
Reddy, M., Borum, R., Berglund, J., Vossekuil, B., Fein, R., & Modzeleski, W. (2001). Evaluating risk for targeted violence in schools: Comparing risk assessment, threat assessment, and other approaches. *Psychology in the Schools, 38,* 157–172.
Schwarz, E. D., & Kowalski, J. M. (1991a). Malignant memories: PTSD in children and adults after a school shooting. *Journal of the American Academy of Child and Adolescent Psychiatry, 30,* 936–944. doi:10.1097/00004583-199111000-00011.
Schwarz, E. D., & Kowalski, J. M. (1991b). Posttraumatic stress disorder after a school shooting: Effects of symptom threshold selection and diagnosis by *DSM-III, DSM-III-R,* or proposed *DSM-IV. American Journal of Psychiatry, 148,* 592–597.
Schwarz, E. D., & Kowalski, J. M. (1992a). Personality characteristics and posttraumatic stress symptoms after a school shooting. *Journal of Nervous and Mental Disease, 180,* 735–737. doi:10.1097/00005053-199211000-00013.
Schwarz, E. D., & Kowalski, J. M. (1992b). Malignant memories: Reluctance to utilize mental health services after a disaster. *Journal of Nervous and Mental Disease, 180,* 767–772. doi:10.1097/00005053-199212000-00005.
Schwarz, E. D., Kowalski, J. M., & McNally, R. J. (1993). Malignant memories: Post-traumatic changes in memory in adults after a school shooting. *Journal of Traumatic Stress, 6,* 545–553. doi:10.1007/BF00974322.
Séguin, M., Chawky, N., Lesage, A., Boyer, R., Guay, S., Bleau, P., … & Roy, D. (2013). Evaluation of the Dawson College Shooting Psychological Intervention: Moving toward a multimodal extensive plan. Psychological Trauma: Theory, Research, Practice, and Policy, 5, 268-276. doi: 10.1037/a0027745.
Sewell, K. W. (1996). Constructional risk factors for post-traumatic stress response after mass murder. *Journal of Constructivist Psychology, 9,* 97–107. doi:10.1080/10720539608404657.
Shultz, J. M., Cohen, A. M., Muschert, G. W., & Flores de Apodaca, R. (2013). Fatal school shootings and the epidemiological context of firearm mortality in the United States. *Disaster Health, 1,* 84–101. doi:10.4161/dish.26897.
Sloan, I. H., Rozensky, R. H., Kaplan, L., & Sanders, S. M. (1994). A shooting incident in an elementary school: Effects of worker stress on public safety, mental health, and medical personnel. *Journal of Traumatic Stress, 7,* 565–574. doi:10.1007/BF02103007.
Stephenson, K. L., Valentiner, D. P., Kumpula, M. J., & Orcutt, H. K. (2009). Anxiety sensitivity and posttrauma stress symptoms in female undergraduates following a campus shooting. *Journal of Traumatic Stress, 22,* 489–496. doi:10.1002/jts.20457.

Suomalainen, L., Haravuori, H., Berg, N., Kiviruusu, O., & Marttunen, M. (2011). A controlled follow-up study of adolescents exposed to a school shooting—psychological consequences after four months. *European Psychiatry, 26,* 490–497. doi:10.1016/j.eurpsy.2010.07.007.

Swanson, J. W. (2011). Explaining rare acts of violence: The limits of evidence from population research. *Psychiatric Services, 62,* 1369–1371. doi:10.1176/appi.ps.62.11.1369.

Trappler, B., & Friednman, S. (1996). Posttraumatic stress disorder in survivors of the Brooklyn Bridge shooting. *American Journal of Psychiatry, 153,* 705–707.

Turunen, T., Haravuori, H., Punamäki, R., Suomalainen, L., & Marttunen, N. (2014).The role of attachment in recovery after a school-shooting trauma. *European Journal of Psychotraumatology, 5,* 22728.doi:10.3402/ejpt.v5.22728.

Vicary, A. M., & Fraley, R. C. (2010). Student reactions to the shootings at Virginia Tech and Northern Illinois University: Does sharing grief and support over the Internet affect recovery? *Personality and Social Psychology Bulletin, 36,* 1555–1563. doi:10.1177/0146167210384880.

Chapter 7
When Man Harms Man: The Interpersonal Ramifications of War Captivity

Jacob Y. Stein, Avigal Snir and Zahava Solomon

> Though there may be no human event that is as without defense as torture, others give rise to the same central question—By what perceptual process does it come about that one human being can stand beside another human being in agonizing pain and not know it, not know it to the point where he himself inflicts it? (Scarry, 1985, p. 61)

> All those norms of human behavior which are inculcated in one from the cradle are subjected to deliberate and systematic destruction…Only by a maximum exertion of will is it possible to retain one's former, normal scale of values. Irina Ratushinskaya, political prisoner (Herman, 1992, pp. 77–78)

Introduction

Warfare exposes combatants to substantial threats to physical and mental integrity. However, as terrible as combat may become, for a certain group of soldiers, combat is but the first step in a protracted traumatic journey. The group of soldiers we are referring to consists of those who fall captive by the enemy during their service—an eventuality dreaded by any soldier, at times dreaded even more than death itself. Such dread is surely justified as prisoners of war (POWs) are exposed to an additional set of traumatic stressors, a second layer of pain and strife that amasses over the already heavy burden of combat's toll. These additional stressors,

J. Y. Stein (✉) · A. Snir · Z. Solomon
Mass Trauma Research Lab, Bob Shapell School of Social Work,
Tel Aviv University, 69978 Tel Aviv, Israel
e-mail: cobisari@gmail.com

A. Snir
e-mail: sniravigal@gmail.com

Z. Solomon
e-mail: solomon@post.tau.ac.il

K. E. Cherry (ed.), *Traumatic Stress and Long-Term Recovery*,
DOI 10.1007/978-3-319-18866-9_7

as will become evident in the course of this chapter, many times consist of significant interpersonal violations and may then lead to subsequent impediments to interpersonal relationships in their aftermath.

The current chapter will then be devoted to the elaboration and explication of the multifarious interpersonal ramifications of war captivity. These will be accompanied by findings from a prospective longitudinal study raging over more than three decades, examining the long-term effects of captivity for repatriated Israeli POWs taken captive in the 1973 Yom Kippur War. In order to explicate the interpersonal aspects of former POWs' (henceforth ex-POWs) experience, the chapter has been divided into two distinct yet strongly interconnected sections, devoted to the trauma and posttrauma of war captivity, respectively.

Chapter Overview

As noted, the first section of this chapter focuses on the trauma at hand and is intended to contextualize the after effects of war captivity in the actual experiences that had brought about their manifestation, namely war and war captivity themselves. Explicating the horrors of war is meant not only as a means for achieving a better understanding of the experiences inveterate in war imprisonment, but also to enable a comparison of the characteristics of traumata sustained on the battlefield and those which may be endured in the incarceration that may follow. Hence, we first situate war captivity within the general context of war stressors, physical, mental, and interpersonal; and then turn to the time of captivity itself and the harsh experiences it entails. Throughout this section, we primarily highlight the interpersonal aspects of captivity, the ramifications of which are further discussed in the next section.

In the second section, indeed the lion's share of the chapter, we discuss the posttraumatic long-term ramifications of war captivity. As noted, we ground these consequences in a prospective longitudinal study of Israeli ex-POWs. Throughout this section, we tie our examinations to broader theoretical frameworks such as attachment theory and loneliness research. By integrating these with one another, we address the greater context of interpersonal deficit. In so doing, we are able to demonstrate how several aspects of ex-POWs' psychosocial realities following repatriation are strongly related to what they have endured in their time of incarceration.

We bring this chapter to a closing by laying forth the implications of the observations made throughout the chapter for future research, clinical practice, and policy making.

Traumatic Stressors of War and War Captivity

It is now time to dive into the two worlds of extreme adversity at hand: war and war captivity.

The Stressors of Combat

When dealing with ex-POWs, one must realize that more often than not these are soldiers who have endured combat to some extent and have subsequently fallen captive by their enemies. This means that they have been exposed to combat stressors prior to captivity and have carried those burdens of war with them as they were marched, usually blindfolded, humiliated, and bruised, into their captors' dungeons. Hence, in order to understand the experience of being a POW, it is imperative that one first have some awareness of the context that the POW has come from—that is an understanding of the immediate and ongoing implications of combat.

As Scarry (1985, p. 61) most poignantly notes, "The most obvious analogue to torture is war." Both cases represent a reality in which human beings deliberately harm other human beings, and both very often leave scars on both body and soul. The person participating in combat is faced with many adversities. The most obvious of these are the constant threats to one's physical integrity and indeed to one's life. These include a multitude of physical deficits such as a dearth of sleep, nutrition, hygiene, and shelter. Additionally, on the battlefield, combatants are under continuous exposure to life-threatening circumstances as all around them bullets buzz and strike, and bombs explode and demolish. Naturally, these give rise to devastating sensations of fatigue, deterioration in health, feelings of uncertainty, helplessness, and dread. Indeed, combat entails a kind of continuous anticipated dread, a constant fear that something terrible is just on the verge of happening. All of these come together and take their toll not only on the combatant's body but also on his psychological state (Solomon, 1993). But there are additional, less conspicuous yet no less significant aspects involved that are worthy of attention.

Combatants must often face interpersonal deficits such as loneliness (Dasberg, 1976; Solomon, Mikulincer, & Hobfoll, 1986), lack of social support, and the denial of any sense of privacy (Solomon, 2001). Combatants are further exposed to severe violence as they are condemned to witness the death and injuries of others, often their own friends and comrades. Moreover, they must often also behold the gruesome demise of the enemy, as they find themselves taking the role of the perpetrator, engaged in the aggressive and violent acts of killing. Furthermore, in the face of this reality, many soldiers may come to question whether they have betrayed "what's right" (Shay, 1994) in the process of fighting for their country, thus sustaining what has been termed *moral injury* (Litz et al., 2009; Shay, 2014;).

Subsequent captivity then continues to drain the remaining vitality that the combatant has managed to retain, as it occurs after the soldier may be quite battered, tired, lethargic, and devoid of much of what has kept him going up to that point.

It is imperative that we keep this in mind as we begin to examine the hardship of captivity within the depths of the captors' dungeons.

In the Captors' Dungeons: The Dreadful Experience of War Captivity

Soldiers who fall captive by the enemy continue to be exposed to even more extreme interpersonal traumatic experiences than those sustained on the battlefield. It is important to take note of the fact that there is no "one" experience of war imprisonment, and experiences may vary as the captors vary. For instance, one might expect to see different forms of torture manifest in the Vietnamese camps, than in the Nazi concentration camps, the Soviet gulag, or the Japanese or the *Islamic State of Iraq and Syria* (ISIS) captivities.

Take for instance the population that is the focus of this chapter, namely Israeli POWs who were held captive in Arab countries. During the 1973 Yom Kippur War, 240 infantry Israeli soldiers fell captive on both the Syrian and Egyptian fronts. POWs held in Egypt were released after a relatively short period of time extending slightly more than a month. However, POWs in Syria were held for as long as 8 months. One significant difference between these two captivities is that during captivity in Egypt, the prisoners were held in separate cells, while in Syria, after a period of rigorous interrogations, POWs were held in two groups, each situated in a large shared room. While sharing a conjoint cell may be expected to somewhat alleviate POWs' loneliness, it has also been reported by ex-POWs to have been a source of new stress due to lack of privacy and intense unregulated contact with other POWs (Avnery, 1982; Lieblich, 1994). These experiences gave rise to feelings of humiliation, guilt, frustration, and shame—all significant stressors.

However, some attributes are similar in many instances of war captivity and are less bound to the captors' identity. Many times for instance, the abuse begins long before arriving at the enemy's captivity facilities. Israeli POWs on either front disclose being subjected to humiliation and beating from the moment they lay down their weapons and throughout their journey to their location of imprisonment. They attest to being denied any opportunity for orientation as they were led to their destination blind folded and tied up. Indeed, the actual moment of falling captive is a stressor on its own merit.

Upon arriving and during one's captivity, the POW is usually held in poor conditions of sanitation, is set in a climate of extensive maltreatment, and is continuously deprived of sufficient amounts of food and water (e.g., Hunter, 1993). Whereas deprivation in combat is a matter of environmental and logistic constraints, deprivation in captivity is intentional, deliberate, and easily attributed to malicious human conduct. Various methods of control and coercion are employed by captors in order to deprive POWs of their most elementary sense of autonomy and replace it with a sense of humiliation, horror, and helplessness. Thus, it is of utmost importance to realize that captivity does not only include harsh conditions but is also characterized by vile and many times sadistic and pernicious interpersonal interactions between captive and captors (Avnery, 1982; Herman, 1992).

Indeed, learning of the horrors of captivity bears with it the realization that there is no limit to the innovation, ingenuity, and creativity of human evil and torture. Instigated by a guard's boredom, bad day, or sadistic nature, brutal beatings for no particular reasons may be a matter of course in the routine environment of captivity. According to POWs' reports, torture during interrogation sessions often entailed, the usage of electric shocks, beatings, whipping, and many other methods for inflicting pain. POWs sustained burns, severe blows, and mutilation. However, bearing witness to POWs' testimonies, one very rapidly comes to the understanding that torture and misconduct exceed the brutality of interrogations, and were extended to all realms of captivity. For instance, POWs disclose instances where they were forced to stand for days in their cells, facing the wall, and in full awareness that any failure to remain erect would result in brutal beatings. Or they attest of being deprived of any kind of liquid substance, literally in a state of scorched throats all dried up and longing for water. And in those moments, a guard would enter the cell, a bucket of water in his hand. As hope begins to well up, the guard would spill the water on the floor, just out of the prisoner's reach. Or then again, they tell of mock executions designed to give the prisoner the sense that he is about to be executed by a firing squad—indeed that he *is* executed, as the trigger is pulled and no bullet is shot. We commonly think that a person may die only once. However, in the face of these firing squads, POWs have experienced their executions and deaths, time and time again. POWs recount being urinated on, or then again of those moments in which they realized that they are expected to urinate and defecate in their garments, and they tell of doing so. They tell of being thrown into an empty cell, deprived of any light or mental stimulation for days on end. They confessed their confusion as they sensed the walls of their cells are moving, just to realize that the sense of motion is due to the fact that their cell is infested with swarms of blood thirsty flees. Many POWs note that one of the most difficult experiences in captivity has been to see their friends being tortured and witness their agony, or otherwise the experience of hearing their screams echo within the dungeon's corridors. It is both the horror of bearing witness to such torture and the terror of knowing that your turn is coming that made these experiences extremely intolerable.

We may learn of yet another technique, one that was also evident in the Israeli POWs experience and has become part and parcel of the attempt to break the POWs' spirit, namely the use of false propaganda. Recall that combatants have fallen captive in the course of combat. Hence, their knowledge of "the big picture" of both the war efforts and their state's faring was extremely limited. This was of great import for their captors who knew very well how to use this piece of information against them. In fact, during the Yom Kippur War, Israeli POWs were repeatedly exposed to anti-Israeli propaganda, misinformed of the death of Israel's leaders, the triumph of Arab states over Israel, and the Arab occupation of Israel altogether. At times, captives were informed that their homes were destroyed and their loved ones and relatives were killed. These acts of misinformation then served to exacerbate feelings of hopelessness and despair. Far from being an exhaustive account of the horrors of captivity, the above may provide a preliminary notion of what the experience may be like.

Deprivation of a benevolent human interaction may enhance the captive's dependency upon his captors and strengthen these distorted and harmful relationships. How confusing is it when the person on whom you depend for food and for relieving body wastes is at the same time the person who is in charge of your most agonizing experiences? These confusions are apparent, for instance, in certain attributions made by POWs vis-à-vis their captors (Avnery, 1982). POWs tell of categorizing guards as "the good guard" and the "bad guard" as they compared their captors' cruelty. It is noteworthy that it is not that the "good" ones were kind, but rather that they were not as cruel as others. Nevertheless, the attempt to infuse some meaning of goodness even in those menacing times is noteworthy.

Questions Deriving from the Interpersonal Dimensions of War Captivity

Given all of the above, it then becomes quite clear that war captivity bears extensive multilayered and multifarious interpersonal aspects. Taking these into account, several questions arise regarding the impact of war captivity on interpersonal perceptions, experiences, and actual relationships in postwar quotidian life:

- One may come to ask, whether ex-POWs maintain a clear separation between the traumatic interpersonal experiences (in the battlefield and in captivity) and the interpersonal world in daily lives once the war is over? Or is the experiential divide breached?
- One may also ponder, if the interpersonal violation does permeate one's perceptions after captivity, what form does such a penetration take in the veterans' interpersonal experiences and relationships after repatriation? How do these perceptions manifest in one's everyday interpersonal reality?
- Specifically, in terms of internalized representations of others, what might the effects of captivity be on basic and early developmental interpersonal constructs (such as attachment working models)?
- In terms of actual relationships, what effects might these short lived, but intense distorted relationships with one's captures have on the long-term relationships with families, wives, and children? In other words, what are the long-lived interpersonal ramifications and damages of the aforementioned short-lived abuse?

(Incarcerated) Johnny Comes Home: What Comes After War Captivity

While the gates of imprisonment may have opened years ago, and the shackles lie behind, all eroded and rusty, many ex-POWs are left to face the pathogenic effects of captivity on a daily basis (see Chap. 23, this volume). Studies have found that posttraumatic stress disorder (PTSD) is the most common pathological psychological outcome of war captivity (e.g., Dikel, Engdahl, & Eberly, 2005; Speed, Engdahl, Schwartz, & Eberly, 1989; Sutker, Allain Jr, & Winstead, 1993). However, the diagnosis of PTSD does not take into account the complexity of adaptation to trauma. It has been suggested that, following repeated abuse in captivity, victims tend to develop not only PTSD but also a unique form of posttraumatic sequela that penetrates and consumes their personality, often referred to as complex PTSD (e.g., Herman, 1992) or disorders of extreme stress not otherwise specified (DESNOS; e.g., van der Kolk, 2001; van der Kolk, Roth, Pelcovitz, Sunday, & Spinazzola, 2005).

Additionally, ex-POWs often suffer from a myriad of psychiatric comorbidities, including anxiety disorders and depression (e.g., Neria, Solomon, & Dekel, 1998; Solomon & Dekel, 2005). Furthermore, the literature concerning the aftermath of war captivity identified ex-POWs as a high-risk group for various psychiatric disorders, including schizophrenia (Beebe, 1975), hysteria (Sutker, Bugg, & Allain, 1991), paranoia (Ursano, Boydstun, & Wheatley, 1981), and alcoholism (Beebe, 1975).

Although many ex-POWs may suffer from PTSD symptoms, these symptoms may fluctuate over time. According to Zeiss and Dickman (1989), time can either heal or intensify the psychological wounds of captivity, depending on an ex-POW's internal and external resources as well as life experiences after repatriation.

Whereas previous studies have shown the severe physical and psychological consequences of captivity, consequences in the interpersonal domain are greatly unexplored. These aspects are of great import as interpersonal resources and relationships are known to have robust effects on the development of other psychological disorders, on well-being, adjustment, and functioning (Cloitre, Miranda, Stovall-McClough, & Han, 2005).

The Longitudinal Study of Ex-POW's in Israel

In light of the aforementioned, distinct attributes of war captivity, Solomon and her colleagues set out to prospectively examine the long-term impact of war captivity on interpersonal relationships among Israeli ex-POWs. The study targeted all Israeli land forces soldiers who had been captured by Syria and Egypt in the 1973 Yom Kippur War. The study then followed these ex-POWs over the course of a 35-year period, summoning them in for follow-up assessments in 1991, 2003, and 2008 (See Solomon, Horesh, Ein-Dor, & Ohry, 2012).

Veterans were then divided into two groups: (a) ex-POWs and (b) a control group consisting of combat veterans, who fought in the same fronts as the ex-POWs but were not taken captive. Controls were matched with the ex-POWs in personal and military backgrounds. In this comprehensive study, both groups were assessed and compared across an array of intrapersonal and interpersonal domains. Among these, were psychopathologies (e.g., PTSD, depression, anxiety) comorbidities, and psychosocial aspects, along with a wide gamut of other variables. In the current chapter, we focus on those findings relating to the interpersonal aspects that were found significant in the aftermath of war captivity.

One variable involved concerns ex-POWs' attachment patterns. Indeed, as will become evident below, a significant implication of the interpersonal violations in captivity for the time that is to follow may be the detrimental effect on one's capacity to draw upon his attachment resources in times of need. In order to address these ramifications, we first provide the theoretical foundations of attachment theory and its significance for understanding traumatic aftermaths.

War Captivity as an Attachment Injury

> …Prolonged captivity disrupts all human relationships and amplifies the dialectic of trauma. The survivor oscillates between intense attachment and terrified withdrawal. (Herman 1992, p. 93).

According to attachment theory (Bowlby, 1982), human beings are born with a psychobiological system (i.e., the attachment behavioral system) that motivates them to seek proximity to supportive others (i.e., attachment figures) in times of need. This is done for the sake of gaining a sense of safety and security (see Chaps. 8 and 22, for related discussion). However, people differ in their inclination to activate this attachment system. That is to say that while the predisposition to seek proximity and to rely on others as a source for protection and security is a universal phenomenon, nevertheless, some people are more reluctant than others to do so. According to attachment theorists, these varying inclinations in adulthood are a result, primarily but not exclusively of the person's history of interactions with attachment figures throughout his or her developmental stages in infancy and early childhood (Bowlby, 1982). Interactions with figures that exhibit availability, sensitivity, and responsiveness in times of need promote effective proximity-seeking strategies and encourage the development of a stable sense of security. This sense of security includes implicit beliefs that the world is generally safe, that other people are "well-intentioned and kind-hearted" (Hazan & Shaver, 1987; Mikulincer & Shaver, 2007), that one is valued, loved, understood, accepted, and cared for by others, and that one can explore the environment with interest and engage rewardingly with other people. These beliefs are associated with and rooted in positive mental representations of self and others, which Bowlby (1973) called "internal working models." Such internal models shape the person's expectations regarding future interactions with the same or other relationship partners over time, especially in times of need.

Unfortunately, when a person's attachment figures have not been reliably and consistently available, sensitive, and supportive in the critical early years of one's life, he or she learns that seeking proximity to others does not relieve distress. Under these circumstances, negative working models are formed and a representation of self as not sufficiently lovable develops along with a representation of others as unaccepting, unreliable, and unresponsive, if not downright abusive or cruel. Conversely, affect-regulation strategies other than secure-based proximity seeking may develop. Attachment theory refers to these alternative patterns as "attachment-anxious" and "attachment-avoidant" orientations. According to the theory, individual differences in working models and distress-regulation strategies eventually become trait-like attachment "styles" or orientations–characteristic patterns of relational expectations, emotions, and behavior (Bowlby, 1982; Fraley & Shaver, 2000).

In times of stress, a secure-based attachment pattern can constitute a source of power and comfort. This seems to be the case when facing traumatic experiences (for an overview, see Mikulincer & Shaver, 2007, pp. 387–391). Indeed, previous studies have shown that attachment security can have healing effects for people suffering from PTSD and can improve their response to treatment (e.g., Forbes, Parslow, Fletcher, McHugh, & Creamer, 2010). For those who fell captive, where no actual comforting and supporting figures are present, internalized positive and stable attachment figures might enable better adjustment and coping, during captivity and in the years after the war.

Solomon, Ginzburg, Mikulincer, Neria, and Ohry (1998) examined the implications of attachment in both immediate coping and long-term adjustment of Israeli ex-POWs. In this study, as expected, individuals with secure attachment retrospectively reported less suffering and helplessness in the time they were captive, compared to attachment-insecure persons. They also demonstrated the use of more active coping strategies and exhibited better long-term adjustment. In contrast, attachment-avoidant POWs reported feeling helplessness and hostility, and anxious individuals reported feeling abandoned and vulnerable. Both avoidant and anxious individuals reported long-term maladjustment following captivity. Secure attachment style then serves as a stress-regulation resource and revealed the important role that attachment style plays in adjustment following traumatic stress (See also Zakin, Solomon, & Neria, 2003).

Whereas the protective effect of secure attachment against psychological distress is well documented, there remains the question regarding the possible effects of traumatic experiences on the attachment system. Although attachment orientations are initially formed in relationships with primary caregivers (usually parents) during infancy and early childhood (Bowlby, 1982), as confirmed by several decades-long longitudinal studies (reviewed in Cassidy & Shaver, 2008); Bowlby (1988) also argued that relationships formed later in one's ontogeny (e.g., friends, romantic partners, and therapists) can alter the sense of security in attachment. In fact, research indicates that a person's sense of attachment security can change, subtly, or dramatically, depending on naturally occurring or experimentally induced contexts (Mikulincer & Shaver, 2007).

As is quite well established at this point, war captivity is indeed an extreme extraordinary context involving malicious interpersonal interactions. It is therefore not surprising that a deep relationship between the captive and the captor may develop in which the captor is transformed into an omnipotent source of all good and evil. This repeated abuse and infliction during war captivity might lead to an *attachment injury*, which may foster grave repercussions for the attachment system.

Attachment injury is a concept adopted from couple's therapy (Johnson, Makinen, & Millikin, 2001). It is used to denote the unrepairable damage to human relationships that results from a severe violation of expected trust and care on the part of significant others. As captivity shatters all senses of human decency, it is therefore expected that ex-POWs' confidence in others' good will and their availability and responsiveness in times of need would be affected by the traumatic experiences of captivity.

Solomon, Dekel, and Mikulincer (2008) conducted a first attempt to explore such changes in attachment orientations over time. This study examined the aforementioned Yom Kippur ex-POWs in two time points—18 and 30 years after the war. The findings indicated that, whereas attachment anxiety and avoidance remained stable over time among control veterans, these forms of insecurity increased over time among ex-POWs. Moreover, increases in attachment anxiety and avoidance were associated with increases in PTSD symptoms.

In a subsequent wave of this longitudinal study, Mikulincer, Ein-Dor, Solomon, and Shaver (2011) recontacted the ex-POWs and control veterans 35 years after the war, and once again assessed PTSD severity and attachment orientations. Findings revealed that attachment anxiety and avoidance continued to increase among ex-POWs. Here, again, PTSD severity was associated with attachment insecurities at each of the three time points. On the other hand, among former combatants who did not undergo captivity, a decline in attachment anxiety and avoidance was found. Among other things, this decline seems to reflect normative age-related processes whereby a person moves towards greater security in the course of midlife (Klohnen & John, 1998; Zhang & Labouvie-Vief, 2004). The increase in attachment insecurities among ex-POWs over the 17-year study period then suggests that the aftereffects of war captivity persist not only in the form of greater attachment-related insecurity over time, but also in inhibiting and indeed reversing the normative age-related improvement in emotion regulation and interpersonal relationships.

The results from these studies indicate that among ex-POWs, attachment security has eroded over time and that this erosion was particularly strong in cases of more severe PTSD. It seems that traumatic interpersonal relations with captors may damage ex-POWs' trust and confidence in other people's goodwill in ways that undermine their ability to establish and sustain secure attachments after returning home. Hence, even ex-POWs who once had secure attachments may become significantly less secure and more anxious or avoidant as a result of their time in captivity, and may defensively avoid interpersonal intimacy following their extremely traumatic experience.

In sum, we can see that attachment helps to downregulate distress and inhibit posttraumatic symptoms (Mikulincer, Shaver, & Horesh, 2006). However, this ability can be disrupted by traumatic events, and such a disruption can then contribute to the perpetuation of emotional problems following the trauma. The findings obtained to date imply a reciprocal, recursive, amplifying cycle of PTSD and attachment insecurities: attachment concerns, worries, and doubts contribute to the development of PTSD over time, and heightened PTSD, in turn, can further erode the sense of security and reduce the chances of an ex-POW to achieve a secure mental state.

It is then simple to see how an attachment injury as severe as that sustained in captivity may lead to impaired interpersonal deficit. Such deficit may be represented by yet another concept—loneliness. Loneliness is an experience associated with many unhealthy effects in its own right (Cacioppo & Cacioppo, 2014; Hawkley & Cacioppo, 2010). According to attachment theory, "loneliness is a form of separation distress that results from failure to have one's basic attachment needs fulfilled" (Mikulincer & Shaver, 2007, p. 280). Thus, it has been shown throughout innumerous research endeavors linking attachment and loneliness that anxious and avoidant attachment styles are associated with greater loneliness (for a review, see Mikulincer & Shaver, 2007, pp. 280–282). The question we turn to now is how loneliness is inflected by trauma of war captivity and in what manner it affects concentric relational circles of family, friends, society, and state.

Loneliness Following Combat and Captivity: Estrangement, Alienation, and Experiential Isolation

Loneliness is a very diverse phenomenon, and one that may resist definition. Nevertheless, it may be said that any experience worthy of the name "loneliness" entails a sense of painful isolation which harbors a subjectively experienced deficiency of relational needs and some desire that these needs be more adequately satisfied within given relationships (Stein & Tuval-Mashiach, 2015b). Indeed, loneliness is a multifarious umbrella concept which entails many diverse phenomena such as perceived social isolation (i.e., the sense that one is devoid of social connections such as peers, friends, colleagues, etc.), perceived emotional isolation (i.e., the sense that one lacks a close intimate relationship such as a spouse), perceived collective isolation (the sense of a lack of belonging to a designated group such as family or state; Cacioppo & Cacioppo, 2012), and existential isolation (the sense that one is an inherently isolated being (Ettema, Derksen, & van Leeuwen, 2010; Mijuskovic, 2012). Many cases of loneliness are multilayered and may include a sense of failed intersubjectivity (Wood, 1986). The latter refers to the sense that the commonality of the taken-for-granted meanings and mutual experience within a relationship has been shattered. Indeed, Wood claims that failed intersubjectivity *is* loneliness.

As noted, loneliness and isolation may play an important role in the experience of war captivity. Prisoners are often kept in solitary confinement, sometimes for very long periods of time. In such conditions, wherein the prisoner is deprived of all human contact and is subjected to extreme isolation and boredom, thoughts of his terrible conditions penetrate his consciousness, and he lacks any exterior stimulation that may distract him from his horrifying predicament (Avnery, 1982). As one POW once told the first author,[1] in those times of confinement he dreaded his isolation so much that he would rather be tortured than remain in such confined desolation. This is what Frieda Fromm-Reichman (1990) in her seminal work on loneliness has addressed as the feeling of "real loneliness" which is "such a painful, frightening experience that people will do practically everything to avoid it" (p. 306).

Loneliness is experienced by many ex-POWs both in the short-term and long-term aftermaths of captivity. Hence, loneliness may have dire implications concerning several aspects of one's social life. Several phenomena relating to dysfunctional interpersonal cognitions and behaviors may contribute to this feeling. For one, symptoms of withdrawal and avoidance which are typical of posttraumatic experiences may bring the repatriated POW to refrain from human contact, thus exacerbating his loneliness. Second, as attachment mechanisms may be damaged, one may become less secure in the presence of others as these no longer represent figures worthy of trust. Laub and Uerhahn's (1989) notion of "failed empathy" may be appropriate in this regard. Laub and Uerhahn have coined this term as they addressed the harsh reality of the concentration camps in the Holocaust (see Chap. 23, this volume). Accordingly, the captors' persisting display of apathetic responses in the face of their captives' suffering may develop into a generalized enduring mistrust towards other people, which may in turn lead to a negative self-perception that hinders interpersonal relationships. This is tantamount to the notion of attachment injury discussed earlier. In yet another explanatory vein, the impact of loneliness on PTSD symptoms may be explained by feelings of shame and guilt that may promote a sense of inferiority that may in turn inhibit the propensity to seek help or share ones experience with others. Taken as a whole, these abound to a lack of much needed social support which has been identified as "the most important risk factor of all" which may indeed "protect trauma-exposed individuals from developing PTSD" (Friedman, Resick, & Keane, 2007, p. 8), a finding found repeatedly in PTSD risk factor meta-analyses (Brewin, Andrews, & Valentine, 2000; Ozer, Best, Lipsey, & Weiss, 2003).

Attempting to understand post-captivity loneliness from the ex-POWs' perspective, Stein and Tuval-Mashiach (2015a) have conducted a phenomenological study exploring the narratives of Israeli veterans of combat and captivity. The researchers scrutinized the narratives for descriptions of painful modes of isolation (i.e., loneliness) and attempted to identify and characterize these modes of isolation and the deficient relational needs lying in their infrastructure. The researchers found that POWs have spoken mostly of being alone with their traumatic experiences, having practically no one around with whom they can share their past and, in cases

[1] Unless otherwise specified, all references to accounts by veterans have been made in testimonies given at the testimonial project at the Israel Center for Victims of Terror and War (NATAL) and have been part of a previous project of the first author.

of PTSD, also their present experiences. Hence, the researchers suggest that this mode of isolation is best realized when referred to as *experiential loneliness*.

What is it that makes ex-POWs feel that they must bear their unbearable experiences alone? There are many answers to this question. For one, as we normally perceive people who have undergone the same situation as us to be more likely to understand what it is like (Hodges, 2005), the realization that war captivity is perceived as "no man's experience" may be expected to foster a sense of never truly being understood. Second, ex-POWs may feel that they wish to spare their close ones the agony of learning of their suffering. As one POW has attested, for 25 years, he abstained from disclosing his experiences and has kept them even from his wife for the simple reason that he did not wish for her to suffer. Another ex-POW attested, "I've never told my parents the details because I felt that they have suffered enough. All I told them was that I made a stop in hell and came back." Hence, the ex-POW may feel that he is the only one feeling what he feels and is therefore alone with his suffering. Such isolation may go beyond the experiencing individual and permeate concentric circles of interpersonal relationships.

The Multiple Contexts of Interpersonal Deficit: Marital, Social, and National

So far, we have discussed the deep and long-term internal psychological costs of war captivity, from injury to attachment working models, to feelings of loneliness many years following repatriation. These internal injuries may then permeate several realms of interpersonal relationships. From this point of view, it is easily understandable why trauma in general, and human-made trauma in particular, are believed to undermine the ability to create and maintain intimate relationships (Mills & Turnbull, 2004).

Loneliness, just like attachment, may have dire ramifications on one's intimate relationships. Indeed, studies of spousal relations have consistently revealed that war captivity has deleterious effects on marital life (e.g., Cook, Riggs, Thompson, Coyne, & Sheikh, 2004; Neria et al., 2000). In their longitudinal study, Solomon and Dekel (2008) found that ex-POWs reported lower levels of marital adjustment than veterans that have not endured captivity. However, interestingly enough, loneliness has been found to mediate the relation between PTSD symptomatology and marital adjustment as a whole.

An additional series of studies from our group has longitudinally showed that Israeli ex-POWs face difficulties in maintaining satisfied relationships with their spouses and their children. It was found that in addition to the lower martial adjustment, ex-POWs exhibit also lower sexual satisfaction in their martial relationships compared with combatants that were not captured (Zerach, Anat, Solomon, & Heruti, 2010). In another study, the results indicated that 20 years after the war, former ex-POW couples exhibited lower rates of self-disclosure in their marital relationship and higher verbal abuse in comparison to control couples (Dekel,

Enoch, & Solomon, 2008). However, it remains to be determined whether these effects are due to the captivity experience or whether they are due to PTSD, which only some of the prisoners develop after captivity. Dekel and Solomon (2006) have examined martial relations among Israeli ex-POW's and showed that PTSD and related behaviors such as verbal aggression and sexual dissatisfaction contributed significantly to the variance in marital relations. These results highlight the detrimental impact of features that are associated with PTSD but that are not part of the PTSD diagnosis on the marital adjustment of former POWs.

Unsurprisingly, ex-POWs may find that they are struggling with difficulties also with parenting. Although studies on the impact of war captivity on parenting are scarce, we can learn from the literature about Holocaust survivors documenting direct manifestations of intrusive memories and numbing responsiveness as well as indirect manifestations of loneliness experiences among their offspring as a result of an inability to provide emotional care and protection (Wiseman, 2008).

Similar to Holocaust survivors, ex-POWs have been known to alternate between fear of intimacy and the need to compensate and be overprotective in their relations with their children (Cohen, Dekel, Solomon, & Lavie, 2003). One important, albeit somewhat expected, finding from the longitudinal study is that ex-POWs reported lower levels of positive parenting, compared to war veterans who were not held in captivity (Zerach, Greene, Ein-Dor, & Solomon, 2012).

Ex-POWs seem to be caught in an unfortunate vicious cycle, in which the difficulties to maintain intimacy, and close relationships may subsequently generate an even stronger sense of isolation, while hindering their families' ability to be supportive. Marital relationships, are initially founded upon the presumption that spouses will be there for one another, and understand one another in their hard times, "in sickness and in health." These presuppositions are shattered and become saturated with feelings of failed intersubjectivity and loneliness. Thus, one may face the unfortunate eventuality wherein he feels that his own wife and children do not and practically cannot understand what he has been through. These negative feelings may lead to a deterioration in ex-POWs' relationship with their closest most valued people.

Another realm of interpersonal relationships is the social circle of friends. Such is the story recounted by Aherenfeld (Bachar & Aherenfeld, 2010, pp. 220–221), himself an ex-POW of the Yom Kippur War. Aherenfeld and his "brothers in arms" (fellow soldiers) were commanded by their superior officer to surrender as their post was overtaken by the Egyptian forces. Upon his return from captivity, he explains that his friends from before the war, before captivity, seemed to no longer pose any interest for him after repatriation.

> Unexpectedly, with my frieds – some of which were close friends, childhood friends, it was more difficult for me. Even somewhat strange. Truly, I was happy to meet them and spend time in their company but I felt, as if there is a distance continually growing between me and them. Some of them have never even participated in the fighting in the Yom Kippur War and in the secrecy of my heart I scorned them. Sometimes I would ask myself, actually, what do we have in common? In the most important event of our time, an event that fashioned our souls forever, they were absent. And if they weren't there, then they will never understand what happened there. They won't understand me. I was there. In the dungeon,

> alone. And here too, when I am with friends, I am actually alone.they are not really with me. They cannot be with me. I witnessed friends continuing with the routines of their lives as usual. . . . and I felt a bit stuck. A bit outside. I began losing interest in them. . . . as if an invisible hand had disintegrated the intimate relationship we had for years.

The third and broadest circle of isolation is formed vis-à-vis ones society and state. As noted, ex-POWs may feel that they are no longer a part of society as this society as a people do not share their experiences (Stein & Tuval-Mashiach, 2015a). One may then feel that the society from where he was sent into battle has forsaken him. Indeed, as life at the home front goes on as if nothing has happened, the ex-POW may feel that no one cares about what he has been through, about the suffering he has endured, and indeed the suffering he keeps enduring in the form of PTSD and complex PTSD symptoms. These symptoms make captivity, for him, very much alive and kicking. Realizing the manner in which society may be perceived in the post-captivity reality, we can begin to apprehend how loneliness manifests, and how in turn it gives rise to a sense of betrayal.

Conversely, the reality that POWs face upon repatriation is not always one of welcoming. Instead, they may face allegations of dereliction of duty for falling captive in the first place, or accusations of upright betrayal as they are suspected of giving valuable information to the enemy. In this respect, ex-POWs may themselves feel that they were betrayed by their state—that the contract has been breached (Gavriely, 2006). Subsequently, they may feel estranged and lose all faith in the state and its institutions.

Concluding Remarks: Looking Back Looking Forward

It has long been realized that trauma inflicted by another human being is worse than that inflicted by nature and that this severity may have detrimental ramifications for prospective human bonds (Charuvastra & Cloitre, 2008). This chapter serves to strengthen this realization. Throughout this chapter, we have highlighted the manner in which various dimensions of interpersonal malicious conduct during captivity are weaved into a tapestry of dysfunctional interpersonal relationships thereafter. As we have seen, war captivity can take a complex and painful toll on the course of the traumatized individual's life. Moreover, the deleterious effects of the traumatic experience often extend beyond the individual personal lives, impacting concentric circles of family, friends, society, and state. Where once attachment was, detachment now resides, and where connection has reigned now loneliness and isolation rule. It is then our duty both as members of the society from which veterans are sent to the front lines of battle to defend, and as clinicians and researchers to find paths for mending these fractures in interpersonal bonds.

As researchers, we must work to further understand the experiences at hand from the perspective of those who have endured captivity (Stein, Tuval-Mashiach, & Solomon, under review). That is to say that we must find ways to explore these experiences qualitatively and phenomenologically and give voice to the atrocities of torture as authentic witnesses (Felman & Laub, 1992). As Shay (2002, p. 144, italics in original) notes:

> When trauma survivors hear that enough of the truth of their experience has been understood, remembered, and retold—no cone who did not experience their trauma can ever grasp *all* of this truth—then the circle of communalization is complete.

In examining ex-POWs stories, we then not only advance our knowledge of their conditions but also work towards the communalization of their trauma and towards reinstating interpersonal ties. In so doing, we may work to breech the walls of ex-POWs' experiential isolation and loneliness (Stein & Tuval-Mashiach, 2015a). This may be a point of import also for clinicians.

Findings from previous studies have shown that, compared with non-captive combatants, approximately twice as many ex-POWs felt that they needed psychotherapy and as much as five times more actually sought and obtained it (Neria et al., 2000). The finding that war captivity trauma plays a role in attachment orientation, loneliness, marital maladjustment, and parenting, suggests that close attention should be paid to interpersonal aspects in treatment. This is important both for the actual relationships of ex-POWs, and for the alleviation of other aftereffects such as PTSD symptomatology (Tarrier et al., 1999).

Indeed, when treating ex-POWs, one cannot ignore the associated attachment worries and doubts. Increasing a sense of security in the client-therapist relationship through the evocation of memories or images of security-enhancing attachment figures can have a soothing effect that may facilitate a good therapeutic outcome. It is the clinicians' task to work with patients to reinstate the shattered trust in others and mend attachment injuries. Due to their professional knowledge and understanding, clinicians may gain the trust of the traumatized individual before closer circles (e.g., wife and family) do. As such, they are bestowed with the opportunity to become a relational home for the traumatic pain, thus bridging otherwise incommensurable experiential worlds (e.g., Carr, 2011; Stolorow, 2007, 2011). It is possible that providing experiences of security within the therapeutic setting can reestablish attachment security, reduce loneliness, and altogether promote healing.

It is then up to therapists to broaden the circles of trust and expand interpersonal connection in ex-POWs' relational domains. To this end, therapists should attempt to identify and foster additional sources of security in the patient's environment (e.g., family members, friends, a religious community), which are often also damaged following the war. As interpersonal relationships seem to be compromised following captivity, efforts to explain the extreme traumatic experiences and the ramifications of captivity, using psycho-educational methods, could go a long way in helping ex-POWs once again be accepted and understood by their various support systems. Naturally, all of these beneficial prospects of therapy must be systematically investigated before we can make any generalizations or claim that therapy accomplishes such a reinstatement of relational bonds.

Finally, we may address implications for society and state. Soldiers rarely go to war of their own accord. They are sent by their governments, who employ them as instruments in the pursuit of some national goal. The responsibility to alleviate the pain caused by war trauma rests not only with the traumatized person but also with society at large. One would therefore expect those who send men to war, endangering their lives and their physical and mental health, to take responsibility for them upon their return and to offer them treatment that would address the wide range of difficulties they face. Policy makers must find a way to uproot any accusation of betrayal and treat repatriated POWs not as traitors but as the victims they are. Only in so doing may the circle of interpersonal malattunement be broken, and healing may begin.

References

Avnery, A. (1982). *Coping and adjustment to war captivity*. Unpublished Master's thesis, Hebrew University, Jerusalem.

Bachar, I., & Aherenfeld, U. (2010). *Prisoner by command! The story of Uri Aherenfeld Yom Kippur prisoner in Egypt*. Tel Aviv: Ma'ariv Books.

Beebe, G. W. (1975). Follow-up studies of World War II and Korean war prisoners. II. Morbidity, disability, and maladjustments. *American Journal of Epidemiology, 101*(5), 400–422.

Bowlby, J. (1973). *Attachment and loss. Vol. 2: Separation: Anxiety and anger*: New York, NY: Basic Books.

Bowlby, J. (1982). *Attachment and loss. Vol. 1: Attachment* (2nd ed.). New York: Basic Books.

Bowlby, J. (1988). *A secure base: parent-child attachment and healthy human development*. New York, NY: Basic Books.

Brewin, C. R., Andrews, B., & Valentine, J. D. (2000). Meta-analysis of risk factors for posttraumatic stress disorder in trauma-exposed adults. *Journal of Consulting and Clinical Psychology, 68*(5), 748–766.

Cacioppo, J. T., & Cacioppo, S. (2012). The phenotype of loneliness. *European Journal of Developmental Psychology, 9*(4), 446–452.

Cacioppo, J. T., & Cacioppo, S. (2014). Social relationships and health: the toxic effects of perceived social isolation. *Social and Personality Psychology Compass, 8*(2), 58–72.

Carr, R. B. (2011). Combat and human existence: Toward an intersubjective approach to combat-related PTSD. *Psychoanalytic Psychology, 28*(4), 471–496.

Cassidy, J., & Shaver, P. (2008). *Handbook of attachment: Theory, research, and clinical applications*. New York: Guilford.

Charuvastra, A., & Cloitre, M. (2008). Social bonds and posttraumatic stress disorder. *Annual Review of Psychology, 59*, 301–328. doi:10.1146/annurev.psych.58.110405.085650.

Cloitre, M., Miranda, R., Stovall-McClough, K. C., & Han, H. (2005). Beyond PTSD: Emotion regulation and interpersonal problems as predictors of functional impairment in survivors of childhood abuse. *Behavior Therapy, 36*(2), 119–124.

Cohen, E., Dekel, R., Solomon, Z., & Lavie, T. (2003). Posttraumatic stress symptoms and fear of intimacy among treated and non-treated survivors who were children during the Holocaust. *Social Psychiatry and Psychiatric Epidemiology, 38*(11), 611–617.

Cook, J. M., Riggs, D. S., Thompson, R., Coyne, J. C., & Sheikh, J. I. (2004). Posttraumatic stress disorder and current relationship functioning among World War II ex-prisoners of war. *Journal of Family Psychology, 18*(1), 36–45.

Dasberg, H. (1976). Belonging and loneliness in relation to mental breakdown in battle: With some remarks on treatment. *Israel Annals of Psychiatry & Related Disciplines, 14*(4), 307–321.

Dekel, R., & Solomon, Z. (2006). Marital relations among former prisoners of war: Contribution of posttraumatic stress disorder, aggression, and sexual satisfaction. *Journal of Family Psychology, 20*(4), 709–712.

Dekel, R., Enoch, G., & Solomon, Z. (2008). The contribution of captivity and post-traumatic stress disorder to marital adjustment of Israeli couples. *Journal of Social and Personal Relationships, 25*(3), 497–510.
Dikel, T. N., Engdahl, B., & Eberly, R. (2005). PTSD in former prisoners of war: Prewar, wartime, and postwar factors. *Journal of Traumatic Stress, 18*(1), 69–77.
Ettema, E. J., Derksen, L. D., & van Leeuwen, E. (2010). Existential loneliness and end-of-life care: a systematic review. *Theoretical Medicine and Bioethics, 31*(2), 141–169.
Felman, S., & Laub, D. (1992). *Testimony: Crises of witnessing in literature, psychoanalysis, and history*. Florence: Routledge.
Forbes, D., Parslow, R., Fletcher, S., McHugh, T., & Creamer, M. (2010). Attachment style in the prediction of recovery following group treatment of combat veterans with post-traumatic stress disorder. *The Journal of Nervous and Mental Disease, 198*(12), 881–884.
Fraley, R. C., & Shaver, P. R. (2000). Adult romantic attachment: Theoretical developments, emerging controversies, and unanswered questions. *Review of General Psychology, 4*(2), 132–154.
Friedman, M. J., Resick, P. A., & Keane, T. M. (2007). PTSD: Twenty-five years of progress and challenges. In M. J. Friedman, T. M. Keane, & P. A. Resick (Eds.), *Handbook of PTSD: Science and practice* (pp. 3–18). New York: Guilford.
Fromm-Reichmann, F. (1990). Loneliness. *Contemporary Psychoanalysis, 26*(2), 305–330.
Gavriely, D. (2006). Israel's cultural code of captivity and the personal stories of Yom Kippur war ex-POWs. *Armed Forces & Society, 33*(1), 94–105.
Hawkley, L. C., & Cacioppo, J. T. (2010). Loneliness matters: A theoretical and empirical review of consequences and mechanisms. *Annals of Behavioral Medicine, 40*(2), 218–227.
Hazan, C., & Shaver, P. (1987). Romantic love conceptualized as an attachment process. *Journal of Personality and Social Psychology, 52*(3), 511–524.
Herman, J. L. (1992). *Trauma and recovery*. New York: Basic Books.
Hodges, S. D. (2005). Is how much you understand me in your head or mine? In B. F. Malle & S. D. Hodges (Eds.), *Other minds: How humans bridge the divide between self and others* (pp. 298–309). New York: Guilford.
Hunter, E. J. (1993). The Vietnam prisoner of war experience. In J. P. Wilson & B. Raphael (Eds.), *International handbook of traumatic stress syndromes* (pp. 297–303). New York, NY: Plenum Press.
Johnson, S. M., Makinen, J. A., & Millikin, J. W. (2001). Attachment injuries in couple relationships: A new perspective on impasses in couples therapy. *Journal of marital and family therapy, 27*(2), 145–155.
Klohnen, E. C., & John, O. P. (1998). Working models of attachment: A theory-based prototype approach. In J. A. Simpson & W. S. Rholes (Eds.), *Attachment theory and close relationships* (pp. 115–140). New York: Guilford Press.
Laub, D., & Auerhahn, N. C. (1989). Failed empathy–a central theme in the survivor's holocaust experience. *Psychoanalytic Psychology, 6*(4), 377–400.
Lieblich, A. (1994). Seasons of captivity: The experience of POWs in the Middle East. New York: New York University Press.
Litz, B. T., Stein, N., Delaney, E., Lebowitz, L., Nash, W. P., Silva, C., & Maguen, S. (2009). Moral injury and moral repair in war veterans: A preliminary model and intervention strategy. *Clinical Psychology Review, 29*, 695–706. doi:10.1016/j.cpr.2009.07.003.
Mijuskovic, B. L. (2012). *Loneliness in philosophy, psychology, and literature*. Bloomington, IN: iUniverse Books.
Mikulincer, M., & Shaver, P. R. (2007). *Attachment in adulthood: Structure, dynamics, and change*. New York, NY: Guilford Press.
Mikulincer, M., Shaver, P. R., & Horesh, N. (2006). Attachment bases of emotion regulation and posttraumatic adjustment. In D. K. Snyder, J. A. Simpson, & J. N. Hughes (Eds.), *Emotion regulation in families: Pathways to dysfunction and health* (pp. 77–99). Washington, DC: American Psychological Association.
Mikulincer, M., Ein-Dor, T., Solomon, Z., & Shaver, P. R. (2011). Trajectories of attachment insecurities over a 17-year period: A latent growth curve analysis of the impact of war captivity and posttraumatic stress disorder. *Journal of Social and Clinical Psychology, 30*(9), 960–984.

Mills, B., & Turnbull, G. (2004). Broken hearts and mending bodies: The impact of trauma on intimacy. *Sexual and Relationship Therapy, 19*(3), 265–289.

Neria, Y., Solomon, Z., & Dekel, R. (1998). An eighteen-year follow-up study of Israeli prisoners of war and combat veterans. *The Journal of Nervous and Mental Disease, 186*(3), 174–182.

Neria, Y., Solomon, Z., Ginzburg, K., Dekel, R., Enoch, D., & Ohry, A. (2000). Posttraumatic residues of captivity: A follow-up of Israeli ex-prisoners of war. *Journal of Clinical Psychiatry, 61*(1), 39–46.

Ozer, E. J., Best, S. R., Lipsey, T. L., & Weiss, D. S. (2003). Predictors of posttraumatic stress disorder and symptoms in adults: A meta-analysis. *Psychological Bulletin, 129*(1), 52–73.

Scarry, E. (1985). *The body in pain: The making and unmaking of the world.* New York, NY: Oxford University Press.

Shay, J. (1994). *Achilles in Vietnam: Combat trauma and the undoing of character.* New York: Atheneum.

Shay, J. (2002). *Odysseus in America: Combat trauma and the trials of homecoming.* New York, NY: Scribner.

Shay, J. (2014). Moral injury. *Psychoanalytic Psychology, 31*(2), 182–191.

Solomon, Z. (1993). *Combat stress reaction: The enduring toll of war.* New York, NY: Plenum.

Solomon, Z. (2001). The impact of posttraumatic stress disorder in military situations. *Journal of Clinical Psychiatry, 62*(Suppl 17): 11–15.

Solomon, Z., & Dekel, R. (2005). Posttraumatic stress disorder among Israeli ex-prisoners of war 18 and 30 years after release. *Journal of Clinical Psychiatry, 66*(8), 1031–1037.

Solomon, Z., & Dekel, R. (2008). The contribution of loneliness and posttraumatic stress disorder to marital adjustment following war captivity: A longitudinal study. *Family Process, 47*(2), 261–275.

Solomon, Z., Mikulincer, M., & Hobfoll, S. E. (1986). Effects of social support and battle intensity on loneliness and breakdown during combat. *Journal of Personality and Social Psychology, 51*(6), 1269–1276.

Solomon, Z., Ginzburg, K., Mikulincer, M., Neria, Y., & Ohry, A. (1998). Coping with war captivity: The role of attachment style. *European Journal of Personality, 12*(4), 271–285.

Solomon, Z., Dekel, R., & Mikulincer, M. (2008). Complex trauma of war captivity: A prospective study of attachment and post-traumatic stress disorder. *Psychological Medicine, 38*(10), 1427–1434.

Solomon, Z., Horesh, D., Ein-Dor, T., & Ohry, A. (2012). Predictors of PTSD trajectories following captivity: A 35-year longitudinal study. *Psychiatry Research, 199*(3), 188–194.

Speed, N., Engdahl, B., Schwartz, J., & Eberly, R. (1989). Posttraumatic stress disorder as a consequence of the POW experience. *The Journal of Nervous and Mental Disease, 177*(3), 147–153.

Stein, J. Y., & Tuval-Mashiach, R. (2015a). Loneliness and isolation in life-stories of Israeli veterans of combat and captivity. *Psychological Trauma: Theory, Research, Practice, and Policy, 7*(2), 122–130. doi: 10.1037/a0036936.

Stein, J. Y., & Tuval-Mashiach, R. (2015b). The social construction of loneliness: An integrative conceptualization. *Journal of Constructivist Psychology, 28*(3), 210–227. doi: 10.1080/10720537.2014.911129.

Stein, J. Y., Tuval-Mashiach, R., & Solomon, Z. (under review). Considering intersubjective needs in trauma research: Advocating hermeneutically and phenomenologically oriented qualitative research.

Stolorow, R. D. (2007). *Trauma and human existence: Autobiographical, psychoanalytic, and philosophical reflections.* New York: Analytic Press/Taylor & Francis Group.

Stolorow, R. D. (2011). *World, affectivity, trauma: Heidegger and post-Cartesian psychoanalysis.* New York: Routledge/.

Sutker, P. B., Bugg, F., & Allain, A. N. (1991). Psychometric prediction of PTSD among POW survivors. *Psychological Assessment: A Journal of Consulting and Clinical Psychology, 3*(1), 105.

Sutker, P. B., Allain Jr., A. N., & Winstead, D. K. (1993). Psychopathology and psychiatric diagnoses of World War II Pacific theater prisoner of war survivors and combat veterans. *American Journal of Psychiatry, 150*, 240–245.

Tarrier, N., Pilgrim, H., Sommerfield, C., Faragher, B., Reynolds, M., Graham, E., et al. (1999). A randomized trial of cognitive therapy and imaginal exposure in the treatment of chronic post-traumatic stress disorder. *Journal of Consulting and Clinical Psychology, 67*(1), 13–18.
Ursano, R. J., Boydstun, J. A., & Wheatley, R. D. (1981). Psychiatric illness in US Air Force Viet Nam prisoners of war: A five-year follow-up. *The American Journal of Psychiatry, 138*(3), 210–314.
van der Kolk, B. A. (2001). The assessment and treatment of complex PTSD. In R. Yehuda (Ed.), *Treating trauma survivors with PTSD* (pp. 127–156). American Psychiatric Press.
van der Kolk, B. A., Roth, S., Pelcovitz, D., Sunday, S., & Spinazzola, J. (2005). Disorders of extreme stress: The empirical foundation of a complex adaptation to trauma. *Journal of Traumatic Stress, 18*(5), 389–399.
Wiseman, H. (2008). On failed intersubjectivity: Recollections of loneliness experiences in offspring of Holocaust survivors. *American Journal of Orthopsychiatry, 78*(3), 350–358.
Wood, L. A. (1986). Loneliness. In R. Harré (Ed.), *The social construction of emotions* (pp. 184–209). New York, NY: Basil Blackwell.
Zakin, G., Solomon, Z., & Neria, Y. (2003). Hardiness, attachment style, and long term psychological distress among Israeli POWs and combat veterans. *Personality and Individual Differences, 34*(5), 819–829.
Zeiss, R. A., & Dickman, H. R. (1989). PTSD 40 years later: Incidence and person-situation correlates in former POWs. *Journal of Clinical Psychology, 45*(1), 80–87.
Zerach, G., Anat, B. D., Solomon, Z., & Heruti, R. (2010). Posttraumatic symptoms, marital intimacy, dyadic adjustment, and sexual satisfaction among ex-prisoners of war. *The Journal of Sexual Medicine, 7*(8), 2739–2749.
Zerach, G., Greene, T., Ein-Dor, T., & Solomon, Z. (2012). The relationship between posttraumatic stress disorder symptoms and paternal parenting of adult children among ex-prisoners of war: A longitudinal study. *Journal of Family Psychology, 26*(2), 274–284.
Zhang, F., & Labouvie-Vief, G. (2004). Stability and fluctuation in adult attachment style over a 6-year period. *Attachment & Human Development, 6*(4), 419–437.

Chapter 8
Does Extreme Trauma Transfer? The Case of Three Generations of the Holocaust

Abraham Sagi-Schwartz

Introduction

Our field has always expressed interest in exploring whether and how transmission of trauma might take place across generations. Maltreating families can teach us a great deal about the cross-generational transmission of trauma. Scholars have long suspected that parents who were abused as children, in turn, abuse their own children and that patterns of abusive caregiving in general are transmitted from one generation to the next. The mechanism of this process has been discussed by Cicchetti, Toth, and Maughan (2000), who described an ecological model of transmission which suggests how maltreatment is transmitted across generations. This type of trauma, though, is inflicted by trusted attachment figures within the family.

In this chapter, we address the consequences of severe trauma that children experienced *not* within the family but of trauma inflicted by anonymous social and destructive forces external to the normative family. Toward that end, we focus on World War II Holocaust survivors and their offspring. We feel we can say rather clearly that the Holocaust was the most traumatic catastrophe ever designed by "civilized" human beings, with other humans being subjected to horrifying slaughters.

The Holocaust began in Germany in the well-known "Crystal Night" (Kristallnacht in German), November 9–10, 1938, when approximately 7,500 Jewish shops were destroyed and 400 synagogues were burnt down. The onset of massive slaughter of Jews began on that night and expanded rapidly over all Europe until 1945, resulting in the industrialized murder and extermination of six million Jews.

A tragic consequence of such atrocious events is that Holocaust survivors provide an opportunity for studying the enduring effects of massive trauma and extremely stressful experiences (Carmil & Breznitz, 1991). Insights that can be gained

A. Sagi-Schwartz (✉)
Center for the Study of Child Development,
University of Haifa, 6035 Rabin Building, Haifa 31905, Israel
e-mail: sagi@psy.haifa.ac.il

K. E. Cherry (ed.), *Traumatic Stress and Long-Term Recovery*,
DOI 10.1007/978-3-319-18866-9_8

from the current study concerning the long-term consequences of the Holocaust on survivors may extend to adaptational challenges for survivors of other, more recent genocides, each characterized by its distinctive feature. As the systematic extermination during the Holocaust began in the early 1940s of the previous century, there has been a sense of urgency about the research because even the youngest survivors who have any memory of the event are today in their mid-to-late 70s. Although there is ample documentation of many aspects of the events and consequences of the Holocaust, the window for first-hand empirical studies of survivors, involving sufficient numbers to recruit proper samples, is rapidly narrowing and, in the not-too-distant future, will be shut forever. This is all the more true of studies involving the assessment of survivors over an extended period of time. We took advantage of this narrowest of intervals, when three generations are simultaneously at hand, including the first generation of survivors and the third generation still in its infancy, to produce findings that shed light on vulnerability and resilience in general and that are applicable to other traumatic and catastrophic life events, of which genocide is only one.

In this regard, two main questions are addressed: (1) Do child survivors of extreme Holocaust trauma show marks of their traumatic experiences even 60 or more years later? (2) Was the trauma passed on to the next generations? Within this context, the notion of transmission gap of trauma and breaking the cycle of trauma is discussed. The discussion draws on our programmatic research conducted over the past two decades with three generations of Holocaust survivors, research that incorporates personal stories as well as psychological, interpersonal, genetic, physiological, and epidemiological data. Because we draw a lot of our discussion on attachment theory and research, in the next section, we begin with a brief overview of major attachment concepts, and then we introduce the notion of transmission of trauma to contextualize our findings.

Attachment, Attachment Security/Insecurity, and Transmission of Trauma

Perhaps the best way the basic tenet of attachment theory can be described is to use the words of John Bowlby, the founder of the theory: "To say of a child that he is attached to, or has an attachment to someone, means that he is strongly disposed to seek proximity to and contact with a specific figure, and to do so in certain situations, notably when he is frightened, tired or ill" (Bowlby, 1984, p. 371). According to Bowlby, there is an innate bias to become attached to a primary caregiver regardless of the specific cultural niche. This is an enduring, long-lasting, emotional tie to a special person, and in fact, "all of us, from the cradle to the grave, are happiest when life is organized as a series of excursions, long or short, from the secure base provided by our attachment figure(s)" (Bowlby, 1988, p. 62). When a child is exposed to sensitive parenting, he/she is likely to form a secure attachment relationship with the attachment figure. When insensitive care is experienced, then the likelihood for insecure attachment is heightened. It should be emphasized that both secure and insecure attachments are considered normative, with longitudinal studies demonstrating that secure and insecure attachment can be seen as protective and risk factors, respectively, for later adaption and functioning (see, e.g., Sagi-Schwartz & Aviezer, 2005). There is also ample cumulative cross-cultural evidence for the universality of the theory and findings across many cultures and ethnic groups (see for a review, Van IJzendoorn & Sagi-Schwartz, 2008).

Sometimes, however, such a secure base and safe haven may be in jeopardy. Using the insights of attachment theory, we can describe the cross-generational transmission of trauma as a vicious circle of "fright without solution," in the words of Hesse and Main (1999), where frightened or frightening parental behavior prevents children from developing trust and dependence on their caregiver, and it causes them to withdraw into disorganized behavior. This is most characteristic of abused and maltreated children (Van IJzendoorn & Bakermans-Kranenburg, 2009).

At the same time, many maltreated individuals succeed in breaking the cycle of abuse. To understand how traumatized people may manage to do this, we examined the transmission patterns of World War II Holocaust survivors, members of normative families who experienced severe trauma. Holocaust survivors were exposed to an unexpected, harsh separation from parents in early childhood, loss of parents in early childhood, and traumatic, inhumane atrocities suffered by themselves and by people in their environment (for example, see Chap. 23, this volume).

We have good reason to assume that if loss of a dear relative occurred, it can be expected that the loss may not be psychologically resolved and that the unresolved loss should result in prolonged trauma. This is because many of the grief mechanisms that help people to resolve the loss of loved ones under natural life trajectories were simply not available to Holocaust survivors who were, at times, even exposed directly to the murder of their parents, often under terrifying circumstances, and sometimes also extermination of the entire family. In many cases, there was a significant gap between the time of the parents' death and the time when the children were informed about it, and they were never able to learn the exact time of their parents' death or its location. Moreover, there are no burial places or graves for the loved ones. Many survivors also felt guilt for not being able to help their parents, for staying alive, and simultaneously felt anger for being left alone. Under such horrific circumstances, which we consider to go against "the laws of nature," we expect to find prolonged unresolved loss and trauma. By contrast, people who experience loss in the natural course of their lives have access to all the necessary markers or symbols that facilitate the mourning process: the death is natural, the time of death is known, there is a designated grave, there are no guilt feelings concerning the death, etc. In the context of our study, the question arises whether the effects of such atrocious experiences are transmitted to the next generations?

Our Holocaust Project Across Three Generations

Based on prior trauma research and literature, we anticipated the severe trauma sustained by the first generation of Holocaust survivors to be transmitted to the next one. In the case of trauma inflicted within the family, when the child has no caregiver to turn to in times of stress, there is clear evidence of attachment disorganization. Because it is beyond the scope of this chapter to address in length the issues of adversity within the family, the reader is advised to look into the effect of maltreatment of children growing up with abusive parents, amidst domestic violence, or in multiple-risk families or institutions, in a review article by Van IJzendoorn and Bakermans-Kranenburg (2009; see also Chap. 9 of this volume for related discussion). But, whether extreme trauma that originates outside the family—within normative families—also leads to insecure-disorganized attachment, still needs to be answered.

We hypothesize that normative families subjected to external trauma have several characteristics that may ease the consequences that we observe when anguish takes place within the family. From an attachment perspective, the first such characteristic has to do with the existence of a secure emotional infrastructure before trauma occurred and before the experience of separation and loss.

For the less familiar reader, we provide here, first, a brief description of two classical attachment measures so that further descriptions and discussions below will be better understood. In the strange situation procedure (SSP; Ainsworth, Blehar, Waters, & Wall, 1978), infant behavior during reunion with the mother after two 3-min separations is classified into three main categories of attachment. Securely attached infants (B classification) may or may not be upset when their mother leaves, but her return has a calming effect, and they show minimal resistant and avoidant behavior. Avoidant infants (A classification) do not seek proximity or contact with their returning caregiver, but instead they show avoidant behavior. Resistant or ambivalent infants (C classification) seek contact, but at the same time, resist the caregiver; some resistant infants are unable to settle within the duration of the 3-min reunion episodes. A fourth category of attachment classification, most pertinent to the discussion in this chapter, refers to disorganized infants (D classification; Main & Solomon, 1990). In this category, "the infant displays disorganized and/or disoriented behaviors in the parent's presence, suggesting a temporary collapse of behavioral strategies…the infant may freeze with a trancelike expression, hands in air" (Hesse, 1999, p. 399).

The Adult Attachment Interview (AAI; Hesse, 2008) assesses current mental representations of childhood attachment experiences, including loss and trauma experiences. Five attachment classifications are coded as follows: (1) secure: autonomous, coherent in exploring past experiences whether positive or negative (*F* classification); (2) insecure: dismissive of past relationships with attachment figures and attachment experiences (*DS* classification); (3) insecure: preoccupied with past experiences and angry toward attachment figures (*E* classification); (4) insecure: disoriented with regard to attachment because of the lack of resolution of loss/trauma (labeled as *U* and is most pertinent to this chapter); (5) insecure: cannot classify (CC; a mixture of diverging mental representations of attachment so that no single representation seems to dominate the participant's thinking about the past; Hesse, 2008).

We can imagine the outcomes that would have been expected if, for example, the SSP or the AAI had been available in the 1930s, before the World War II Holocaust. It is reasonable to assume that infants and adults in Amsterdam, Antwerp, Paris, and Berlin would have achieved typical outcomes in the SSP and AAI similar to those we find today in normative families.

The second characteristic associated with normative families that were caught in the Holocaust is that they did not always personally experience or witness traumatizing events; we know about many families that, for a certain period of time, remained united while they were escaping and hiding.

Another factor we must take into account is the availability of support systems. During the Holocaust, the trauma was not inflicted on the children by parents or trusted attachment figures but by anonymous destructive social forces. Unfortunately, and upon harsh separations from their beloved parents, many children experienced terrifying hostilities with German Schutzstaffel (SS) officers who examined them to determine whether they qualify as "Aryan" (in a very simplistic translation for this chapter = master race, but, of course, the term Aryanism is much more complicated historically and symbolically).

Under these horrifying circumstances, is it possible to find a source for a strong feeling of hope? We explored the role played by social support systems, such as the legitimizing of prolonged grief, a collective national identity, and feelings of safety from anti-Semitism (Solomon & Chaitin, 2007). Other sources of support can be found in the meaning ascribed to the new generation (Frankl, 1997), in the resources found in fellow survivors, in public Holocaust memorials, and in the continued bond with the deceased parents (Silverman & Nickman, 1996).

In fact, as can be seen next, our findings eventually revealed only limited cross-generational transmission of trauma. Therefore, the question arises whether we are observing transmission of trauma or perhaps instead also posttraumatic growth (Tedeshi & Calhoun, 2004; see also Chap. 17, this volume) ? At the time that we conducted the study, the first and second generations (grandmothers and mothers) were adults. Therefore, in order to assess cross-generational transmission of the trauma sustained by the grandmothers, from an attachment perspective, we examined the adult mental representations with regard to early attachment relationships in child survivors (grandmothers) and their daughters (mothers), using the AAI. Moreover, we were able to administer the SSP to the third generation with a focus on disorganized attachment in infancy. These special circumstances have resulted in a unique three-generation study, which makes the present research different from other attachment studies.

According to some Holocaust experts (for review see Bar-On et al., 1998), the parental styles of Holocaust survivors may be dependent upon the need for their children, and the survivors are also described as anxious and conflictual, frightened and frightening, helpless and unexpected, and emotionally unavailable. Would it then lead to attachment insecurity, to attachment disorganization? What can be learned about the risk of children from normative families living in peace, until their world suddenly collapsed without any comprehensible reason? And what are the consequences for the children's attachment when unexpectedly they lose entirely their attachment figures, seemingly against all "laws of nature"?

In such context, we set out to examine two issues: The first is regarding the first generation, namely what are the implications of the accumulated traumatic experiences before, during, and after the Holocaust on survivors. In other words, does the concept of "sequential traumatization" apply here for first generation (Keilson, 1992)? The second issue concerns secondary and tertiary traumatization and loss, that is, traumatic effects of events and loss that did not take place in the lives of the second and third generations themselves, but only in those of their parents who may or may not have communicated their experiences—in a verbal or nonverbal way (Wiseman et al. 2002). Taken together, we asked whether sequential traumatization for first generation necessarily leads to transmission across generations (i.e., secondary and tertiary traumatization). Or, maybe we observe here a "transmission gap"?

Holocaust research is inconclusive with regard to cross-generational transmission of traumatic experiences. The reasons may be methodological, having to do with massive reliance on convenience samples and also clinical samples, both of which may result in negatively biased results. To avoid such bias, we used a different methodology as described next, aimed at examining the effects of catastrophic trauma, separation, and loss, as well as uncovering the hidden reserves of human stamina and resilience.

Method

First Phase

First Generation We recruited a non-convenience sample of Holocaust child survivors (now grandmothers) and a comparison group without Holocaust experience in their childhood (Sagi-Schwartz et al., 2003). We made sure that the two groups are well matched in the post-World War II macro life events and stresses they experienced, so this variable was well controlled. The complete details of the study are described in Sagi-Schwartz et al. (2003). Our measures and assessments included observations in the home and laboratory, standard psychological tests, semi-structured interviews and inventories, and physiological, genetic, and epidemiological data.

Even 55 years after the events, we found significant differences between the two groups in the domain of traumatic stress. The Holocaust group showed elevated markers of post-traumatic stress disorder (PTSD), more signs of unresolved stress, and more expressions of traumatic stress and anxiety. Child survivors also displayed a significantly higher rate of unresolved classifications (U) on the AAI, which reflects trauma resulting from unresolved loss and a breakdown in organization associated with that loss.

Moreover, we examined separately child survivors who experienced severe risk factors, such as being exposed directly to the murder of their parents, or those who experienced uncontrolled separation from the parent. We found in the AAI that child survivors who were exposed to the brutal murder of their mothers or to frightening separation from them had significantly higher lack of resolution of mourning (LRM) scores than did child survivors who did not observe the murder of their mothers and those whose mothers were in position to control the separation from them. The same was true for the loss and separation that child survivors experienced from their fathers.

We also assessed protective factors, in the form of time spent with significant others after the loss of parents or final separation from them. Child survivors who benefitted from longer periods spent with a support system, showed lower levels of LRM than those who did not benefit from such support, but the statistical difference was only marginally significant. It is possible that the marginal difference that the protective factors seem to have made is the result of measurement problems and of statistical power, but it is also possible that the trauma was of such magnitude that significant others were not able to compensate for it.

Another aspect of our observations highlighted a unique adult attachment classification that was detected in those individuals who experienced catastrophic parental loss in childhood. In two cases, using the AAI, we identified an absence of attachment representations (AAR) in adult years (Koren-Karie, Sagi-Schwartz, & Joels, 2003). In both cases, the relationship with the parents lasted only for the first 4–5 years of life, with no opportunity thereafter to develop new close relations. The result of the traumatic interruption of the parental relationship, alongside a pervasive absence of substitute attachment figures, was an unrecoverable destruction of an already established pattern of attachment, leading to inability to form any type of meaningful attachment in adulthood. In one of the cases, the adult daughter was classified as one with dismissing state of mind with regard to attachment relationships (DS3, namely a subcategory of the DS described before) and her infant as avoidantly attached (A2 which is a subcategory of the general avoidant category defined before); in the other case, the adult daughter was also classified as dismissing (DS3) and her infant as securely attached (B3, a subcategory of the general secure-B category). There are different ways of interpreting the meaning of these extreme cases. On the one hand, becoming a DS3 in the second generation may be the best possible adaptation strategy—but at least with an organized pattern—given a mother who had no attachment representations at all. On the other hand, in one of the two cases, we detected further transmission to the third generation (avoidantly attached) but not so in the other case (securely attached). Naturally, we cannot derive conclusive evidence from two case studies.

Finally, looking at the adaptation-related measures of the first generation, we found that Holocaust child survivors (the grandmothers) did well in their marital lives, were successful in caring for their children, and felt good about their own well-being (Sagi-Schwartz et al., 2003).

Second and Third Generation Similarly to the first generation, we also matched the second-generation mothers who had Holocaust background with a comparison group without such background, and we applied the same measures and assessments that we used for the first generation. Our findings indicate that the second generation did not differ from the control group on measures of attachment, traumatic stress, and unresolved attachment, nor did they differ on measures of anxiety, perceived well-being, caregiving of their mothers, and interaction with their infants (the third generation; Sagi-Schwartz et al., 2003). Next, we matched the third generation (infants) with a comparison group and applied the SSP to both groups. We found that the grandchildren of Holocaust survivors did not differ from the control group in their attachment patterns (Sagi-Schwartz, van IJzendoorn, Bakermans-Kranenburg, 2008).

Second Phase

To study the very long-term effects of early trauma, we conducted phase 2 of the study 11 years later, close to 70 years after the Holocaust. This phase was important also because in their more advanced age, Holocaust survivors are facing new challenges. Therefore, we retested both the first and the second generation for trauma-related effects. We found that the child survivors (grandmothers) showed more dissociative symptomatology and more signs of traumatic stress than did the control group with no Holocaust background. By contrast, the second generation (mothers) again did not differ from controls on any of the measures, including dissociative symptoms, mental and physical health, cognitive functioning, satisfaction with life, reported life stress, and number of stressful life events (Fridman, Bakermans-Kranenburg, Sagi-Schwartz, & van IJzendoorn, 2011).

Meta-Analyses

Overall, we feel confident that our carefully controlled study, conducted in Israel, shows no evidence of cross-generational transmission in either phase 1 or phase 2. Although we are certain that our methodology was rigorous, our findings needed further corroboration, which we believed would be best accomplished by means of a meta-analysis, a quantitative study of all empirical studies for evidence-based conclusions on that topic.

With regard to the first generation, the overall picture that emerged from the cumulative studies is that Holocaust survivors in both convenience and non-convenience samples are performing less well than controls on total adjustment, and that they show a higher prevalence of posttraumatic stress (Barel, van IJzendoorn, Sagi-Schwartz, & Bakermans-Kranenburg, 2010). This effect, however, was more prominent when examined with convenience samples. At the same time, Holocaust survivors in general did not lag much behind controls on several measures such as physical health and cognitive functioning. This attests to remarkable resilience, consistent with the work of Bonanno and Mancini (2012), on coping with grief and trauma, which also demonstrates a host of outcomes people show when exposed to extreme adversity, including the salutary role and moderating impact of various aspects in people's lives.

With regard to the second generation, in the select group (convenience sample), we found overall more mental health problems, posttraumatic stress symptoms, and psychopathological symptoms than we did in the control group, but this was not the case in the non-select group (non-convenience samples; Van IJzendoorn, Bakermans-Kranenburg, & Sagi-Schwartz, 2003). Therefore, when we controlled for quality of design, the detected effect appeared only in convenience and clinical samples; we found no cross-generational effect in random and nonclinical samples. It is possible, therefore, that the secondary traumatization revealed by measures of posttraumatic stress symptoms, general mental health, and psychopathological symptomatology is an artifact of the design of Holocaust studies. This may have important implications on (inappropriate and misleading) conclusions that emerge from many studies that claim for intergenerational transmission of trauma in second-generation offspring of Holocaust survivors. Finally, we detected no third-generation effects, irrespective of the nature of the samples (Sagi-Schwartz et al., 2008).

"Under the Skin" Effects

First Generation We also looked for long-term, second-generation effects that might be concealed "under the skin" of the neurobiological system, so to speak. We searched for remnants of traumatic experiences that may surface only after stressful events. We checked whether latent long-term effects of primary or secondary traumatization might be detectable in stress regulation, as measured by hypothalamic-pituitary-adrenal (HPA) axis functioning and its end-product cortisol level (see Chap. 9, this volume, for related discussion). To this end, in phase 2 of the study, we collected saliva in order to assess daily cortisol and stress reactivity cortisol levels from child survivors. We also collected DNA samples (via buccal swabs) from the first generation in search for gene×environment interaction effects. There is a growing literature now about the moderating role of various unique genetic polymorphisms toward differentially better and worse outcomes in different people who experience the same positive or negative life events respectively (gene×environment interaction; Belsky & Pluess, 2013). Therefore, Holocaust survivors may also respond differently when subject to the same traumatic experiences, and thus further influencing factors such as gene–environment interactions should be examined. The ADRA2B gene was used in a study with Rwandan Civil War refugees in which it was found that the *deletion* variant of this gene compared with the *wild* type of the same gene was associated with more vividly reexperiencing traumatic events in these victims (De Quervain et al., 2007). Along a similar line, we examined the potential moderating role of ADRA2B on the long-term effects of the Holocaust on HPA-axis functioning of survivors, and we also found a gene×environment interaction effect with daily cortisol levels (Fridman, Bakermans-Kranenburg, Sagi-Schwartz, & van IJzendoorn, 2012). Wild type ADRA2B carriers among Holocaust survivors showed higher stress reactivity cortisol levels than comparisons, but no difference was found between Holocaust survivors and their comparisons who were deletion carriers. The same pattern was found for stress reactivity cortisol. Thus, although both groups had been exposed to the same massive genocidal trauma, the ADRA2B gene seems to play an important moderating role in posttraumatic stress dysregulation, as carriers of the wild type and deletion ADRA2B gene display different levels of cortisol secretion. Specifically, in the long term, carriers of the deletion variant may have resolved their vividly remembered experiences, so that at present, they show less stress dysregulation, as evident from their cortisol levels.

Another extensively studied gene in the area that seeks for gene×environment interaction is the DRD4 (Belsky & Pluess, 2013). Our DNA samples have also provided evidence of gene×environment interaction when comparing carriers of the 7-repeat long and short DRD4 alleles. We found that survivors carrying the long allele scored significantly higher than did carriers of the short allele on trauma-related indices including the Impact of Event Scale (IES) which is a posttraumatic stress measure that purports to assess the intensity of intrusion and avoidance responses that follow exposure to extreme stress (Horowitz, Wilner, & Alvarez, 1979) and the Berkeley–Leiden Adult Attachment Questionnaire for Unresolved (BLAAQU) which constitutes two major scales: unresolved states of mind and unusual beliefs (Main, van IJzendoorn, & Hesse, 1993; Sagi, van IJzendoorn, Joels, & Scharf, 2002). When compared to survivors carrying the short DRD4 allele, those carrying the long allele also showed more LRM on the AAI and (marginally significant) higher dissociation scores on the Dissociative Experiences Scale (DES) which assesses the frequency of dissociative experiences (Carlson & Putnam, 1993). All these findings suggest that the short DRD4 allele moderates the negative effects of trauma.

Second Generation We also explored "under-the-skin" effects for the second generation, and in phase 2, we collected cortisol and stress reactivity cortisol from the mothers as well. When we compared the second generation with the control group, we found that they did not show elevated levels of daily saliva cortisol secretion, and that the daughters of survivors and the daughters of controls showed similar curves in cortisol reactivity. Thus, overall, cortisol reactivity to stress did not show secondary traumatization effects (Fridman et al., 2012).

Inspired by the findings of two studies, we also explored whether the effects of traumatic experiences in childhood are detectable in offspring only under highly stressful life circumstances. In one study (Solomon, Kotler, & Mikulincer, 1988), soldiers who were children of Holocaust survivors exhibited more markers of long-term combat reactions after the 1982 Lebanon War—which was an extreme life event for all combat soldiers—than did soldiers without a Holocaust background. The second study (Baider et al. 2000) found that patients with breast cancer—by all means a very stressful situation—who were children of Holocaust survivors, exhibited more extreme psychological distress than did patients with breast cancer without a Holocaust background. Along similar line, we also found a significant group × dissociation interaction in the second generation (Van IJzendoorn, Fridman, Bakermans-Kranenburg, & Sagi-Schwartz, 2013). Specifically, the children of Holocaust survivors showed lower daily cortisol secretion only when their surviving parents displayed greater dissociation.

We can conclude that in the case of genocidal trauma, primary traumatization gets under the skin, but secondary traumatization appears to be restricted to adult children whose parents showed more intense levels of dissociation. Therefore, in the second generation, the absence of differences in response to stress between adult offspring of Holocaust survivors and controls corresponds to meta-analytic findings. Although the survivors display posttraumatic symptoms, unbiased samples show no evidence that they transmitted the trauma to their children. Cortisol levels confirm this conclusion. Thus, the Holocaust, and genocide in general, leave their imprint on the behavior and psychology of survivors for many years after the traumatic event, but there is no cross-generational transmission as revealed by cortisol reaction, except under circumstances of extreme stress.

Posttraumatic Growth

Prosocial Propensities We also explored the positive side of the coin. That is, some scholars have raised the possibility of altruism born of suffering (ABS) (Staub & Vollhardt, 2008), where individuals who have experienced profound suffering may become particularly motivated to help others, not despite their adverse experiences but precisely because of them. Others have suggested that altruism can be viewed as one possible manifestation of posttraumatic growth (Tedeshi & Calhoun, 2004). Based on findings concerning the patterns of communication about the Holocaust in families (Wiseman et al., 2002), we examined patterns of involvement with the mother's Holocaust background (Alkalay, Sagi-Schwartz, & Wiseman, 2015). We identified two groups: those with high verbal knowledge of the Holocaust (HVKH; $n=20$) and those with low verbal knowledge, indeed, silence (LVKH; $n=22$). We also included into the analysis those with no Holocaust background ($n=36$) and assessed empathy and helping behavior (Alkalay et al. 2015). We did not find attachment classification to be significantly associated with empathy toward mothers in distress or with helping mothers in need. But, we found that communication pattern mattered: Daughters with HVKH were significantly more empathic and helping than controls with no Holocaust background and also than those with LVKH.

Life-Expectancy In a different study with national-based data (Sagi-Schwartz, Bakermans-Kranenburg, Linn, van IJzendoorn, 2013), we explored whether surviving genocidal experiences, like the Holocaust, may lead to shorter life expectancy. This might be the initial expectation given that most survivors not only suffered psychosocial trauma but also malnutrition, restriction in hygienic and sanitary facilities, and lack of preventive medical and health services, with potentially damaging effects for later health and life expectancy. Therefore, in a population-based, retrospective cohort study of the Holocaust, based on the entire population of immigrants from Poland to Israel ($N = 55{,}220$), we explored whether genocidal survivors have a higher risk to die younger than comparisons without such background. Data were derived from the population-wide official database of the National Insurance Institute of Israel for all immigrants from Poland, 4–20 years of age, when the World War II Holocaust started (1939). Those who immigrated to Israel between 1945 and 1950 comprised the Holocaust group and those immigrated before 1939 comprised the comparison group, that is, not exposed to the Holocaust. Hazard of death—a statistical term used in epidemiology and biostatistics—was derived by a Cox regression showing that the risk of death was reduced by 6.5 months for Holocaust survivors compared to non-Holocaust comparisons. More specifically, the lower hazard of death was most substantial in males who were at the onset of the Holocaust between 10–15 years of age (adolescents) and 16–20 years of age (late adolescents and emerging adults), namely for the adolescent group, the life expectancy of Holocaust survivors was increased with 10 months, and for the late adolescent and emerging adult group it was increased with 18 months. In other words, we found that against all odds, as most literature might not suggest, genocidal survivors were likely to live longer and not shorter. As for females, it appears that their usual survival advantage (Leon, 2011) compared to the males sustained itself across all age cohorts, but this advantage was not increased by their Holocaust experiences, namely we did not find a difference in life expectancy between female Holocaust and non-Holocaust survivors. We suggested two explanations for the finding that male survivors live longer: Differential mortality during the Holocaust and posttraumatic growth associated with protective factors in Holocaust survivors or in their environment after World War II (for more details, see Sagi-Schwartz et al. 2013).

Conclusion and Future Directions

In this chapter, we have addressed two global goals: First, examining the debilitating effects of catastrophic trauma, separation, and loss in the Holocaust context; second uncovering untold reserves of human stamina and resilience. We have shown that Holocaust survivors continue to show signs of having been traumatized, even 70 years after the event, but at the same time, they were not impaired in other adaptation measures. The second and third generations, however, are doing well in all domains, with one exception of the second generation doing less well only under circumstances of extreme stress. Moreover, daughters of Holocaust child survivors who reported high verbal knowledge of the Holocaust in their family demonstrated elevated expressions of empathy and more prosocial behavior toward their mother, and they invested more time in psychological support for their mother than did participants who reported low verbal knowledge of the Holocaust in their family or those who had no Holocaust background. The study suggests that the psychological gains of open family communication patterns regarding the Holocaust can be discussed in the context of posttraumatic growth resulting in positive outcomes in second generation, namely elevated levels of prosocial propensities. The notion of posttraumatic growth was also used to provide an explanatory model for the surprising finding showing that Holocaust survivors have long life expectancy than those without such an experience, which of course, goes against all odds.

The various findings reviewed in this chapter attest to signs of resilience on the part of child survivors, and decades later, many are able to cope effectively with the consequences of exposure to inhumane trauma and loss. Holocaust survivors may have been able to protect their offspring from their awful war experiences, although they themselves still suffer from the effects of the Holocaust. The possible explanations of this remarkable resilience are yet to be studied. We attempted to provide some preliminary interpretations and explanations for such resilience, and the question remains intriguing, especially with regard to lack of transmission across generations.

Future studies may further investigate the underlying mechanisms of protective and risk factors of developing posttraumatic symptoms after extreme experiences. We proposed that normative families who experienced the Holocaust have several characteristics that may alleviate the outcomes that we observe when adversity takes place within the family. One is associated with a solid, secure, emotional infrastructure prior to the Holocaust time and prior to separation and loss. Another attribute associated with such normative families is that not always had been there personal experiences or witnessing of traumatizing events. We know about many families who hid in various locations, and for some time, they were even still united while escaping and hiding. Also, and not less important, is the fact that the trauma was not inflicted by parents or trusted attachment figures but by brutal inhumane agents from outside the family boundaries. Moreover, we also proposed that we should explore the role of social supports and expressed legitimacy for prolonged grief that may include elements such as support systems, collective national identity, and safe feeling against anti-Semitism (Solomon & Chaitin, 2007), search for meaning and hope with the new generation (Frankl 1997), fellow-survivors resources, public Holocaust memorials, and continued bond with the deceased parent (Silverman & Nickman, 1996). We hypothesized that all these could produce a strong feeling of hope and to give rise to posttraumatic growth. Other possible mechanisms may be associated with what reside in the epigenetics of trauma (McGowan et al., 2009) or in gene–environment interactions underlying the emergence of posttraumatic stress reactions (Belsky & Pluess, 2013). All these set of explanations await further scientific inquiry, and in future studies one is advised to follow the proposed heterogeneity in outcomes for those experiencing trauma (Bonanno & Mancini, 2012).

Acknowledgments The research projects on which this chapter is based involved the active engagement and contribution of the following coworkers: Sarit Alkalay, Efrat Barel, Ayala Fridman, Tirtsa Joels, Nina Koren-Karie, Shai Linn, Miri Scharf, and Hadas Wiseman (University of Haifa, Israel); Marian J. Bakermans-Kranenburg and Marinus H. van IJzendoorn (Leiden University, The Netherlands); Karin Grossmann and Klaus E. Grossmann (Regensburg University, Germany).

This chapter was made possible thanks to the author's tenure as a Phyllis Greenberg Heideman and Richard D. Heideman Fellow, Center for Advanced Holocaust Studies, United States Holocaust Memorial Museum (Washington DC, USA).

References

Ainsworth, M. D. S., Blehar, M. C., Waters, E., & Wall, S. (1978). *Patterns of attachment: A psychological study of the strange situation*. Hillsdale: Erlbaum.

Alkalay, S., Sagi-Schwartz, A., & Wiseman, H. (2015). *Pro-social orientation towards mothers in adult daughters of Holocaust child-survivors*. Manuscript submitted for publication.

Baider, L., Peretz, T., Hadani, P. E., Perry, S., Avramov, R., & De Nour, A. K. (2000). Transmission of response to trauma? Second generation Holocaust survivors' reaction to cancer. *American Journal of Psychiatry, 157,* 904–910.

Barel, E., van IJzendoorn, M. H., Sagi-Schwartz, A., & Bakermans-Kranenburg, M. J. (2010). Surviving the Holocaust: A meta-analysis of the long-term sequelae of a genocide. *Psychological Bulletin, 136,* 677–698.

Bar-On, D., Eland, J., Kleber, R.J., Krell, R., Moore, Y., Sagi, A., et al. (1998). Multigenerational perspectives of coping with the Holocaust experience: On the developmental sequelae of trauma across generations. *International Journal of Behavioral Development, 22,* 315–338.

Belsky, J., & Pluess, M. (2013). Beyond risk, resilience and dysregulation: Phenotypic plasticity and human development. *Development and Psychopathology, 25,* 1243–1261.

Bonanno, G. A., & Mancini, A. D. (2012). Beyond resilience and PTSD: Mapping the heterogeneity of responses to potential trauma. *Psychological Trauma, 4,* 74–83.

Bowlby J. (1984). *Attachment and Loss, Vol I: Attachment* (2nd ed.). London: Pelican.

Bowlby, J. (1988). *A secure base*. New York: Basic Books.

Carlson, E. B., & Putnam, F. W. (1993). An update on the dissociative experiences scale. *Dissociation, 6,* 16–27.

Carmil, D., & Breznitz, S. (1991). Personaltrauma and world view—Are extremely stressful experiences related to political attitudes, religion beliefs, and future orientation? *Journal of Traumatic Stress, 4,* 393–405.

Cicchetti, D., Toth, S. L., & Maughan, A. (2000). An ecological-transactional model of child maltreatment. In A. Sameroff, M. Lewis & S. Miller (Eds.), *Handbook of developmental psychopathology* (2nd ed., pp. 689–722). New York: Kluwer Academic/Plenum Publishers.

De Quervain, D. J. F., Kolassa, I. T., Ertl, V., Onyut, P. L., Neuner, F., Elbert, T., et al. (2007). A deletion variant of the a2b-adrenoceptor is related to emotional memory in Europeans and Africans. *Nature Neuroscience, 10,* 1137–1139.

Frankl, V. E. (1997). *Man's search for ultimate meaning*. New York: In-sight Books/Plenum.

Fridman, A., Bakermans-Kranenburg, M. J., Sagi-Schwartz, A., & van IJzendoorn, M. H. (2011). Coping in old age with extreme childhood trauma: Aging Holocaust survivors and their offspring facing new challenges. *Aging and Mental Health, 15,* 232–242.

Fridman, A., Bakermans-Kranenburg, M. J., Sagi-Schwartz, A., & van IJzendoorn, M. H. (2012). Genetic moderation of cortisol secretion in Holocaust survivors: The role of ADRA2B. *International Journal of Behavioral Development, 36,* 79–84.

Hesse, E. (1999). The adult attachment interview: Historical and current perspectives. In J. Cassidy & P. Shaver (Eds.), *Handbook of attachment: Theory, research and clinical applications* (pp. 395–433). New York: Guilford Press.

Hesse, E. (2008). The adult attachment interview: Protocol, method of analysis, and empirical studies. In J. Cassidy & P. Shaver (Eds.), *Handbook of attachment: Theory, research and clinical applications* (2nd ed., pp. 552–598). New York: Guilford Press.

Hesse, E., & Main, M. (1999). Second generation effects of unresolved trauma in nonmaltreating parents: Dissociation, frightening and threatening parental behavior. *Psychoanalytic Inquiry, 19,* 481–540.

Horowitz, M. J., Wilner, N., & Alvarez, W. (1979). Impact of event scale: A measure of subjective stress. *Psychosomatic Medicine, 4,* 209–218.

Keilson, H. (1992). *Sequential traumatization in children.* Jerusalem: Magnes.

Koren-Karie, N., Sagi-Schwartz, A., & Joels, J. (2003). Absence of attachment representations (AAR) in the adult years: The emergence of a new AAI classification in catastrophically traumatized Holocaust child survivors. *Journal of Attachment and Human Development, 5,* 381–397.

Leon, D. A. (2011). Trends in European life expectancy: A salutary view. *International Journal of Epidemiology, X,* 1–7.

Main, M., & Solomon, J. (1990). Procedures for identifying infants as disorganized/disoriented during the Ainsworth Strange Situation. In M. T. Greenberg, D. Cicchetti & E. M. Cummings (Eds.), *Attachment in the preschool years: Theory, research and intervention* (pp. 121–160). Chicago: University of Chicago Press.

Main, M., van IJzendoorn, M. H., & Hesse, E. (1993, March). Unresolved/unclassifiable responses to the Adult Attachment Interview: Predictable from unresolved states and anomalous beliefs in the Berkeley–Leiden Adult Attachment Questionnaire. Paper presented at *Adolescent attachment organization: Findings from the BLAAQ self- reportinventory, and relations to absorption and dissociation.* Symposium conducted at the 60th Anniversary Meeting of the Society for Research in Child Development, New Orleans, LA.

McGowan, P., Sasaki, A., D'Alessio, A. C., Dymov, S., Labonte′, B., Szyf, M., et al. (2009). Epigenetic regulation of the glucocorticoid receptor in human brain associates with childhood abuse. *Nature Neuroscience, 12,* 342–348.

Sagi-Schwartz, A., & Aviezer, O. (2005). Correlates of attachment to multiple caregivers in Kibbutz children from birth to emerging adulthood: The Haifa Longitudinal Study. In K. E. Grossmann, K. Grossmann & E. Waters (Eds.), *Attachment from infancy to adulthood* (pp. 165–197). New York: Guilford Press.

Sagi, A., van IJzendoorn, M. H., Joels, T., & Scharf, M. (2002). Disorganized reasoning in Holocaust survivors: An attachment perspective. *American Journal of Orthopsychiatry, 72,* 194–203.

Sagi-Schwartz, A., van IJzendoorn, M. H., Grossmann, K. E., Joels, T., Grossmann, K., Scharf, M., et al. (2003). Attachment and traumatic stress in female Holocaust child survivors and their daughters, *American Journal of Psychiatry, 160,* 1086–1092.

Sagi-Schwartz, A., van IJzendoorn, M. H., & Bakermans-Kranenburg, M. J. (2008). Does intergenerational transmission of trauma skip a generation? No meta-analytic evidence for tertiary traumatization with third generation of Holocaust survivors. *Attachment and Human Development, 10,* 105–121.

Sagi-Schwartz A., Bakermans-Kranenburg M. J., Linn S., & van IJzendoorn, M. H. (2013). Against all odds: Genocidal trauma is associated with longer life-expectancy of the survivors. *PLoS One, 8*(7), e69179. doi:10.1371/journal.pone.0069179.

Silverman P. R., & Nickman S. L. (1996). Children's construction of their dead parents. In D. Klass, P. R. Silverman & L. Nickman (Eds.), *Continuing bonds: New understandings of grief* (pp. 73–86). Washington, D.C.: Taylor & Francis.

Solomon, Z., & Chaitin, J. (2007). Childhood in the shadow of the Holocaust, survived children and second generation. Tel Aviv: Hakibbutz Hameuchad [Hebrew].

Solomon, Z., Kotler, M., & Mikulincer, M. (1988). Combat related post-traumatic stress disorder among 2nd-generation Holocaust survivors—Preliminary findings. *American Journal of Psychiatry, 145,* 865–868.

Staub, E., & Vollhardt, J. (2008). Altruism born of suffering: The roots of caring and helping after victimization and other trauma. *American Journal of Orthopsychiatry, 78,* 267–280.

Tedeshi, R. G., & Calhoun, L. G. (2004). *Posttraumatic growth: Conceptual foundation and empirical evidence.* Philadelphia: Lawrence Erlbaum Associates.

Van IJzendoorn, M. H., Bakermans-Kranenburg, M. J., & Sagi-Schwartz, A. (2003). Are children of Holocaust survivors less well-adapted? No meta-analytic evidence for secondary traumatization. *Journal of Traumatic Stress, 16,* 459–469.

Van IJzendoorn, M. H., & Bakermans-Kranenburg, M. J. (2009). Attachment security and disorganization in maltreating families and orphanages. In: R. E. Tremblay, M. Boivin & R. D. Peters (Eds.), *Encyclopedia on early childhood development* [online] (pp. 1–7). Montreal: Centre of Excellence for Early Childhood Development and Strategic Knowledge Cluster on Early Child Development.

Van IJzendoorn, M. H., & Sagi-Schwartz, A. (2008). Cross cultural patterns of attachment: Universal and contextual dimensions. In J. Cassidy & P. R. Shaver (Eds.), *Handbook of attachment* (2nd ed., pp. 880–905). NewYork: Guilford Press.

Van IJzendoorn, M. H., Fridman, A., Bakermans-Kranenburg, M. J., & Sagi-Schwartz, A. (2013). Holocaust survivors' dissociation moderates offspring level of cortisol. *Journal of Loss and Trauma, 18,* 64–80.

Wiseman, H., Barber, J. P., Raz, A., Yam, I., Foltz, C., & Livne-Snir, S. (2002). Parental communication of Holocaust experiences and interpersonal patterns in offspring of Holocaust survivors. *International Journal of Behavioral Development, 26,* 371–381.

Part II
Consequences of Trauma Exposure

Chapter 9
Physiological Consequences: Early Hardship and Health Across the Life Span

Jennifer N. Morey and Suzanne C. Segerstrom

Introduction

A substantial body of research accumulated over the past three decades provides strong evidence that early childhood adversity (ECA) has a detrimental impact on physical health and health-promoting behaviors across the life span. However, there are challenges for trauma researchers reviewing this literature. First, as ECA research is rapidly expanding across multiple disciplines, it can be difficult to synthesize across studies to identify how and under what conditions ECA impacts physical health. Second, inconsistency in the operationalization and measurement of ECA leads to difficulties in comparisons across studies and outcomes. Finally, even though some studies do include developmental factors, many do not examine timing, duration, cohort, or other considerations that may impact the trauma–health relation. In this chapter, we broadly summarize the impact of childhood trauma across several domains of physiological health throughout the life span, with a focus on the long-reaching implications into adulthood. This is examined first in terms of the specific health outcomes tied to ECA and then in relation to ECA's impact on health-related behaviors. Measurement trends and individual differences relevant to ECA are briefly discussed, and future research directions are suggested.

J. N. Morey (✉) · S. C. Segerstrom
Department of Psychology, University of Kentucky, 115 Kastle Hall, Lexington, KY 40506-0044, USA
e-mail: jennifer.morey@uky.edu

S. C. Segerstrom
e-mail: segerstrom@uky.edu

K. E. Cherry (ed.), *Traumatic Stress and Long-Term Recovery*,
DOI 10.1007/978-3-319-18866-9_9

Overview and Definitions

ECA is a broad construct that lacks a clear conceptualization and measurement strategy (Wegman & Stetler, 2009). In many studies, examples are provided of what constitutes ECA exposure (e.g., physical abuse) rather than operationalizing ECA per se. A recent critical review posited that ECA experiences include those that are "harmful, chronic, distressing, cumulative, and varying in severity" (Kalmakis & Chandler, 2014, p. 2). The American Psychiatric Association (APA, 2013) defines traumatic experiences as involving either experiences or threats of death, sexual violence, and/or severe injury. These experiences can occur to the individual or to others (i.e., witnessing or hearing about the event or being exposed to its aftermath). While some aspects of ECA as studied do fit this conceptualization (such as physical and sexual abuse), other types of ECA align less clearly with this definition of trauma.

Despite a general lack of consistency, many studies purporting to measure ECA examine common factors, including abuse (physical, sexual, or emotional) or neglect (physical or emotional). Other oft-measured stressors include parental divorce or loss, living with a substance-abusing or mentally ill parent, or witnessing violence. The lack of positive experiences, supportive relationships, and nurturance may also be considered a subtype of ECA. Finally, poverty or low socioeconomic status (SES) is widely studied and is highly predictive of health, though SES is less often studied in conjunction with other forms of adversity. Most past studies have aggregated exposures to examine their cumulative influence, which is an empirically supported strategy (Anda et al., 2006; Felitti et al., 1998). However, recent work has called for a micro-level assessment of early life stressors, to better elucidate causal mechanisms in how stress affects long-term health (Odgers & Jaffee, 2013).

A potentially useful but relatively uncommon approach to measuring ECA is to categorize stressors into either abuses or adversities (Odgers & Jaffee, 2013). Abuse is more commonly measured but occurs less often, while adversities are generally more common and encompass a wide range of proximal and distal stressors that can impact children's development. Abuses and adversities might be conceptualized as degrees of trauma. For example, physical punishment is a common adversity and is related to but less severe than physical abuse, and therefore, the former has similar but less extreme effects on health than the latter (Afifi, Brownridge, Cox, & Sareen, 2006). In addition, abuses may be more acute (although certainly not in all cases) while adversities are often chronic or systemic in nature (Odgers & Jaffee, 2013). Another possible distinction might be that abuses often function on the micro-level, with one or a small number of perpetrators committing acts specifically against the child. Adversities are often macro-level problems that involve many players and are tied to the economic conditions and structural inequalities present in society. Background stress which compounds the effects of other stressors may prove analogous here, with chronic adversities compounding the effects of abuses. Frequent adversity may also make abuses more likely to occur or more impactful when they do occur (due to lack of support from close others associated with adversity). Therefore, it is likely that abuses and adversities are conceptually distinct and interact with one another to predict physical health in adulthood.

ECA exposure has been found both prospectively and retrospectively to relate to a range of physical health issues. In a meta-analysis linking ECA and physical health, a small-to-medium association was found across multiple domains of health (Wegman & Stetler, 2009). In past studies, ECA has been conceptualized both as a main effect impacting physical health and as an indirect effect via its influence on health behaviors. Inclusion of all literature linking ECA and physical health and health behaviors is beyond the scope of the present review; however, more comprehensive reviews into specific body systems or diseases are available (e.g., Coelho, Viola, Walss-Bass, Brietzke, & Grassi-Oliveira, 2014; Wegman & Stetler, 2009). In the sections that follow, we briefly summarize the state of empirical knowledge across several dimensions of health and health behaviors to illustrate the far-reaching effects of this type of trauma.

Links to Physiological Health

The Hypothalamic–Pituitary–Adrenal Axis

ECA exposure, like exposure to other types of stressors, stimulates the hypothalamic–pituitary–adrenal (HPA) axis to respond to the threat and ultimately help the body maintain homeostasis. In many studies, the HPA axis has been identified as one mechanism that can explain how stress "gets under the skin" to impact health and disease (Miller, Chen, & Zhou, 2007). To cope with threats, the HPA axis releases hormones (glucocorticoids), including the oft-studied cortisol. Cortisol has an important regulatory function across several body systems, including the metabolic, central nervous, and immune systems. Typically, cortisol is released in response to an immediate stressor and then subsides once the stressor has passed. However, in situations that are plagued by stress (such as exposure to low-SES or chronic abuse), the cortisol stress response does not subside because the stressor itself does not subside (see Chap. 10, this volume, for a related discussion). While this may be adaptive in that it allows the individual to survive and cope with environmental demands, chronic stress exposure can have a disruptive effect on the body. For example, chronic stress has been shown to dysregulate cortisol including leading to elevated or blunted cortisol patterns, as well as alterations in response to specific stressors or challenges. This dysregulation can lead to organ or tissue damage as well as to increasing disease risk across multiple body systems. In those exposed to ECA, evidence for disruption of cortisol output across the life span and in response to myriad early stressors has been found (e.g., Hunter, Minnis, & Wilson, 2011).

Cumulative Adversity Many researchers aiming to understand the physiological effects of ECA have used a measure of cumulative adversity by counting the types of ECA individuals have experienced (e.g., physical abuse, emotional abuse) and aggregating the exposures for analysis. In these studies, exposure to a larger number of adverse events in childhood has been shown to predict cortisol dysregulation. Cortisol alterations have been found early in the life span in samples of maltreated youth. For example, cortisol secretion levels were elevated (and C-peptide levels lower) in 5-year-old children exposed to high levels of family stress when compared with control children (Carlsson, Frostell, Ludvigsson, & Faresjo, 2014). In a study of young adolescents with and without substantiated ECA histories that examined cortisol reactivity to a social stressor, those exposed to ECA (especially physical or sexual abuse) had a blunted cortisol response when compared with controls (Trickett, Gordis, Peckins, & Susman, in press).

In addition to the disrupted patterns evident in children, cortisol patterns have also been shown to be irregular in adults exposed to ECA. In a large longitudinal study reporting associations between ECA and cortisol in middle-aged adults (Power, Thomas, Li, & Hertzman, 2012), high levels of ECA exposure predicted lower morning cortisol levels, and ECA (especially neglect) predicted lower morning cortisol levels and a less steep decline in cortisol levels for women. Cortisol at 3–4 h post awakening was also elevated for men with three or more ECA exposures compared with those unexposed to ECA. Similarly, Heim and colleagues employed standardized challenges to the HPA axis in a sample of adult women and found that abused women with current depression had blunted adrenocorticotropic hormone (ACTH, another element of the HPA axis) responses, as did depressed women without ECA exposure, when compared with controls. However, abused women that were not depressed had elevated ACTH responses in comparison with controls (Heim, Newport, Bonsall, Miller, & Nemeroff, 2001). Finally, salivary cortisol was examined in a longitudinal sample of older adults, and evidence was found for blunted cortisol stress reactivity for those with ECA exposure coupled with adult psychological distress when compared with non-ECA exposed controls. Higher and more sustained cortisol stress reactivity was also found for those with ECA exposure but little distress (Goldman-Mellor, Hamer, & Steptoe, 2012). These studies suggest that greater ECA exposure, quantified as a count of total exposures, dysregulates (either by elevating or blunting) the cortisol response from childhood through older age. This work also demonstrates the importance of considering psychological factors, including distress, when examining the ECA–cortisol relation.

Independent Effects of Specific Stressors Understanding cortisol patterns in relation to specific ECA stressors, either in isolation from other forms of ECA or as possible independent factors that might be interrelated, is a recent research foci. For example, in a study of young adults, evidence was found for a relation between parental warmth, cortisol, and stress. Specifically, on days marked by higher levels of stress, those who experienced low levels of parental warmth (compared with greater warmth) in childhood had higher cortisol levels (measured as area under the curve or AUC; Hanson & Chen, 2010). Luecken and Appelhans (2006) examined a sample of young adults (some of whom experienced parental loss in childhood) and found that those who had loss coupled with early abuse or conflict had higher mean cortisol levels than those who experienced only parental loss without abuse or did not experience loss. Finally, early emotional abuse has been associated with dampening of cortisol reactivity in adults, even when adjusting for the effects of other forms of ECA (Carpenter et al., 2009). These studies suggest a disrupting effect of ECA on cortisol patterns and indicate that specific factors (or interactions of individual risk factors) may drive this effect. More research to address subtypes of ECA for their unique or interactive effects on cortisol is needed, however, to establish the reliability of outcomes.

Low SES Although low SES has been extensively linked to poorer general health, some studies have specifically examined how poverty in childhood impacts cortisol levels. In a sample of children followed for 2 years, AUC cortisol output increased over time for low-SES children but not for high SES children. This relation was partially mediated by other risk factors, including children's reports of chaos in the family (Chen, Cohen, & Miller, 2010). In another study children (aged 6–10) from low-SES backgrounds had higher morning cortisol levels than high SES children, but this difference was no longer evident at the transition to high school (Lupien, King, Meaney, & McEwen, 2001). In a sample of adolescents, lower neighborhood SES was related to lower afternoon cortisol levels even when controlling for family-level SES (Chen & Paterson, 2006). Despite these relations, evidence linking cumulative SES and cortisol has generally been mixed (Dowd, Simanek, & Aiello, 2009). In one examination of childhood SES in relation to adult cortisol levels (i.e., 45-min post awakening, 3-h after, and AUC), it was found that childhood SES may impact adult cortisol patterns largely through its relation with adult SES (Li, Power, Kelly, Kirschbaum, & Hertzman, 2007). It is possible that low-SES impacts physical health (in this case, cortisol) by making it more likely that individuals will be exposed to other types of risk (i.e., adversity or abuse; Evans & Kim, 2010). This idea will require further testing by integrating SES and abuse/adversity into studies concurrently.

Summary The literature linking ECA and HPA axis functioning (specifically cortisol patterns) demonstrates the many ways that cortisol can be dysregulated by adverse early environments. As demonstrated, there is evidence for both HPA hyperreactivity and hyporeactivity in those exposed to ECA. In a meta-analytic review of the HPA axis and broader stress literature, a negative relation was described between the length of time since the stressor began and HPA activity, indicating that cortisol levels (including morning cortisol, ACTH, and other markers) may be higher in immediate response to a stressor but below the normal level after the trauma has passed (Miller et al., 2007). This pattern was also reported in the empirical ECA literature. Specifically, Trickett and colleagues examined nonstress morning cortisol in a sample of abused and control females through childhood, adolescence, and into early adulthood, and they found that cortisol growth rates increased more slowly for those exposed to ECA, and that this pattern began with attenuation in adolescence (Trickett, Noll, Susman, Shenk, & Putnam, 2010). However, when cortisol was examined proximally to the abuse (i.e., closer to the time of disclosure), evidence for higher secretion and a less steep slope over time was found, suggesting that initially those abused were hyperreactive and then become hyporeactive over time. Although not all studies exhibit these patterns (i.e., higher cortisol levels or reactivity in ECA-exposed children and attenuated cortisol in ECA-exposed adults), it still provides one possible example of how ECA's effects on health may change over time. SES may also function in this manner, with those exposed to poverty for a short time exhibiting higher cortisol levels proximal to exposure or greater cortisol reactivity to stress, and those exposed for a longer duration showing lower cortisol levels and blunted cortisol reactivity to stress. Therefore, these findings may help not only to bridge disparate findings in the ECA–cortisol literature but also speak to the importance of considering developmental trajectories and of prospective, longitudinal studies in general when assessing the impact of ECA on HPA axis functioning.

Immune Functioning

When exposed to stress or pathogens, the body mounts an inflammatory response, which differs by stressor characteristics, including duration. Similar to the cortisol response, acute inflammation is often beneficial whereas chronic inflammation (like that associated with adversity or poverty) can have a substantial adverse effect on bodily systems. Chronic stress can lead to heightened systemic inflammation (also referred to as a pro-inflammatory phenotype) that is well recognized as a major hallmark of disease, frailty, and aging (Ershler & Keller, 2000). To understand how ECA exposure is related to immune functioning, many studies have examined the relation between ECA and inflammatory markers including the cytokines interleukin 6 (IL-6), tumor necrosis factor-alpha (TNF-α), and C-reactive protein (CRP). In addition, studies have quantified antibody responses to latent viruses (e.g., Epstein–Barr virus (EBV) and the herpes simplex virus) as a marker of immune system functioning and examined these responses in relation to ECA experience. Higher antibodies are a marker of more latent virus reactivation, worse cellular control of the virus, or both. For more information on the immune system and its relation to stress, see Segerstrom and Miller (2004).

Cumulative Adversity Researchers measuring ECA in terms of cumulative exposure have found evidence that ECA negatively impacts immune system functioning. In children, dysregulation of the immune system (i.e., low spontaneous immune activity as well as an increased immune response to in vitro stimulation) has been found in 5-year-olds exposed to high levels of stress (Carlsson et al., 2014) and in 12-year-old depressed victims of maltreatment who exhibited a higher mean elevation in their CRP levels when compared with control children (Danese et al., 2011), suggesting that ECA's effects on inflammatory markers are evidenced early in the life span. Cumulative ECA has also been shown to predict immune response in adults. In a longitudinal study, childhood maltreatment was associated with higher inflammatory markers (CRP, fibrinogen, and white blood cells) in adults, even after controlling for health behaviors, current stress, and other indicators of early life risk (Danese, Pariante, Caspi, Taylor, & Poulton, 2007). Higher levels of several inflammatory markers (IL-6, fibrinogen, soluble intercellular adhesion molecule-1, and endothelial leukocyte adhesion molecule-1) were also predicted by early adversity exposure in African-American (but not Caucasian) middle-aged adults, though some relations were attenuated by health behaviors, depression, and later-life stressors (Slopen et al., 2010). In addition, in a sample of adult colorectal cancer patients, ECA exposure was linked to higher TNFα and CRP, yet no relation was found in patients with head and neck cancer (Archer, Hutchison, Dorudi, Stansfeld, & Korszun, 2012). Cumulative ECA has also been shown to relate to the manner in which individuals respond to other stressors in adulthood. Specifically, child maltreatment is associated with adults' heightened IL-6 in response to a social stressor (Carpenter et al., 2010) as well as in response to daily stressors (Gouin, Glaser, Malarkey, Beversdorf, & Kiecolt-Glaser, 2012). In sum, cumulative ECA exposure is associated with immune disruption in children and adults, demonstrating that greater exposure to adversity is a risk factor for the pro-inflammatory phenotype.

Independent Effects of Specific Stressors The immune response in relation to specific ECA stressors is another research foci. For example, researchers disaggregated types of ECA and found that women with breast cancer who had a history of emotional neglect or emotional abuse had lower levels of natural killer cell activity (NKCA, the cytotoxic capacity of cells that may kill some kinds of cancer cells) at baseline that persisted over a 9-month follow-up. In addition, those with lower levels of physical neglect had a more pronounced decline in their IL-6 levels over the study period (Witek Janusek, Tell, Albuquerque, & Mathews, 2013). In a study of the independent and interactive effects of abuse and adversity in older adults, experience of at least one type of abuse or of multiple adversities also predicted higher IL-6 levels (Kiecolt-Glaser et al., 2011). Even though independent effects of ECA subtypes are not measured as often as cumulative exposure, measuring ECA in a more sophisticated or complete manner may help to elucidate the complex associations between ECA and inflammatory markers.

Low SES Experience of low childhood SES has also been shown to predict disrupted immune functioning in several studies. First, in a large sample of children aged 6–16 years, income under the poverty line was shown to predict higher cytomegalovirus antibody titers (CMV, a herpes virus) in CMV-positive children (Dowd, Palermo, & Aiello, 2012). Lower SES in childhood predicted higher levels of fibrinogen in a sample of adults, even when controlling for adult SES (Brunner et al., 1996). Finally, Slopen and colleagues considered effects of timing and frequency of exposure as well as SES and adversity in tandem. They measured EBV antibody titers in a sample of young adults. They found some evidence that low-SES as well as sexual abuse occurring 10+ times was associated with higher EBV antibody titers, and that among those who were physically abused, those exposed in the preschool period also had higher EBV antibody titers than those exposed later (Slopen, McLaughlin, Dunn, & Koenen, 2013). These studies suggest that the well-identified link between low SES and physical health may in part be attributable to the immune dysregulation associated with growing up in poverty.

Associations with Health Behaviors Other researchers have conceptualized health-related behaviors (smoking, alcohol consumption, and overeating/overweight) as potential mediators of the ECA and inflammation relationship (e.g., Raposa, Bower, Hammen, Najman, & Brennan, 2014), demonstrating the complexity in determining the precise mechanisms linking ECA, overall health, and inflammatory markers. For example, low-SES and risky family environment were associated with higher CRP in a sample of young adults through associations with BMI as well as psychological functioning (Taylor, Lehman, Kiefe, & Seeman, 2006). In a recent study examining the association between low-SES and CRP levels in young adults, BMI and smoking mediated several associations between SES indicators and CRP differentially by race and sex (Brummett et al., 2013). In a sample of adult women, ECA was directly associated with elevated overall CRP levels as well as greater increases in CRP over a 7-year period, but multiple indicators of ECA were also associated with CRP indirectly via their association with BMI (Matthews, Chang, Thurston, & Bromberger, 2014). Finally, low childhood SES predicted heightened inflammatory markers (e.g., CRP, fibrinogen), yet these associations were mediated in Caucasians by BMI and smoking (among other factors, such as cholesterol; Pollitt et al., 2007). Therefore, extrapolating from the empirical evidence linking ECA with markers of inflammation, it is possible that ECA has a direct effect on immune dysregulation that begins early in life and that is exacerbated by health-compromising behaviors, and it eventually leads to additional physical ailments later in life. This is consistent with Miller, Chen, and Parker's (2011) Biological Embedding of Childhood Adversity model, which posits that ECA permanently alters immune cells to have chronic pro-inflammatory profiles, which are then further heightened by behaviors, ultimately contributing to the development of disease over time.

Summary The literature linking ECA exposure and immune disruption across the life span is robust, suggesting associations between ECA and altered immunity in children and adults that may occur in part through health behaviors. Utilizing different measurement approaches and populations, researchers have demonstrated that adverse experiences negatively impact several indices of the immune system, leading to higher systemic pro-inflammatory cytokines as well as to indications of latent virus activation. Given the well-identified health problems associated with these immune alterations, interventions targeting multiple forms of ECA are likely to have a major impact on physical health overall.

Cardiovascular Health

ECA has been identified as a powerful predictor of multiple indicators of clinical and subclinical cardiovascular disease (CVD). Although rates of death from CVD are on the decline overall, it is still implicated in a substantial number of deaths each year in the USA (Go et al., 2014), so even minor increases in one's risk profile attributable to ECA are likely to have major health consequences. Components of the cardiovascular system include the heart, blood, and blood vessels, and stress from

ECA can impede functioning of each of these components. Researchers have examined multiple indicators and risk factors of CVD, including atherosclerosis, ischemic heart disease, lipid levels, blood pressure/hypertension, heart rate, myocardial infarctions, and carotid intima-media thickness (CIMT). More detailed descriptions of these risk factors are available elsewhere (e.g., Wilson et al., 1998). Heightened inflammatory markers have also been associated with CVD risk (Pearson et al., 2003) demonstrating how ECA-based disruptions in one bodily system can affect other systems as well.

Cumulative Adversity As is the case with many studies examining health effects of ECA, the most common method of examining the impact of early adversity on cardiovascular risk has been through the use of cumulative adversity measures. In one study of children aged 11–14 years, it was found that parent-reported trauma exposure of four or more events was related to several risk factors, including elevated resting heart rate (Pretty, O'Leary, Cairney, & Wade, 2013). In a large-scale study of ten countries, experiencing three or more adversities in childhood predicted hypertension in adulthood, even when accounting for psychological risk factors (i.e., depression, anxiety; Stein et al., 2010). Exposure to ECA has been found to increase risk of ischemic heart disease in adults in a dose-response manner (Dong et al., 2004). In a recent study on blood pressure (among other markers for metabolic syndrome) in adults with mood disorders, greater exposure to ECA predicted higher systolic and diastolic blood pressure, as well as lower high-density lipoprotein (HDL, a potentially protective factor) cholesterol levels (McIntyre et al., 2012). In another study, lipid levels related to ECA in minority and low-SES adults, though results only held for males. Specifically, males with a history of child abuse had lower HDL levels and a lower HDL/low-density lipoproteins (LDL) ratio (Spann et al., 2013).

Other works have examined the impact of health behaviors on the link between ECA and cardiovascular risk. In a recent study, Loucks et al. (2014) found that experiencing a "risky family" environment, characterized by conflict and low levels of nurturance, was associated with increased CIMT (a measure of atherosclerosis) in a sample of Caucasian (but not African-American) adults, though some relations differed when individual items tapping ECA were examined. Cigarette smoking was found to mediate this association. In another recent study, ECA (cumulative exposure and child maltreatment specifically) predicted acute myocardial infarction (AMI) in a large sample of age-heterogeneous adults, but this association was again mediated by smoking (Morton, Mustillo, & Ferraro, 2014). Therefore, the available evidence suggests that the experience of higher levels of cumulative ECA has a detrimental impact on multiple indices of cardiovascular functioning, but may function at least in part through health behaviors.

Independent Effects of Specific Stressors Although the majority of studies reviewed report ECA in terms of cumulative exposure, other researchers have examined specific factors that may play a role in the development of CVD. For example, Ford and Browning (2014) found that hypertension risk was elevated in a prospective sample of adults who were exposed to violence perpetrated with the use of guns or knives (for men only) or were the victim of a weapons-related crime (women only) during their adolescence. In addition, child physical abuse was found in another study to relate to adult heart disease when controlling for health behaviors, other ECA types, and additional risk factors (Fuller-Thomson, Brennenstuhl, & Frank, 2010). Finally, sexual abuse (i.e., a forced sexual encounter) in childhood was related to greater risk for MI when controlling for multiple social and health risk factors in adult men but not women (Fuller-Thomson, Bejan, Hunter, Grundland, & Brennenstuhl, 2012). Therefore, evidence suggests that examining stressors in isolation may provide additional evidence into the conditions under which ECA affects CVD risk.

Low SES A large body of empirical evidence illuminates the association between poverty in childhood and cardiovascular risk. For example, in a review of the relation between childhood SES and CVD risk, Galobardes, Smith, and Lynch (2006) reported that 80 % of the prospective studies reviewed demonstrated a link between low childhood SES and indicators of CVD. In another review of the literature linking SES and cardiovascular outcomes, experiencing low childhood SES was found to have a modest impact on CVD risk (but was often affected by health behaviors or other risk factors), while experiencing low lifetime SES had a more consistent relation with CVD risk (Pollitt, Rose, & Kaufman, 2005).

Links between early SES and CVD risk have also been reported in other studies. For example, in a large prospective study of children, those raised in a low-SES environment experienced worse cardiovascular health (Poulton et al., 2002). In another study, higher baseline blood pressure as well as change in systolic blood pressure over a 10-year period was found to be predicted by the risky family environment and especially low SES in a sample of adults (Lehman, Taylor, Kiefe, & Seeman, 2009). Heart attack risk was also predicted by early disadvantage (encompassing multiple dimensions of low SES) in a large sample of older adults (O'Rand & Hamil-Luker, 2005). In addition, physicians from low-SES backgrounds had a greater risk of developing coronary heart disease before but not after the age of 50 (Kittleson et al., 2006). Therefore, the available evidence does suggest that low SES in childhood has a modest effect on CVD risk in adulthood.

Summary Overall, despite differences in measurement of ECA and the inclusion of various cardiovascular outcomes, the extant literature in this area suggests an association between ECA and multiple (sub)clinical indicators of CVD. However, there is also evidence that this association is mediated by health behaviors in adults, particularly smoking. More research will be needed in this area to further examine ECA characteristics in relation to risk for CVD, especially at younger ages and with consideration of behavioral and psychological mediators.

Chronic Disease and Disability Prevalence

The prevalence of disability and several chronic diseases has been linked to ECA exposure. In fact, SES has been stated to "influence mortality and morbidity rates in almost every disease" (Calixto & Anaya, 2014, p. 643). In one quantitative review of the literature linking ECA and health (Wegman & Stetler, 2009), it was reported that child abuse predicted numerous health outcomes, with the largest effect sizes found for neurological and musculoskeletal problems. As chronic diseases and disability represent a major health burden, reducing risk for their acquisition or their progression poses a significant public health concern.

Cumulative Maltreatment Cumulative ECA exposure has been shown to predict disease and disability. Felitti et al. (1998) found that people who experienced ECA had a greater risk of reporting lower self-rated health and a dose-response risk of having chronic diseases including cancer, liver disease, heart and lung diseases, and bone fractures. Similarly, Scott et al. (2011) found evidence for a dose-response relation between disease and ECA, in that being exposed to three or more adversities was associated with greater risk of multiple health conditions in adulthood, including heart disease, asthma, arthritis, and diabetes.

ECA has also been found to relate to specific diseases. In a large sample of African-American women, abuse (especially sexual abuse) in childhood, but not adolescence, predicted rates of uterine leiomyomata (also called fibroids, a major cause of hysterectomy; Wise, Palmer, & Rosenberg, 2013). Cumulative ECA exposure predicted lung cancer in adults though this relation was partially attenuated by cigarette smoking (Brown et al., 2010). Chronic fatigue syndrome is also predicted in a graded manner by cumulative ECA exposure (Heim et al., 2006). In a study of adults, McIntyre et al. (2012) did not find evidence to support a relation between ECA exposure and some components of metabolic syndrome. However, in other studies, cumulative ECA exposure has been shown to predict greater metabolic syndrome risk, with adult SES, responses to stress, and health behaviors partially explaining the relation (Lee, Tsenkova, & Carr, 2014). In a recent study, a relation between incident metabolic syndrome and abuse in a sample of adult women was found, but this only held for physical abuse (not sexual or emotional; Midei, Matthews, Chang, & Bromberger, 2013). Not all studies support a relation between ECA exposure and disease prevalence, however. In addition to null findings in some of the reviewed studies of metabolic syndrome, in another study no relation was found between irritable bowel syndrome symptoms in adults and prospectively assessed childhood adversity (Goodwin, White, Hotopf, Stansfeld, & Clark, 2013).

Cumulative ECA has also been linked to disability. In a large sample of adults, ECA exposure was related in a graded manner to higher levels of self-reported disability including limitation in activities or use of assistive devices, even when controlling for physical and mental health (Schüssler-Fiorenza Rose, Xie, & Stineman, in press). Disability weights have also been examined as a measure of health condition severity in adults to calculate the disease burden of childhood adversity and mental illness (Cuijpers et al., 2011), and a larger disability burden was found for cumulative ECA than for all mental illnesses combined. Finally, a link between allostatic load (an indicator of multiple types of functioning, including HPA axis, cardiovascular, and metabolic factors) and ECA has been reported in several studies. In one longitudinal prospective study, allostatic load in adolescence was predicted by ECA exposure, but this association was mediated by smoking (Doan, Dich, & Evans, in press). Higher levels of child abuse and lower levels of parental warmth were also shown to predict multisystem health risks (allostatic load) in adults. An interaction between abuse and warmth was found such that those experiencing low warmth and high abuse had the largest multisystem risk (Carroll et al., 2013). Overall, the available evidence is suggestive that ECA exposure in childhood predicts the development of numerous diseases in adulthood, perhaps in a graded or dose-response manner.

Independent Effects of Specific Stressors Independent effects of subtypes of ECA on disease and disability have also been identified. For example, Greenfield and Marks (2009) quantified nine profiles of early violence exposure in their sample of adults, and they found that participants exposed to both frequent physical and psychological violence (compared with those unexposed to either) had lower self-rated health, a higher number of functional limitations, and a higher number of chronic conditions over a 10-year period. Cuijpers et al. (2011) measured cumulative ECA exposure as it relates to disease, but they also examined individual ECA subtypes. They found that abuse and neglect were the most heavily associated with disability weights, while death of a parent was not independently associated with disease. In a large sample of Swedish adults, experiencing parental death in childhood was unassociated with total cancer risk, but it was associated with the risk of human papillomavirus-related and pancreatic cancers (Kennedy et al., 2014). Physical abuse has also been shown to predict rates of medical diagnoses, bronchitis/emphysema, and ulcers in adults, but health behaviors and gender modified these relations (Springer, 2009). Results of these studies lend support to the view that specific types of ECA exposure may independently predict disease prevalence; however, more work is needed to examine these factors in conjunction (and possibly interaction) with additional risk factors.

Low SES Finally, growing up in poverty has been linked empirically with some aspects of chronic disease. For example, in a review of the literature, Calixto and Anaya (2014) found that SES related to the prevalence and presentation of several forms of autoimmune disease, including rheumatoid arthritis and multiple sclerosis. Experiencing low SES in childhood (as well as low SES in adulthood) has also been linked to arthritis in a large sample of adults, partially through its influence on BMI (Baldassari, Cleveland, & Callahan, 2013). Finally, a relation was found between residing in a single-parent household and asthma hospitalization in a sample of children aged 1–16; however, this relation was completely attenuated by household income, demonstrating that lower income is associated with higher levels of asthma-related health-care utilization (Moncrief, Beck, Simmons, Huang, & Kahn, 2014).

Summary In sum, ECA has been shown to relate to several aspects of disease and disability. Although not all researchers have reported links between ECA exposure and morbidity or mortality (e.g., White & Widom, 2003), available evidence does suggest that children exposed to these hardships are more likely to develop chronic disease or disability as they age. Life course prospective studies are needed to examine how these diseases develop in trauma-exposed youth. Mechanisms may differ depending on the disease studied but could include behaviors (such as smoking or substance use), societal factors (e.g., exposure to hazardous chemicals in the environment), or physiological wear and tear on the body. For example, the allostatic load theory of stress helps to explain why stressors encountered early in life may be especially impactful for disease. Chronic stress such as that experienced with exposure to abuse or adversity dysregulates several body systems, and over time, this dysregulation leads to a heightened risk for developing disease. Identifying the precise mechanisms linking ECA and disease prevalence will require a more detailed and specific assessment of ECA experiences early in life, but it is a worthwhile endeavor so that hopefully diseases can be prevented or their impact lessened.

Summary of Physiological Risk

So far, this review has examined the impact of ECA experiences on HPA axis functioning, inflammation, CVD risk, and chronic disease. The overwhelming weight of the empirical evidence suggests that ECA is a powerful destructive force in the health and lives of children that extends throughout the life span. Several of the reviewed studies indicate a direct relation between ECA experiences and physical health. However in many studies, as described in the previous sections, the association between ECA and health was mediated by risky health behaviors (e.g., Morton et al., 2014). Therefore, these health behaviors will be reviewed briefly.

Health Risks and Behaviors

ECA exposure has been shown to increase the likelihood of engaging in health-compromising behaviors, namely smoking, alcohol and other substance abuse, and risky sexual behaviors. Exposure to ECA is also related to being overweight or obese. ECA can impact health behaviors directly, and these behaviors can also indirectly effect the relation between ECA and multiple physical health domains. For example, health-related behaviors accounted for approximately 10% of the difference in adult health outcomes between those of low and high childhood SES in one study (van de Mheen, Stronks, Looman, & Mackenbach, 1998). Therefore, it is important to identify how early adversity can lead individuals to make health-relevant choices and how these choices impact their physiology.

Cigarette Smoking

Cigarette smoking has been associated with ECA in several studies, including Felitti et al. (1998) who found greater risk for smoking among adults who experienced at least four types of trauma in childhood. Adults' risk of cigarette smoking (currently or ever) increased in a graded manner with their exposure to ECA (Ford et al., 2011). In addition, smoking persistence (among those already dependent at baseline) in a large prospective sample of adults was found to be predicted by childhood maltreatment (Elliott et al., 2014). Smoking has also been found to mediate the association between ECA and several physical health conditions. For example, smoking mediated the relation between ECA and AMI in adults (Morton et al., 2014). Support for cigarette smoking as a mediator between ECA and allostatic load was found in a longitudinal study of 9-year-olds followed through adolescence (Doan et al., in press). Finally, low childhood SES predicted smoking in adulthood in another study. Smoking also directly predicted mortality, and it had a substantial indirect effect on the relation between low SES and mortality (Giesinger et al., 2014). Therefore, smoking behavior is likely exacerbated by ECA and intimately related to the development of further health problems.

Alcohol and Other Substance Use/Abuse

Felitti et al. (1998) found that ECA exposure predicted greater risk of alcoholism and illicit drug abuse. Following this study, others have also found evidence for higher alcohol or drug use among those who experienced trauma in childhood. In a sample of adolescents with substance abuse disorders, the majority (60 %) were exposed to either sexual or physical abuse in childhood (Danielson et al., 2009), and a dose-response relationship was found between abuse and substance abuse characteristics, with those experiencing both physical and sexual abuse having the greatest risk. In a sample of adult men, a greater risk of binge drinking and being drunk at least once/week was identified among those that experienced historically reported (i.e., when participants were children) ECA, but this association was attenuated by low childhood SES (Kauhanen, Leino, Lakka, Lynch, & Kauhanen, 2011). Retrospectively reported ECA exposure to at least three adversities was also associated with binge drinking in this sample. Exposure to physical punishment, as well as abuse, has been found to heighten the likelihood of alcohol use/abuse in adulthood (Afifi et al., 2006). Evidence was also found for a relation between alcohol use persistence and childhood maltreatment in a large sample of adults (Elliott et al., 2014). Abuse and exposure to violent crime in childhood, as well as growing up in a home where substance use or smoking were present, also predicted substance dependence (i.e., alcohol, cocaine, or opioid) in adults, with mood/anxiety disorders mediating the relation between ECA and dependence (Douglas et al., 2010). Emotional maltreatment (beyond the effects of other ECA types) was found to be a strong predictor of alcohol dependence severity in a treatment-seeking sample of adults, with some evidence of mediation by borderline personality symptoms (Potthast, Neuner, & Catani, 2014). Finally, in an interesting study, alcohol abuse (as well as traumatic intrusions or unwanted thoughts about past trauma) was found to mediate the relation between early trauma exposure and risky sexual behavior in young adults (Walsh, Latzman, & Latzman, 2014). In general, the available evidence does suggest that alcohol and other substance abuse is more likely to occur in those with a history of ECA, but this relation may be impacted by concurrent psychological symptoms.

Risky Sexual Behaviors

Another cluster of health-related behaviors that is affected by ECA exposure involves risky sexual behaviors. Evidence suggests that exposure to adverse environments in childhood predicts earlier menarche, early age at first intercourse, and sexual risk taking (Anda et al., 2006; Belsky, Steinberg, Houts, & Halpern-Felsher, 2010). ECA exposure has been associated empirically with having a greater number of sexual partners and positive history of sexually transmitted diseases (Felitti et al., 1998). In a sample of Mexican-American and African-American adolescents, those with a history of abuse were more likely to engage in sexual risk behaviors, including having sex earlier, with more partners, and being exposed to sexually transmitted diseases more often (Champion et al., 2005). In a sample of adults, greater exposure to ECA was strongly related to higher rates of teenage pregnancy and also poorer fetal outcomes (Hillis et al., 2004). As mentioned, Walsh et al. (2014) found evidence that ECA heightened several aspects of risky sexual behavior through its influence on alcohol and intrusive thought. In a sample of young adult women, ECA exposure predicted sexual risk, and those experiencing 3+ types of ECA reported the highest levels of sexual risk behavior (Hahm, Lee, Ozonoff, & Van Wert, 2010). Engaging in risky sexual behaviors can have myriad outcomes both physiologically and psychologically, one of which (unintended pregnancy and parenting) can directly impact future generations. Therefore, prevention of ECA is an important challenge with implications for public health via the reduction of risky sexual behaviors and adverse outcomes.

Overweight or Obesity

Obesity is a well-recognized health epidemic in many developed nations, and it is a major cause of numerous health problems. Obesity risk is impacted by some health conditions and is intimately related to chronic stress-induced changes in the immune and metabolic systems (Kyrou, Chrousos, & Tsigos, 2006). However, obesity and being overweight are also likely products of a sedentary lifestyle and/or consuming excess calories. Some researchers have specifically examined these latter behaviors for their relation with ECA exposure. For example, Felitti et al. (1998) found evidence linking ECA exposure with physical inactivity in adults. Relatedly, in another study of multiple health risk behaviors, physical activity was most related to early SES (van de Mheen et al., 1998). In an interesting study on children's consumption of unhealthy foods, it was found that greater traumatic stress symptoms predicted higher consumption of most types of unhealthy foods and beverages

(Vilija & Romualdas, 2014). Stress-induced eating has also been identified as a pathway linking women's ECA exposure to their metabolic syndrome risk (Lee et al., 2014). Other work has suggested that, in low-SES environments, safe opportunities for physical exercise and for healthy food choices can be limited (e.g., Cohen, Janicki-Deverts, Chen, & Matthews, 2010).

In addition to these behavioral links with ECA, many studies have examined the more general relation between ECA exposure and overweight/obesity. In a meta-analysis, 81% of the reviewed studies supported a link between obesity and a form of ECA (Midei & Matthews, 2011). Empirically, heightened obesity risk has been found in children exposed to chronic intimate partner violence (Boynton-Jarrett, Fargnoli, Suglia, Zuckerman, & Wright, 2010) and in young adolescents with a

Table 9.1 Common self-report retrospective measures for examining ECA exposure

Name of and citation for measure	Includes	Scoring	Benefits	Possible drawbacks
Adverse Childhood Experiences Questionnaire (Dube, Williamson, Thompson, Felitti, & Anda, 2004)	Emotional, sexual, and physical abuse; household and family dysfunction	Frequency count of exposures	Relatively comprehensive, easy to score	No SES information
Child Abuse and Trauma scale (Kent & Waller, 1998; Sanders & Becker-Lausen, 1995)	Three subscales (negative home environment, sexual abuse, and punishment); fourth subscale added later for emotional abuse	Score reflects subscale mean	Questions asked in a sensitive manner, relatively comprehensive	Focuses largely on exposures in the family/home, no SES information
Childhood Trauma Questionnaire (Bernstein et al., 1994, 2003)	Emotional, sexual, and physical abuse; emotional and physical neglect	Summed for total and subscale scores, validity questions included	Most highly cited measure of ECA (Thabrew et al., 2012), easy to compare across populations	No assessment of adversities or trauma characteristics (i.e., age of onset)
Early Trauma Inventory, Self-Report (Bremner, Bolus, & Mayer, 2007)	Emotional, sexual, and physical abuse; general trauma	Different methods were explored, counting number of events is recommended	Also assesses frequency, onset, perpetrator, and impact of trauma, includes a variety of trauma types	Longer to administer due to depth of questions; however, a short form is available
Risky Families Questionnaire (Taylor, Lerner, Sage, Lehman, & Seeman, 2004)	Family dysfunction and conflict	Summed to derive a cumulative exposure index	Focus on family-level factors including affection and maltreatment	Not a comprehensive measure of ECA

SES socioeconomic status, *ECA* early childhood adversity

dose-response relation evident between ECA and elevated BMI and waist circumference (Pretty et al., 2013). Children's experience of more frequent and chronic negative events predicted greater likelihood of overweight/obesity in adolescence (Lumeng et al., 2013). Lower SES (at both the family and the neighborhood level) has also been related to adolescents' higher BMI (Chen & Paterson, 2006). Substantial evidence also suggests that exposure to adversity in childhood puts one at risk for obesity in adulthood (Anda et al., 2006; Boynton-Jarrett, Rosenberg, Palmer, Boggs, & Wise, 2012; Carpenter et al., 2010; Felitti et al., 1998; McIntyre et al., 2012). For example, a relation between greater ECA exposure and central obesity (but not BMI) in middle-aged adults was identified even when controlling for health risk factors (Davis et al., 2014). More studies are needed to clarify the mechanisms by which different forms of ECA exposure are linked to increases in adiposity over time, which, given the detrimental and pervasive effects of obesity, are likely to have a tremendous health impact.

Challenges and Conclusions

Measurement Challenges

There is a great deal of variability in how ECA is measured across studies. Because many studies examining physical health are conducted with adults, measurement is necessarily retrospective. In addition, due to their ease of administration, self-report questionnaire measures are often utilized. Information about five commonly used retrospective self-report measures is provided in Table 9.1. A full review of all measures of ECA is beyond the scope of this chapter; however, this topic has been approached by others (Burgermeister, 2007; Strand, Sarmiento, & Pasquale, 2005; Thabrew, de Sylva, & Romans, 2012).

Studies carried out on the physical health effects of low-SES exposure quantify SES in several ways. Many studies include only one indicator of childhood SES or use crude or broad categorizations for SES (Cohen et al., 2010). Father's occupation (Brunner et al., 1996; van de Mheen et al., 1998) is a very common indicator. Other indicators include parents' education level, conditions of the family home, self-reported low SES, residential crowding, and being raised by a single parent (Galobardes et al., 2006). Calixto and Anaya (2014) list education, income, ancestry, and occupational and social class as the most important SES factors. Overall, many studies do not measure SES in a way that is conducive for examining within-person change over time starting in childhood nor in a manner that is comprehensive (i.e., by including many indicators of SES).

Importantly, none of the measures available are comprehensive in measuring abuse, neglect, common adversities, SES, and parental warmth. To compensate, researchers have combined or added to existing measures or developed their own surveys. This practice, coupled with the lack of operational definition of ECA present in most studies, can lead to a fragmented research base. In addition, examining the impact of early trauma exposure across the life span is inherently a developmental undertaking, yet past measurement of ECA has been less than attentive to developmental factors. In part, this may be due to issues with measurement equivalence across ages and cohorts and the difficulty in retrospectively disentangling whether health is being affected by proximal or distal exposure to stressful events (or some combination of the two). Efforts should be made to increase the scope and the precision of current measurement, including assessing understudied adversities (e.g., frequent moving, foster care entry, natural disasters—see Chap. 10, this volume).

The Influence of Individual Differences

The ECA literature suggests that early trauma exposure is salient and detrimental for most of those who experience it. However, some people who are exposed to ECA do not experience notable physical or psychological consequences, and there appears to be evidence for some heterogeneity in individual responses (Shonkoff, Boyce, & McEwen, 2009). Individual differences might impact the relation between ECA and physical health and contribute to this heterogeneity, including resilience, education and/or intelligence, and social support.

Resilience is a well studied and complex protective factor and comprises the ability to respond in an adaptive manner when faced with trauma (see Chap. 16, this volume, for related discussion). Some aspects of resiliency are considered to be individual-level factors, such as coping skills and IQ, while other protective factors are external, including parental monitoring, appropriate family functioning, and having a larger number of adults in one's home (Tiet et al., 1998). Individuals higher in resilience experience fewer problems after ECA exposure. For example, resilience has been shown to reduce the tendency for hazardous alcohol and illicit drug use in those exposed to ECA (Wingo, Ressler, & Bradley, 2014). However, recognition of the protectiveness of individual resiliency should not serve to alleviate society's role in the reduction of ECA nor its obligation to victims. In fact, even in those youth labeled as resilient, evidence can still be found to suggest physiological effects of ECA exposure (Brody et al., 2013). Therefore, although resilience may help individual children weather the storm of adversity, it is important to also consider broader societal factors that contribute both to the prevalence and consequences of ECA exposure.

Higher intelligence or higher levels of education have also been shown to impact ECA exposure consequences. For example, higher IQ and higher educational aspirations were associated with better adjustment in youth (Tiet et al., 1998). However, other studies have suggested that education is not enough to ameliorate the risks associated with ECA. For example, Montez and Hayward (2014) found that higher education did not remove all consequences of early disadvantage, in that those with disadvantaged childhoods still lived shorter and more impaired lives. However, evidence was found for the benefit of upward mobility, in that those from a disadvantaged background that obtained higher education experienced similar or better outcomes on average than advantaged individuals with lower educational attainment. In addition, in a study of male medical doctors, it was found that those raised in a low-SES household had a greater risk of developing coronary heart disease before the age of 50 (Kittleson et al., 2006).

Finally, social support or the presence of a supportive adult, is a major factor influencing the physiological effects of ECA. Whereas the lack of a supportive adult can be considered an adversity, the presence of at least one stable and healthy relationship with an adult can protect against the harmful effects of ECA (see Chap. 1, this volume, for related discussion). These relationships have been termed safe, stable, nurturing relationships (or SSNRs, see Schofield, Lee, & Merrick, 2013). As one example in a recent study, the presence of a supportive role model in children of low-SES backgrounds predicted lower IL-6, though this relation was partially explained by patterns of optimistic thought (Chen, Lee, Cavey, & Ho, 2013). In addition, because so many adversities are predicated on the dysfunction of close adults, a more stable adult influence may ameliorate these negative effects, including by stopping the abuse or neglect altogether or simply by providing the child with material needs or affection. Therefore, the presence or absence of a supportive relationship is a very important individual difference impacting how children might respond to ECA exposure.

Future Directions

The literature linking ECA and physical health is both compelling and complex; however, avenues for improvement exist. Although the evidence provides substantial support for a linkage between ECA and poor health, evidence is often presented piecemeal and without a consideration of interactions among mental and physical health. In addition, more precision should be instituted into the measurement of ECA. Categorizing stressors into whether they constitute a form of abuse or adversity may provide greater insight into exactly which kinds of trauma are predictive of which outcomes. A greater focus on developmental factors including "age, timing, severity, and duration" of exposure (Odgers & Jaffee, 2013, p. 36) is needed. Next, a greater understanding of individual and intergenerational trajectories is important. This literature has repeatedly shown that the experience of ECA can lead to continued adversity exposure over time. In one study (Kiecolt-Glaser et al., 2011) the authors summarize their findings by stating that "childhood adversities cast a very long shadow" (p. 16) on the individual. The literature suggests that this shadow, for some, may be even longer, compromising their lifetime health and creating risky or hostile environments that shape future generations' health much like their own. Finally, movement beyond description of the manifold ways in which ECA exposure is detrimental to health is needed; trauma researchers must continue to put these findings into action to reduce health-related disparities. As Braveman and Barclay (2009) note, it may appear as though society cannot afford to target child poverty, but with its (and other forms of ECA's) far-reaching implications, we cannot afford to ignore it. Due to its origins in early life, ECA may serve as a physiological and psychological foundation for coping responses to all other forms of trauma an individual will experience in their life span, demonstrating its paramount importance for well (or ill)-being.

Acknowledgments Support for this research was provided by a grant from the National Institute on Aging (AG026307-R01 and AG028383-P30).

References

Afifi, T. O., Brownridge, D. A., Cox, B. J., & Sareen, J. (2006). Physical punishment, childhood abuse and psychiatric disorders. *Child Abuse and Neglect, 30*(10), 1093–1103.

American Psychiatric Association (APA). (2013). *Diagnostic and statistical manual of mental disorders* (5th ed. Text Revised). Washington, D.C.: American Psychiatric Association

Anda, R., Felitti, V., Bremner, J., Walker, J. D., Whitfield, C., Perry, B. D., et al. (2006). The enduring effects of abuse and related adverse experiences in childhood: A convergence of evidence from neurobiology and epidemiology. *European Archives of Psychiatry and Clinical Neuroscience, 256*(3), 174–186.

Archer, J. A., Hutchison, I. L., Dorudi, S., Stansfeld, S. A, & Korszun, A. (2012). Interrelationship of depression, stress and inflammation in cancer patients: A preliminary study. *Journal of Affective Disorders, 143*(1–3), 39–46.

Baldassari, A. R., Cleveland, R. J., & Callahan, L. F. (2013). Independent associations of childhood and current socioeconomic status with risk of self-reported doctor-diagnosed arthritis in a family-medicine cohort of North-Carolinians. *BMC Musculoskeletal Disorders, 14,* 327.

Belsky, J., Steinberg, L., Houts, R. M., & Halpern-Felsher, B. L. (2010). The development of reproductive strategy in females: Early maternal harshness → earlier menarche → increased sexual risk taking. *Developmental Psychology, 46*(1), 120–128.

Bernstein, D. P., Fink, L., Handelsman, L., Foote, J., Lovejoy, M., Wenzel, K., et al. (1994). Initial reliability and validity of a new retrospective measure of child abuse and neglect. *The American Journal of Psychiatry, 151*(8), 1132–1136.

Bernstein, D. P., Stein, J. A., Newcomb, M. D., Walker, E., Pogge, D., Ahluvalia, T., et al. (2003). Development and validation of a brief screening version of the childhood trauma questionnaire. *Child Abuse and Neglect, 27*(2), 169–190.

Boynton-Jarrett, R., Fargnoli, J., Suglia, S. F., Zuckerman, B., & Wright, R. J. (2010). Association between maternal intimate partner violence and incident obesity in preschool-aged children: Results from the fragile families and child well-being study. *Archives of Pediatrics and Adolescent Medicine, 164*(6), 540–546.

Boynton-Jarrett, R., Rosenberg, L., Palmer, J. R., Boggs, D. A., & Wise, L. A. (2012). Child and adolescent abuse in relation to obesity in adulthood: The Black Women's Health Study. *Pediatrics, 130*(2), 245–253.

Braveman, P., & Barclay, C. (2009). Health disparities beginning in childhood: A life-course perspective. *Pediatrics, 124,* S163–S175.

Bremner, J. D., Bolus, R., & Mayer, E. A. (2007). Psychometric properties of the early trauma inventory—Self report. *The Journal of Nervous and Mental Disease, 195*(3), 211–218.

Brody, G. H., Yu, T., Chen, E., Miller, G. E., Kogan, S. M., & Beach, S. R. H. (2013). Is resilience only skin deep? Rural African Americans' socioeconomic status-related risk and competence in preadolescence and psychological adjustment and allostatic load at age 19. *Psychological Science, 24*(7), 1285–1293.

Brown, D. W., Anda, R. F., Felitti, V. J., Edwards, V. J., Malarcher, A. M., Croft, J. B., et al. (2010). Adverse childhood experiences are associated with the risk of lung cancer: A prospective cohort study. *BMC Public Health, 10,* 20.

Brummett, B. H., Babyak, M. A, Singh, A., Jiang, R., Williams, R. B., Harris, K. M., et al. (2013). Socioeconomic indices as independent correlates of C-reactive protein in the National Longitudinal Study of Adolescent Health. *Psychosomatic Medicine, 75*(9), 882–893.

Brunner, E., Smith, G. D., Marmot, M., Canner, R., Beksinska, M., & O'Brien, J. (1996). Childhood social circumstances and psychosocial and behavioural factors as determinants of plasma fibrinogen. *Lancet, 347*(9007), 1008–1013.

Burgermeister, D. (2007). Childhood adversity: A review of measurement instruments. *Journal of Nursing Measurement, 15*(3), 163–176.

Calixto, O.-J., & Anaya, J.-M. (2014). Socioeconomic status. The relationship with health and autoimmune diseases. *Autoimmunity Reviews, 13*(6), 641–654.

Carlsson, E., Frostell, A., Ludvigsson, J., & Faresjo, M. (2014). Psychological stress in children may alter the immune response. *The Journal of Immunology, 192*(5), 2071–2081.

Carpenter, L. L., Tyrka, A. R., Ross, N. S., Khoury, L., Anderson, G. M., & Price, L. H. (2009). Effect of childhood emotional abuse and age on cortisol responsivity in adulthood. *Biological Psychiatry, 66*(1), 69–75.

Carpenter, L. L., Gawuga, C. E., Tyrka, A. R., Lee, J. K., Anderson, G. M., & Price, L. H. (2010). Association between plasma IL-6 response to acute stress and early-life adversity in healthy adults. *Neuropsychopharmacology, 35*(13), 2617–2623.

Carroll, J. E., Gruenewald, T. L., Taylor, S. E., Janicki-Deverts, D., Matthews, K. A, & Seeman, T. E. (2013). Childhood abuse, parental warmth, and adult multisystem biological risk in the coronary artery risk development in young adults study. *Proceedings of the National Academy of Sciences of the United States of America, 110*(42), 17149–17153.

Champion, J. D., Piper, J. M., Holden, A. E. C., Shain, R. N., Perdue, S., & Korte, J. E. (2005). Relationship of abuse and pelvic inflammatory disease risk behavior in minority adolescents. *Journal of the American Academy of Nurse Practitioners, 17*(6), 234–241.

Chen, E., & Paterson, L. Q. (2006). Neighborhood, family, and subjective socioeconomic status: How do they relate to adolescent health? *Health Psychology, 25*(6), 704–714.

Chen, E., Cohen, S., & Miller, G. E. (2010). How low socioeconomic status affects 2-year hormonal trajectories in children. *Psychological Science, 21*(1), 31–37.

Chen, E., Lee, W. K., Cavey, L., & Ho, A. (2013). Role models and the psychological characteristics that buffer low-socioeconomic-status youth from cardiovascular risk. *Child Development, 84*(4), 1241–1252.

Coelho, R., Viola, T. W., Walss-Bass, C., Brietzke, E., & Grassi-Oliveira, R. (2014). Childhood maltreatment and inflammatory markers: A systematic review. *Acta Psychiatrica Scandinavica, 129*(3), 180–192.

Cohen, S., Janicki-Deverts, D., Chen, E., & Matthews, K. A. (2010). Childhood socioeconomic status and adult health. *Annals of the New York Academy of Sciences, 1186,* 37–55.

Cuijpers, P., Smit, F., Unger, F., Stikkelbroek, Y., Ten Have, M., & de Graaf, R. (2011). The disease burden of childhood adversities in adults: A population-based study. *Child Abuse and Neglect, 35*(11), 937–945.

Danese, A., Pariante, C. M., Caspi, A., Taylor, A., & Poulton, R. (2007). Childhood maltreatment predicts adult inflammation in a life-course study. *Proceedings of the National Academy of Sciences of the United States of America, 104*(4), 1319–1324.

Danese, A., Caspi, A., Williams, B., Ambler, A., Sugden, K., Mika, J., et al. (2011). Biological embedding of stress through inflammation processes in childhood. *Molecular Psychiatry, 16*(3), 244–246.

Danielson, C. K., Amstadter, A., Dangelmaier, R. E., Resnick, H. S., Saunders, B. E., & Kilpatrick, D. G. (2009). Does typography of substance abuse and dependence differ as a function of exposure to child maltreatment? *Journal of Child and Adolescent Substance Abuse, 18*(4), 323.

Davis, C. R., Dearing, E., Usher, N., Trifiletti, S., Zaichenko, L., Ollen, E., et al. (2014). Detailed assessments of childhood adversity enhance prediction of central obesity independent of gen-

der, race, adult psychosocial risk and health behaviors. *Metabolism: Clinical and Experimental, 63*(2), 199–206.
Doan, S. N., Dich, N., & Evans, G. W. (in press). Childhood cumulative risk and later allostatic load: Mediating role of substance use. *Health Psychology*. Advance online publication.
Dong, M., Giles, W. H., Felitti, V. J., Dube, S. R., Williams, J. E., Chapman, D. P., et al. (2004). Insights into causal pathways for ischemic heart disease: Adverse childhood experiences study. *Circulation, 110*(13), 1761–1766.
Douglas, K., Chan, G., Gelernter, J., Arias, A. J., Anton, R. F., Weiss, R. D., et al. (2010). Adverse childhood events as risk factors for substance dependence: Partial mediation by mood and anxiety disorders. *Addictive Behaviors, 35*(1), 7–13.
Dowd, J. B., Simanek, A. M., & Aiello, A. E. (2009). Socio-economic status, cortisol and allostatic load: A review of the literature. *International Journal of Epidemiology, 38*(5), 1297–1309.
Dowd, J. B., Palermo, T. M., & Aiello, A. E. (2012). Family poverty is associated with cytomegalovirus antibody titers in U.S. Children. *Health Psychology, 31*(1), 5–10.
Dube, S. R., Williamson, D. F., Thompson, T., Felitti, V. J., & Anda, R. F. (2004). Assessing the reliability of retrospective reports of adverse childhood experiences among adult HMO members attending a primary care clinic. *Child Abuse and Neglect, 28*(7), 729–737.
Elliott, J. C., Stohl, M., Wall, M. M., Keyes, K. M., Goodwin, R. D., Skodol, A. E., et al. (2014). The risk for persistent adult alcohol and nicotine dependence: The role of childhood maltreatment. *Addiction, 109*(5), 842–850.
Ershler, W. B., & Keller, E. T. (2000). Age-associated increased interleukin-6 gene expression, late-life diseases, and frailty. *Annual Review of Medicine, 51,* 245–270.
Evans, G. W., & Kim, P. (2010). Multiple risk exposure as a potential explanatory mechanism for the socioeconomic status-health gradient. *Annals of the New York Academy of Sciences, 1186,* 174–189.
Felitti, V. J., Anda, R. F., Nordeberg, D., Williamson, D. F., Spitz, A. M., Edwards, V., et al. (1998). Relationship of childhood abuse and household dysfunction to many of the leading causes of death in adults: The Adverse Childhood Experiences (ACE) study. *American Journal of Preventive Medicine, 14*(4), 245–258.
Ford, J. L., & Browning, C. R. (2014). Effects of exposure to violence with a weapon during adolescence on adult hypertension. *Annals of Epidemiology, 24*(3), 193–198.
Ford, E. S., Anda, R. F., Edwards, V. J., Perry, G. S., Zhao, G., Li, C., et al. (2011). Adverse childhood experiences and smoking status in five states. *Preventive Medicine, 53*(3), 188–193.
Fuller-Thomson, E., Brennenstuhl, S., & Frank, J. (2010). The association between childhood physical abuse and heart disease in adulthood: Findings from a representative community sample. *Child Abuse and Neglect, 34*(9), 689–698.
Fuller-Thomson, E., Bejan, R., Hunter, J. T., Grundland, T., & Brennenstuhl, S. (2012). The link between childhood sexual abuse and myocardial infarction in a population-based study. *Child Abuse and Neglect, 36*(9), 656–665.
Galobardes, B., Smith, G. D., & Lynch, J. W. (2006). Systematic review of the influence of childhood socioeconomic circumstances on risk for cardiovascular disease in adulthood. *Annals of Epidemiology, 16*(2), 91–104.
Giesinger, I., Goldblatt, P., Howden-Chapman, P., Marmot, M., Kuh, D., & Brunner, E. (2014). Association of socioeconomic position with smoking and mortality: The contribution of early life circumstances in the 1946 birth cohort. *Journal of Epidemiology and Community Health, 68*(3), 275–279.
Go, A. S., Mozaffarian, D., Roger, V. L., Benjamin, E. J., Berry, J. D., Blaha, M. J., et al. (2014). Heart disease and stroke statistics—2014 update: A report from the American Heart Association. *Circulation, 129,* e28–e292.
Goldman-Mellor, S., Hamer, M., & Steptoe, A. (2012). Early-life stress and recurrent psychological distress over the lifecourse predict divergent cortisol reactivity patterns in adulthood. *Psychoneuroendocrinology, 37*(11), 1755–1768.

Goodwin, L., White, P. D., Hotopf, M., Stansfeld, S. A., & Clark, C. (2013). Life course study of the etiology of self-reported irritable bowel syndrome in the 1958 British birth cohort. *Psychosomatic Medicine, 75*(2), 202–210.

Gouin, J.-P., Glaser, R., Malarkey, W. B., Beversdorf, D., & Kiecolt-Glaser, J. K. (2012). Childhood abuse and inflammatory responses to daily stressors. *Annals of Behavioral Medicine, 44*(2), 287–292.

Greenfield, E. A., & Marks, N. F. (2009). Profiles of physical and psychological violence in childhood as a risk factor for poorer adult health: Evidence from the 1995–2005 National Survey of Midlife in the United States. *Journal of Aging and Health, 21*(7), 943–966.

Hahm, H. C., Lee, Y., Ozonoff, A., & Van Wert, M. J. (2010). The impact of multiple types of child maltreatment on subsequent risk behaviors among women during the transition from adolescence to young adulthood. *Journal of Youth and Adolescence, 39*(5), 528–540.

Hanson, M. D., & Chen, E. (2010). Daily stress, cortisol, and sleep: The moderating role of childhood psychosocial environments. *Health Psychology, 29*(4), 394–402.

Heim, C., Newport, D. J., Bonsall, R., Miller, A. H., & Nemeroff, C. B. (2001). Altered pituitary-adrenal axis responses to provocative challenge tests in adult survivors of childhood abuse. *The American Journal of Psychiatry, 158*(4), 575–581.

Heim, C., Wagner, D., Maloney, E., Papanicolaou, D. A., Solomon, L., Jones, J. F., et al. (2006). Early adverse experience and risk for chronic fatigue syndrome: Results from a population-based study. *Archives of General Psychiatry, 63*, 1258–1266.

Hillis, S. D., Anda, R. F., Dube, S. R., Felitti, V. J., Marchbanks, P. A., & Marks, J. S. (2004). The association between adverse childhood experiences and adolescent pregnancy, long-term psychosocial consequences, and fetal death. *Pediatrics, 113*(2), 320–327.

Hunter, A., Minnis, H., & Wilson, P. (2011). Altered stress responses in children exposed to early adversity: A systematic review of salivary cortisol studies. *Stress: The International Journal on the Biology of Stress, 14*(6), 614–626.

Kalmakis, K. A., & Chandler, G. E. (2014). Adverse childhood experiences: Towards a clear conceptual meaning. *Journal of Advanced Nursing, 70*(7), 1489–1501.

Kauhanen, L., Leino, J., Lakka, H.-M., Lynch, J. W., & Kauhanen, J. (2011). Adverse childhood experiences and risk of binge drinking and drunkenness in middle-aged Finnish men. *Advances in Preventive Medicine, 2011,* 478741.

Kennedy, B., Valdimarsdóttir, U., Sundström, K., Sparén, P., Lambe, M., Fall, K., et al. (2014). Loss of a parent and the risk of cancer in early life: A nationwide cohort study. *Cancer Causes and Control : CCC, 25*(4), 499–506.

Kent, A., & Waller, G. (1998). The impact of childhood emotional abuse: An extension of the child abuse and trauma scale. *Child Abuse and Neglect, 22*(5), 393–399.

Kiecolt-Glaser, J. K., Gouin, J.-P., Weng, N.-P., Malarkey, W. B., Beversdorf, D. Q., & Glaser, R. (2011). Childhood adversity heightens the impact of later-life caregiving stress on telomere length and inflammation. *Psychosomatic Medicine, 73*(1), 16–22.

Kittleson, M. M., Meoni, L. A., Wang, N.-Y., Chu, A. Y., Ford, D. E., & Klag, M. J. (2006). Association of childhood socioeconomic status with subsequent coronary heart disease in physicians. *Archives of Internal Medicine, 166*(21), 2356–2361.

Kyrou, I., Chrousos, G. P., & Tsigos, C. (2006). Stress, visceral obesity, and metabolic complications. *Annals of the New York Academy of Sciences, 1083,* 77–110.

Lee, C., Tsenkova, V., & Carr, D. (2014). Childhood trauma and metabolic syndrome in men and women. *Social Science and Medicine, 105,* 122–130.

Lehman, B. J., Taylor, S. E., Kiefe, C. I., & Seeman, T. E. (2009). Relationship of early life stress and psychological functioning to blood pressure in the CARDIA study. *Health Psychology, 28*(3), 338–346.

Li, L., Power, C., Kelly, S., Kirschbaum, C., & Hertzman, C. (2007). Life-time socio-economic position and cortisol patterns in mid-life. *Psychoneuroendocrinology, 32*(7), 824–833.

Loucks, E. B., Taylor, S. E., Polak, J. F., Wilhelm, A., Kalra, P., & Matthews, K. A. (2014). Childhood family psychosocial environment and carotid intima media thickness: The CARDIA study. *Social Science and Medicine, 104,* 15–22.

Luecken, L. J., & Appelhans, B. M. (2006). Early parental loss and salivary cortisol in young adulthood: The moderating role of family environment. *Development and Psychopathology, 18*(1), 295–308.
Lumeng, J. C., Wendorf, K., Pesch, M. H., Appugliese, D. P., Kaciroti, N., Corwyn, R. F., & Bradley, R. H. (2013). Overweight adolescents and life events in childhood. *Pediatrics, 132*(6), e1506–e1512.
Lupien, S. J., King, S., Meaney, M. J., & McEwen, B. S. (2001). Can poverty get under your skin? Basal cortisol levels and cognitive function in children from low and high socioeconomic status. *Development and Psychopathology, 13*(3), 653–676.
Matthews, K. A., Chang, Y.-F., Thurston, R. C., & Bromberger, J. T. (2014). Child abuse is related to inflammation in mid-life women: Role of obesity. *Brain, Behavior, and Immunity, 36,* 29–34.
McIntyre, R. S., Soczynska, J. K., Liauw, S. S., Woldeyohannes, H. O., Brietzke, E., Nathanson, J., et al. (2012). The association between childhood adversity and components of metabolic syndrome in adults with mood disorders: Results from the international mood disorders collaborative project. *International Journal of Psychiatry in Medicine, 43*(2), 165–177.
Midei, A. J., & Matthews, K. A. (2011). Interpersonal violence in childhood as a risk factor for obesity: A systematic review of the literature and proposed pathways. *Obesity Reviews, 12*(5), e159–e172.
Midei, A. J., Matthews, K. A., Chang, Y.-F., & Bromberger, J. T. (2013). Childhood physical abuse is associated with incident metabolic syndrome in mid-life women. *Health Psychology, 32*(2), 121–127.
Miller, G. E., Chen, E., & Zhou, E. S. (2007). If it goes up, must it come down? Chronic stress and the hypothalamic-pituitary-adrenocortical axis in humans. *Psychological Bulletin, 133*(1), 25–45.
Miller, G. E., Chen, E., & Parker, K. J. (2011). Psychological stress in childhood and susceptibility to the chronic diseases of aging: Moving towards a model of behavioral and biological mechanisms. *Psychological Bulletin, 137*(6), 959–997.
Moncrief, T., Beck, A. F., Simmons, J. M., Huang, B., & Kahn, R. S. (2014). Single parent households and increased child asthma morbidity. *The Journal of Asthma, 51*(3), 260–266.
Montez, J. K., & Hayward, M. D. (2014). Cumulative childhood adversity, educational attainment, and active life expectancy among U.S. Adults. *Demography, 51*(2), 413–435.
Morton, P. M., Mustillo, S. A., & Ferraro, K. F. (2014). Does childhood misfortune raise the risk of acute myocardial infarction in adulthood? *Social Science and Medicine, 104,* 133–141.
Odgers, C. L., & Jaffee, S. R. (2013). Routine versus catastrophic influences on the developing child. *Annual Review of Public Health, 34,* 29–48.
O'Rand, A. M., & Hamil-Luker, J. (2005). Processes of cumulative adversity: Childhood disadvantage and increased risk of heart attack across the life course. *Journals of Gerontology: Series B, 60B*(SI–II), 117–124.
Pearson, T. A., Mensah, G. A., Alexander, R. W., Anderson, J. L., Cannon III, R. O., Criqui, M., et al. (2003). Markers of inflammation and cardiovascular disease: Application to clinical and public health practice: A statement for healthcare professionals from the Centers for Disease Control and Prevention and the American Heart Association. *Circulation, 107*(3), 499–511.
Pollitt, R. A., Rose, K. M., & Kaufman, J. S. (2005). Evaluating the evidence for models of life course socioeconomic factors and cardiovascular outcomes: A systematic review. *BMC Public Health, 5,* 7.
Pollitt, R. A., Kaufman, J. S., Rose, K. M., Diez-Roux, A. V., Zeng, D., & Heiss, G. (2007). Early-life and adult socioeconomic status and inflammatory risk markers in adulthood. *European Journal of Epidemiology, 22*(1), 55–66.
Potthast, N., Neuner, F., & Catani, C. (2014). The contribution of emotional maltreatment to alcohol dependence in a treatment-seeking sample. *Addictive Behaviors, 39*(5), 949–958.
Poulton, R., Caspi, A., Milne, B. J., Thomson, W. M., Taylor, A., Sears, M. R., & Moffitt, T. E. (2002). Association between children's experience of socioeconomic disadvantage and adult health: A life-course study. *Lancet, 360*(9346), 1640–1645.

Power, C., Thomas, C., Li, L., & Hertzman, C. (2012). Childhood psychosocial adversity and adult cortisol patterns. *The British Journal of Psychiatry, 201*(3), 199–206.

Pretty, C., O'Leary, D. D., Cairney, J., & Wade, T. J. (2013). Adverse childhood experiences and the cardiovascular health of children: A cross-sectional study. *BMC Pediatrics, 13,* 208.

Raposa, E. B., Bower, J. E., Hammen, C. L., Najman, J. M., & Brennan, P. A. (2014). A developmental pathway from early life stress to inflammation: The role of negative health behaviors. *Psychological Science, 25*(6), 1268–1274.

Sanders, B., & Becker-Lausen, E. (1995). The measurement of psychological maltreatment: Early data on the Child Abuse and Trauma scale. *Child Abuse and Neglect, 19*(3), 315–323.

Schofield, T. J., Lee, R. D., & Merrick, M. T. (2013). Safe, stable, nurturing relationships as a moderator of intergenerational continuity of child maltreatment: A meta-analysis. *The Journal of Adolescent Health, 53*(4 Suppl), S32–S38.

Schüssler-Fiorenza Rose, S. M., Xie, D., & Stineman, M. (in press). Adverse childhood experiences & disability in U.S. adults. *PM & R*. Advance online publication.

Scott, K. M., Von Korff, M., Angermeyer, M. C., Benjet, C., Bruffaerts, R., de Girolamo, G., et al. (2011). Association of childhood adversities and early-onset mental disorders with adult-onset chronic physical conditions. *Archives of General Psychiatry, 68*(8), 838–844.

Segerstrom, S. C., & Miller, G. E. (2004). Psychological stress and the human immune system: A meta-analytic study of 30 years of inquiry. *Psychological Bulletin, 130*(4), 601–630.

Shonkoff, J. P., Boyce, W. T., & McEwen, B. S. (2009). Neuroscience, molecular biology, and the childhood roots of health disparities: Building a new framework for health promotion and disease prevention. *JAMA, 301*(21), 2252–2259.

Slopen, N., Lewis, T. T., Gruenewald, T. L., Mujahid, M. S., Ryff, C. D., Albert, M. A., et al. (2010). Early life adversity and inflammation in African Americans and Whites in the midlife in the United States survey. *Psychosomatic Medicine, 72*(7), 694–701.

Slopen, N., McLaughlin, K. A., Dunn, E. C., & Koenen, K. C. (2013). Childhood adversity and cell-mediated immunity in young adulthood: Does type and timing matter? *Brain, Behavior, and Immunity, 28,* 63–71.

Spann, S. J., Gillespie, C. F., Davis, J. S., Brown, A., Schwartz, A., Wingo, A., et al. (2013). The association between childhood trauma and lipid levels in an adult low-income, minority population. *General Hospital Psychiatry, 36*(2), 150–155.

Springer, K. W. (2009). Childhood physical abuse and midlife physical health: Testing a multi-pathway life course model. *Social Science and Medicine, 69*(1), 138–146.

Stein, D. J., Scott, K., Abad, J. M. H., Aguilar-Gaxiola, S., Alonso, J., Angermeyer, M., et al. (2010). Early childhood adversity and later hypertension: Data from the World Mental Health Survey. *Annals of Clinical Psychiatry, 22*(1), 19–28.

Strand, V. C., Sarmiento, T. L., & Pasquale, L. E. (2005). Assessment and screening tools for trauma in children and adolescents: A review. *Trauma, Violence and Abuse, 6*(1), 55–78.

Taylor, S. E., Lerner, J. S., Sage, R. M., Lehman, B. J., & Seeman, T. E. (2004). Early environment, emotions, responses to stress, and health. *Journal of Personality, 72*(6), 1365–1393.

Taylor, S. E., Lehman, B. J., Kiefe, C. I., & Seeman, T. E. (2006). Relationship of early life stress and psychological functioning to adult C-reactive protein in the coronary artery risk development in young adults study. *Biological Psychiatry, 60*(8), 819–824.

Thabrew, H., de Sylva, S., & Romans, S. E. (2012). Evaluating childhood adversity. *Advances in Psychosomatic Medicine, 32,* 35–57.

Tiet, Q. Q., Bird, H. R., Davies, M., Hoven, C., Cohen, P., Jensen, P. S., & Goodman, S. (1998). Adverse life events and resilience. *Journal of the American Academy of Child and Adolescent Psychiatry, 37*(11), 1191–1200.

Trickett, P. K., Noll, J. G., Susman, E. J., Shenk, C. E., & Putnam, F. W. (2010). Attenuation of cortisol across development for victims of sexual abuse. *Development and Psychopathology, 22*(1), 165–175.

Trickett, P. K., Gordis, E., Peckins, M. K., & Susman, E. J. (in press). Stress reactivity in maltreated and comparison male and female young adolescents. *Child Maltreatment*. Advance online publication.

van de Mheen, H., Stronks, K., Looman, C. W. N., & Mackenbach, J. P. (1998). Does childhood socioeconomic status influence adult health through behavioural factors? *International Journal of Epidemiology, 27*(3), 431–437.

Vilija, M., & Romualdas, M. (2014). Unhealthy food in relation to posttraumatic stress symptoms among adolescents. *Appetite, 74,* 86–91.

Walsh, K., Latzman, N. E., & Latzman, R. D. (2014). Pathway from child sexual and physical abuse to risky sex among emerging adults: The role of trauma-related intrusions and alcohol problems. *The Journal of Adolescent Health, 54*(4), 442–448.

Wegman, H. L., & Stetler, C. (2009). A meta-analytic review of the effects of childhood abuse on medical outcomes in adulthood. *Psychosomatic Medicine, 71*(8), 805–812.

White, H. R., & Widom, C. S. (2003). Does childhood victimization increase the risk of early death? A 25-year prospective study. *Child Abuse and Neglect, 27*(7), 841–853.

Wilson, P. W. F., D'Agostino, R. B., Levy, D., Belanger, A. M., Silbershatz, H., & Kannel, W. B. (1998). Prediction of coronary heart disease using risk factor categories. *Circulation, 97*(18), 1837–1847.

Wingo, A. P., Ressler, K. J., & Bradley, B. (2014). Resilience characteristics mitigate tendency for harmful alcohol and illicit drug use in adults with a history of childhood abuse: A cross-sectional study of 2024 inner-city men and women. *Journal of Psychiatric Research, 51,* 93–99.

Wise, L. A., Palmer, J. R., & Rosenberg, L. (2013). Lifetime abuse victimization and risk of uterine leiomyomata in Black women. *American Journal of Obstetrics and Gynecology, 208*(4), 272.e1–272.e13.

Witek Janusek, L., Tell, D., Albuquerque, K., & Mathews, H. L. (2013). Childhood adversity increases vulnerability for behavioral symptoms and immune dysregulation in women with breast cancer. *Brain, Behavior, and Immunity, 30 Suppl*, S149–S162.

Chapter 10
Severe Stress and Anxiety Disorders in Adolescence: The Long-Term Effects of Disasters

Carl F. Weems and Donice M. Banks

Introduction

While susceptibility may vary greatly depending on the geographic region, the lifetime risk of disaster exposure among children and adolescents has been estimated to be above 13% for youth in the United States (Blease, Turner, & Finkelhor, 2010). Research suggests that exposure to both human-caused and natural disasters is associated with a number of posttraumatic stress (PTS) reactions in youth, including symptoms of several mental disorders (e.g., Aber, Gershoff, Ware, & Kotler, 2004; Eisenberg & Silver, 2011; La Greca, Silverman, Vernberg, & Roberts, 2002; Norris, Friedman, & Watson, 2002; Osofsky, Osofsky, Kronenberg, Brennan, & Hansel, 2009; Weems & Overstreet, 2008). This chapter provides an overview of research conducted on the emotional consequences of stress exposure in youth, focusing on the development of anxiety and related problems among youth exposed to disasters.

This chapter primarily reviews research conducted on Hurricane Katrina-exposed youth to illustrate findings and further emphasizes research on the long-term consequences and trajectories of symptoms over time. To understand the long-term effects, researchers have begun to define and identify multiple trajectories and the importance of identifying resilient subsamples in trauma and disaster-exposed individuals (Masten & Obradovic, 2008; see also Chap. 1, this volume). For example, in important syntheses of the literature, Bonanno, Brewin, Kaniasty, and La Greca (2010) and Bonnano, Westphal, and Mancini (2011) have identified four prototypical trajectories: chronicity, characterized by a sharp elevation in symptoms and functional impairment leading to chronic dysfunction; resilience or healthy adjust-

C. F. Weems (✉)
Department of Human Development and Family Studies, Iowa State University, 2330C Palmer, Ames, IA 50011-4380, USA
e-mail: cweems@iastate.edu

D. M. Banks
Department of Psychology, University of New Orleans, New Orleans, LA 70148, USA
e-mail: dmbanks1@uno.edu

K. E. Cherry (ed.), *Traumatic Stress and Long-Term Recovery*,
DOI 10.1007/978-3-319-18866-9_10

ment, indicated by transient symptoms and minimal impairment; recovery, characterized by initial elevations in symptoms and distress that gradually decrease over months; and delayed distress, exemplified by moderate elevations in symptoms and distress following a traumatic event that gradually worsen over time (see also Masten & Obradovic, 2008). This chapter attempts to build upon these reviews to identify potential predictors of the various long-term outcomes across multiple levels of analysis within an integrative perspective drawn from contextual/ecological theories of human development (see Weems & Overstreet, 2008, 2009).

A contextual perspective emphasizes that disasters exert multiple levels of influence on emotional development through the interference of several basic human needs. In the proceeding sections, an overview of the perspective is presented that draws upon the reviews in Weems and Overstreet (2008, 2009). The perspective is then used as a framework to review research on the long-term consequences of severe stress on anxiety and related disorders.

Ecological Needs-Based Perspective

The perspective is based most directly upon Bronfenbrenner's ecological systems theory. This theory posits that individuals function within multiple contexts, or "ecologies," that influence each other and human development (Bronfenbrenner, 1979; see also Chap. 12, this volume), including the macrosystem, which is the most distal ecology and includes the government, culture, cultural values, and beliefs; the exosystem, which consists of processes taking place between two or more contexts, one of which does not directly involve the child, but has implications for the individual child (e.g., parents' workplace); the mesosystem, which represents the linkages between proximal ecologies (e.g., school and home, parental participation in the child's school); and the microsystem, which represents the proximal ecologies within which the child develops, including the family and school environments and peer relationships. The ontogenic level is the ecology of the individual and represents factors within the individual that influence developmental adaptation. In addition to these contexts, ecological systems also emphasize the chronosystem, which concerns time frames such as when events occur in one's life and changes over time. The role of time is emphasized across studies in this chapter.

The ecological needs-based perspective (Weems & Overstreet, 2008) also posits that disasters impact emotional development by threatening basic human needs and goals. When needs are met, an individual is more likely to be resilient in the face of adversity (see Hobfoll, 1989; Sandler, 2001 for expanded discussion). The ecological needs-based model highlights that in the case of disasters and their aftermath, threats to basic needs and the depletion of resources may come from every ecology surrounding the child, increasing the risk for negative emotional outcomes. Conversely, factors that are protective or that may promote resilience may occur within each ecology. These effects may change over time. Thus, an ecological needs-based perspective can be used to integrate data and knowledge by showing how various factors within different ecologies surrounding the child act alone and/or in conjunction with other ecologies to either impede (protect) or foster (increase the risk of) the development of psychopathology and organizes our review of the long-term consequences (effects of time or chronosystem).

In a meta-analysis of disaster-exposed youth, Furr, Comer, Edwards, and Kendall (2010) reported that the timing of assessment was a salient factor as those studies that were conducted within a year of disaster exposure yielded a stronger dose–response effect (i.e., greater exposure associated with worse outcomes) than studies conducted more than 1 year after disaster exposure. For instance, among adolescents in New York City who were assessed 15 months following the 9/11 terrorist attacks, only small dose–response effects were found for mental health symptomatology (Gershoff, Aber, Ware, & Kotler, 2010). This finding lends to the possibility that recovery may have already occurred for many of the study's participants (Masten & Narayan, 2012). Other researchers suggest that youths' post-disaster symptomatology typically remits over time (La Greca et al., 2002). According to Vogel and Vernberg (1993), youth symptomatology post disaster often decreases rapidly, typically within 9–14 months, and symptoms remit within a period of 18 months to 3 years. However, factors such as life threat or long-term disruption in contexts such as the family and community have the potential to affect recovery. As implied by the ecological needs-based model, there may be multiple levels of influence on the development of emotional and behavioral problems following a disaster following from disruptions to contexts or ecologies which results in long-term distress. While the long-term effects of disaster exposure are relatively understudied, researchers have suggested that many youth continue to experience symptoms of distress, such as symptoms of post-traumatic stress disorder (PTSD), anxiety, and depression, for extended periods after the traumatic event (e.g., Norris, Perilla, Riad, Kaniasty, & Lavizzo, 1999; Weems et al., 2010), even as long as 5 years post disaster (Goenjian et al., 2005).

Table 10.1 summarizes 16 longitudinal studies that examined the effects of Hurricane Katrina on youth symptoms or related outcomes over time frames 12 months or greater after the event. The table provides information regarding study characteristics, mental health outcomes, and the ecologies examined in each study. The studies listed in the table are referenced throughout the text to exemplify each ecology's influence on post-disaster outcomes. The findings from the studies of long-term disaster effects suggest that youth are continuing to experience long-term distress following the Katrina disaster. For example, in a longitudinal study of youth exposed to Hurricane Katrina, Abramson, Park, Stehling-Ariza, and Redlener (2010) found that in 2010, more than 4 years post disaster, 40.8 % of parents in Louisiana and 49.1 % of parents in Mississippi reported that their children were experiencing emotional and/or behavioral problems that developed after experiencing the disaster, and the cumulative prevalence rate of diagnosed mental health conditions (i.e., anxiety, depression, or behavioral disorder) across 4 years post disaster was more than 37 %.

Ontogenic Influences

The ontogenic level is the ecology of the individual and represents factors within the individual that influence developmental adaptation. First at this level is what the literature indicates about the course of mental health following disasters. As

Table 10.1 Summary of longitudinal studies examining long-term outcomes following Hurricane Katrina (over 12 months)

Study	*N*	Time frame	Sample	Outcomes	Predictors and correlates	Ecologies examined
Abramson et al. (2010)	283	Four annual waves from Jan–Aug 2006 (5–12 months post Katrina) to Nov. 2009–2010 (50–54 months)	Community/displaced; age: 4–17 years Gender and ethnicity not given	Serious emotional disturbance (SED; psychological, emotional, and behavioral dysfunction)	Multiple individual, social, and contextual factors (e.g., Parental mental health, living situation); parental and child's prior mental health; hurricane exposure	Microsystem, mesosystem
Banks and Weems (2014)	191	24 and 30 months post Katrina	School age: 8–15 years; 55 % male; 99 % minority	PTSD, anxiety, and depression	Parent and peer social support	Microsystem
Hensley-Maloney and Varela (2009)	302	6.5 and 17.5 months post Katrina	School age: 10–15; 61 % female; 60 % minority	Panic symptoms at T1 and T2	Child's age, gender, parent level of education, family income, ethnicity, and panic at T1; anxiety sensitivity at T1 and T2; Hurricane trauma exposure	Ontogenic
Kelley et al. (2010)	381	5 and 15.5 months post Katrina	Community; age: 8–16 years;76 % minority; gender not given	PTSD symptoms at T2	PTSD symptoms at T1; hurricane exposure and violence exposure	Microsystem
Kilmer et al. (2009)	68	12 and 24 months post Katrina	Community age: 7–10 years 54 % female; 85 % minority	Posttraumatic growth at T2	Hurricane exposure; posttraumatic growth at T1; PTSD symptoms at T1and T2	Ontogenic
Kilmer and Gil-Rivas (2010)	66	12 and 24 months post Katrina	Community age: 7–10 years; 56 % female; 85 % minority	Child's posttraumatic growth at T2	Child report of multiple cognitive factors; PTSD symptoms and posttraumatic growth at T1; parent report of parenting behaviors, parental posttraumatic growth, and parental mental health at T1, PTSD symptoms at T1 and T2	Ontogenic, microsystem

Table 10.1 (continued)

Study	*N*	Time frame	Sample	Outcomes	Predictors and correlates	Ecologies examined
Kronenberg et al. (2010)	387	24 and 36 months post Katrina	School/displaced age: 9–18 years; 54.5 % female; 27 % minority	PTSD and depression symptoms at T2; Individual symptom recovery patterns from T1 to T2	Hurricane exposure; multiple cognitive, social, and contextual factors; previous trauma, multiple life stressors (e.g., school problems), PTSD and depression symptoms at T1	Ontogenic, microsystem
McLaughlin et al. (2009)	797	Longitudinal/cross-sectional analyses only; three annual waves from Mar to Nov 2007 and Aug to Nov 2008 (18–27 months post Katrina)	Community age: 4–17 years; gender and ethnicity not given	Parent report of child's hurricane- and non-hurricane-related serious emotional disturbance (psychological, emotional, and behavioral dysfunction)	Multiple demographic (age, gender, ethnicity, etc.) and contextual factors; Parent report of child's hurricane exposure (e.g., death of a loved one), child's hurricane-related stress, parent's mental health	Ontogenic, microsystem, exosystem
McLaughlin et al. (2010)	576	Three annual waves from Mar–Nov 2007 and Aug–Nov 2008 (18–39 months post Katrina)	Community age: 4–17 years; gender and ethnicity not given	Parent report of child's hurricane- and non-Hurricane-related serious emotional disturbance (SED; psychological, emotional, and behavioral dysfunction) at T1 and T2	Multiple demographic (e.g., age, gender, ethnicity, etc.) and contextual factors, parent report of child's pre-hurricane functioning (parent retrospective report); hurricane-related stress at T1 and T2	Exosystem, ontogenic, microsystem
Rohrbach et al. (2009)	280	13 months pre-Rita and follow-ups at 7 and 19 months post Rita	School age: ninth graders (M=14.4 years); 68 % female; 32 % minority	Substance abuse at T2 and T3	Age, gender, and ethnicity; substance abuse at T1; hurricane exposure, life disruption, negative life events and PTSD symptoms at T2	Microsystem, ontogenic, exosystem

Table 10.1 (continued)

Study	*N*	Time frame	Sample	Outcomes	Predictors and correlates	Ecologies examined
Ward et al. (2008)	[a]	Academic years: 2004–2005 (pre-Katrina), 2005–2006 (post Katrina), and 2006–2007 (post Katrina)	School/displaced age: Pre-K to grade 12	Ethnicity, SES, school attendance, disciplinary problems (e.g., suspension, expulsion), achievement, grade retention, and dropout rates at T2 and T3	School attendance, disciplinary problems (e.g., suspension, expulsion), achievement, grade retention, and dropout rates at T1	Microsystem
Weems et al. (2010, 2013)	191	24 and 30 months post Katrina	School age: 8–15 years; 55 % male; 99 % minority	PTSD symptoms and PTSD severity Group membership at T2; test anxiety; academic achievement	Age, gender, hurricane exposure, life events, PTSD symptoms, PTSD severity group Membership at T1	Ontogenic, microsystem, macrosystem
Weems and Graham (2014) and Weems et al. (2012)	141	24 and 30 months post Katrina and 1 month post Gustav	Grades fourth through eighth	Identified trajectories of PTSD symptoms; PTSD symptoms	Subsequent exposure, non-avoidant coping; TV viewing of Gustav	Ontogenic; macrosystem
Weems et al. (2014)	94 and 141	Sample 1: 13, 20, and 26 months post Katrina and 5 months post Hurricane Gustav Sample 2: Time 1; 24 months post Katrina) and 1 month and 8 months post Gustav	Sample 1; (initial grade 9th followed to 11th Sample 2; grades 4th through 8th	Memories of Katrina		Ontogenic

[a] School database population study of over 50,000 youth
PTSD post-traumatic stress disorder, *SED* serious emotional disturbance

noted earlier, while there appear to be general declines over time, researchers have begun to define and identify multiple trajectories of symptoms following disasters (Bonanno et al., 2010, 2011; see Chap. 1, this volume) and the importance of identifying resilient subsamples (Masten & Obradovic, 2008). In other words, there may not be just one single course but a set of potential long-term outcomes. Conceptually, resilience emphasizes "that some children facing adversity nonetheless do well (or return to positive functioning following a period of maladaptation)" (Sroufe, 1997, p. 256). Resilience then is defined by (1) exposure to some risk (e.g., facing disaster-related adversity) as well as (2) the relatively positive functioning of some compared to others. As a subcomponent of (1), the "resilient" should have the same level of risk exposure as the non-resilient (for related discussion, see Luthar, Cicchetti, & Becker, 2000). Clearly, exposure to a disaster represents risk, but samples of disaster-exposed youth can be very heterogeneous with regard to the level of exposure. Thus, a group with a stable low trajectory may seem "resilient" but in fact may simply be relatively less exposed to traumatic experiences.

Weems and Graham (2014) followed up at a third assessment point (right after Hurricane Gustav) in a study of the stability of PTSD symptoms among ethnic minority youth in grades 4 through 8 who were assessed at 24 and 30 months post Hurricane Katrina. The investigators initially found a generally high level of stability in PTSD symptoms and that younger age, being female, and continued disrepair to the child's home were predictive of stable, elevated PTSD symptoms (Weems et al., 2010). Weems and Graham found that there were general declines in symptoms. However, subsamples of youth with increasing, decreasing, chronic, and stable low levels of PTSD symptoms were identified, consistent with previous theorizing. High subsequent Gustav exposure was associated with more chronic symptoms, while low Gustav exposure was associated with declines in symptoms. A relatively large group (43 % of the sample) with a stable low trajectory was identified. The stable low trajectory group had significantly fewer exposure experiences, although the level of exposure was not homogeneous. A subsample of the stable low group was defined as resilient. The identification of this resilient group was made according to commensurability in level of risk exposure (total sample average or higher levels of disaster experiences) with the non-resilient group (i.e., chronic/stable high). In this case, a much smaller portion ($n = 16\,\%$) was considered resilient. Moreover, comparison of all stable low with stable high would have led to an erroneous conclusion about the use of avoidant coping strategies. It was the truly resilient (low symptoms and high exposure) who reported the lowest levels of avoidant coping strategies.

Kronenberg et al. (2010) assessed youth aged 9–18 years for symptoms of PTSD and depression at 2 and 3 years following Hurricane Katrina and classified youth into the outcome trajectories of stress resistant, normal response and recovery, delayed breakdown, and breakdown without recovery. One encouraging finding was that overall symptomatology decreased between the 2nd and 3rd years, and the majority (72.3 %) of participants were classified as either stress resistant or having a normal response and recovery. However, the remaining participants, who reported higher hurricane exposure, continued to report significant symptoms of PTSD and depression, and were classified as breakdown without recovery or delayed breakdown. Younger age, being female, and the presence of family concerns (e.g., parent still unemployed following the storm) were all associated negative responses to the disaster and poor recovery patterns.

Disaster experiences that involve life threat can challenge one's sense of control and self-efficacy in containing the threat, leading to emotional reactions that may be difficult to regulate (Norris et al., 2002) and ultimately increasing the risk for the development of psychopathology. Theoretically, at the individual level, direct exposure to life threat in a disaster increases activity of the hypothalamic–pituitary–adrenal (HPA) axis as part of a normative fight–flight reaction (see Chap. 9, this volume). Fear reactions are associated with elevations in the secretion of cortisol, a corticosteroid hormone produced by the adrenal cortex that can be assayed from blood, urine, or saliva samples (see Nadar & Weems, 2011, for a review). The intense taxing of this system in disasters may lead to dysregulation of the system. Dysregulation in this system has been associated with a number of emotional and behavioral disorders (Weems & Carrión, 2009; Yehuda, 2006). Research suggests that after a period of relative cortisol hypersecretion, elevated levels may reverse in trauma-exposed individuals (Weems & Carrión, 2007) to relatively low levels of cortisol (Yehuda, 2006). For example, Pfeffer, Altemus, Heo, and Jiang (2007) examined cortisol levels among bereaved youth following the September 11 attacks, finding that while bereaved youth had higher cortisol levels, those with PTSD had relatively lower evening cortisol levels than those without PTSD. This low cortisol may result from an enhanced negative feedback loop at the pituitary–adrenal level of the HPA axis (Yehuda et al., 1995). One mechanism for this sensitization may be an increased number of glucocorticoid receptors in the HPA axis that facilitates the negative feedback loop (Yehuda, 2006).

The experience of traumatic stress has been associated with atypical brain development in youth, including attenuated volume in brain regions that are involved in cognitive emotional processing such as the hippocampus (Carrión, Weems, & Reiss, 2007). Changes in neural structure and function following stress (Carrión et al., 2007; Carrión, Garrett, Menon, Weems, & Reiss, 2008; Carrión, Weems, Richert, Hoffman, & Reiss, 2010), and susceptibility to dysregulation in the normative stress response may characterize individual risk for mental health problems among disaster victims. Recently, La Greca, Lai, Joormann, Auslander, and Short (2013) found molecular genetic evidence for susceptibility, in that they showed that while greater exposure to hurricane stressors was related to more symptoms of PTSD and depression in a sample of youth, this effect was stronger for children with the met allele of the brain-derived neurotrophic factor (BDNF). There is also some evidence to suggest that differential brain activation may occur between trauma and non-trauma-exposed youth. Yang et al. (2011) examined a sample of Taiwanese adolescents using functional magnetic resonance imaging (fMRI) 14 months after exposure to a severe earthquake. Following the presentation of traumatic reminders (words) of the earthquake, the PTSD participants demonstrated activation in the bilateral visual cortex, bilateral cerebellum, and left parahippocampal gyrus; such activation was not present among the control participants.

Research has suggested that preexisting characteristics of the child can influence the impact of disaster exposure on mental health outcomes. In particular, previous research has documented that pre-hurricane trait anxiety and negative affect levels predict PTSD symptoms above and beyond exposure to the trauma (La Greca, Silverman, & Wasserstein, 1998; Weems et al., 2007). Anxiety sensitivity is another trait that has been studied in relation to hurricane exposure and panic (Hensley-Maloney & Varela, 2009). The authors assessed youth at 5–8 months and 17–18 months post Katrina and found that while hurricane exposure and anxiety sensitivity did predict panic symptoms at the initial assessment, the association between exposure and panic was not significant when youth were assessed at 17–18 months post disaster. The authors theorized that the temporal association between the trauma and panic symptoms could be due to an elevation in anxiety sensitivity following trauma which then generalizes to non-trauma-related cues and ultimately results in anxiety sensitivity having an association with panic over time.

One important consideration with regard to post-disaster outcomes over time is disaster-related secondary stressors (Silverman & La Greca, 2002). These stressors may function as cascading or cumulative events which then have the potential to promote the persistence of long-term psychopathology. For example, McLaughlin et al. (2010) found that several Hurricane Katrina-exposed children and adolescents developed new serious emotional disturbance (SED) during the period between baseline (18–27 months post Katrina) and follow-up 12–18 months later, and the onsets of SED during this period were more frequent among participants reporting high stress following from disaster-related secondary adversities. Additionally, post-hurricane negative life events such as family illness, financial strain, and arguments with parents have been found to be significant predictors of adolescents' increased substance use (i.e., alcohol, marijuana, and cigarettes) from 13 months pre Hurricane Rita to 19 months post disaster (Rohrbach, Grana, Vernberg, Sussman, & Sun, 2009). This finding is in line with the extant literature indicating that adverse life events are associated with psychological distress, which may lead to substance use in an effort to alleviate the distress (Newcomb, Huba, & Bentler, 1986; Wills, 1986; Wills, Vaccaro, & McNamara, 1992).

Microsystem Influences

The microsystem is the next level up from the individual child and represents the proximal ecologies within which the child develops, including the family/home and school environments and peer relationships (see Chap. 12, this volume). Disasters can affect youth adaptation by causing stress and disruptions in the family, school, and neighborhood environments. Disaster research on the microsystems impacted by disaster has tended to focus on the family environment, with studies showing that marital stress, domestic violence, and parental psychopathology increase after disasters (Larrance, Anastario, & Lawry, 2007; Norris et al., 2002). Research by Scheeringa and Zeanah (2008) and Spell et al. (2008) shows the importance of parental mental health for child functioning at two distinct developmental points. For preschool children, Scheeringa and Zeanah (2008) found that the onset of new mental health problems in preschool children was significantly correlated with the onset of new mental health problems in their caregivers. For school-age children (8–16 years), Spell et al. (2008) obtained a similar finding among a sample of 260 displaced mother–child dyads impacted by Katrina with maternal psychological distress a significant predictor of child mental health.

Focusing on long-term outcomes, Abramson et al. (2010) reported that data collected in a longitudinal study across 4 years post Katrina showed that youth whose parents reported mental health illness were more than five times as likely to have serious emotional disturbance than youth whose parents did not suffer from such distress. As noted by Scaramella, Sohr-Preston, Callahan, and Mirabile (2008), parental emotional distress and mental illness undermine parenting efficacy, resulting in increases in parental irritability and decreases in consistent discipline, both of which increase the risk for child mental health problems. In a longitudinal study, Kelley et al. (2010) found that youth who reported greater hurricane exposure had parents who reported more maladaptive coping; these parents were then more likely to employ the use of corporal punishment, which was associated with youths' PTSD symptoms at both 3–7 and 14–17 months post disaster.

Disasters may also result in the disruption of the school microsystem. There is evidence to suggest an indirect effect of disaster exposure (i.e., indirectly through PTSD symptoms fostering increased test anxiety) on youths' academic achievement (standardized test scores), a full 30 months following Katrina (Weems et al., 2013). Disasters may also necessitate relocation to another school. Ward, Shelley, Kaase, and Pane (2008) conducted a longitudinal study to examine the differences in achievement and school-related behavior between displaced and non-displaced students in Mississippi 2 years after Hurricane Katrina. The results indicated that displaced students were more likely to have disciplinary problems (i.e., suspension and expulsion) and had lower academic achievement than their non-displaced peers. Based on data collected 1 year before Hurricane Katrina, the authors determined that there were preexisting differences in behavior and achievement between the two groups before the storm, but there was an increase in suspension and expulsion post disaster for both displaced and non-displaced students. Additionally, displaced students had greater odds of being suspended or expelled, suggesting that not only were the students previously demonstrating disciplinary problems but that the forced relocation may also have amplified the effects of the trauma and been associated with the increase in disciplinary problems.

A critical factor of youths' microsystems is the social support received. Banks and Weems (2014) found that higher levels of social support from family and peers were associated with lower levels of psychological distress (i.e., symptoms of PTSD, anxiety, and depression) in a large sample of minority youth when assessed 36–65 months after Hurricane Katrina. The results from the study also showed that there was an association between lower social support and higher psychological distress longitudinally, similar to other studies that have examined longitudinal associations between social support and post-disaster distress in youth (e.g., Jaycox et al., 2010; La Greca, Silverman, Vernberg, & Prinstein, 1996; La Greca, Silverman, Lai, & Jaccard, 2010). Peer social support, in particular, showed multiple associations with lower distress concurrently and longitudinally in Banks and Weems' study, which makes theoretical sense as peer relationships become more salient across the developmental range of youth included in the study and so youth may have turned to peers more so than family for assistance in coping and decreasing isolation following the disaster (e.g., Pynoos & Nader, 1988; Vernberg & Vogel, 1993). Importantly, however, the findings from the study suggested the possibility that high hurricane exposure may potentially overwhelm the benefit of peer social support against the development of PTSD symptoms for some youth.

Increased risk created by disasters within microsystem environments may be offset by the presence of protective factors within the other microsystems surrounding the child. For example, school-based mental health services represent a protective factor within the school microsystem that can offset the negative developmental outcomes associated with disaster exposure (Abramson & Garfield, 2006; Pynoos, Goenjian, & Steinberg, 1998). Salloum and Overstreet (2008) and Weems et al. (2009, 2015) demonstrate the effectiveness of school-based interventions for children in post-disaster environments. Weems et al. (2009, 2015) tested the effects of a school-based test anxiety intervention on reducing PTS symptoms in which Hurricane Katrina-exposed youth with elevated test anxiety completed a primarily behavioral (e.g., relaxation training combined with gradual exposure to anxiety-provoking test-related stimuli) group-administered, test-anxiety-reduction intervention. Their findings yielded a statistically significant effect of the intervention on test anxiety levels and academic performance with evidence of positive secondary effects on PTS symptoms. Moreover, change in test anxiety predicted change in PTS, and there appeared to be no negative effects on natural PTS symptom decline. Test anxiety was highly associated with anxiety and depressive symptoms and was also predictive of PTSD symptoms.

Mesosystem Influences

The mesosystem is an intermediary system and represents linkages between more proximal (microsystems) ecologies. For example, parental participation in the child's school such as parent–teacher association meetings is a mesosystem connection between the microsystems of school and home. Disasters may sever these mesosystem ties between the various microsystems in children's lives (e.g., a longer commute to work or increased workplace demands may make attending school-based meetings more difficult). Salloum and Overstreet's (2008) school-based intervention study illustrates the potential to repair mesosystem connections in post-disaster environments. The intervention design included parent meetings, but most parents of the children receiving the intervention found it difficult to come to the school for a meeting, so the intervention incorporated a community-based parent meeting (i.e., at the parent's home or work) scheduled at the parent's convenience.

This flexibility in service provision resulted in successful parent meetings for 73 % of the sample, which allowed the opportunity to strengthen connections and ensure consistency between the home and school environments. Youth in the intervention groups had statistically significant reductions in PTS symptoms, depression, and traumatic grief.

Abramson et al. (2010) assessed the prevalence of serious emotional disturbance (i.e., both mental health distress and social, behavioral, or functional impairment) among youth in Louisiana and Mississippi more than 4 years post Hurricane Katrina and found that the three contexts of parents, household, and neighborhood were interrelated in contributing to youths' SED, such that pre-disaster poverty and post-disaster neighborhood social disorder each had a direct effect on post-disaster household stressors. These contexts, in turn, exerted a combined effect on parents which then was associated with youth SED. The authors theorized that the ongoing instability in the parental, household, and neighborhood contexts may have resulted in youths' sense of decreased social relatedness and control, and thus contributed to youths' long-term post-disaster mental health.

Exosystem Influences

The exosystem is the next level up from the micosystems in which the child develops, and involves the influences on youth adaptation that originate in contexts that do not directly involve the child, such as parent's workplace. Theoretically, they exert their effects by creating disruptions in contexts that do involve the child (e.g., family, school). These indirect effects are potentially insidious risk factors for mental health problems among youth. Parent's loss of work, financial difficulties, or work-related stress may translate to increased parental mental health problems or ineffective parenting, which in turn may increase risk for child mental health problems. For example, a longer work commute compared to before Hurricane Katrina was associated with PTSD symptoms in the New Orleans workforce (DeSalvo et al., 2007). Scheeringa and Zeanah (2008) found that workplace demands were the primary reason for parent–child separations during the evacuation and recovery periods following Katrina. Similarly, McLaughlin et al. (2009, 2010) found that lower family income among youth assessed from 18 to 39 months post Katrina was associated with increased risk for hurricane-attributable serious emotional disturbance.

Macrosystem Influences

Disasters may impact youth emotional problems at the broadest level. These may include geographic characteristics, broad government policies, national infrastructure, cultural values, and regional and national norms (see Bobo, 2006; Bourque, Siegel, Kano, & Wood, 2006). In particular, national infrastructure and wealth including socioeconomic and demographic characteristics are related to disaster-related deaths and injuries (Haque, 2003), and national wealth is related to less damage and death (i.e., countries with higher income and higher educational attainment experience fewer losses following disaster; see Toya & Skidmore, 2007). As an example of national norms, following the September 11 attacks, Gil-Rivas, Silver, Holman, McIntosh, and Poulin (2007) surveyed a large national sample of adolescents at 2 weeks and again at 7 months post attacks, and despite the distance from the attacks and the fact that exposure was indirect, links to PTS symptoms in youth were found (see also Schlenger et al., 2002; Schuster et al., 2001).

One mechanism for finding links between distal exposure and stress symptoms is media coverage (Comer & Kendall, 2007; Pfefferbaum et al., 2003). A macrosystem context which includes 24-hours-a-day/7-days-a-week news coverage and constant media exposure may thus broaden the effects of any particular disaster. Research suggests that watching more television (TV) coverage of a disaster is associated with more negative stress responses, including PTSD symptoms (Comer & Kendall, 2007; Pfefferbaum et al., 2003). Similar results have been found following the 9/11 attacks and Hurricane Gustav (e.g., Lengua, Long, Smith, & Meltzoff, 2005; Schuster et al., 2001; Weems, Scott, Banks, & Graham, 2012). An additional consideration is youth with preexisting distress symptoms, as the association between TV viewing and post-disaster symptomatology may be stronger for these youth compared to those without preexisting symptoms (Weems et al., 2012). Thus, the interaction between the macrosystem and individual factors may result in heightened risk for distress following trauma.

Conclusions

The research we have reviewed indicates that there are substantial effects of disaster exposure on youth. While the long-term effects of disaster exposure are relatively understudied, the extant literature suggests that many youth continue to experience symptoms of psychological distress long after a traumatic event. To understand the long-term effects, researchers have begun to define and identify multiple trajectories and the importance of identifying resilient subsamples in trauma and disaster-exposed individuals (see also Chap. 1, this volume). The ecological needs-based perspective can be used to integrate data and knowledge by showing how various factors within different ecologies surrounding the child act alone and/or in conjunction with other ecologies to either impede (protect) or foster (increase the risk of) the development of psychopathology.

Finally, it is important to highlight that effective interventions are available to youth experiencing mental health difficulties following disasters. Cognitive behavioral therapies (CBT) have extensive empirical support (e.g., Chemtob, Nakashima, & Hamada, 2002; see Silverman et al., 2008, for review and meta-analysis). CBT interventions are typically exposure based, and include various additional specific techniques such as psychoeducation, cognitive coping strategies, and relapse prevention (see Silverman et al., 2008). The research to date for disaster-exposed youth indicates reductions in youths' PTS symptoms from pre- to posttreatment, as well as maintenance of treatment gains at follow-up (Chemtob et al., 2002; Salloum & Overstreet, 2008; Taylor & Weems, 2011). However, as noted by several reviewers and reports, there is limited intervention research available and there is a need for further research on what interventions may best address the needs of disaster-exposed youth (Masten & Narayan, 2012).

Acknowledgment Correspondence concerning this chapter can be addressed to Carl F. Weems, Department of Human Development and Family Studies, Iowa State University, 2330C Palmer, Ames, IA 50011-4380, USA.
Electronic mail may be sent to cweems@iastate.edu

References

Aber, J. L., Gershoff, E. T., Ware, A., & Kotler, J. A. (2004). Estimating the effects of September 11th and other forms of violence on the mental health and social development of New York City's youth: A matter of context. *Applied Developmental Science, 8,* 111–129.

Abramson, D. M., & Garfield, R. (2006). On the edge—A report of the Louisiana child and family health study. www.ncdp.mailman.columbia.edu/files/marshall_plan.pdf. Accessed Dec 2006.

Abramson, D. M., Park, Y. S., Stehling-Ariza, T., & Redlener, I. (2010). Children as bellwethers of recovery: Dysfunctional systems and the effects of parents, households, and neighborhoods on serious emotional disturbance in children after Hurricane Katrina. *Disaster Medicine and Public Health Preparedness, 4*(S1), S17–S27.

Banks, D. M., & Weems, C. F. (2014). Family and peer social support and their links to psychological distress among hurricane-exposed minority youth. *American Journal of Orthopsychiatry, 84*(4), 341–352.

Becker-Blease, K. A., Turner, H. A., & Finkelhor, D. (2010). Disasters, victimization, and children's mental health. *Child Development, 81*(4), 1040–1052.

Bobo, L. D. (2006). Katrina: Unmasking race, poverty, and politics in the 21st century. *Du Bois Review, 3,* 1–6.

Bourque, L. B., Siegel, J. M., Kano, M., & Wood, M. M. (2006). Weathering the storm: The impact of hurricanes on physical and mental health. *The Annals of the American Academy of Political and Social Science, 604,* 129–151.

Bonanno, G. A., Brewin, C. R., Kaniasty, K., & La Greca, A. M. (2010). Weighing the costs of disaster consequences, risks, and resilience in individuals, families, and communities. *Psychological Science in Public Interest, 11,* 1–49.

Bonanno, G. A., Westphal, M., & Mancini, A. D. (2011). Resilience to loss and potential trauma. *Annual Review of Clinical Psychology, 7,* 1–25.

Bronfenbrenner, U. (1979). *The ecology of human development.* Cambridge: Harvard University Press.

Carrión, V. G., Weems, C. F., & Reiss, A. L. (2007). Stress predicts brain changes in children: A pilot longitudinal study on youth stress, PTSD, and the hippocampus. *Pediatrics, 119,* 509–516.

Carrión, V. G., Garrett, A., Menon, V., Weems, C. F., & Reiss, A. L. (2008). Posttraumatic stress symptoms and brain function during a response-inhibition task: An fMRI study in youth. *Depression and Anxiety, 25,* 514–526.

Carrión, V. G., Weems, C. F., Richert, K., Hoffman, B., & Reiss, A. L. (2010). Decreased prefrontal cortical volume associated with increased bedtime cortisol in traumatized youth. *Biological Psychiatry, 68,* 491–493.

Chemtob, C. M., Nakashima, J. P., & Hamada, R. S. (2002). Psychosocial intervention for post-disaster trauma symptoms in elementary school children. *Archives of Pediatric and Adolescent Medicine, 156,* 211–216.

Comer, J. S., & Kendall, P. C. (2007). Terrorism: The psychological impact on youth. *Clinical Psychology: Science and Practice, 14,* 179–212.

DeSalvo, K. B., Hyre, A. D., Ompad, D. C., Menke, A., Tynes, L. L., & Muntner, P. (2007). Symptoms of posttraumatic stress disorder in a New Orleans workforce following Hurricane Katrina. *Journal of Urban Health, 84,* 142–152.

Eisenberg, N., & Silver, R. C. (2011). Growing up in the shadow of terrorism: Youth in America after 9/11. *American Psychologist, 66,* 468.

Furr, J. M., Comer, J. S., Edmunds, J. M., & Kendall, P. C. (2010). Disasters and youth: A meta-analytic examination of posttraumatic stress. *Journal of Consulting and Clinical Psychology, 78*(6), 765.

Gershoff, E. T., Aber, J. L., Ware, A., & Kotler, J. A. (2010). Exposure to 9/11 among youth and their mothers in New York City: Enduring associations with mental health and sociopolitical attitudes. *Child Development, 81*(4), 1142–1160.

Gil-Rivas, V., Silver, R. C., Holman, E. A., McIntosh, D. N., & Poulin, M. (2007). Parental response and adolescent adjustment to the September 11, 2001 terrorist attacks. *Journal of Traumatic Stress, 20*(6), 1063–1068. doi:10.1002/jts.20277.

Goenjian, A. K., Walling, D., Steinberg, A. M., Karayan, I., Najarian, L. M., Pynoos, R. (2005). A prospective study of posttraumatic stress and depressive reactions among treated and untreated adolescents five years after a catastrophic disaster. *American Journal of Psychiatry, 162,* 2302–2308.

Haque, C. E. (2003). Perspectives of natural disasters in East and South Asia, and the Pacific Island States: Socio-economic correlates and needs assessment. *Natural Hazards, 29*(3), 465–483.

Hensley-Maloney, L., & Varela, R. (2009). The influence of hurricane exposure and anxiety sensitivity on panic symptoms. *Child and Youth Care Forum, 38*(3), 135–149.

Hobfoll, S. E. (1989). Conservation of resources: A new attempt at conceptualizing stress. *American Psychologist, 44,* 513–524.

Jaycox, L. H., Cohen, J. A., Mannarino, A. P., Walker, D. W., Langley, A. K., Gegenheimer, K. L., et al. (2010). Children's mental health care following Hurricane Katrina: A field trial of trauma-focused psychotherapies. *Journal of Traumatic Stress, 23*(2), 223–231.

Kelley, M. L., Self-Brown, S., Le, B., Bosson, J. V., Hernandez, B. C., & Gordon, A. T. (2010). Predicting posttraumatic stress symptoms in children following Hurricane Katrina: A prospective analysis of the effect of parental distress and parenting practices. *Journal of Traumatic Stress, 23*(5), 582–590.

Kilmer, R. P., & Gil-Rivas, V. (2010). Exploring posttraumatic growth in children impacted by Hurricane Katrina: Correlates of the phenomenon and developmental considerations. *Child Development, 81*(4), 1211–1227.

Kilmer, R. P., Gil-Rivas, V., Tedeschi, R. G., Cann, A., Calhoun, L. G., Buchanan, T., & Taku, K. (2009). Use of the revised posttraumatic growth inventory for children. *Journal of Traumatic Stress, 22*(3), 248–253.

Kronenberg, M. E., Hansel, T., Brennan, A. M., Osofsky, H. J., Osofsky, J. D., & Lawrason, B. (2010). Children of Katrina: Lessons learned about postdisaster symptoms and recovery patterns. *Child Development, 81*(4), 1241–1259. doi:10.1111/j.1467-8624.2010.01465.x.

La Greca, A. M., Silverman, W. K., Vernberg, E. M., & Prinstein, M. J. (1996). Symptoms of posttraumatic stress in children alter Hurricane Andrew: A prospective study. *Journal of Consulting and Clinical Psychology, 64,* 712–723.

La Greca, A. M., Silverman, W. K., & Wasserstein, S. B. (1998). Children's predisaster functioning as a predictor of posttraumatic stress following Hurricane Andrew. *Journal of Consulting and Clinical Psychology, 66,* 883–892.

La Greca, A. M., Silverman, W. K., Vernberg, E. M., & Roberts, M. C. (Eds.). (2002). *Helping children cope with disasters and terrorism*. Washington, DC: American Psychological Association.

La Greca, A. M., Silverman, W. K., Lai, B., & Jaccard, J. (2010). Hurricane-related exposure experiences and stressors, other life events, and social support: Concurrent and prospective impact on children's persistent posttraumatic stress symptoms. *Journal of Consulting and Clinical Psychology, 78*(6), 794.

La Greca, A. M., Lai, B. S., Joormann, J., Auslander, B., & Short, M. (2013). Children's risk and resilience following a natural disaster: Genetic vulnerability, posttraumatic stress, and depression. *Journal of Affective Disorders*. doi:10.1016/j.jad.2013.07.024.

Larrance, R., Anastario, M., & Lawry, L. (2007). Health status among internally displaced persons in Louisiana and Mississippi travel trailer parks. *Annals of Emergency Medicine, 49,* 590–601.

Lengua, L. J., Long, A. C., Smith, K. I., & Meltzoff, A. N. (2005). Pre-attack symptomatology and temperament as predictors of children's responses to the September 11 terrorist attacks. *Journal of Child Psychology and Psychiatry, 46*(6), 631–645.

Luthar, S. S., Cicchetti, D., & Becker, B. (2000). The construct of resilience: A critical evaluation and guidelines for future work. *Child Development, 71*(3), 543–562.

Masten, A. S., & Narayan, A. J. (2012). Child development in the context of disaster, war, and terrorism: Pathways of risk and resilience. *Psychology, 63,* 227–257.

Masten, A. S., & Obradovic, J. (2008). Disaster preparation and recovery: Lessons from research on resilience in human development. *Ecology and Society, 13*(1), 9.

McLaughlin, K. A., Fairbank, J. A., Gruber, M. J., Jones, R. T., Lakoma, M. D., Pfefferbaum, B., et al. (2009). Serious emotional disturbance among youths exposed to Hurricane Katrina 2 years postdisaster. *Journal of the American Academy of Child and Adolescent Psychiatry, 48*(11), 1069–1078.

McLaughlin, K. A., Fairbank, J. A., Gruber, M. J., Jones, R. T., Osofsky, J. D., Pfefferbaum, B., et al. (2010). Trends in serious emotional disturbance among youths exposed to Hurricane Katrina. *Journal of the American Academy of Child and Adolescent Psychiatry, 49*(10), 990–1000.

Nader, K. O., & Weems, C. F. (2011). Understanding and assessing cortisol levels in children and adolescents. *Journal of Child and Adolescent Trauma, 4,* 318–338.

Newcomb, M. D., Huba, G. J., & Bentler, P. M. (1986). Life change events among adolescents: An empirical consideration of some methodological issues. *Journal of Nervous and Mental Disease, 174,* 280–289.

Norris, F. H., Perilla, J. L., Riad, J. K., Kaniasty, K., & Lavizzo, E. A. (1999). Stability and change in stress, resources, and psychological distress following natural disaster: Findings from Hurricane Andrew. *Anxiety, Stress, and Coping, 12,* 363–396.

Norris, F. H., Friedman, M. J., & Watson, P. J. (2002). 60,000 disaster victims speak: Part II. Summary and implications of the disaster mental health research. *Psychiatry, 65,* 240–260.

Osofsky, H. J., Osofsky, J. D., Kronenberg, M., Brennan, A., & Hansel, T. C. (2009). Posttraumatic stress symptoms in children after Hurricane Katrina: Predicting the need for mental health services. *American Journal of Orthopsychiatry, 79*(2), 212–220. doi:10.1037/a0016179.

Pfeffer, C. R., Altemus, M., Heo, M., & Jiang, H. (2007). Salivary cortisol and psychopathology in children bereaved by the September 11, 2001 terror attacks. *Biological Psychiatry, 61,* 957–965. doi:10.1016/j.biopsych.2006.07.037.

Pfefferbaum, B., Seale, T., Brandt, E., Pfefferbaum, R., Doughty, D., & Rainwater, S. (2003). Media exposure in children one hundred miles from a terrorist bombing. *Annals of Clinical Psychiatry, 15,* 1–8.

Pynoos, R. S., & Nader, K. (1988). Psychological first aid and treatment approach to children exposed to community violence: Research implications. *Journal of Traumatic Stress, 1,* 445–473.

Pynoos, R. S., Goenjian, A. K., & Steinberg, A. M. (1998). A public mental health approach to the postdisaster treatment of children and adolescents. *Child and Adolescent Psychiatric Clinics of North America, 7*(1), 195.

Rohrbach, L. A., Grana, R., Vernberg, E., Sussman, S., & Sun, P. (2009). Impact of Hurricane Rita on adolescent substance use. *Psychiatry: Interpersonal and Biological Processes, 72*(3), 222–237. doi:10.1521/psyc.2009.72.3.222.

Salloum, A., & Overstreet, S. (2008). Evaluation of individual and group grief and trauma interventions for children post disaster. *Journal of Clinical Child and Adolescent Psychology, 37,* 495–507.

Sandler, I. (2001). Quality and ecology of adversity as common mechanisms of risk and resilience. *American Journal of Community Psychology, 29,* 19–61.

Scaramella, L. V., Sohr-Preston, S. L., Callahan, K. L., & Mirabile, S. P. (2008). A test of the Family Stress Model on toddler-aged children's adjustment among Hurricane Katrina impacted and non-impacted low income families. *Journal of Clinical Child and Adolescent Psychology, 37,* 530–541.

Scheeringa, M. S., & Zeanah, C. H. (2008). Reconsideration of harm's way: Onsets and comorbidity patterns of disorders in preschool children and their caregivers following Hurricane Katrina. *Journal of Clinical Child and Adolescent Psychology, 37,* 508–518.

Schlenger, W. E., Caddell, J. M., Ebert, L., Jordan, B. K., Rourke, K. M., Wilson, D., et al. (2002). Psychological reactions to terrorist attacks: Findings from the National Study of Americans' Reactions to September 11. *Journal of the American Medical Association, 288*(5), 581–588.

Schuster, M. A., Stein, B. D., Jaycox, L. H., Collins, R. L., Marshall, G. N., Elliott, M. N., et al. (2001). A national survey of stress reactions after the September 11, 2001, terrorist attacks. *New England Journal of Medicine, 345*(20), 1507–1512.

Silverman, W. K., & La Greca, A. M. (2002). Children experiencing disasters: Definitions, reactions, and predictors of outcomes. In A. M. La Greca, W. K. Silverman, E. M. Vernberg, & M. C. Roberts (Eds.), *Helping children cope with disasters* (pp. 11–34). Washington, DC: American Psychological Association.

Silverman, W. K., Oritz, C. D., Viswesvaran, C., Burns, B. J., Kolko, D. J., Putnam, F. W., & Amaya-Jackson, L. (2008). Evidence based treatments for children and adolescents exposed to traumatic events. *Journal of Clinical Child and Adolescent Psychology, 37*(1), 156–183.

Spell, A. W., Kelley, M. L., Self-Brown, S., Davidson, K., Pellegrin, A., Palcic, J., Meyer, K., Paasch, V., & Baumeister, A. (2008). The moderating effects of maternal psychopathology on children's adjustment post-Hurricane Katrina. *Journal of Clinical Child and Adolescent Psychology, 37,* 553–563.

Sroufe, L. A. (1997). *Emotional development: The organization of emotional life in the early years*. Cambridge: Cambridge University Press.

Taylor, L. K., & Weems, C. F. (2011). Cognitive-behavior therapy for disaster exposed youth with posttraumatic stress: Results from a multiple-baseline examination. *Behavior Therapy, 42,* 349–363.

Toya, H., & Skidmore, M. (2007). Economic development and the impacts of natural disasters. *Economics Letters, 94*(1), 20–25.

Vernberg, E. M., & Vogel, J. M. (1993). Part 2: Interventions with children after disasters. *Journal of Clinical Child Psychology, 22*(4), 485–498.

Vogel, J. M., & Vernberg, E. M. (1993). Part 1: Children's psychological responses to disasters. *Journal of Clinical Child Psychology, 22*(4), 464–484.

Ward, M. E., Shelley, K., Kaase, K., & Pane, J. F. (2008). Hurricane Katrina: A longitudinal study of the achievement and behavior of displaced students. *Journal of Education for Students Placed at Risk, 13*(2–3), 297–317.

Weems, C. F., & Carrión, V. G. (2007). The association between PTSD symptoms and salivary cortisol in youth: The role of the time since the trauma. *Journal of Traumatic Stress, 20,* 903–907.

Weems, C., & Carrión, V. (2009). Diurnal salivary cortisol in youth: Clarifying the nature of posttraumatic stress dysregulation. *Journal of Pediatric Psychology, 34,* 389–395.

Weems, C. F., & Graham, R. A. (2014). Resilience and trajectories of posttraumatic stress among youth exposed to disaster. *Journal of Child and Adolescent Psychopharmacology, 24*(1), 2–8.

Weems, C. F., & Overstreet, S. (2008). Child and adolescent mental health research in the context of Hurricane Katrina: An ecological-needs-based perspective and introduction to the special section. *Journal of Clinical Child and Adolescent Psychology, 37,* 487–494.

Weems, C. F., & Overstreet, S. (2009). An ecological-needs-based perspective of adolescent and youth emotional development in the context of disaster: Lessons from Hurricane Katrina. In Katie E. Cherry (Ed.), *Lifespan perspectives on natural disasters: Coping with Katrina, Rita and other storms* (pp. 27–44). New York: Springer.

Weems, C. F., Piña, A. A., Costa, N. M., Watts, S. E., Taylor, L. K., & Cannon, M. F. (2007). Predisaster trait anxiety and negative affect predict posttraumatic stress in youth after Hurricane Katrina. *Journal of Consulting and Clinical Psychology, 75,* 154–159.

Weems, C. F., Taylor, L. K., Costa, N. M., Marks, A. B., Romano, D. M., Verrett, S. L., & Brown, D. M. (2009). Effect of a school-based test anxiety intervention in ethnic minority youth exposed to Hurricane Katrina. *Journal of Applied Developmental Psychology, 30,* 218–226.

Weems, C. F., Taylor, L. K., Cannon, M. F., Marino, R., Romano, D. M., Scott, B. G., Perry A. M., & Triplett, V. (2010). Posttraumatic stress, context, and the lingering effects of the Hurricane Katrina disaster among ethnic minority youth. *Journal of Abnormal Child Psychology, 38,* 49–56.

Weems, C. F., Scott, B. G., Banks, D. M., & Graham, R. A. (2012). Is TV traumatic for all youths? The role of pre-existing posttraumatic stress symptoms on the link between disaster coverage and stress. *Psychological Science, 23,* 1293–1297.

Weems, C. F., Scott, B. G., Taylor, L. K., Cannon, M. F., Romano, D. M., & Perry A. M. (2013). A theoretical model of continuity in anxiety and links to academic achievement in disaster exposed school children. *Development and Psychopathology, 25,* 729–738.

Weems, C. F., Russell, J.D., Banks, D. M., Graham, R. A., Neill, E. L., & Scott, B. G. (2014). Memories of traumatic events in childhood fade after experiencing similar less stressful events: Results from two natural experiments. *Journal of Experimental Psychology: General,* 143, 2046–2055. doi: 10.1037/xge0000016

Weems, C. F., Scott, B. G., Graham, R. A., Banks, D. M., Russell, J. D., Taylor, L. K., et al. (2015). Fitting anxious emotion-focused intervention into the ecology of schools: Results from a test anxiety program evaluation. *Prevention Science, 16,* 200–210. DOI: 10.1007/s11121-014-0491-1.

Wills, T. A. (1986). Stress and coping in early adolescence: Relationships to substance use in urban school samples. *Health Psychology, 5*(6), 503–529.

Wills, T. A., Vaccaro, D., & McNamara, G. (1992) The role of life events, family support, and competence in adolescent substance use: A test of vulnerability and protective factors. *American Journal of Community Psychology, 20*(3), 349–374.

Yang, P., Yen, C. F., Tang, T. C., Chen, C. S., Yang, R. C., Huang, M. S., et al. (2011). Posttraumatic stress disorder in adolescents after Typhoon Morakot-associated mudslides. *Journal of Anxiety Disorders, 25*(3), 362–368.

Yehuda, R. (2006). Advances in understanding neuroendocrine alterations in PTSD and their therapeutic implications. *Annals of the New York Academy of Sciences, 1071,* 137–166.

Yehuda, R., Kahana, B., Binder-Brynes, K., Southwick, S. M., Mason, J. W., & Giller, E. L. (1995). Low urinary cortisol excretion in Holocaust survivors with posttraumatic stress disorder. *American Journal of Psychiatry, 152,* 982–986.

Chapter 11
Psychosocial Consequences: Appraisal, Adaptation, and Bereavement After Trauma

Edward E. Waldrep and Charles C. Benight

Introduction

In an ideal world, traumatic life events would be rare and limited to only things outside the capacity for human intervention (i.e., accidents, natural disasters). Unfortunately, that is not the world we live in. Traumatic events have been found to be more common than anyone would prefer. Prevalence rates of trauma exposure can range from anywhere between 50 and 90% of the population (Kessler, Sonnega, Bromet, Hughes, & Nelson, 1995; Breslau et al., 1998).

The effects of experiencing a trauma on an individual can be devastating and fundamentally change the way one perceives his/her self and the world (Ehlers & Clark, 2000; Foa & Rothbaum, 1998; Janoff-Bulman, 1992). Negative outcomes following direct exposure to traumatic events have been studied extensively (Norris et al., 2002) and include a variety of negative outcomes including post-traumatic stress disorder (PTSD; Brewin, Andrews, & Valentine, 2000), negative coping behaviors (Kilpatrick et al., 2000), and disrupted social functioning (Guay, Billette, & Marchand, 2006). Positive change following trauma has also been studied including benefit finding (Helgeson, Reynolds, & Tomich, 2006), stress-related growth (Park, Cohen, & Murch, 1996), meaning making (Park & Ai, 2006), and posttraumatic growth (Tedeschi & Calhoun, 2004). More specific details of traumatic events and how they can change lives are detailed in Sect. I of this book and beyond the scope of this chapter. The purpose of this chapter is to focus on the process of human adaptation to a variety of traumatic stress contexts.

E. E. Waldrep (✉)
Department of Psychology, Kent State University, Kent, OH 44242, USA
e-mail: ewaldrep@kent.edu

C. C. Benight
Department of Psychology, Trauma Health & Hazards Center, University of Colorado at Colorado Springs, 4017 Columbine Hall, Colorado Springs, CO 80918, USA
e-mail: benight@uccs.edu

K. E. Cherry (ed.), *Traumatic Stress and Long-Term Recovery*,
DOI 10.1007/978-3-319-18866-9_11

To do so, we start by describing cognitive models of stress and adaptation to psychological trauma and then incorporate those models within the theoretical framework of social cognitive theory (SCT; Bandura, 1997). SCT is a practical, empirically supported theoretical framework that is able to account for the various features observed in posttraumatic adaptation, both negative and positive responses. In addition, the theory provides a fertile ground to generate testable hypotheses to further our understanding of how human beings react to life's most tragic events. The essential components of the theory are described as well as studies that have highlighted the effectiveness of this approach.

Cognitive and Resource Models of Traumatic Stress

Before we launch into a deeper description of the coping process related to traumatic stress, it is important to define the use of the terms stress versus traumatic stress. We argue that the human adaptation processes are the same and stress versus traumatic stress are on a continuum ranging from a mild stressor or annoyance (e.g., being late for a business meeting) to-life threatening stress (e.g., being in a severe car accident). The adaptation demands are clearly more severe for a life-threatening event, yet the cognitive processes involved in self-regulation are the same. For the purpose of this chapter, stressful events refer to traumatic stress.

Coping with stressful events is a dynamic process that changes over time (Benight & Bandura, 2004; Folkman & Lazarus, 1985). Successful adaptation to traumatic stressors requires the person to recognize the nature of the traumatic stressor, determine what needs to be done in response, and then engaging in behaviors determined to bring about desired results (Bandura, 1997). Lazarus and Folkman's (1984) transactional theory of stress delineates the cognitive elements thought to mediate the relationship between environmental conditions and coping behaviors (see also Chap. 3, this volume). Stress results from the perception that environmental demands are greater than the resources one is able to apply. This threatens one's well-being and is experienced as stressful (Lazarus & Folkman, 1984). The essential cognitive elements in the coping process are primary and secondary appraisals of a stress-evoking event (for a review, see: Folkman & Moskowitz, 2004).

Primary appraisals refer to the initial evaluation of how relevant specific situational demands are for personal well-being (Folkman, 1984). For less severe stress, this includes appraisals that are deemed to be irrelevant, benign, and positive. Traumatic stress, by definition, is appraised to be stressful. Stressors perceived to be a challenge are characterized by the potential for growth and more pleasurable emotions (Lazarus & Folkman, 1984). More recent research on traumatic stress has suggested opportunities for growth are important to consider (Tedeschi & Calhoun, 2004). Such encounters may elicit heightened physiological activation, but the energy is guided into effort to overcome the perceived challenge (Tomaka, Blascovich, Kelsey, & Leitten, 1993). Limited research has looked at specific appraisals of challenge versus threat in trauma survivors, yet the evidence for resilience (Bonanno & Mancini, 2012) in trauma survivors suggests more work in this area is needed.

Negative affectivity, such as anger and fear, are associated with harm/loss and threat perceptions (Folkman, 1984). Within this model, personal factors are considered to be essential elements of how stressful encounters are perceived. Relevant personal factors include preexisting beliefs (e.g., religious, cultural), situational (i.e., perceived ability to exert some control over the situation), and commitments (e.g., parenthood, occupation) that may influence the individual's well-being (Folkman, 1984).

Following the primary appraisal process, secondary appraisal is the process that evaluates available resources and possible courses of action (Lazarus & Folkman, 1984). Available coping resources can include things such as social support, physical capabilities, material resources, psychological factors, as well as perceived situational control (Folkman, 1984). The coping process involves the dynamic integration of the initial appraisal of the stressful event with the various coping resources that the individual perceives that they are able to employ at a given point in time.

Another model of psychological stress is the conservation of resources (COR) theory (Hobfoll, 1989, 1991, 2001; see also Chap. 1, this volume). In contrast to Lazarus and Folkman's (1984) transactional theory of stress, COR theory attempts to conceptualize how humans experience stress in a more objective manner by focusing on resources considered to be more available to measurement. The primary tenet of the theory is that people work to obtain, retain, and protect resources (Hobfoll, 2001). Loss of valued resources is suggested to be the determining factor of the human experience of stress. Resources are identified as objects (e.g., material possessions), conditions (e.g., marriage, work), personal characteristics (e.g., self-esteem, social effectiveness), and energies (e.g., knowledge, insurance). Stress is the result of resources being threatened or lost (Hobfoll, 1991). Stress is also considered to occur when there is a lack of resource gain following an investment of possessed resources (Hobfoll, 1991).

Within this model, humans actively identify what resources they value and work to obtain those resources. Once resources have been obtained, individuals will strive to preserve the resources they have or invest them in opportunities to acquire more. Further, available resources can be used to either protect or compensate from a potential loss (Hobfoll, 1991). Loss spirals can be one of the consequences of traumatic events. An individual caught in a loss spiral will not have the same amount of resources to invest to offset further loss. Within this framework, traumatic stress can result from a rapid loss of resources (Hobfoll, 1991). The traumatic event results in a rapid loss of resources because of its unexpected nature, excessive demands, and strategies have not been developed to use available resources to lessen the impact of the loss (Hobfoll, 1991). COR theory's focus on objective resources has demonstrated strong empirical associations with posttraumatic stress (Hobfoll, 2001). However, intrapersonal factors have been shown to mediate the relationship between resource loss and posttraumatic distress (Benight, Swift, Sanger, Smith, & Zeppelin, 1999b).

There are other models that focus more specifically on the development and maintenance of PTSD such as the dual representation theory (Brewin, Dalgleish, & Joseph, 1996), shattered assumptions about the world and one's self (Janoff-Bulman,

1992), emotional processing theory (Foa, Steketee, & Rothbaum, 1989), and cognitive appraisal-based approach (Ehlers & Clark, 2000) among others (see Brewin & Holmes, 2003).

The preceding discussion highlights the interactional process between the individual and a traumatic stress experience. The importance of cognitive processes in managing the often sudden and extreme demands of traumatic stress is central in most of the theoretical approaches. SCT provides a useful framework for understanding human behavior in the throes of traumatic stress and points to the importance of self-regulation.

Social Cognitive Theory

SCT is a wide-ranging model of human behavior (Bandura, 1997). SCT proposes that human behavior is the result of the bidirectional influence of three primary determinants (see Fig. 11.1): environmental, behavior, and internal personal factors (Bandura, 1997). Bandura (1997) refers to the dynamic influence of these factors upon each other as *triadic reciprocal causation.* Human agency and self-regulation are essential elements of the theory. Human agency refers to the capacity for one to act intentionally to bring about a desired outcome (Bandura, 2001). Self-regulation refers to the human ability to incorporate forethought to plan behavior and use available resources to achieve those outcomes (Bandura, 1997; Maddux, 1995). Agency facilitates the self-regulative behavior necessary to successfully adapt to stressful situations (Bandura, 2001; Benight & Bandura, 2004; Folkman, 1984). Therefore, humans are more than reactionary animals attempting to meet environmental demands. Humans are agents directly shaping environments because of the capacity to act intentionally and envision desired outcomes (Bandura, 1997).

Self-efficacy beliefs are integral to self-regulation and serve as a key psychological construct within SCT (Bandura, 1997; Maddux, 1995). Self-efficacy beliefs refer to the perceived ability to engage in the necessary behaviors to bring

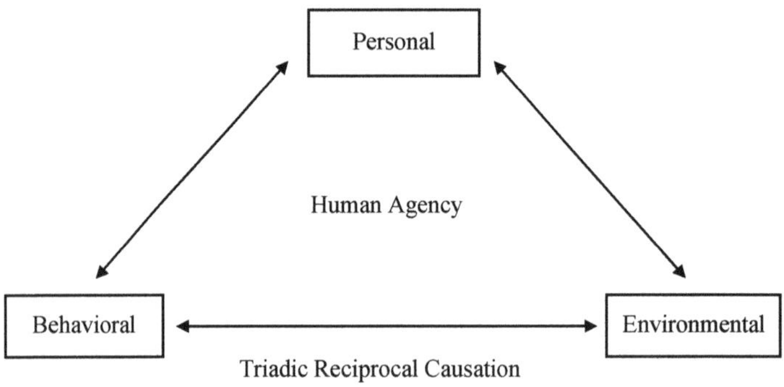

Fig. 11.1 Triadic reciprocal causation model representing the bi-directional influence of intrapersonal (cognitive, affective, physiological), behavioral, and environmental factors

about desired results (Bandura, 1997). Self-efficacy beliefs have been investigated rigorously in a wide range of human behaviors (see Bandura, 1997) and garnered outstanding empirical support (Cervone, 2000). According to Bandura (1997), self-efficacy beliefs are the most direct, proximal predictors of human behavior in a specific domain. Although more general self-efficacy beliefs have demonstrated reliable and significant associations with a wide range of outcome variables and cultural contexts (Luszczynska, Scholz, & Schwarzer, 2005), they are not considered to be as powerful in predicting critical outcomes as situationally specific self-efficacy beliefs. In the context of traumatic stress, specific self-efficacy beliefs associated with posttraumatic adaptation are referred to as coping self-efficacy (CSE; Benight & Bandura, 2004).

Coping Self-Efficacy

CSE beliefs refer to the perceived ability to meet the demands imposed on an individual by experiencing a traumatic event (Benight & Bandura, 2004). Traumatic events comprise situations that include physical threat to oneself or loved ones and can happen in a wide variety of contexts including military combat, physical assault, sexual assault, natural disasters, and man-made disasters among others (Breslau et al., 1998; Norris, 1992). Each different type of event may have unique recovery demands. For example, motor vehicle accident (MVA) survivors may have to deal with physical injuries, challenges with insurance companies, and loss of transportation, whereas sexual assault survivors may have to deal with physical injuries, fear of becoming pregnant if the victim is female, decision making related to reporting the crime, as well as the challenge of intimacy after the event. Neither one of these examples exhaust the potential challenges anyone may face after such experiences. They merely highlight some of the psychological and social demands trauma can impose on an individual. It is important to note that many, if not most, of the posttraumatic recovery demands for many individuals are completely foreign, compounding the coping challenges. Of course, this may not be the case for survivors of repeated trauma such as child abuse or soldiers who have been repeatedly deployed to combat zones, for example (see Chap. 7, this volume). Multiple exposures create additional posttraumatic burdens that complicate the coping process.

The duration of the traumatic exposure can vary greatly as well. Some events may be acute and time-limited stressors such as a MVA, whereas others may persist for months or even years (e.g., the aftermath of a natural disaster; see Chaps. 10, 12, and 13, this volume). Whether acute or chronic, recovering from a traumatic event challenges an individual's capacity to cope. Thus, it is important to understand the evolving posttraumatic coping difficulties that an individual must navigate.

Self-efficacy beliefs play a critical role during this adaptation process (Bandura, 1997; Benight & Bandura, 2004). Indeed, the process of recovering from a traumatic event can push an individual's capacity to cope to the limits and beyond

(Bandura, 1997; Benight & Bandura, 2004). The novel coping demands require that the individual draw upon previous coping experiences in different domains (Bandura, 1997; Benight & Bandura, 2004). CSE beliefs are then developed through self-evaluation and self-regulative processes throughout recovery (e.g., success or failure feedback).

These feedback systems are described in the triadic reciprocal process (see Fig. 11.1). Individuals evaluate successes or failures as they engage in coping behaviors (e.g., seeking social support, managing intrusive thoughts) targeted to help recover from the tragic event. Indeed, as SCT posits, through our ability to use forethought and self-reflection, humans are able to influence the posttraumatic recovery environment through the skillful application of strategic planning and resource utilization. Successful coping experiences after the traumatic event can foster a sense of personal mastery, a powerful source of self-efficacy beliefs. Over time, perceived successful management of critical posttraumatic demands enhances personal beliefs in one's coping capabilities, promotes effective posttraumatic adaptation, and may potentiate posttraumatic growth (Benight & Bandura, 2004; Cieslak, Benight, & Lehman, 2008). Conversely, many survivors experience a sense of complete personal failure due to a perfect storm of intrusive thoughts related to the trauma, serious on-going environmental challenges, and social isolation. Such thoughts drive a deeper sense of one's inability to cope, increasing distress, and feelings of despair.

Research investigating the association between CSE beliefs and posttraumatic adaptation has been conducted with a variety of different populations and traumatic events including natural disaster (Benight, Antoni, Kilbourn, & Ironson, 1997; Benight & Harper, 2002; Benight et al., 1999b; Hirschel & Schulenberg, 2009), physical assault (Johansen, Wahl, Eilertsen, & Weisaeth, 2007); inter-partner violence (Benight, Harding-Taylor, Midboe, & Durham, 2004; Lambert, Benight, Wong, & Johnson, 2013), military combat (Solomon, Benbenishty, & Mulkulincer, 1991), reintegration of veterans after combat deployment (Smith, Benight, & Cieslak, 2013), terrorist attack (Benight et al., 2000), MVAs (Benight, Cieslak, Molton, & Johnson, 2008), and bereavement (Benight, Flores, & Tashiro, 2001). Studies have consistently demonstrated the predictive power of CSE beliefs with a variety of posttraumatic outcomes (Benight & Bandura, 2004; Luszczynska, Benight, & Cieslak, 2009b). The following sections briefly describe the results of various studies investigating the association between CSE beliefs and psychosocial outcomes in different traumatic stress settings.

Coping Self-Efficacy in Various Posttrauma Environments

Natural Disaster

Natural disasters can have significant mental and physical health implications (Lowe, Tracy, Cerdá, Norris, & Galea, 2013; Norris, Slone, Baker, & Murphy, 2006; Norris, Friedman Watson, Byrne, Diaz, & Kaniasty, 2002). Although most will recover with time, the coping challenges with a major disaster are significant (see Chaps. 5, 10, 12, and 13, this volume). Benight and colleagues investigated the role of CSE beliefs following a series of natural disasters including Hurricane Andrew (Benight et al., 1997, 1999a), Hurricane Opal (Benight et al., 1999b), and a dual wildfire and flood (Benight & Harper, 2002).

Benight et al. (1999a) demonstrated that acute CSE perceptions after the hurricane mediated the effect of resource loss on both acute and longer-term (approximately 1 year later) distress. Also, following Hurricane Andrew, Benight et al. (1997) examined the role of CSE beliefs of human immunodeficiency virus positive (HIV+) gay male disaster survivors and healthy male controls. CSE demonstrated a significant negative relationship with posttraumatic stress symptoms. In the HIV+ sample, CSE accounted for 51 % of the variance of posttraumatic stress symptoms after controlling for the estimated damage, perceived life threat, education, income, and cluster of differentiation (CD)4 cell count (Benight et al., 1997). The results were similar when predicting general psychological distress, accounting for an additional 27 % of the variance. The same pattern was replicated in the healthy control sample as well. CSE accounted for an additional 30 % of posttraumatic stress symptoms and 25 % of general distress after controlling for other variables.

Similarly, following Hurricane Opal, Benight et al. (1999b) found that CSE accounted for 34 % of general psychological distress over and above resource loss and gender in this cross-sectional study. This study also demonstrated that CSE beliefs mediated the relationship between resource loss and posttraumatic stress symptoms, optimism and general distress, as well as social support (for predictors of PTSD, see Ozer, Best, Lipsey, & Weiss, 2003) and distress (Benight et al., 1999b).

Following a devastating wildfire and subsequent deadly flash flood, Benight and Harper (2002) assessed the longitudinal predictive capacity of CSE beliefs. The community was initially threatened with a wildfire that engulfed 12,000 acres of land and took several homes and left much of the landside charred and bare. Soon after, a flash flood claimed two fatalities and disrupted essential community resources (e.g., water, transportation, communications) for months. CSE beliefs significantly predicted posttraumatic stress symptoms and general distress immediately following the disasters after controlling for age, gender, and acute stress responses. Further, CSE beliefs, assessed at time 1, mediated the relationship between acute stress responses and general distress on posttraumatic stress symptoms at 1 year.

Taken together, these studies highlight the central role of CSE beliefs during the process of disaster recovery. Individuals who perceive the ability to exert some control in the posttraumatic environment can offset the effects of lost resources and facilitate protective factors such as social support. Benight and Bandura (2004) argue that social support is more than a tangible resource. It requires the development, and maintenance, of social networks facilitated by an individual who is confident in his or her ability to develop them (Bandura, 1997). In addition, social support may come in many forms ranging from people willing to listen to material resources delivered after mass destruction. Benight et al. (1999a) point out that regardless of the available resources, their effective utilization is dependent upon the requisite knowledge and skills to use them once obtained. CSE perceptions are also important to consider when an individual is trying to cope with the myriad of challenges related to domestic violence, as discussed in the following section.

Intimate Partner Violence

Intimate partner violence (IPV) poses a substantial risk for developing PTSD as well as a range of negative health outcomes (Dutton et al., 2006; Golding, 1999). In addition to symptoms of PTSD, IPV survivors may be faced with a wide range of challenges including embarrassment, housing concerns, parenting, as well as the direct physical consequences of the abuse (i.e., black eye, strained neck). Benight et al. (2004) developed the Domestic Violence Coping Self-Efficacy Scale (DV-CSE) to assess the perceived ability to manage specific cognitive and behavioral aspects of posttraumatic adaptation following IPV. As predicted, higher DV-CSE beliefs were associated with reduced posttraumatic stress symptoms and higher levels of well-being (Benight et al., 2004), whereas lower DV-CSE beliefs were associated with increased levels of posttraumatic distress. Interestingly, in a sample of undergraduate women who responded to a hypothetical domestic violence scenario, Rhatigan, Shorey, and Nathanson (2011) demonstrated that self-efficacy perceptions were an important aspect to decision making regarding domestic violence situations.

Lambert et al. (2013) investigated the role of DV-CSE beliefs in a sample of 55 women exposed to IPV. Consistent with SCT, DV-CSE beliefs demonstrated a strong negative relationship with both posttraumatic stress symptoms as well as depression. The study also investigated an additional source of self-efficacy, the interpretation of physiological and affective states (Bandura, 1997). Maladaptive appraisals of physiological sensations during the recovery process may signal ineffective coping strategies and undermine CSE (Benight & Bandura, 2004). Consistent with SCT, the authors found that CSE beliefs mediated the relationship between the negative interpretation of physiological sensations and posttraumatic distress (Lambert et al., 2013). Military combat and post-deployment adaptation, whereas clearly different from IPV, also challenges one's perception of posttraumatic coping capabilities.

Military Combat and Reintegration

The objectively violent nature of military combat affects a wide range of psychosocial consequences (see Chap. 7, this volume). Estimates of PTSD prevalence among troops deployed to the recent wars in Iraq and Afghanistan have varied considerably, likely due to methodological and measurement differences (Ramchand et al., 2010). Sundin et al. (2010) recently conducted a comprehensive review of prevalence studies published from 2004 to 2008, each of which utilized large ($N > 300$), nontreatment-seeking samples. These authors found that among these methodologically sound studies, rates of PTSD ranged from 10 to 17% in nonrandom studies with samples of line infantry units, and, from 2.1 to 11.6%, in random population-based studies. PTSD prevalence among treatment-seeking samples appears to be considerably higher with rates ranging from 12 (Erbes, Westermeyer, Engdahl & Johnsen, 2007) to 37.8% (Jakupcak, Luterek, Hunt, Conybeare, & McFall, 2008). Depression and substance abuse are also problematic among this population (Thomas et al., 2010; Seal et al., 2009).

Solomon et al. (1988, 1991) examined the role of perceived self-efficacy for combat situations of Israeli soldiers following their combat experiences. Soldiers were assessed at 12, 24, and 36 months after participating in combat operations. One year after combat, perceived self-efficacy was associated with performance during combat (combat stress reactions) and subsequent posttraumatic stress symptoms. Soldiers who reported low perceived self-efficacy to engage in a combat capacity reported more posttraumatic stress symptoms and were more likely to have impaired performance during combat. At 24 months, low combat self-efficacy was associated with higher posttraumatic stress and global distress symptoms. Interestingly, at 36 months, the pattern changed somewhat. Low combat self-efficacy continued to be associated with higher overall distress, but it was no longer significantly associated with posttraumatic stress symptoms (Solomon et al., 1991). The focus on combat-specific self-efficacy beliefs may account for why the relationship among the variables changed over time (see also Chap. 7, this volume).

These studies also showed that soldiers who were treated and returned to the frontline as soon as possible reported higher self-efficacy and lower subsequent distress than soldiers removed from the line for treatment (Solomon et al., 1988). Consistent with SCT, soldiers who were triaged and returned to their combat units were able to gain additional mastery experiences to bolster their perceived combat self-efficacy.

However, assessing additional self-efficacy determinants related to the specific demands of psychosocial adaptation after combat are needed. Recently, investigators have focused on the self-efficacy beliefs following combat and its impact on soldiers after they return home. Smith et al. (2013) assessed post-deployment coping self-efficacy (PD-CSE) beliefs of US operations Iraqi Freedom and Enduring Freedom (OIF/OEF) veterans after they returned home. The measure included 18 items related to the social reintegration of soldiers and post-combat adaptation. As predicted, PD-CSE demonstrated a strong negative relationship with posttraumatic stress and depression symptoms. This study also demonstrated the important mediating role of PD-CSE between social support and subsequent post-deployment distress and depression symptoms (Smith et al., 2013). Soldiers are trained to manage combat and the reintegration home. In stark contrast, terrorist attacks are by their intent sudden unpredictable actions meant to induce terror and fear in the targeted population. CSE perceptions have also been investigated under these conditions.

Terrorist Attack

In 1995, the Oklahoma City federal building was the target of a terrorist attack. A bomb decimated the building, killing 168 people and injuring many more. Benight et al. (2000) examined CSE beliefs focused on meeting the specific demands of recovery after the bombing. Individuals who worked nearby the building, many of whom were directly affected, were recruited and assessed 2 and 12 months after the attack. Two months after the attack, CSE was a significant predictor of global distress and posttraumatic stress symptoms after controlling for the threat of death, income, social support, and loss of resources. Including CSE in the model accounted for an additional 23 % of the variance of global distress, 22 % intrusive thoughts and memories of the event, and 28 % of the frequency of trauma-specific symptoms. CSE assessed 1 year after the attack remained a significant preceptor of global distress, intrusive thoughts and memories, and posttraumatic stress symptom severity after controlling for social support and loss of resources (Benight et al., 2000).

Thompson et al. (2006) studied 501 adults living in southern California 2 years following the September 11 attacks. Through qualitative interviews, the researchers found that personal control/mastery was associated with less reported distress. Dealing with the aftermath of a terrorist attack undoubtedly challenges existing coping capacities. The two studies just described suggest that perceptions of coping capability may be important to consider. Support for the predictive value of CSE beliefs following an MVA has also been reported.

Motor Vehicle Accident

MVAs may be one of the most frequently occurring traumatic events (Breslau et al., 1998). As mentioned previously, MVA survivors are confronted with not only the potential of developing PTSD but also a myriad of other consequences. Benight et al. (2008) longitudinally investigated MVA coping self-efficacy (MVA-CSE). Survivors were assessed at 1 week, 1 month, and 3 months after the accident.

In this sample, MVA-CSE demonstrated a significant negative relationship with posttraumatic stress symptoms. In addition, early change in MVA-CSE, between time 1 and time 2, was a significant predictor of 90-day posttraumatic stress symptoms after controlling for accident responsibility, involvement in litigation, peritraumatic dissociation, and posttraumatic distress at time 1 (Benight et al., 2008). They also found that the influence of time 1 posttraumatic distress on time 3 posttraumatic distress was mediated by MVA-CSE assessed at time 2.

Bereavement

The death of a loved one is a tremendously stressful event for the surviving partner. Citing differential outcomes for bereaved spouses, Benight et al. (2001) examined the role of bereavement-coping self-efficacy (B-CSE) beliefs in a sample of cancer widows. B-CSE was positively associated with psychological well-being, health, spiritual well-being, and negatively associated with emotional distress. Further, B-CSE was also a significant predictor of emotional distress after controlling for age, income, education, time since death, anticipatory grief, social support, life event stress, and marital satisfaction accounting for an additional 20 % of the variance alone (Benight et al., 2001).

Bauer and Bonanno (2001) examined relationship of self-efficacy and other self-evaluations following the death of a spouse. Self-efficacy beliefs were not directly assessed but were coded from taped interviews. Comments that referred to a perceived capability were coded as indicators of self-efficacy. Participants in the study were interviewed 6, 14, and 25 months after the death of their spouse. Self-efficacy beliefs at 14 and 25 months were negatively associated with grief (Bauer & Bonanno, 2001). Individuals who made statements indicating strong self-efficacy reported significantly less grief over time. Higher levels of self-efficacy were also found to be a significant predictor of grief in regression analyses.

Health Outcomes

Self-efficacy beliefs have also been shown to influence physical health (Bandura, 1997). It is important to understand how self-regulation processes influence physical health outcomes for both healthy individuals and those who are suffering from chronic illnesses when confronted with traumatic stress. Chronic stress associated with the long-term posttraumatic distress can lead to overactivation of neuroendocrine systems and result in immunosuppressive effects (Segerstrom & Miller, 2004; see also Chap. 9, this volume). Further, the PTSD has been linked to several chronic medical conditions and immunological alterations (Pace & Heim, 2011).

Several studies have looked at the importance of CSE beliefs and health-related outcomes in healthy individuals coping with significant stress and trauma (Benight et al., 2001; Cieslak, Benight, Luszczynska, & Laudenslager, 2011; Wiedenfeld, O'Leary, Bandura, Brown, Levine, & Raska, 1990). In addition, several investigations have focused on CSE perceptions in trauma survivors who are also coping with a major illness (Benight et al., 1997; Cieslak et al., 2008). A meta-analytic review of the relationship between self-efficacy and health-related outcomes following collective trauma showed medium-to-large effect sizes in cross-sectional studies and large effect sizes in longitudinal studies (Luszczynska, Benight, & Cieslak, 2009a). Consistent with these findings, CSE following bereavement showed a strong positive relationship with good physical health in a non-ill sample (Benight et al., 2001).

In an attempt to elucidate the importance of CSE in understanding neuroendocrine connections with posttraumatic distress, Cieslak, Benight, Luszczynska, and Laudenslager (2011) conducted a longitudinal study of healthy MVA survivors. CSE beliefs 1 week after the accident predicted salivary cortisol collected at 3 months after the trauma indirectly through 1 month posttraumatic stress symptoms (Cieslak et al., 2011).

CSE perceptions appear to also be important for chronic illness individuals coping with trauma. Benight et al. (1997) found that HIV+ men with lower CSE to meet the demands of recovering from a hurricane displayed different, potentially maladaptive neuroendocrine profiles than those with higher CSE. Also, investigating men with HIV, Cieslak et al. (2008) found CSE perceptions to be influential in promoting posttraumatic growth in individuals with higher PTSD symptoms.

Conclusion and Future Directions

Traumatic life events are by definition extremely distressing events. They have the potential to impose tremendous changes to the psychological status, physical health, financial status, and interpersonal relationships of survivors. Comprehensive models of human adaptation are needed to account for the wide range of psychosocial consequences that result from trauma exposure. Several theoretical models elucidate the important role of cognition in the human response to traumatic stress (cf. Lazarus & Folkman, 1984; Folkman & Moscowitz, 2004). Evidence from a wide range of traumatic events converges to support the primary role of CSE beliefs in the adaptation to traumatic events. Based on this evidence, one can argue that self-efficacy beliefs serve as a focal point for self-regulation. Indeed, SCT can account for a wide range of observations related to posttraumatic recovery (Benight & Bandura, 2004) as well as make falsifiable predictions of human behavior.

Lastly, self-efficacy beliefs are modifiable, making them an ideal target for intervention (Bandura, 1997). Enactive mastery experiences, observing the success or failures of others, verbal persuasion, and the interpretation of physiological sensations are all sources of self-efficacy. Identifying and modifying maladaptive patterns that negatively influence self-efficacy beliefs after trauma may serve to offset the development of long-term distress. Further, developing a sense of mastery and empowerment may enhance the capacity for positive outcomes from life's most devastating experiences.

References

Bandura, A. (1997). *Self-efficacy. The exercise of control*. New York: W. H. Freeman and Company.

Bandura, A. (2001). Social cognitive theory: An agentic perspective. *Annual Review of Psychology, 52,* 1–26.

Bauer, J. J., & Bonanno, B. A. (2001). I can, I do, I am: The narrative differentiation of self-efficacy and other self-evaluations while adapting to bereavement. *Journal of Research in Personality, 35,* 424–448.

Benight, C. C., & Bandura, A. (2004). Social cognitive theory of posttraumatic recovery: The role of perceived self-efficacy. *Behaviour Research and Therapy, 42,* 1129–1148.

Benight, C. C., & Harper, M. L. (2002). Coping self-efficacy perceptions as a mediator between acute stress response and long-term distress following natural disasters. *Journal of Traumatic Stress, 15,* 177–186.

Benight, C. C., Antoni, M. H., Kilbourn, K., Ironson, G., Kumar, M. A., Fletcher, M. A., Redwine, L., Baum, A., & Scheiderman, N. (1997). Coping self-efficacy buffers psychological and physiological disturbances in HIV-infected men following a natural disaster. *Health Psychology, 16*(3), 248–255.

Benight, C. C., Ironson, G., Klebe, K., Carver, C., Wynings, C., Greenwood, D., et al. (1999a). Conservation of resources and coping self-efficacy predicting distress following a natural disaster: A causal model analysis where the environment meets the mind. *Anxiety, Stress, and Coping, 12,* 107–126.

Benight, C. C., Swift, E., Sanger, J., Smith, A., & Zeppelin, D. (1999b). Coping self-efficacy as a prime mediator of distress following a natural disaster. *Journal of Applied Social Psychology, 29,* 2443–2464.

Benight, C. C., Freyaldenhoven, R. W., Hughes, J., Ruiz, J. M., & Zoschke, T. A. (2000). Coping self-efficacy and psychological distress following the Oklahoma City bombing. *Journal of Applied Social Psychology, 30*(7), 1331–1344.

Benight, C. C., Flores, J., & Tashiro, T. (2001). Bereavement coping self-efficacy in cancer widows. *Death Studies, 25,* 97–125.

Benight, C. C., Harding-Taylor, A., Midboe, A. M., & Durham, R. (2004). Psychometric validation of a domestic violence coping self-efficacy measure. *Journal of Traumatic Stress, 17,* 505–508.

Benight, C. C., Cieslak, R., Molton, I. R., & Johnson, L. E. (2008). Self-evaluative appraisals of coping capability and posttraumatic distress following motor vehicle accidents. *Journal of Counsulting and Clinical Psychology, 76,* 677–685.

Bonanno, G. A. & Mancini, A. D. (2012). Beyond resilience and PTSD: Mapping the heterogeneity of responses to potential trauma. *Psychological Trauma: Theory, Research, Practice, and Policy, 4,* 74–83.

Breslau, N., Kessler, R. C., Chilcoat, H. D., Schultz, L. R., Davis, G. C., Andreski, P. (1998). Trauma and posttraumatic stress disorder in the community: The 1996 Detroit area survey of trauma. *Archives of General Psychiatry, 55,* 626–632.

Brewin, C. R., & Holmes, E. B. (2003). Psychological theories of posttraumatic stress disorder. *Clinical Psychology Review, 23,* 339–376.

Brewin, C. R., Dalgeish, T., & Joseph, S. (1996). A dual representation theory of posttraumatic stress disorder. *Psychological Review, 103*(4), 670–686.

Brewin, C. R., Andrews, B., & Valentine, J. D. (2000). Meta-analysis of risk factors for posttraumatic stress disorder in trauma exposed adults. *Journal of Consulting and Clinical Psychology, 68*(5), 748–766.

Cervone, D. (2000). Thinking about self-efficacy. *Behavior Modification, 24,* 30–56.

Cieslak, R., Benight, C. C., & Lehman V. C. (2008). Coping self-efficacy mediates the effects of negative cognitions on traumatic distress. *Behaviour Research and Therapy, 46,* 788–798.

Cieslak, R., Benight, C. C., Luszczynska, A., & Laudenslager, M. L. (2011). Longitudinal relationships between self-efficacy, posttraumatic distress and salivary cortisol among motor vehicle accident survivors. *Stress and Health, 27*(3), 261–268.

Dutton, M. A., Green, B. L., Kaltman, S. I., Roesch, D. M., Zeffiro, T. A., & Krause E. D. (2006). Intimate partner violence, PTSD, and adverse health outcomes. *Journal of Interpersonal Violence, 21*(7), 955–968.

Ehlers, A., & Clark, D. M. (2000). A cognitive model of posttraumatic stress disorder. *Behaviour Research and Therapy, 38,* 319–345.

Erbes, C., Westermeyer, J., Engdahl, B., & Johnsen, E. (2007). Posttraumatic stress disorder and service utilization in a sample of service members from Iraq and Afghanistan. *Military Medicine, 172,* 359–363.

Foa, E. B., & Rothbaum, B. O. (1998). *Treating the trauma of rape: Cognitive behavioral therapy for PTSD.* New York: Guilford.

Foa, E. B., Steketee, G., & Rothbaum, B. O. (1989). Behavioral/cognitive conceptualizations of posttraumatic stress disorder. *Behavior Therapy, 20,* 155–176.

Folkman, S. (1984). Personal control and stress and coping processes: A theoretical analysis. *Journal of Personality and Social Psychology, 46*(4), 839–852.

Folkman, S., & Lazarus, R. S. (1985). If it changes it must be a process: Study of emotion and coping during three stages of a college examination. *Journal of Personality and Social Psychology, 48*(1), 150–170.

Folkman, S., & Moskowitz, J.F. (2004). Coping: Pitsfalls and promise. *Annual Review of Psychology, 55,* 745–774.
Golding, J. M. (1999). Intimate partner violence as a risk factor for mental disorders: A meta-analysis. *Journal of Family Violence, 14*(2), 99–132.
Guay, S., Billette, V., & Marchand. A. (2006). Exploring the links between posttraumatic stress disorder and social support: Processes and potential research avenues. *Journal of Traumatic Stress, 19*(3), 327–338.
Helgeson, V. S., Reynolds, K. A., & Tomich, P. L. (2006). A meta-analytic review of benefit finding and growth. *Journal of Consulting and Clinical Psychology, 74*(5), 797–816.
Hirschel, M. J., & Schulenberg, S. E. (2009). Hurricane Katrina's impact on the Mississippi Gulf Coast: General self-efficacy's relationship to PTSD prevalence and severity. *Psychological Services, 6*(4), 293–303. doi:10.1037/a0017467
Hobfoll, S. E. (1989). Conservation of resources: A new attempt at conceptualizing stress. *American Psychologist, 44*(3), 513–524.
Hobfoll, S. E. (1991). Traumatic stress: A theory based on rapid loss of resources. *Anxiety Research, 4,* 187–197.
Hobfoll, S. E. (2001). The influence of culture, community, and the nested-self in the process: Advancing conservation of resources theory. *Applied Psychology: An International Review, 50,* 337–421.
Jakupcak, M., Luterek, J., Hunt, S., Conybeare, D., & McFall, M. (2008). Posttraumatic stress and its relationship to physical health functioning in a sample of Iraq and Afghanistan war veterans seeking postdeployment VA health care. *The Journal of Nervous and Mental Disease, 196*(5), 425–428.
Janoff-Bulman, R. (1992). *Shattered assumptions: Towards a new psychology of trauma.* New York: Free Press.
Johansen, V. A., Wahl, A. K., Eilertsen, D., & Weisaeth, L. (2007). Prevalence and predictors of posttraumatic stress disorder (PTSD) in physically injured victims of non-domestic violence: A longitudinal study. *Social Psychiatry and Psychiatric Epidemiology, 42*(7), 583–593. doi:10.1007/s00127-007-0205-0
Kessler, R. C., Sonnega, A., Bromet, E., Hughes, M., & Nelson, C. B. (1995). Posttraumatic stress disorder in the National Comorbidity Survey. *Archives of General Psychiatry, 52,* 1048–1060.
Kilpatrick, D. G., Acierno, R., Saunders, B., Resnick, H. S., Best, C. L., & Schnurr, P. P. (2000). Risk factors for adolescent substance abuse and dependence: Data from a national sample. *Journal of Consulting and Clinical Psychology, 68,* 19–30.
Lambert, J. E., Benight, C. C., Wong, T., & Johnson, L. E. (2013). Cognitive bias in the interpretation of physiological sensations, coping self-efficacy, and psychological distress after intimate partner violence. *Psychological Trauma: Theory, Research, Practice, and Policy, 5*(5), 494–500.
Lazarus, R. S., & Folkman, S. (1984). *Stress, appraisal, and coping.* New York: Springer.
Lowe, S. R., Tracy, M., Cerdá, M., Norris, F. H., & Galea, S. (2013). Immediate and longer-term stressors and the mental health of Hurricane Ike survivors. *Journal of Traumatic Stress, 26*(6), 753–761. doi:10.1002/jts.21872
Luszczynska, A., Scholz, U., & Schwarzer, R. (2005). The general self-efficacy scale: Multicultural validation studies. *The Journal of Psychology, 139*(5), 439–457.
Luszczynska, A., Benight, C. C., & Cieslak, R. (2009a). Self-efficacy and health-related outcomes of collective trauma. *European Psychologist, 14*(1), 51–62.
Luszczynska, A., Benight, C. C., Cieslak, R., Kissinger, P., Reilly, K. H., & Clark, R. A. (2009b). Self-efficacy mediates effects of exposure, loss of resources, and life stress on posttraumatic distress among trauma survivors. *Applied Psychology: Health and Well- Being, 1*(1), 73–90.
Maddux, J. E. (1995). Self-efficacy theory: An introduction. In J. E. Maddux (Ed.) *Self-efficacy, adaptation, and adjustment* (pp. 3–36). New York: Plenum.
Norris, F. H. (1992). Epidemiology of trauma: Frequency and impact of different potentially traumatic events on different demographic groups. *Journal of Consulting and Clinical Psychology, 60*(3), 409–418.

Norris, F. H., Friedman, M. J., Watson, P. J., Byrne, C. M., Diaz, E., & Kaniasty, K. (2002). 60,000 disaster victims speak: Part I. An empirical review of the empirical literature, 1981–2001. *Psychiatry: Interpersonal and Biological Processes, 65*(3), 207–239.

Norris, F. H., Slone, L. B., Baker, C. K., & Murphy, A. D. (2006). Early physical health consequences of disaster exposure and acute disaster-related PTSD. *Anxiety, Stress & Coping: An International Journal, 19*(2), 95–110. doi:10.1080/10615800600652209.

Ozer, E. J., Best, S. R., Lipsey, T. L., & Weiss, D. S. (2003). Predictors of posttraumatic stress disorder and symptoms in adults: A meta-analysis. *Psychological Bulletin, 129*(1), 52–73.

Pace, T. W. W., & Heim, C. M. (2011). A short review on the psychoneuroimmunology of posttraumatic stress disorder: From risk factors to medical comorbidities. *Brain, Behavior, and Immunity, 25,* 6–13.

Park, C. L., & Ai, A. L. (2006). Meaning making and growth: New directions for research on survivors of trauma. *Journal of Loss and Trauma, 11,* 389–407.

Park, C. L., Cohen, L. H., & Murch, R. L. (1996). Assessment and prediction of stress-related growth. *Journal of Personality, 64*(1), 71–105.

Ramchand, R., Schell, T. L., Karney, B. R., Osilla, K. C., Burns, R. M., & Calderone, L. B. (2010). Disparate prevalence estimates of PTSD among service members who served in Iraq and Afghanistan: Possible explanations. *Journal of Traumatic Stress, 23*(1), 59–68.

Rhatigan, D. L., Shorey, R. C., & Nathanson, A. M. (2011). The impact of posttraumatic symptoms on women's commitment to a hypothetical violent relationship: A path analytic test of posttraumatic stress, depression, shame, and self-efficacy on investment model factors. *Psychological Trauma: Theory, Research, Practice, and Policy, 3*(2), 181–191. doi:10.1037/a0020646

Seal, K. H., Metzler, T. J., Gima, K. S., Bertenthal, D., Maguen, S., & Marmar, C. (2009). Trends and risk factors for mental health diagnoses among Iraq and Afghanistan veterans using Department of Veteran Affairs health care, 2002–2008. *American Journal of Public Health, 99,* 1651–1658.

Segerstrom, S. C., & Miller, G. E. (2004). Psychological stress and the human immune system: A meta-analytic study of 30 years of inquiry. *Psychological Bulletin, 130*(4), 601–630.

Smith, A. J., Benight, C. C., & Cieslak, R. (2013). Social support and postdeployment coping self-efficacy of distress among combat veterans. *Military Psychology, 25*(5), 452–461.

Solomon, Z., Weisenberg, M., Schwarzwald, J., & Mikulincer, M. (1988). Combat stress reaction and posttraumatic stress disorder as determinants of perceived self-efficacy in battle. *Journal of Social and Clinical Psychology, 6,* 356–370.

Solomon, Z., Benbenishty, B. B., & Mikulincer, M. (1991). The contribution of wartime, pre- war, and post-war factors to self-efficacy: A longitudinal study of combat stress reaction. *Journal of Traumatic Stress, 4,* 345–361.

Sundin, J., Fear, N. T., Iversen, A., Rona, R. J., & Wessely, S. (2010). PTSD after deployment to Iraq: Conflicting rates, conflicting claims. *Psychological Medicine, 40,* 367–282.

Tedeschi, R. G., & Calhoun, L., G. (2004). Posttraumatic growth: Conceptual foundations and empirical evidence. *Psychological Inquiry, 15*(1), 1–18.

Thomas, J. T., Wilk, J. E., Riviere, L. A., McGurk, D., Castro, C. A., & Hoge, C. W. (2010). The prevalence of mental health problems and functional impairment among active component and national guard soldiers 3 and 12 months following combat in Iraq. *Archives of General Psychiatry, 67,* 614–623.

Thompson, S. C., Schlehofer, M. M., Bovin, M. J., Dougan, B. T., Montes, D., & Trifskin, S. (2006). Dispositions, control strategies, and distress in the general public after the 2001 terrorist attack. *Anxiety, Stress & Coping: An International Journal, 19*(2), 143–159. doi:10.1080/10615800600615891.

Tomaka, J., Blascovich, J., Kelsey, R. M., & Leitten, C. L. (1993). Subjective, physiological, and behavioral effects of threat and challenge appraisal. *Journal of Personality and Social Psychology, 65*(2), 248–260.

Wiedenfeld, S. A., O'Leary, A., Bandura, A., Brown, S., Levine, S., & Raska, K. (1990). Impact of perceived self-efficacy in coping with stressors on components of the immune system. *Journal of Personality and Social Psychology, 59*(5), 1082–1094. doi:10.1037/0022-3514.59.5.1082.

Chapter 12
When Neighborhoods Are Destroyed by Disaster: Relocate or Return and Rebuild?

Keri L. Kytola, Katie E. Cherry, Loren D. Marks and Trevan G. Hatch

Introduction

The 2005 Atlantic hurricane season brought two category 3 storms, Katrina and Rita, within 4 weeks of each other. These treacherous hurricanes left a trail of immeasurable losses across the US Gulf Coast. When homes, neighborhoods, and communities are destroyed by disaster, survivors must relocate to habitable geographic regions. Depending on the individual and his or her circumstances, temporary or permanent new living arrangements become a necessity. Following a disaster, uncertainties driven by environmental destruction may be overwhelming and possibly frightening, although survivors find traction to move ahead despite the hardships of displacement and catastrophic damage to homes and communities. Understanding how environmental factors affect personal as well as community-wide recovery in the years after a disaster is a timely and urgent challenge for social scientists. Greater awareness and insight into disaster survivors' experiences may

K. E. Cherry (✉)
Department of Psychology, Louisiana State University, 236 Audubon Hall, Baton Rouge, LA 70803-5501, USA
e-mail: pskatie@lsu.edu

K. L. Kytola
Department of Psychology, Oklahoma State University, Stillwater, OK 74078, USA
e-mail: keri.kytola@okstate.edu

L. D. Marks
School of Family Life, Brigham Young University, 2092C Joseph F. Smith Building, Provo, Utah 84602, USA
e-mail: loren_marks@byu.edu

T. G. Hatch
School of Social Work, Louisiana State University, 335 Long Fieldhouse, Baton Rouge, LA 70803-5501, USA
e-mail: thatch8@lsu.edu

K. E. Cherry (ed.), *Traumatic Stress and Long-Term Recovery,*
DOI 10.1007/978-3-319-18866-9_12

be key to the development of successful interventions to lessen suffering in future storms and natural disasters.

In this chapter, we focus on the role that the post-disaster environment plays in long-term recovery for Hurricane Katrina and Rita survivors at least 5 years after these events. Our goal is to present an insiders' perspective on post-disaster adjustment based on the experiences of people who relocated permanently and those who returned to their storm-devastated homes to rebuild and re-establish lifestyles. We begin with an overview of Bronfenbrenner's (1979) ecological systems theory which has been adapted to study the psychological impact of natural disasters (Kilmer & Gil-Rivas, 2010; Weems & Overstreet, 2009); see also Chap. 10, this volume). An ecological systems approach, among other contextual theories, provides a useful conceptual framework for thinking about individuals nested within the broader social contexts of family, community, and cultural traditions and heritage. In the second section, we describe our qualitative methodology, which was modeled after our earlier work with indirectly affected older adults in Louisiana Healthy Aging Study (LHAS) 4–14 months after the storms (Cherry et al., 2011; Silva Brown et al., 2010. This chapter is based on interviews conducted with directly affected coastal residents between 5 and 7 years after the 2005 storms. All had experienced catastrophic hurricane damage and losses, which are reported elsewhere (Cherry et al., 2015). Here we present two emergent themes that provide insight into the frustrations and forced environmental changes after the 2005 storms. The remaining themes are presented in Chap. 13 (this volume). In the last section, we focus on adjustment and new life circumstances in the years after natural disaster.

Conceptual Framework and Literature

Nested Ecologies

Recent theorizing on post-disaster psychological reactions from a child developmental perspective traces its origins to Bronfenbrenner's (1977, 1979) ecological systems theory, which offers an integrative conceptual framework for studying factors that affect adaptation and well-being after a disaster (Kilmer & Gil-Rivas, 2010; Weems & Overstreet, 2009). In brief, the ecological systems theory holds that children function within multiple nested contexts or ecologies that vary in proximity to the individual. Proximal ecologies include family, school, and peers, among other influences close to a person. Distal ecologies include the farthest sources of influence, such as government, sociocultural values, and beliefs. Proximal and distal ecologies are assumed to exert bidirectional influence, where changes in one ecology may influence another as well as an individual's development (see Chap. 10, this volume).

Bronfenbrenner's original formulation of ecological systems theory, which emphasized multiple nested ecologies at increasing levels of abstraction, later gave rise to his bioecological model with greater focus on characteristics of the individual over time as a critical determinant of development (Bronfenbrenner & Morris, 2006). An ecological framework for disaster research, which emphasizes proximal and distal factors that affect well-being in children and families, has motivated research on topics as diverse as childhood wellness and community resilience after disaster (Pfefferbaum, Pfefferbaum & Norris, 2010) to the emotional consequences of destruction and loss after Hurricane Katrina for disaster-exposed youth in New Orleans (Weems & Overstreet, 2009; for review, see Chap. 10, this volume) and coping behaviors and well-being among Katrina-displaced older adults (Kamo, Henderson, & Roberto, 2011). Here we adopt an ecological systems perspective to guide our work on psychosocial consequences of Hurricanes Katrina and Rita for a primarily older sample of adults directly affected by these storms.

Disrupted Ecologies and Psychosocial Consequences

On August 29, 2005, residents of Louisiana held their collective breath in anticipation of the massive, category 5 hurricane churning in the Gulf of Mexico. Hurricane Katrina (and Rita, 1 month later) was on an unstoppable path of destruction. Louisianans in the coastal parish (county) of St. Bernard, just 5 miles southeast of the great city of New Orleans, were sent into a flight of panic, shock, and fear as the local government issued a mandatory evacuation order just hours before the storm made landfall.

Without ample time to prepare for evacuation, many people faced the reality of staying behind to bear witness to Katrina's destruction of their homes, community, and way of life. Residents who evacuated in advance of the storm avoided having to experience Katrina's wrath firsthand, yet most witnessed the storm's devastating effects via television or radio transmission. In nearby Baton Rouge, LA, an estimated 200,000 evacuees arrived overnight from storm-ravaged coastal areas, resulting in immediate infrastructure challenges and disruptions in daily life (Cherry, Allen, & Galea, 2010). These storms brought many challenges at the time, although the adverse effects were longer lasting than initially foreseen. Those who experienced the hurricanes were fully aware that normal living would be temporarily suspended, but they did not know it would be completely lost. Hurricane Katrina spared no one in her comprehensive swath of destruction. Homes, neighborhoods, schools, shopping centers, businesses, places of worship, and entire geographic regions were destroyed (Cherry, 2009).

In the present research, we compared former residents who relocated permanently to non-coastal communities after the 2005 storms and current coastal residents who had returned to rebuild and re-establish lives in St. Bernard and Plaquemines parishes in south Louisiana. Based on an ecological systems perspective, we reasoned that proximal and distal ecologies would be impoverished in areas where community resources (e.g., social networks, schools, businesses, places of worship) were severely damaged or destroyed by the storm. Those who returned to devastated areas to rebuild their homes would therefore be exposed to a longer duration of adversity than former residents who relocated to non-coastal communities after the storms. One might expect that the experiences and needs among former and current coastal residents would differ in the immediate post-disaster period and in the years since 2005 (see also Chap. 13, this volume). Such a pattern of outcomes would provide new evidence concerning proximal and distal ecological influences on post-Katrina recovery.

To summarize, participants responded to open-ended questions designed to examine different, but complementary aspects of post-Katrina recovery: (a) challenges, obstacles, and setbacks after the storms, (b) establishing a new daily routine, (c) the return of "normal living," and (d) what others should know about their hurricane experiences. These open-ended questions were given to provide greater breadth and depth of responses than would have been possible with a strictly quantitative assessment. Taken together, participants' responses to these questions yielded narrative data that were analyzed for recurring concepts and emergent themes. We expected that responses for both groups would be similar concerning lost property, disrupted social and professional networks, and difficulties with insurance claims (see also Chap. 13, this volume). In contrast, current residents' responses may qualitatively differ from those of former residents due to a longer duration of adversity driven by disruption and losses in proximal and distal ecologies, including limited community resources and social milieu.

Method

Participants and Procedure

A total of 125 adults were interviewed between March, 2010, and November, 2012. They were former and current residents of St. Bernard and Plaquemines parishes in south Louisiana, with catastrophic Hurricane Katrina damage. Former residents consisted of 62 persons who were displaced and relocated permanently to non-coastal communities after the storm (*M* age = 58.4, SD = 17.1 years; age range: 18–89 years; 21 males, 41 females). Current residents were 63 directly affected persons who were also displaced but returned to rebuild and restore their lives in their coastal parish communities (*M* age = 60.7, SD = 15.0 years, age range: 20–83 years; 26 males, 37 females). A more thorough description of the sample and procedure is given elsewhere (Cherry et al., 2015).

Participants were tested individually in their homes or in a community location across two (or more) sessions separated by at least a week. The procedures used in this study were reviewed and approved by the Institutional Review Board of Louisiana State University in Baton Rouge, LA. To preserve anonymity, all participants were assigned a three-digit number, with former residents in the 100s (101–162) and current residents in the 200s (201–263), as referenced throughout this chapter.

In the first session, informed consent was obtained and quantitative measures were administered (see Cherry et al., 2015). Participants were given a prepared page with seven open-ended questions in all, which were reviewed briefly and left with them to reference later, if desired. In the second session, these questions were presented to participants in turn on individually prepared cards. Their oral responses were digitally recorded and transcribed verbatim. Transcriptions were audited for accuracy and print copies were produced for the purpose of qualitative coding by an independent group of research assistants. In this chapter, we focus on participants' responses to the following four questions:

1. "People who lived through Hurricanes Katrina and Rita experienced a variety of challenges, obstacles, and setbacks. Please tell us how you coped with the challenges you faced after the storms."
2. "What kinds of things did you do to establish a new daily routine?"
3. "When did 'normal living' come back for you?"
4. "What would you like others to know about your experiences with Hurricanes Katrina and Rita?"

Analysis and Coding

Participants' narrative data were open coded and content analyzed in a manner consistent with grounded theory methodology (Strauss & Corbin, 1998). In brief, two research teams, consisting of one graduate student and three undergraduate students per team (eight coders total), performed independent open coding (identifying recurring themes and concepts in the text) on an interview-by-interview basis. One team coded former residents' narratives (100s series), while the other team coded current residents' narratives (200s series).

To promote rigor, every interview was independently coded in its entirety by two coders, referred to as "coding partners" or "coding pairs." Each coding pair met weekly to review and discuss their independently assigned codes. Coding partners would compare and contrast their independent open coding from the previous week on a line-by-line, page-by-page basis with each other, alternatively "leading out" by discussing her/his personal open coding of a given page. Following presentation of one's independent coding of a given page, the other coding partner would discuss similarities and differences from their coding. Each team member provided a numeric content analysis (NCA) of his/her open coding for each interview, similar to Miles and Huberman's (1994) "data accounting sheet" (p. 80). Similarities and discrepancies between individual coders were noted.

Following the weekly "coding pair" meeting, full "team" (two coding pairs) meetings were held to compare and contrast emerging themes across interviews. The two teams met separately on a weekly basis for several months until the open coding and content analysis was completed for all interviews. At this point, we collected all NCAs for each interview, offering multiple "at-a-glance" perspectives of the concepts and themes expressed in each of the interviews (Marks, Cherry, &

Silva, 2009). Each team member identified her/his top central themes based on two factors: *prevalence* (within and across interviews) and *salience*. To strengthen inter-rater reliability and minimize idiosyncratic bias, all central themes were reviewed and discussed within each team until a consensus was reached. By doing so, the team-based analysis revealed both relevant data segments that may have been overlooked and peripheral excerpts that were deemed "a stretch."

A final combined team meeting (with all eight coders) was held to identify similarities and differences among the central themes that had emerged from former and current residents' narratives. To ensure that the final central themes were verifiable and clearly supported by the data, team members then revisited all of the interviews and copied and pasted all data that had been directly identified with a given theme into a specific file. Each team member was assigned one prospective "core" theme which they were asked to confirm. Ultimately, in order to be deemed "core" or central, a given theme required several pages of supporting data—consistent with Patton's (2002) suggestion of creating a data "audit trail" (p. 93). Although many themes were identified during the team-based, open-coding analyses, the "core" themes presented here were identified by *consensus* (see also Chaps. 4, 13, 14, 18, 20, and 21, this volume). In other words, the themes featured in our related work were not merely emergent or noticeable. Indeed, to be identified as a "core" theme, *every* member of the coding team must have identified the theme many times across interviews and must have produced the NCA trail to document the theme as core and central. The themes presented shortly met these rigorous criteria.

Findings

Five major themes emerged from our team-based analysis. Two themes are presented here, which include: (1) *There's No Going Back: The "Old Normal" is Gone Forever* and (2) *You Don't Understand Unless You Were There.* The remaining themes are discussed in Chap. 13 (this volume). Illustrative and supportive excerpts from the participants' interviews are provided in connection with each of these major themes.

Theme 1: There's No Going Back: The "Old Normal" Is Gone Forever

Coastal residents faced countless challenges in an uncertain and chaotic post-disaster environment. One pressing dilemma is where to live when one's home and way of life has been washed away in the floodwaters of Katrina. Over a million displaced US Gulf Coast residents faced an exceedingly difficult decision of whether to relocate permanently and start over somewhere else, or return home and rebuild despite the catastrophic devastation, hardships, and crippled infrastructure. For many people, interpersonal, economic, and historical factors likely influenced the decision to relocate or go back to their coastal homes (see Henry, 2013, for a related discussion). At least 5 years later, former and current residents alike repeatedly made the point that their life today does not resemble what it was like prior to August of 2005. The next quotes, from a former (151) and two current residents (253, 227), illustrate differences in the length of displacement for those who relocated permanently versus those who returned to rebuild, although the sense of loss and painful steps of moving on in a world that has changed appear remarkably similar:

> **151** (65-year old male)**:** Life was never, ever going to be the same. Oftentimes people will say to us, "But look at the beautiful home you have. You all have everything you could possibly want." And that's true. But what we don't have is life as we knew it before Katrina. So although you can go out and buy furniture, the loss—it never, ever goes away. When I say loss, what I mean is your life is never the same.

> **253** (21-year old male)**:** Normal living…I could tell you probably when it came back the most, but I'm not sure that I can really say that we ever got back to full, normal living because so much of what we had known before the storm had changed. We were able to get back into our old house, you know, two years after the storm had hit. It was, but even then it was renovated, so it was new. And, I was able to go back to the same school that I had gone to before the storm, but the people who were there were different. You know, some people had left. Some new people had come in. So it was always this process of getting re-familiarized with everything, because nothing was normal. So I mean, I guess the, the most normal was when we were finally able to get back into our house and go back to my old school. But even then I, I think there was never a point when things were fully normal because things had changed too much for that.

There is a sense of comfort in the familiar, yet transformed and now different home and school environments 2 years after the storm for this adolescent (253) who was a high school student at the time of the 2005 hurricanes. One may sense a similar sentiment in the next quote of a middle-aged man (227) when he returned to his former home and reopened his business 3 years after the storm:

> **227** (54-year old male)**:** I guess normal could be different, could be different for everybody. As far as completely normal, I don't think my life ever did get completely back the way it was, doesn't mean that I don't have a normal routine and I don't have a life that's—it's different, but yet it's consistent. And what was normal then and what was normal now, I feel is different. But as far as being normal to some consistency, I would say it took about three years to get the businesses reopened and be back in a home and at least feel like things would get back to some type of normalcy where I could live within my own home and have my businesses running again and that kind of felt probably more normal than anything else at that point.

As this man notes, "normal could be different for everybody." Most would agree that what constitutes "normal" is subjective and may also evolve over time, so it may not be possible to quantify this term for strictly research purposes. Nonetheless, our participants shed some light on what "normal living" means to them, what it was considered before the storms, and why it never fully returned after the 2005 hurricanes. Based on the participants' direct storm experiences, "normal living" would appear to mean living one's life as he or she so chooses, being close to and seeing immediate and extended family members regularly, having access to necessary establishments (schools, shopping centers, hospitals, etc.), participating in local activities, and feeling a sense of home and belonging. After Katrina and Rita swept through the US Gulf Coast region, this idea of what was "normal" has reportedly disappeared.

Both former and current residents of St. Bernard and Plaquemines parishes spoke of *the loss of a way of life.* Their comments provide a unique insiders' perspective on why their lives will never again be "normal" in the pre-Katrina sense:

160 (65-year old female)**:** Well, the loss wasn't a material loss so much as losing our sense of home, family, community, and plans for the future. And we feel that will never be the same. All of our families lived in close together, and we felt even if we went back to St. Bernard it could never…everybody wasn't going back for one reason or another, so that way of life, we'll never have again.

215 (77-year old female)**:** I lost my neighbors. I lost my neighborhood. I lost my church. I lost my parish priest. I lost everything. I lost my way of life. My life today is not the same as it was before Katrina. It will never be the same and I know one of your questions I have to look at, it says, "When did your life get back to normal?" My life has never been normal. It's not going to be because I can't get my normal life back. It's not there anymore. I have made a new life, a new normalcy.

Despite the effort and time spent restoring their homes, "normal living," which today is referenced as the "pre-Katrina normal," was taken abruptly away by the 2005 storms. The "old normal" way of life may not ever fully return. Both former and current residents recognize this ecological transition and acknowledge that their lives will never be the same because of the many changes after the hurricanes. They are coping with the loss of the pre-Katrina "old normal" and adapting to the "new normal" that came about many years later, as illustrated in the following quotes:

222 (66-year old male)**:** I don't think it will ever be normal.I think that's just something you have to live with and deal with, you know.And try to understand what happened. And what could be done about it and just hope it don't happen again.If it did happen again I would probably have a negative attitude about coming back, and trying to have to re-do it again. Doing it once was hard. I don't regret it, but I wouldn't want to do it again.

For older participants, one can also sense a strong and possibly regretful feeling that they will never get to experience the old normal in their lifetimes:

260 (64-year old female)**:** It will never be normal again. What was normal before is not normal now. And normal for me was, you know, now I had all these people living with me, where before it was just my husband and I. Now we have people living with us because they have no place else to go. They need to fix up their homes, family and friends are gone. Community destroyed. So it's a new normal. Not one that I like because it's really hard to, it's hard every day to know what was. And you've got to kind of hope it will be. But will you be around to see it? Family had moved away. Friends have moved away, neighbors, I was in my home for forty years. Neighbors moved away. Now we don't know who our neighbors are. The closeness, that was a real close knot, was, a real close-knit community. And that part is gone.

On the other hand, three current residents reported that finding a new normal in a sea of chaos was easier once they returned to St. Bernard because they were able to come back to their home town and rebuild their lives even though it was emotionally and financially challenging. These current residents' remarks reflect a more positive outlook on transitioning from the old normal to the new normal:

256 (54-year old female)**:** As far as our normal living, that new normal for us, I think came from me mentally, emotionally when we got back here. It didn't feel right any place else that we were and when we came back here, it finally…it did. And we quickly established routines, things that we still follow now that now we call it, everyone does your new normal, you know? You know, here's the new normal. It's not the old normal, but it is the new normal and that's what we follow now. It's as normal as it's going to be and I think we've reached a level of acceptance.

242 (46-year old male)**:** You know the old, the saying here, you know, in St. Bernard, I got it on the back. [Referring to the idea of "Which normal are you talking about, the old normal or the new normal?"] And the old normal is not all bad or all good. And neither is the new normal all bad or all good, you know…. One day you're a part of this community, you know, thriving close-knit neighborhood and then, you know, it's all gone in a day, you know. So there's no getting back to that normal ever…and we're still developing a new normal. And like I said, you know, it was bad on the old normal and good on the normal. This is similar as far as good and bad. But still developing the new normal. You know, those relationships, you know, there's a void there so you're developing new…trying to develop new relationships with people in the same type of fashion. But they're different people so, you know, you're trying to make those connections. That's just a development in process, and there are some successes there and then which are good. New house, new neighborhood…those parts of it are good, you know.

Despite losing the old normal that characterized pre-Katrina coastal life, being there for old and new neighbors alike appeared to contribute to the well-being of current residents. Emergence of a "new normal" for former and current residents included negative experiences that should not be overlooked, such as the difficulty of being a stranger in a new town and a pervasive feeling that other people don't understand the Katrina experience, as discussed more fully in the next section.

Theme 2: "You Don't Understand Unless You Were There"

From an ecological perspective, the experience of disaster translates to a simultaneous collapse of proximal and distal ecologies as friends and family evacuate to distant cities and the familiar routines of school, work, and everyday life are destroyed. The upheaval and multiple layers of chaos after a disaster would be difficult, if not impossible to fathom, unless one has lived through such an experience (see Chap. 13, this volume). The two subthemes appearing later on offer some insight. The first subtheme, "Witness to Tragedy" conveys the horror of what happened in St. Bernard parish from the eyes of three public servants who sheltered in place and carried out their professional obligations through the storm, flooding, and desperate days that followed. The second subtheme "on rebuilding ecologies" offers a glimpse into the long and arduous process of recovery. Participants' stories of hardship, perceived neglect by governmental entities, and assistance through the helping hands of volunteers are highlighted.

"No one gets it" and variations on this sentiment appeared frequently throughout the interviews. Participants often said that people who did not experience Hurricanes Katrina and Rita firsthand in 2005 would not understand the hardships that they and others displaced by the storm faced and continued to struggle with every day. One current resident summed this sentiment up succinctly:

214 (56-year old female)**:** It's just like people just don't…they don't understand. They will never understand. You don't understand unless you're in that situation.

Both former and current coastal residents spoke of frustration related to strangers who were unsympathetic or simply unaware of the plight of the *newly homeless,* a stark and burdensome reality for those directly impacted by the storm. The next quotes provide insight into former residents' negative experiences while looking for a new place to call their home:

> **110** (58-year old female)**:** Since coming to Baton Rouge, I cannot begin to tell you how many times I have been referred to as "a Katrina person." I am so much more than that. I am a person who loves her family dearly and that we are struggling to put our lives back together again, one day at a time.…A lot of my neighbors are victims of Katrina. Someone once referred to my neighborhood as "Katrina Village." I wish the community would be more enlightened to the struggles of displaced victims and how they really feel, and the struggles and obstacles that they have had to overcome…. Some of the comments made right after Katrina and Rita made me sick. Like this one: 'If I have to listen to one more Katrina story, I'm going to scream.' That person is truly clueless or just plain insensitive to the plight of people who are just trying to put their lives back together one day at a time. I can't tell you how many times when I would start to say something about the struggles we…struggles we were going through, only to have someone cut me off in the middle of a sentence…these were health…health care professionals just like myself. How sad.

Participants spoke of feeling unwelcomed by strangers in non-coastal communities, an unsettling and rather disturbing violation of "the golden rule" (i.e., *do unto others as you would have them do unto you):*

> **147** (43-year old male)**:** You know, one of the things we talked about earlier that bothered us…what bothered us was people that, you know, you wasn't as welcome as you thought you would welcome other people, you know, you want to be treated the way you treat people…[You should treat them]…the way you want to be treated.

He went on to describe changes he observed among his friends and family after the storm:

> **147** (43-year old male)**:** I guess one of the things that hurt sometimes more than others is that people that you knew and love and grew up around has changed since then. You know, plenty of it's your own family. They moral, some of their morals and family went to the way side. And that's not the people that would agree to interview with you. I tell you that because they know it.

Another painful reality was the impatience among strangers who were not directly affected, chiding survivors to "get over it," as revealed in this former residents' response:

> **141** (55-year old female)**:** That's really hard. And I guess also you never know what it feels like unless you've been there yourself. You know, you've been through something like this yourself and when people say, "Oh, it's been five years, four years, six years, whatever… Just move on. Get over it." That that really bothers me that people say that.

Current residents also conveyed a feeling of being out of place after the storm, with some having been displaced for up to 2 years before resettling in their original coastal community. One participant, a high school student at the time, described her ordeal. She said her host high school offered "refugee classes" for displaced students. Local students at the host high school noticed regional differences in speech patterns and she was teased about her accent. She said:

261 (20-year old female): We had refugee classes in school…and a lot of kids, because we had a lot of kids, would say that to us, because they heard that from their parents. [I had a friend there] and he always used to go, "Say water, say cucumber, I like when you say things with "er's" at the end. Keep saying them, keep saying them!" So I'd always, you know, sit there and talk to him, and he'd make me say water. I remember the principal come up to me, going, "Don't make her say water, that's a touchy subject for those people." We're those people! I'm like, now I feel like a minority, I feel like I understand what they mean when people get offended with the words, "those people." Like, what is that supposed to mean?

Interestingly, her reflection "now I feel like a minority" is consistent with findings from a quantitative study carried out during the immediate aftermath of Katrina, where being from New Orleans was associated with feelings of discrimination, regardless of one's race (Weems et al., 2007). And she closed with the following summation, sadly insightful of humanity's shortcomings:

261: People don't understand things until they go through it. A lot of people aren't compassionate, and you, you know it's sad that you got to say it like that, but a lot of people don't understand something until it happens to them, and they don't think before they speak, you know?

A gentleman who was in St. Bernard during the agonizing days after the storm reflected on the catastrophic devastation and desperate circumstances in Katrina's immediate aftermath:

230 (49-year old male): People, if they have never lived down here, have no idea. And even now if they come down now they could never imagine what it looked like before. This is clean. The pictures are two dimensional, or even the videos you're looking at, unless you've got high definition TV, it's a two dimensional thing. But what you're missing is the full picture, you're missing the silence. Still it's never come back the way it was before the hurricane. I never want anything like that to ever happen to anybody, but, you know, I think it's something people should see. To get the full measure of something you have to have the full body experience. Somebody come up with a virtual reality where you step in that situation, and you'd never be one of those people in the media or one of our governmental officials saying, "Maybe we shouldn't rebuild." Let them experience that in their own home town setting. See what they feel, you know?

Both former and current residents conveyed the idea that people just don't understand how catastrophic and comprehensive the destruction actually was, *unless they were there*. In the words of a former St. Bernard resident:

117 (61-year old female): They did not know unless they were one of the aid groups that went down there. They did not know that every house was devastated, that the whole community was devastated. That every job, every business, everything was devastated. And I don't think, you know, even though everybody saw the pictures, I think they thought it was like, you know, when you see the flood water in Iowa, where they go down, you know, but we had such a different experience because houses were just totally destroyed.

Although many participants who experienced Hurricanes Katrina and Rita felt that no "outsiders" could possibly understand what went on in south Louisiana following the storms, first responders and others who witnessed the destruction firsthand on August 29, 2005 can shed light on this experience. Their remarks provide a collective image of the devastation, as discussed next.

Subtheme 1: Witnesses to Tragedy: Voices of Professionals Who Were There Serving the Public

Katrina's catastrophic impact and the unprecedented flooding after the levee breaches created a chaotic and desperate set of circumstances. Public servants who stayed behind experienced a greater level of involvement in the chaos as they carried out their professional obligations under desperate circumstances. "It was bad," said one nurse who sheltered in place at a local hospital on August 29, 2005, working tirelessly through the storm and the sweltering heat in the long days that followed. The reality of her situation is captured in the next quote:

> **Nurse (214)** (56-year old female)**:** Once we got out, I mean our basic needs were tended to and all, but being in here (the local hospital) directly after the storm…Then, it wasn't only that you had to worry about yourself; you still had people to take care of. That's what I don't understand about the news media and other concerns or whatever people saying about medical folks that were in here taking care of people. You don't know the circumstances. I don't think anybody intentionally gave anybody medicine that would do them in.
> You know, they don't understand that when a person is incapacitated and really ill and you're not getting the proper nourishment or, you know, it's hot and all…you know they're in…usually you'd be in an air conditioned room or something. You can't metabolize things that you have to take, normally. Things that would normally be a normal course of event might kill you in a certain other circumstance. If you got to take your diabetic medicine, for instance, if you don't eat properly, If you're not getting the proper nourishment, your sugar could bottom out or it's things like that. I don't think the public on basic…you know with news media, they don't understand that.

Similarly, a first responder described his frustrations with the situation, especially the media coverage as briefly mentioned by the nurse:

> **Fire and Rescue (252)** (56-year old male)**:** One thing that stopped me from watching and reading the news was…early on in the disaster—I don't remember if it was the first time I was out or the second time I was out—I was watching the news…in our trailer in north of the lake in Hammond (Louisiana). And this gentleman come on TV and was complaining that it took us sixteen days to find his sister's body. And I just went off on the TV. My wife and my two sons are sitting in the trailer and they looking at me like I'm a madman because I'm yelling at the TV. Because I only have so many people to search twenty-six thousand houses, and at the first search that we did was a sound search. We went from Arabi all the way down to Yscloskey and Delacroix Island (the full length of St. Bernard parish). And on a sound search trying to find as many live people as we could…it wasn't until the second search that we went into buildings and started looking for bodies. My concern in the beginning was people that were still alive. And it took sixteen days for us to find his sister's body. And I yelled at the TV, "How many people do you think I have to be able to search all of these houses, and how long do you think it takes?' And he couldn't hear me….

Finally, a local elected official shared her experience, which included people having unrealistic expectations, despite the comparable situation everyone was in:

> **Local Elected Official (260)** (64-year old female): It was very dark after the storm. The responsibility of being both American Red Cross, which is known for disaster services. Running that job we called, and a responsibility to my voters, and my community, was really, really hard. Because people are expecting so much out of you, not realizing that you lost everything too.

> You know, people expected more from you. And at the same time I think they realized, they didn't realize, or didn't stop to think, "Hey, you know, we're all in the same boat." We literally lost everything [too]. And people sometimes were hostile with the elected officials. And so you know you just tried to…and it was because they were hurting and there wasn't a whole lot you could do to help.
>
> And people as usual expected much of their government. And the government wasn't here. And of course we were here, but we're a local government. And so, and I think that's one of the biggest disappointments. That's, I said it all the time is, that the, our government, being federal, didn't give us the support that we all thought we would get. Because everybody kept saying, you know as soon as the infrastructure starts to get better, meaning traffic and vehicles could start coming in at, you know, the national guard would be here. But I mean it was ten days before we saw anybody. It was very, very lonely and almost abandoned feeling.
>
> And so in my mind I kept saying, "Well, the Red Cross is coming, Red Cross is coming." But it was so overwhelming because all the Red Crosses in southeast Louisiana were wiped out. You know, New Orleans Red Cross, St. Bernard Red Cross, it wasn't just, so, there was no coming. There was no sitting and waiting for something to come. And I tell this all the time, we SOS, we save ourselves. We started doing things and said, "Look, we don't know if and when any helps coming, this is what we have to do." As much as I love this community, it was not a nice place to be. And we had only been in office eighteen months. So it wasn't like we had been there, you know, for years and years and years and could've done anything about the levee breaking….

These quotes offer a glimpse of what happened though the eyes of those who directly witnessed Katrina and her aftermath. Through their observations, perhaps others can sense the desperation and despair among people whose lives have been forever changed by this epic storm. In addition to first responders, among other public officials who were expected to work through the storm, an estimated 6,000 residents of St. Bernard did not evacuate before Hurricane Katrina made landfall. All who sheltered in place found themselves trapped in a surreal nightmare for several days without adequate food, water, and outside assistance (Buuck, 2007; Schaefer, 2007). Sadly, the slow response of federal authorities meant death for some who had survived Katrina's landfall and the horrific flooding. Enduring days on rooftops, flooded shelters of last resort, and other dire circumstances, thousands of stranded citizens and public servants alike were in fear for their lives, as the next quote from another current resident who witnessed the storm directly illustrates:

> **231** (50-year old female)**:** The government was not prepared. People need to know that, to respond to a disaster of this magnitude at all. At all. And people weren't here. It was the truest of most chaos. It was the definition of chaos and instability and unfathomable circumstances. You never thought that…this was the United States of America at all. We kept waiting for the boat to come down the river and the Army to come in and save the day, and every day would go by, and nope. Not here yet. So by Thursday, when we left, I really didn't know if we were going to live or if we were going to die. I really didn't. That was the first day that I thought, we could die. We might die here. If we don't get out of here, we might die.

A crucial point to take away from these firsthand accounts is that more preparation at the state and national level is needed to avoid similar, tragic situations in the future (see Pffeferbaum et al., 2010, for a related discussion). Fortunately, where the government fell short, faith-based communities and volunteers from across the nation and from distant cities all over the world provided aid for devastated residents and public servants (Cain & Barthelemy, 2008; Cherry et al., 2010), a saving grace that many survivors remembered in the years after the storms (see Chap. 14, this volume).

Subtheme 2: The Special Case of Rebuilding Ecologies: On Hardships, Perceived Neglect, and Volunteer Efforts

The coastal parishes (counties) of south Louisiana, among other Gulf Coast communities, are not new to the devastating effects of hurricanes and tropical storms. Older persons spoke of the unnamed storm of 1947 and Hurricane Flossy in September of 1956 (see Chap. 18, this volume). Later came Hurricanes Audrey in 1957, Betsy in 1965, Camille in 1969, Andrew in 1992, and Georges in 1998, among others too numerous to list here. Consistent with an ecological perspective, lifelong residents of geographic regions that are prone to hurricanes have likely developed certain adaptive capacities that build on personal and social resources that facilitate recovery when destructive hurricanes strike. To illustrate, consider these remarks by two lifelong coastal residents on recovery and rebuilding in the wake of Hurricane Katrina:

> **238** (67-year old male)**:** That's what I tell everybody. Do what you have to do, you know. The thing is, you can't depend on everybody else to do it for you. You have to pick up and learn that you have to do for yourself. And you know, at the time of Hurricane Katrina and Rita, everybody was trying to get established, so you couldn't depend on everybody else. You had to do what you had to do for yourself. It's like I tell them all, we've been through it before, so it's not, so it wasn't really a new experience to us.

Arguably, his comment reflects self-sufficiency and prior experience with environmental destruction delivered by forces of nature—"you have to do it for yourself…. we've been through it before…" Perceived social support is another personal resource when faced with disaster-related adversities and the challenges of rebuilding. This lifelong coastal resident's remark is illustrative:

> **235** (43-year old female)**:** It's very important to be around the people and the community right after the storm than be away and not know what's going on. I wanted to see the people and I wanted to be there and hug the people and say, 'I know what you're going through.' And I didn't want to go back to that normal life. I wanted to be where…I wanted to be in the destruction area. I didn't want to leave it but I had nowhere to stay.

Coming back to live in a storm-devastated community in the months after Katrina's catastrophic impact brought layers of difficulty, from the emotional shock of seeing one's home destroyed to finding out whether prior jobs and the means of making a living would be available and viable. Current residents spoke of these and other hardships in these next quotes:

> **204** (62-year old female): Kind of being in a state of limbo at first, until you could feel, "Okay this is where I am going to be for a short time," and then work from there…it was well over a month before they allowed us to come back into St. Bernard Parish, so you even knew what was going on, if your home was still there and then just seeing the devastation when you came in was just overwhelming.

208 (66-year old female): When we came back the first day, I thought my house would be fine, and when I walked in and saw what it looked like, it was hard because, I mean, that was the house I raised my kids in and I had lived in for twenty-something years. And when I saw what it looked like with the front door chopped, and everything all over everywhere and everything ruined, water marks up to the ceiling and holes in the ceiling where the sheet rock fell through, It was horrible. It was just totally, totally horrible.

212 (69-year old female): When I saw my house for the first time I wanted to just leave it. I didn't want to come back. But my husband, we didn't know what was going to happen with his work so we just waited it out, and I said, "Well if we don't know what to do now, something's going to tell us what to do." And something did because they did open his plant again, and we found that out in April of 2006.

Moving forward in the aftermath of 2005 hurricanes proved to be a monumental undertaking for many survivors who tackled obstacles and challenges head on with scant guidance from parish, state, or federal government entities. Consequently, it is not surprising that some current residents who returned after the hurricanes felt a sense of betrayal, mental anguish, and fear of future disasters leading to similar experiences, as this quote illustrates:

260 (64-year old female): I have lost all my trust in the government. That is the one thing that has come out if this for me. I no longer trust my government. And I don't want to be like that, but I've seen it firsthand. Anything happens in this country, we are S.O.L. [sic].

Many participants spoke of negative experiences with the government which adversely impacted their recovery. The next quotes provide additional insight into current residents' angst stemming from their encounters with Federal Emergency Management Agency (FEMA) and programs such as Road Home during the rebuilding and recovery phase of the disaster:

252 (56-year old male): The obstacles and setbacks were basically the Federal Government—trying to get through their forms and the hoops that they made us jump through to get what little money that they did give us.

247 (70-year old male): I think the more you depend on the government, the more you invite delays and technicalities and all this other stuff which just adds to your woes, you know. Had we depended on the Road Home, we'd have been two years or three years getting back in our house instead of back in in a year.

211 (55-year old female): I can't believe the government [can] let so many…they have so much at their disposal that it [could have] been handled in a different kind of way. You know, I mean maybe there's too much red tape. Maybe there are too many chains of command. Whose toes are going to get stepped on? You know, politics has to be set aside. You know, when experiences like this happens in this country, it just seems to me that there was no reason for the…it just didn't seem like things happened fast enough. And like I said, this thing, Katrina, was something that was never expected. It never happened before, and I hope they take everything that happened, and learn from it, and make sure that it doesn't happen to somebody else again when they need help. There's no reason that people couldn't get help immediately.

On the contrary, some current residents had a different opinion on governmental assistance and state recovery programs, such as the Louisiana Recovery Authority (LRA). One current resident reported:

251 (70-year old female): A lot of positive came out of Katrina, a lot of positive. Let me tell you, there was no way that I could come back home and have my house paid for. I had a 30-year mortgage, and my house was only 14-years old. So I came back, my house is paid for. I came back, I mean I know we lost everything, but FEMA and them stepped up. They helped us a heck of a lot….And people complain about it, but they did. But there is no reason for that, no reason for them to complain because FEMA stepped up, LRA stepped up and I mean we got all kind of funds. Just recently I got a hundred and fifty dollar deductible and when I didn't get all of my money, they sent me a check to make up the difference for that. And now they working on this seventy five hundred dollars so that we can get shutters for our house free for Katrina. So it's a lot of positive. I don't understand why people [are] complaining, because we wouldn't be where we [are] at if we wouldn't get all these helps. Just think if we came back and had to do this on our own, you know?

Despite the hardships and challenges after the massive 2005 storms, some current residents spoke of positive experiences. The move back to St. Bernard and Plaquemines parishes after the storms gave current residents an opportunity to call a familiar place home and see some old faces that helped restore something that had been completely destroyed. Volunteer efforts of neighbors assisting each other with clean up, coupled with volunteers from all over the country who came to lend a helping hand, also made a difference for many current residents. We conclude with several heartfelt and positive responses:

210 (57-year old male): The biggest thing would be pretty much everyone that was down here that came down, whether they were coming down to see their own homes or whatever, were always there to try and help their neighbors or whoever else, too. And I think that happened a lot, and you had people coming down at different stages of the recovery. What happened was the people kind of pitched in and would help other people I think a little bit more in their situation even though they had their own problems….

254 (59-year old male): And, those people helped us. Those people helped us. You can count, you know, I can sit here and count everybody that laid a hand on us for the first year after Katrina, you know, helped us in one way or another. And, of course, we try and give back the same as what we got.

254 (59-year old male): And there is any number of positive actions that I saw people do, you know that you don't normally see every day. But, I saw any number of positive activities, things that would make you proud of the human race, go on.

To summarize, the narrative text highlighted here has revealed an undeniable and pervasive theme—namely, the feeling that no one understands the Katrina experience, unless they experienced it for themselves. The voice of one current resident perfectly captures this collective lamentation:

215 (77-year old female): I would like the whole country to really know or comprehend what happened down here. [I want them to know] that we're not a bunch of people hanging out on a roof waiting for the government to come rescue us. Like someone said recently. And he used to be a sports broadcaster down here and he works now I think it's CNN he works with. He made a comment about the people in Nashville being flooded. That they didn't go up on a roof and wait for the government to come. Nashville was a whole different story. Yes, they had water, okay, but they knew it was coming. We didn't know this water was coming here. And there were some people that couldn't leave because they couldn't afford to leave. I don't believe the country really understood what happened down here, and they still don't. [Now], with this oil spill.[1] They all think we a bunch of third world country people waiting for the government to come help us.

[1] Participant 215 is referencing the catastrophic 2010 Deepwater Horizon oil spill in the Gulf Coast (see Chap. 4, this volume).

The voices of the first responders, as documented in the first subtheme, among others who sheltered in place on August 29, 2005, provide direct evidence of the complete destruction of a community by the forces of wind and water and the noble efforts of those who struggled for survival. In the years that followed, further insight into the lengthy and at times, painful process of restoring damaged ecologies was revealed in the second subtheme, from the proximal factors of home and family to the increasingly distal factors of neighborhoods, businesses, local government, and cultural heritage. Others may not know how it feels to experience catastrophic disruptions in familial and social support systems (with evacuations, family, and friends are scattered widely) and the devastating loss of homes and communities (schools, shopping centers, places of worship). However, diverse viewpoints from former and current residents, service personnel, and local government officials provide a step in the direction of helping others understand.

Conclusions and Implications

The findings from our qualitative analysis suggest that differences between former residents who were permanently displaced and current residents who returned to rebuild may be minimal, at least in the two respects we focus on in this chapter. Both groups experienced life changing effects of Hurricanes Katrina and Rita and both mourn the passing of the *old normal*. A pervasive sense of loss among former and current residents was often coupled with the feeling that *no one understands*. These reports were frequent and salient across the 125 interviews considered here—including participants who relocated *and* those who returned and rebuilt. One noteworthy difference was the longer duration of adversity (defined as a period of time without a stable residence and convenient access to goods and services) for current residents who returned to rebuild, compared to former residents who relocated elsewhere. Whether one's challenge was to find a new town in which to live or to rebuild a hurricane-damaged hometown, the fundamental importance of recovering the sense of belonging in a community and having a perceived social support network should be kept in mind. One current coastal resident seemed to capture the feeling of many of our participants when she exclaimed:

> **235** (43-year old female)**:** I want everyone to know that your home community and way of life could be washed away, but it was harder to lose the community than it was my home. You can rebuild the house, but you cannot rebuild the community. It's very hard. You can lose a home, but if you had nowhere to go when you get home then it's not a home. If you don't have a school, you don't have groceries, you don't have neighbors, you don't have family. I wouldn't want to live there so it was much harder to lose my whole way of life more than what it was to see my house gone.

The emergent themes presented here are rich with local and historical color and also have noteworthy implications that warrant further consideration. From a theoretical point of view, our results are consistent with an ecological systems perspective on post-disaster psychological reactions, highlighting the need for further study of individuals nested within multiple ecologies (see Kilmer & Gil-Rivas, 2010; Weems & Overstreet, 2009; Chap. 10, this volume). From an applied perspective, feelings of loss and frustration that persist over time underscore the need for conducting assessments in the years after a catastrophic disaster. We found that those who experienced the devastation directly, including people who now reside outside of the severely damaged areas, are still processing the lifestyle changes imposed by the 2005 storms. The persistence of storm-related feelings among former and current coastal residents alike highlights a need for support services in disaster-affected areas, and indirectly affected communities that have become a new home for those permanently displaced by the storm.

In conclusion, these data provide a unique contribution to the literature on long-term hurricane recovery guided by an ecological systems theory perspective. Addressing the needs of individuals and families who have been directly impacted by disasters in the years after these events remains a pressing challenge for social scientists and those in the helping professions. Disaster survivors' lived experiences also raise awareness of the need to prepare effectively for future disasters on local, state, and national levels.

Acknowledgments We are grateful to Sr. Mary Keefe and Fr. John Arnone of Our Lady of Lourdes Catholic Church in Violet, LA and Gayle Buckley, Judy Chiappetta, and Catherine Serpas for their assistance with recruitment. We thank Susan McNeil of the St. Bernard Council on Aging and Sean Warner of the Gulf Coast Trust Bank in St. Bernard for providing space for interviews. We thank Kelli Broome, Susan Brigman, Ashley Cacamo, Pamela Nezat, and Mary Beth Tamor for their help with data collection and Robert Pressley, Penni Fontenot, Sarah Finney, Lauren Edwards, Allison Kennedy, Amy Goff and Graham Belou for their assistance with transcriptions. We also thank Yaxin Lu, Bethany Pinkston, Sarah Hebert, Savannah Ballard, Trevor Johnson, and Brandon Cohen for assistance with qualitative analyses, and Carl Weems for helpful feedback on an earlier draft of this chapter.

This research was supported by grants from the Louisiana Board of Regents and the BP Gulf of Mexico Research Initiative, Office of Research and Economic Development, Louisiana State University. This support is gratefully acknowledged.

References

Bronfenbrenner, U. (1977). Toward an experimental ecology of human development. *American Psychologist, 32,* 513–531.

Bronfenbrenner, U. (1979). *The ecology of human development.* Cambridge: Harvard University Press.

Bronfenbrenner, U., & Morris, P. A. (2006). The bioecological model of human development. In R. M. Lerner & W. R. Dumon (Eds.), *Handbook of child psychology Vol. 1. Theoretical models of human development* (6th ed., pp. 793–828). Hoboken: Wiley.

Brown, J. S., Cherry, K. E., Marks, L. D., Jackson, E. M., Volaufova, J., Lefante, C., & Jazwinski, S. M. (2010). After Hurricanes Katrina and Rita: Gender differences in health and religiosity in middle-aged and older adults. *Health Care for Women International, 31*(11), 997–1012. doi:http://dx.doi.org/10.1080/07399332.2010.514085.

Buuck, M. M. (2007). *Firestorm: Hurricane Katrina and the St. Bernard Fire Department.* Xlibris Corporation.

Cain, D. S., & Barthelemy, J. (2008). Tangible and spiritual relief after the storm: The religious community responds to Katrina. *Journal of Social Service Research, 34,* 9–42.
Cherry, K. E. (Ed.). (2009). *Lifespan perspectives on natural disasters: Coping with Katrina, Rita and other storms*. New York: Springer.
Cherry, K. E., Allen, P. D., & Galea, S. (2010). Older adults and natural disasters: Lessons learned from Hurricanes Katrina and Rita. In P. Dass-Brailsford (Ed.), *Crisis and disaster counseling: Lessons learned from Hurricane Katrina and other disasters* (pp. 115–130). Thousand Oaks: Sage.
Cherry, K. E., Silva Brown, J., Marks, L. D., Galea, S., Volaufova, J., Lefante, C., et al. (2011). Longitudinal assessment of cognitive and psychosocial functioning after Hurricanes Katrina and Rita: Exploring disaster impact on middle-aged, older, and oldest-old adults. *Journal of Applied Biobehavioral Research, 16,* 187–211.
Cherry, K. E., Sampson, L., Nezat, P. F., Cacamo, A., Marks, L. D., & Galea, S. (2015). Long-term psychological outcomes in older adults after disaster: relationships to religiosity and social support. *Aging & Mental Health, 19*(5), 430–443.
Henry, J. (2013). Return or relocate? An inductive analysis of decision-making in a disaster. *Disaster, 37,* 293–316.
Kamo, Y., Henderson, T. L., & Roberto, K. A. (2011). Displaced older adults' reactions to and coping with the aftermath of Hurricane Katrina. *Journal of Family Issues, 30,* 1346–1370.
Kilmer, R. P., & Gil-Rivas, V. (2010). Introduction: Attending to ecology. In R. P. Kilmer, V. Gil-Rivas, R. G. Tedeschi & L. G. Calhoun (Eds.), *Meeting the needs of children, families, and communities post-disaster: Lessons learned from Hurricane Katrina and its aftermath* (pp. 3–24). Washington, D.C.: American Psychological Association.
Marks, L. D., Cherry, K. E., & Silva, J. L. (2009). Faith, crisis, coping and meaning making after Katrina. In K. E. Cherry (Ed.), *Lifespan perspectives on natural disasters: Coping with Katrina, Rita and other storms* (pp. 195–215). New York: Springer.
Miles, M. B., & Huberman, A. M. (1994). *Qualitative data analysis: An expanded sourcebook.* Thousand Oaks: Sage.
Patton, M. Q. (2002). *Qualitative research & evaluation methods* (3rd ed.). Thousand Oaks: Sage.
Pfefferbaum, B., Pfefferbaum, R. L., & Norris, F. (2010). Community resilience and wellness for children exposed to Hurricane Katrina. In R. P. Kilmer, V. Gil-Rivas, R. G. Tedeschi & L. G. Calhoun (Eds.), *Meeting the needs of children, families, and communities post-disaster: Lessons learned from Hurricane Katrina and its aftermath* (pp. 265–288). Washington, D.C.: American Psychological Association.
Schaefer, M. (2007). *Lost in Katrina.* Gretna: Pelican.
Silva Brown, J., Cherry, K. E., Marks, L. D., Jackson, E. M., Volaufova, J., Lefante, C., & Jazwinski, S. M. (2010). After Hurricanes Katrina and Rita: Gender differences in health and religiosity in middle-aged and older adults. *Health Care for Women International, 31*(11), 997–1012. doi:http://dx.doi.org/10.1080/07399332.2010.514085.
S. M. (2010). *Lost in Katrina*. Gretna: Pelican.
Strauss, A., & Corbin, J. (1998). *Basics of qualitative research: Techniques and procedures for developing grounded theory*. Thousand Oaks: Sage.
Weems, C. F, & Overstreet, S. (2009). An ecological-needs-based perspective of adolescent and youth emotional development in the context of disaster: Lessons from Hurricane Katrina. In K. E. Cherry (Ed.), *Lifespan perspectives on natural disasters: Coping with Katrina, Rita and other storms* (pp. 27–44). New York: Springer.
Weems, C. F., Watts, S. E., Marsee, M. A., Taylor, L. K., Costa, N. M., Cannon, M. F., Carrión, V. G., & Piña, A. A. (2007). The psychosocial impact of Hurricane Katrina: Contextual differences in psychological symptoms, social support, and discrimination. *Behaviour Research and Therapy, 45,* 2295–2306.

Chapter 13
Loss, Chaos, Survival, and Despair: The Storm after the Storms

Trevan G. Hatch, Katie E. Cherry, Keri L. Kytola, Yaxin Lu and Loren D. Marks

Introduction

The 2005 Atlantic hurricane season brought two category 3 hurricanes, Katrina and Rita, which resulted in unparalleled destruction and devastation for the US Gulf Coast residents (see Chaps. 10 and 12, this volume). Lingering signs of the damage from these massive storms in 2005 can still be seen in coastal towns and communities today. Many neighborhoods were completely destroyed, including houses and schools. Some families were separated and many friends moved away. Coastal residents lost their jobs and their religious communities, as businesses and churches were destroyed (Henry, 2013; Kamo, Henderson, & Roberto, 2011).

The psychosocial consequences of disasters, like Hurricanes Katrina and Rita, are well documented in disaster research literature (Neria, Galea, & Norris, 2009;

K. E. Cherry (✉)
Department of Psychology, Louisiana State University, 236 Audubon Hall,
Baton Rouge, LA 70803-5501, USA
e-mail: pskatie@lsu.edu

T. G. Hatch
School of Social Work, Louisiana State University, 335 Long Fieldhouse,
Baton Rouge, LA 70803-5501, USA
e-mail: thatch8@lsu.edu

L. D. Marks
School of Family Life, Brigham Young University, 2092C Joseph F.
Smith Building, Provo, Utah 84602, USA
e-mail: loren_marks@byu.edu

K. L. Kytola
Department of Psychology, Oklahoma State University, Stillwater, OK 74078, USA
e-mail: keri.kytola@okstate.edu

Y. Lu
Louisiana Department of Education, 1201 North Third Street, Baton Rouge, LA 70802, USA
e-mail: Yaxinlu3@gmail.com

K. E. Cherry (ed.), *Traumatic Stress and Long-Term Recovery*,
DOI 10.1007/978-3-319-18866-9_13

Norris et al., 2002; Norris & Elrod, 2006). For instance, disruptions to social networks and heightened prevalence of depression, anxiety, and posttraumatic stress may be observed in the first weeks and months after a disaster. Other evidence has shown that behavioral and mental health consequences of disasters may persist 2 or more years after these events (Galea, Tracy, Norris, & Coffey, 2008; Gleser, Green, & Winget, 1981). From a developmental perspective, short-term and long-term psychological effects have been found in children exposed to natural disasters (i.e., hurricanes, Belter, Dunn, & Jeney, 1991; flooding, Earls, Smith, Reich, & Junk, 1988). For example, McFarlane, Policansky, and Irwin (1987) tested children at several points following a natural disaster. They found that after 8 months, the number of children who were at high risk for psychiatric disorders increased dramatically, and these rates remained high for more than 2 years (see also Green et al., 1991). Adults who experienced a traumatic event have also exhibited psychological effects over time including posttraumatic stress disorder (PTSD), anxiety, depression, and affective disorders (Breslau, Davis, Andreski, & Peterson, 1991; Sharan, Chaudhary, Kavathekar, & Saxena, 1996). Older adults are considered by some to be a special risk group for post-disaster distress (Massey, 1997). However, older adults who survive disaster may be resilient to adverse psychosocial outcomes (Cherry, Galea, & Silva, 2008; Cherry et al., 2011), although further research is needed to evaluate the long-term effects of disaster exposure, especially for frail elderly adults (Cherry, Allen, & Galea, 2010).

Our primary purpose in this chapter is to examine the challenges that survivors faced after Hurricanes Katrina and Rita and highlight their experiences as remembered 5 or more years after these storms. Some challenges seem to have remained in the forefront of our participants' minds while the recollection of other challenges may have faded over time. There is evidence in the research literature to indicate that the vividness and effects of some experiences, such as physical pain or hunger, may diminish over time. For instance, individuals who experience a tremendous amount of pain—a severe ear infection or toothache—may not remember how painful the ear infection or toothache felt several years later (Eich, Reeves, Jaeger, & Graff-Radford, 1985). In contrast, other traumatic life experiences such as crises of health or finances, or the death of a loved one may be remembered with great clarity bringing waves of sorrow and additional challenges that have lasting effects. Similarly, our participants have identified losing personal possessions (e.g., pictures, tools, vehicles, etc.); dealing with insurance companies; or securing the basic necessities of clothes, food, and temporary shelter immediately after the storms as challenging because those were their immediate needs. These challenges, however, may pale in comparison to less tangible, interpersonal challenges that have lingered for 5 years or more.

To summarize, participants' narratives highlighted in this chapter bring into focus the immediate challenges of meeting basic needs and the lingering challenges related to a wide range of post-disaster losses that may be less apparent to those with limited hurricane experience. In particular, our participants have spoken of the loss of friends and colleagues who relocated elsewhere, the diminished sense of community, and lasting sorrow and mental fatigue (in local parlance, "Katrina brain") associated with the burden of surviving a disaster, followed by stress of *rebuilding* a life. In addition to identifying *which* challenges may have been the most difficult to manage over time, this chapter also examines *how* the various proximal and distal challenges affected our participants several years after the storms.

Method

Participants and Interview Procedure

In all, 125 individuals participated in this study. They were 62 former coastal residents relocated to new homes in non-coastal communities (*M* age = 58.4, *SD* = 17.1 years, 21 males, 41 females) and 63 current residents returned to rebuild and restore their lives in their home communities (*M* age = 60.7, *SD* = 15.0 years, 26 males, 37 females). Sociodemographic characteristics of the sample and other individual differences are reported elsewhere (see Cherry et al., 2015). All participants were assigned a three-digit number to protect anonymity; former residents in the 100s (101–162) and current residents in the 200s (201–263), which we reference here and in Chaps. 12, 14, 20, and 21 (this volume).

Interviews were conducted in participants' homes or in a community location in two sessions (or more, if needed). At the end of the first session, participants were given seven open-ended questions on a prepared sheet, which were read aloud and reviewed. In the second session (at least 1 week later), participants answered these questions and their responses were recorded. Digital voice files were transcribed verbatim and double-checked for accuracy. In this chapter, we focus on participants' responses to these questions: (1) "People who lived through Hurricanes Katrina and Rita experienced a variety of challenges, obstacles and setbacks. Please tell us how you coped with the challenges you faced after the storms." (2) "What kinds of things did you do to establish a new daily routine?" (3) "When did 'normal living' come back for you?" (4) "What would you like others to know about your experiences with Hurricanes Katrina and Rita?"

Participants' responses were analyzed using open and axial coding, two techniques from grounded theory methodology (Strauss & Corbin, 1998). We conducted team-based analyses to enhance the reliability and validity of these findings (see Chap. 12, this volume, for description). Five themes pertaining to the challenges current and former coastal residents faced after Hurricanes Katrina and Rita in 2005 were revealed; three are presented next and two appear in Chap. 12 (this volume).

Findings

The themes presented next reflect participants' personal anguish, fatigue, and discouragement after their homes and communities were *devastated* by the 2005 hurricanes. They lost material possessions, their "entire community"—including houses, jobs, neighbors, churches, public buildings, and institutions (Cherry et al., 2015). Many were thrown into a tailspin of sorrow—overwhelmed with the task of trying to adjust to their new circumstances.

Part of the "truth" that has emerged from this study is the remarkable resilience apparent in the interviews. As documented in Chaps. 20 and 21 (this volume), participants seemed to gravitate toward faith, family, and friends for comfort and support. Chapters 20 and 21 deal primarily with healthy and successful coping strategies and efforts—emphasizing the positive and salutogenic. Another portion of the full truth is that, for many, psychological and emotional scars linger—even years later. We are grateful for the opportunity, within this edited volume, to present different facets of participants' reports—thereby conveying a richer, more complete version of the "truth" regarding these 125 participants' experiences.

The themes presented here capture challenges they faced after the storms. These themes are: (1) "I Don't Want to Lose Another Friend:" A Loss of More than Material Possessions, (2) "No Coping, Just Surviving:" Chaos and the Crushing Burden of Survival, and (3) "[Katrina] Made Me a Weaker Person:" Anguish and Despair after the Storms. Primary data are presented in connection with each theme next, consistent with our objective to provide the reader with the opportunity to hear the participants' "voices" (e.g., Gilligan, 1992).

Theme 1: "I Don't Want to Lose Another Friend:" A Loss of More than Material Possessions

A former coastal resident (124) told a new friend after Katrina: "I don't know if I want to get close to you, because I don't want to lose another friend" *(69-year-old female)*. Her lament echoes the voices of many who agreed overwhelmingly that material possessions do not matter as much as relationships (see Chap. 21, this volume). Although participants reported the loss of family heirlooms, photographs, and wedding memorabilia (with profound regret in most cases), many also spontaneously mentioned that relationships with God, family, and friends are what matter *most*. Accordingly, the greatest challenge for many was that, in addition to losing most of their personal possessions, they also lost their entire community and network of friends.

Another former resident explained the context behind this type of statement, as many outsiders are unaware of the life-changing devastation that descended upon the communities embedded in St. Bernard and Plaquemines Parishes of south Louisiana:

> **115** *(48-year old female)*: I would like everybody to know [and]…understand that in the history of America, no county (we call them parishes) has ever been decimated like St. Bernard has. The entire parish was destroyed; with the exception of three to five buildings, everything was destroyed. The way that this parish was…you grew up and you bought a house down the street from your Mom. You didn't move. Certainly some people did, but

most people stayed close to home. So when [Katrina] destroyed the entire parish, you are looking at generations of families being out of some place to live…. You know when they… had the flooding in Tennessee…it was terrible, really terrible…[but] it wasn't an entire… parish [that] was destroyed…. So that's what I would like people to understand: that it was not [just] a neighborhood. New Orleans was not [entirely] destroyed; *neighborhoods* of New Orleans were destroyed. But St. Bernard, an entire parish was destroyed…where pretty much everybody you know was born, raised, and then lived in that same neighborhood. They were destroyed…. That's what I'd like Brad Pitt to know as he's rebuilding those houses in the Ninth Ward; the Ninth Ward is one neighborhood. If you go just a mile down the road, you will run into miles and miles and miles of destruction.

She emphasized to "everybody" outside the community that the hurricanes did not generate a 60–90-day inconvenience consisting of flooding, followed by the hassle of replacing carpet, drywall, and furniture—rather, the storms decimated everything save a few buildings and then forced tens of thousands of people out of their homes in St. Bernard Parish alone. Participants 117 and 252 echo similar details:

117 *(61-year old female)*: Every house was devastated—the whole community was devastated… Every job, every business, everything was devastated. And I don't think, you know, even though everybody saw the pictures, I think they thought it was like…the flood water in Iowa…but we had such a different experience because houses were [not just wet or damaged, they were] just totally destroyed.

252 *(56-year old male)*: I would like them to understand what happened here, that it wasn't just a hurricane [that] came in and then it left and we were alright or we were back on our feet… This parish was 67,000 people before the storm. We are [now] in March of 2011, five and a half years later, and we're only at 35,000 people. When a jurisdiction is one hundred percent wiped out…it takes *years* to go about getting government up and running. We're just five and a half years in, and they just started the hospital. We don't have a hospital. Five and a half years in [and still] we're working out of a clinic.

As illustrated by the three previous reports, individuals who experienced the devastation were adamant that outsiders learn the extent of what happened to their communities. Residents of the region were not just inconvenienced; the infrastructure of their parish and their way of life were obliterated. Their homes, churches, family businesses, government buildings, hospitals, schools, and shops were nothing more than a memory after Hurricanes Katrina and Rita in 2005.

In addition to the loss of physical structures and personal property, individuals lost daily, face-to-face contact with their friends and peers. For example, one man (134) lamented the loss of relationships that had been nurtured for nearly three decades before the storms:

134 *(60-year old male)*: It was a *loss*. It was a feeling of loss, not just loss [of] things but loss [of] community. You know, we lost our community and our friends because our friends moved everywhere. Pretty much, that's it…. We didn't have our church anymore to go to that we had gone to for twenty-seven years. We had to start going to a new church. It was… it was hard. After a while, you get tired of making new friends.

Many participants in the immediate aftermath of the storms would identify employment and housing as the greatest losses because those necessities were highest in priority at the time. However, our sample—individuals who were interviewed between 5 and 7 years after the storms— seemed to agree that personal relationships, faith community, and intimate social circles were missed more than the possessions, houses, or jobs. As an illustration, one participant offered the following insight:

> **210** *(57-year old male)*: You know, when you grow up somewhere, and you go to school, you have friends, you have family, and all the sudden what happened with Katrina was… you know, the houses are one thing. The houses are something physical that can be replaced, *but it scattered families [and] friends*. The schools that you went to…are no longer there or they've…changed into something else…. So *the biggest loss I would say was loss of community*, a group of people, and a way of life down here.

In Theme 1 *("I Don't Want to Lose Another Friend:" A Loss of More than Material Possessions),* the voices of several participants explained that, in many ways, the most profound losses were relational in nature. Five or more years after the storm, the wounds left by having family and friends torn away had not healed fully—and perhaps never will.

Having established that the distress associated with Hurricane Katrina and Hurricane Rita's catastrophic impact still lingers in the present for many, we now present a theme that takes us back to the carnage and devastation in the immediate aftermath of the storms (Buuck, 2007; Schaefer, 2007). If some of the relational scars left by Katrina were indelible and unrelenting, so too were some of the horrific memories of the chaos and the related fight for survival that followed in the immediate but lasting wake of August 29, 2005. In Theme 2 *("No Coping, Just Surviving:" Chaos and the Crushing Burden of Survival),* we convey participants' experiences regarding the struggle for life amidst the chaos and destruction, which we have termed, "The Storm After the Storm."

Theme 2: "No Coping, Just Surviving:" Chaos and the Crushing Burden of Survival

As our research team coded, analyzed, and discussed the interviews, we were struck by the descriptions not only of what people experienced in the immediate aftermath of the storms, but also of the conditions in which they endured their challenges. For many participants, coping with the possession-related losses in the days following the storms was not their most pressing concern; survival was the first priority.

The conditions following Katrina were reportedly so horrid that some people doubted whether they could endure it, and others questioned, even years later, whether they would be able to survive another similar catastrophe. A 64-year-old man (213), after describing the destruction as analogous to a "war zone," commented that the experience was "something that I don't think anybody should live through." Another man described the event in even stronger language:

> **216** *(80-year old male)*: When we think about it, we don't know how we survived. I wouldn't want to go through it again. I'd probably survive it, but I wouldn't want to go through it…because it's *hell*. It really is. You got to go through it to know.

Another participant similarly commented that he would not wish his experience on anybody:

> **230** *(49-year old male)*: People, if they have never lived down here, have no idea.... They cannot imagine the smell...[and] the silence. No birds.... You can't explain the smell. You know, I wish there was a way to capture that, because that was a major part of it, the smell [of death]. *You knew something was dead*.... I never want anything like that to ever happen to anybody.

For participant 230, the morbid smells and the animal-forsaken trees and skies seemed to be the exclamation point on both his horrible experience and of the catastrophe itself. Another man also expressed his sadness as he reflected on the ambiance of death, disease, and stench in their community in the weeks succeeding the storms:

> **134** *(60-year old male)*: I know it was sad to see the animals that people had left. It was [heartbreaking to see] dead dogs, dead cats everywhere. There was a deer [by] the balcony of a house [near us that] was dead.... [There were] dead raccoons, dead nutrias, and dead possums everywhere because we didn't live far from the marsh... And they smelled horrible. They were weeks old. And it was very hot. Ninety degrees, a hundred degrees; it was horrible. I went to my son-in-law's house to check on it because they couldn't come. And when I walked in, there was a snorting sound coming down from the hall. I don't know what the hell that was and these two dogs [were] living in her house...big old dogs. And they weren't mean. They were just hungry. And ah, but that was sad. There were dogs from across the street that...the guy had left them and they got around the back because the door was pushed in. And they came in there to get out [of] the bad weather.... I remember seeing those dogs. I fed them. I felt sorry for them, but we called the guy. He went and got them but it was sad. They were happy to see me. They figured I was coming to help them.

These kinds of experiences reflect intense abhorrence and may resemble the post-traumatic symptoms associated with war. Based on the participants' recollections of the storms' destruction and the chaos that followed, the recurring description "hell" seems apt.

Several participants recalled specific stressors that contributed to the challenge of enduring the storms. For instance, a 57-year-old man (155) explained that he did not sleep well, and some nights did not sleep at all, because he was overwhelmed with fears of not being able to "survive." This next woman also recalled sleeping very little in the days and weeks after the hurricanes:

> **115** *(48-year old female)*: I have to tell you it was being on automatic pilot...[I] slept very little. I knew that...the first thing we needed to do was get some place to live, shelter, the kids needed to be in school, I needed to worry about money to take care of the kids, clothing, and we made a lot of decisions that we're still feeling the effects [of today], that are still affecting us. We did the best that we could at the time. But, truly, I went into survival mode immediately and took care of business, like from the time we woke up until the time we went to bed, but I have got to say it was like being on automatic pilot.

The descriptions of being on "automatic pilot" or in "survival mode" were common among the participants we interviewed, as illustrated by the following four examples:

> **146** *(46-year old female)*: I think you were just in *forward mode*. Like you were just in *survival mode*. And so, you didn't... sit back and wallow, [you didn't have time to.].

147 *(43-year old male)*: How do you cope with them [the challenges]? *I didn't think there was coping.* You had to do what you had to do to *move forward*… it was either move forward or break down. And there is no breakdown [option] when you have children [depending on you], right?

148 *(64-year old female)*: I was in *survival mode* for a long time. There was so much to do, getting set up somewhere else, paperwork, cleaning out our home, and the muck and taking care of my granddaughter that had suffered brain damage from being hit by a car and was also pregnant. I just kept going and going.

149 *(57-year old female)*: I felt like a *machine*. You just woke up, did what you had to do… did a job and you went to sleep…. And the next day you got up and did [another] job.

Memories of slogging through challenge after challenge while in survival mode in those dark days and weeks following the storms were still vivid and disturbing to many of our participants at least 5 years after the storms. The trauma was so severe for some, it was a struggle to even discuss it. Participant 149 (mentioned earlier), for example, wept openly through much of her interview.

Other stressors included unbearable or unsanitary living conditions. One man, whose job required him to remain in the parish during and after the storm, described living in makeshift huts with no air conditioning for three weeks—under additionally primal conditions involving encroachment of myriad animals into the dwelling place:

131 *(56-year old male)*: So, the first three weeks, we made make-shift shelters at the drainage pumping stations, and lived there with our employees…. We had [to] post-guards at night, we had to take turns sleeping at night because of, at least in the first three or four days, because all the animals were just like us, they were trying to get out of the water, so they'd run to habitate with us in the pump stations. So we'd have somebody stay awake and keep the animals away from the people that were sleeping. It was dogs. It was nutria, muskrat, hogs, skunks, all the regular vermin that you think of, plus the domesticated animals because many people had left their pets behind. So you had dogs and cats, and things like that. Actually some of the dogs [eventually] acted like watch dogs for us.

People also found shelter in various buildings or vehicles. The following account vividly portrays extended days and nights without quality rest—or respite from the Gulf Coast heat and humidity:

220 *(63-year old male)*: I'd sit up all night with the windows rolled up in the truck and couldn't lay down or anything in the truck. And, I couldn't open the windows because [then] the mosquitoes would eat me up. And, [I] just sat there in a pool of water sweating, and then [got] up the next day to work again. I didn't have the gasoline to run back and forth either. The roads were still in bad shape with a lot of debris and dead animals and everything else on them.

The following narrative, from a deputy on patrol during the storm, further illustrates some of the sanitation challenges of surviving in the wake of the storms:

213 *(64-year old male)*: The deputies were housed in the courthouse. And when the storm really hit and the…levee broke up the road…the water started coming in, we were trapped there at that time. We had boats and all, but we were all living in the courthouse…in the different offices. All of a sudden there was no more sewer system. And it was *bad*. I'm telling you, it was bad, really bad. And people had to go to the bathroom. Then some people wouldn't eat because they knew they'd have to go to the bathroom. They couldn't go outside because [of] the flood water. So they used garbage bags and things like that….

> We had a problem with a lot, and then we had a couple of dead bodies that we had stored in there… [and] we had to get it out of there because it was hot, and we didn't want it to start decomposing.

Given the wretched array of sights, smells, and experiences layered on top of the quest for survival, it is understandable that some participants had difficulty in coping in the long-term aftermath. To survive these initial horrors for several days— in a physically and psychologically weakened condition—having to then wrestle with the trauma associated with the losses of possessions, community, and one's previous "way of life" is almost too much to contemplate. A 69-year-old female (122), after describing the chaos, chose (above all else) to emphasize the losses of "church community" and friends being "scattered to the four winds." She referenced this catastrophic event as "a *death* of what we knew and loved."

As referenced earlier and demonstrated at length in Chaps. 20 and 21 (this volume), many participants coped remarkably well—as evidenced on both quantitative and qualitative measures. Some, however, were not as fortunate—the hammer of Katrina delivered a blow from which they reportedly have never fully recovered. This reality is captured in our third theme.

Theme 3: "[Katrina] made me a Weaker Person:" Anguish and Despair after the Storms

Many participants were reportedly people of faith (see Chap. 20, this volume) and were likely familiar with the experience of Job, a figure in the Hebrew Bible, who is the paragon of strength and resilience amidst adversity. Rabbi Harold S. Kusher, author of the bestseller, *When Bad Things Happen to Good People,* notes that "The Book of Job is probably the greatest, fullest, most profound discussion of the subject of good people suffering ever written" (Kushner, 1981; p. 42). To summarize briefly, Job lost all of his personal property and assets, his children, and finally his health. Initially, he mourned his losses while acknowledging that life still had meaning. However, even Job reached the precipice of crippling despair and eventually cursed the day on which he was born. His wife and three of his associates suggested that he give up hope and "die." Job did not give up, but endured his trials.

Most of the participants in our study, like Job, experienced life-changing disruptions in the wake of Hurricanes Katrina and Rita. They lost property, their jobs and/or financial security, many of their relationships, and their way of life. While some may have moved on with their lives, recouping lost resources and discovering a *new normal* after Katina (see Chap. 12, this volume), others reportedly did not. They continue to struggle to this day with losses that generated great personal anguish and sorrow. Assurances of some level of stability and structure, as well as a specific vision of the future, are facilitative (if not essential) in fostering positive coping and hope (Covey, 2003; Frankl, 1984). Many of our participants were, instead, mired in uncertainty in the aftermath of the storm. A 43-year-old female (235), for instance, explained that: "Nobody could give us answers…. We didn't know what to do.

We didn't know where we were going to go." Many people were frozen in fear. A 20-year-old female (218) remembered that shortly after the storms, her mother had an emotional breakdown in Wal-Mart and cried inconsolably while "shopping for underwear." The following two reflections further illustrate the chronic interpersonal stress that numerous participants experienced:

> **225** *(68-year old male)*: It took me forty-two years to build what I wanted on my property. *Katrina ruined it all….* It took forty-two years to build what I have! My health is declining, I'm depressed, I can't basically do the things I want to do and enjoy myself.

> **118** *(53-year old female)*: My family, I'm sure, [we] all had posttraumatic stress syndrome. But, the one thing that we said, is that while we were living in close quarters, we…did not all experience it [PTSD] at the same time. That's probably a good thing. But for those people who were living in much closer conditions for a lot longer than we were, I'm sure that there were many individuals that were bordering on sever[ly poor] mental health, the quality of their mental health [was very low]. So, this was truly a test of how easily you could adapt…. But, some people couldn't move past the material, the loss of material aspects, and it became a very big problem for them. And that's why so many people were literally taking depression medicine.

From a clinical perspective, the disaster research literature documents a range of a mental health challenges for survivors, including depression, posttraumatic stress, and more recently, prolonged grief disorder (Neria et al., 2009). Our participants spoke openly of their experiences with traumatic stress (see Chap. 1, this volume) after Katrina, among other threats to mental health and well-being. In addition to the earlier quotes, consider participant 249 who also doubted whether she could endure another catastrophe without suffering a complete mental breakdown. She offered the following comment as an illustration of just how difficult it can be to survive mentally after experiencing a life-changing natural disaster, even several years later:

> **249** *(51-year old female)*: I personally feel *it made me a weaker person* in the end, if that makes any sense to you. It's like it…broke me down. If it happened again, I don't think I could survive it or be as normal afterwards…. It really did something to [my] memory [and] to the stress. And I feel I am much weaker, like I can't hold it together as much. And if it happened again, I wouldn't be able to hold it together. I think I would fall apart; and maybe not come back. I don't feel mentally strong enough to be able to handle it… [I] can't get a grip on everything. It's just like we're putting the house back together when we first built it…in '89…. *I can't, I can't, I can't get me together…* I think it took three months [for me] to make paint decisions, to put paint on the wall…. It was just very, very mind-boggling for me…. [I] just couldn't do it. I couldn't, and I had a friend who couldn't either. She had the same experience.

Another participant (231) explained that she and her and her husband struggled for years after the storms, seeking therapy to relieve their distress, which seemed to bother her because they were not anxious people before the storms:

> **231** *(50-year old female)*: Five years [passing by] does not mean that we are recovered from this. I think that that was probably one of the things that I found myself really, really grappling with…. I thought by five years we were going to be normal again. Five years has come and gone and…. No, we are far from what we think is normal, but we really don't know what normal is going to be…. We're still suffering a degree of anxiety…[and] it just wasn't in our makeup prior to this, you know. We really are [suffering]. So we've tried formal therapy. We've been through…this is the second person that we're seeing.

Previous research indicates that many retired adults, or older adults, experience unique challenges in coping and dealing with stress after natural disasters (Cherry, Silva, & Galea, 2009). The following comment of a 65-year-old male, reporting on his mother's decline, is a prime example both of what many older adults experienced and also of the stress that can consume family members of older adults:

> **152** *(65-year old male)*: Now I will add one thing—probably the *worst thing* that I can think of, personally, from Katrina was I saw my Mom's physical and mental health deteriorate from that point forward, and she was never the same, you know? Besides the fact that after her house flooded she went—basically we had my sister take her to Michigan to live. Here's a person who lived her whole life in New Orleans, eighty years, and all of a sudden she's in a strange environment with strange people, and she's physically deteriorating. So that was probably—in fact it…wasn't even probably—it *was* the most traumatic thing.

We now move to a final account in this chapter that seems to articulate and capture the palpable pain experienced by some. It, perhaps, represents the darkest outcomes of the storms among those we interviewed, and it encompasses all of the major themes addressed in this chapter: *loss, chaos, survival,* and *despair*. Witness to suicide was mentioned more than once in these interviews. Although suicide itself did not emerge as a major theme in our data, the ripple effects of a few referenced suicides were felt by a wide circle of others. These personal tragedies, coupled with the drowning deaths of 35 elderly adults in St. Rita's nursing home in Violet, a small community in southeast St. Bernard, illustrate the unfathomable circumstances that many people faced in the immediate aftermath of the storms (Cherry et al., 2009, 2010). The following narrative reflects the events surrounding the tragic suicide of a family friend. This participant (110) and her husband had relocated to Baton Rouge, LA. Their teenage son stayed with friends during the week to attend Brother Martin, a private (all male) Catholic high school in New Orleans that had reopened in early 2006. She describes the subsequent shock and trauma of many in the community when the host family father took his life in the garage of their home. Here is what she said:

> **110** *(58-year old female)*: I'll never forget that night I got the phone call, and my son, Peter was hysterical and I kept saying, "What's wrong? What's wrong?" And he goes, "You got to come get me," and I said, "What [do] you mean I have to come get you?" And he goes, "Billy's daddy hung himself."
>
> And you know…at the funeral…I was taken aback by the comments, and it kind of upset Peter, and when we left the funeral home and had driven…back to Baton Rouge, my son said to me, "You know somebody said something at the funeral, I'm kind of really upset about it." And I said, "Well let's talk about it. What did they say?" And he goes, "They turned around and…it was one of the [dads of one of the other] boys, and [this other dad] said, 'Man, what an asshole! How could this guy commit suicide and do this to his son? What an asshole!'" So Peter was really upset about that.
>
> And Peter goes, "Why did he say such a stupid thing?" And I said, "Because, Peter, technically suicide's a very selfish thing." And I said…"[But] I think there's a fine line where someone gets pushed over the edge." I said, "What keeps them from going over the edge is for one split second they get to think, 'I cannot do this to my son. I cannot do this to my family because they're going to suffer dearly." And I said, "I think that's what pulls them back." But I said, "I think for Billy's dad, he must have been in such a deep, deep, dark place that never, unfortunately, [those thoughts did not] cross his mind." And I said, "It's sad because prior to his death," and I learned this at the funeral home, "prior to his suicide, his

> wife told me that she had found out…there was a couple of days that he was late for work, or he would leave work early. And one day, the partner confronted him and apparently he was going back to [his old home] and he would just sit outside of his house that was destroyed…. She confronted him and said, 'Okay I want you to go get help,' because the partners were concerned."
> That was not a good thing—that he would go and park himself in front of this [destroyed] house and just sit there for hours…. And so Peter on the drive coming back to Baton Rouge said, "But, you know, Billy's mom was saying that he [was] seeing a psychiatrist, and the psychiatrist said he wasn't suicidal." And I said, "Well, Peter …something really pushed him off the edge."

Theme 3, and especially the previous excerpt, highlights the reality that several people not only had to endure the effects of a natural disaster but also subsequent tragedies, like witnessing family and friends suffer, or even coping with a severe mental breakdown, or suicide of a family member, friend, or acquaintance.

As we have seen in the aforementioned comments, many people still struggle with profound losses of their property, community, friends, and way of life. The storms, and the chaos and challenges that followed, required many to fight to survive. Some people are still reeling from the storms and are burdened with despair, anguish, and sorrow over 5 years later.

Conclusion and Future Directions

In this chapter, we focused on the challenges participants' faced in the wake of the 2005 hurricanes. Three emergent themes identified in the primary data indicate that these challenges and painful memories of storm-related losses remain relevant in daily life today. As mentioned at the outset of this chapter on "Loss, Chaos, Survival, and Despair" following Hurricanes Katrina and Rita, our participants' reflections offer a stark and perhaps even striking contrast to the narratives presented in Chaps. 14 and 21 (this volume), which emphasize facilitative coping patterns and supports. It is vital, however, to have an informed awareness of the breadth of psychosocial consequences of disasters for those directly affected by these events, which include positive and negative coping responses. Perhaps surprising, but equally important, is the reality of *no coping, just surviving* as illuminated here by current and former coastal residents who were directly affected by the 2005 hurricanes, Katrina and Rita.

For convenience in exposition, we consider first the early days after Katrina made landfall on August 29, 2005. Participants who evacuated in advance of Katrina may have witnessed the devastation by television, popular press, and through social media. In contrast, participants who remained behind experienced the hurricane devastation and horrific flooding after the levee breaches directly. By choice or by circumstance, these participants faced life-threatening circumstances in sweltering heat with little provisions, no clean water, and no outside assistance for days. Our sample included state employees and local officials whose job duties required them to work through the storm (see also Chap. 12, this volume). They spoke of foraging for basic necessities to survive in the early days. The stench of dead animals and the fetid floodwaters that covered their community were among the darkly unpleasant memories which remained vivid many years later.

Public schools had only been in session for a few weeks when Katrina made landfall. Parents with dependent children who evacuated to non-coastal communities faced the challenges of getting their kids into a new school while simultaneously dealing with insurance companies and shuffling from one temporary living situation to the next until they found a stable residence. Coastal residents could not get back to their devastated homes to check on their property for weeks, given the restricted access, which was enforced by the National Guard. The experiences that our participants related were a source of great anguish and sorrow. Some hinted that the Katrina experience pushed them to their limits of endurance, implying that if another natural disaster hit or another major trial arose, they would not be able to "keep it together."

Looking back over the years that had passed since August and September of 2005, participants' descriptions of the losses of community and lifelong friends and neighbors seemed to be greater sources of sorrow and despair than their tangible losses (e.g., homes, property, and personal possessions) which are documented elsewhere (Cherry et al., 2015). Certainly, the loss of material possessions of great sentimental value was painful, especially family photos and memorabilia. However, the present findings center around less tangible losses; people spoke of the chaos that ensued, the burden of surviving, and finally the feelings of personal anguish and despair that some continued to experience in their present-day lives. At least 5 years after Katrina and Rita, participants commented that they lost much more than their personal materials and possessions—they lost their entire community including businesses, schools, government buildings, and even the hospital. Our participants stressed that the community, the way of life, and the infrastructure of the parish as they knew it for 40 years or more was obliterated. Many of their friends, neighbors, and fellow churchgoers left for good. Sorrow associated with these losses seemed to linger much more than sorrow from the loss of houses, furniture, and automobiles.

On a broader note, the clinical implications of lasting grief associated with post-disaster losses, which are evidenced in this chapter, warrant further consideration. Epidemiological research points to the occurrence of psychological distress after disaster, which is understandable, highlighting a critical role for disaster mental health professionals and interventions to address the psychosocial consequences of disaster exposure for survivors. Our participants' voices provide authentic images of post-disaster losses, coupled with the lingering and pervasive sense of sorrow. From a layman's point of view, their descriptions are reminiscent of bereavement over the death of a loved one. Taken together, the three themes presented here underscore a pressing need for further research and clinical work in the area of complicated grief (Shear et al., 2011; see Chap. 22, this volume) and prolonged grief disorder (Maguen, Neria, Conoscenti, & Litz, 2009). We did not formally assess grief reactions in this study, so interpretative caution is warranted. Nonetheless, our findings indicate that further research to examine the long-term trajectories of grief is needed for disaster-affected populations.

The themes presented here and elsewhere in this volume (Chaps. 4, 12, 14, 18, 20, and 21) should be interpreted in light of at least three methodological limitations. First, these qualitative interviews were conducted at one point in time; longitudinal assessments are desirable to examine trajectories of resilience (Cherry & Galea, 2015). Second, a selection bias may limit the generalizability of these findings, because people in poor health or marginal living circumstances may not choose to participate in a study on disaster recovery. Third, the emergent themes are based on personal accounts of storm experiences, which are subject to possible biases and unintentional distortions.

In closing, our findings encourage further research on the psychosocial consequences of natural disasters in the years after these events. Given that future storms are likely, especially in disaster-prone areas, identifying factors associated with resilience and long-term recovery is an urgent and timely challenge.

Acknowledgments We are grateful to Sr. Mary Keefe and Fr. John Arnone of Our Lady of Lourdes Catholic Church in Violet, LA, and Gayle Buckley, Judy Chiappetta, and Catherine Serpas for their assistance with recruitment. We thank Susan McNeil of the St. Bernard Council on Aging and Sean Warner of the Gulf Coast Trust Bank in St. Bernard for providing space for interviews. We thank Kelli Broome, Susan Brigman, Ashley Cacamo, Pamela Nezat, and Mary Beth Tamor for their help with data collection and Robert Pressley, Penni Fontenot, Sarah Finney, Lauren Edwards, Allison Kennedy, Amy Goff, and Graham Belou for their assistance with transcriptions. We also thank Bethany Pinkston, Sarah Hebert, Savannah Ballard, Trevor Johnson, and Brandon Cohen for assistance with qualitative analyses.

This research was supported by grants from the Louisiana Board of Regents and the BP Gulf of Mexico Research Initiative, Office of Research and Economic Development, Louisiana State University. This support is gratefully acknowledged.

References

Belter, R., Dunn, S., & Jeney, P. (1991). The psychological impact of hurricane Hugo on children: A needs assessment. *Advances in Behavior Research and Therapy, 13,* 155–161.

Breslau, N., Davis, G. C., Andreski, P., & Peterson, E. (1991). Traumatic events and post-traumatic stress disorder in an urban population of young adults. *Archives of General Psychiatry, 48,* 216–222.

Buuck, M. M. (2007). *Firestorm: Hurricane katrina and the St. Bernard fire department.* Xlibris Corporation.

Cherry, K. E., & Galea, S. (2015). Resilience after trauma. In D. Ajdukovic, S. Kimhi, & M. Lahad (Eds.), *Resiliency: Enhancing coping with crisis and terrorism* (pp. 35-40). NATO Science for Peace and Security Series. Netherlands: IOS Press.

Cherry, K. E., Galea, S., & Silva, J. L. (2008). Successful aging and natural disasters: Role of adaptation and resiliency in late life. In M. Hersen & A. M. Gross (Eds.), *Handbook of clinical psychology: Volume 1* (pp 810–833). NJ: Wiley.

Cherry, K. E., Silva, J., Galea, S. (2009). Natural disasters and the oldest-old: A psychological perspective on coping and health in late life. In K. E. Cherry (Ed.), *Lifespan perspectives on natural disasters: Coping with Katrina, Rita and other storms* (pp. 171–193). New York: Springer.

Cherry, K. E., Allen, P. D., & Galea, S. (2010). Older adults and natural disasters: Lessons learned from Hurricanes Katrina and Rita. In P. Dass-Brailsford (Ed.), *Crisis and disaster counseling: Lessons learned from Hurricane Katrina and other disasters* (pp. 115–130). Thousand Oaks: Sage.

Cherry, K. E., Silva Brown, J., Marks, L. D., Galea, S., Volaufova, J., Lefante, C., et al. (2011). Longitudinal assessment of cognitive and psychosocial functioning after Hurricanes Katrina and Rita: Exploring disaster impact on middle-aged, older, and oldest-old adults. *Journal of Applied Biobehavioral Research, 16,* 187–211.

Cherry, K. E., Sampson, L., Nezat, P. F., Cacamo, A., Marks, L. D., & Galea, S. (2015). Long-term psychological outcomes in older adults after disaster: relationships to religiosity and social support. *Aging & Mental Health, 19*(5), 430–443.

Covey, S. R. (2003). *The 7 habits of highly effective people*. New York: Free Press.

Earls, F., Smith, E., Reich, W., & Junk, K. (1988). Investigating psychopathological consequences of a disaster in children: A pilot study incorporating a structured diagnostic interview. *Journal of American Academic Child and Adolescent Psychiatry, 27,* 90–95.

Eich, E., Reeves, J. L., Jaeger, B., & Graff-Radford, S. B. (1985). Memory for pain: relation between past and present pain intensity. *Pain, 23,* 375–380.

Frankl, V. (1984). *Man's search for meaning*. New York: Washington Street Press.

Galea, S., Tracy, M., Norris, F., & Coffey, S. E. (2008). Financial and social circumstances and the incidence and course of PTSD in Mississippi during the first two years after Hurricane Katrina. *Journal of Traumatic Stress, 21,* 357–368.

Gilligan, C. (1992). *In a different voice*. Cambridge: Harvard University Press.

Gleser, G. C., Green, B., & Winget, C. (1981). *Prolonged psychosocial effects of disaster: A study of buffalo creek*. New York: Academic.

Green, B. L., Korol, M., Grace, M., Vary, M., Leonard, A., Gleser, G., et al. (1991). Children and disaster: Age, gender, and parental effects on PTSD symptoms. *Journal of the American Academy of Child and Adolescent Psychiatry, 30,* 945–951.

Henry, J. (2013). Return or relocate? An inductive analysis of decision-making in a disaster. *Disaster, 37,* 293–316.

Kamo, Y., Henderson, T. L., & Roberto, K. A. (2011). Displaced older adults' reactions to and coping with the aftermath of hurricane katrina. *Journal of Family Issues, 30,* 1346–1370.

Kushner, H. S. (1981). *When bad things happen to good people*. New York: Anchor Books.

Maguen, S., Neria, Y., Conoscenti, L. M., & Litz, B. T. (2009). Depression and prolonged grief in the wake of disasters. In Y. Neria, S. Galea, & F. H. Norris (Eds). *Mental health and disasters* (pp. 116–130). New York: Cambridge University Press.

Massey, B. A. (1997). Victims or survivors? A three-part approach to working with older adults in disaster. *Journal of Geriatric Psychiatry, 30,* 193–202.

McFarlane, A. C., Polincansky, S. K., & Irwin, C. (1987). A longitudinal study of the psychological morbidity in children due to a natural disaster. *Psychological Medicine, 17,* 727–738.

Neria, Y., Galea, S., & Norris, F. H. (Eds.). (2009). *Mental health and disasters*. New York: Cambridge University Press.

Norris, F. H., & Elrod, C. L. (2006). Psychosocial consequences of disaster: A review of past research. In F. H. Norris, S. Galea, M. J. Friedman, & P. J. Watson (Eds.), *Methods for disaster mental health research* (pp. 20–42). New York: Guilford.

Norris, F. H., Friedman, M. J., & Watson, P. J., Byrne, C. M., Diaz, E., & Kaniasty, K. (2002). 60,000 disaster victims speak: Part I. An empirical review of the empirical literature, 1981–2001. *Psychiatry, 65,* 207–239.

Schaefer, M. (2007). *Lost in Katrina*. Gretna: Pelican Publishing Company.

Sharan, P., Chaudhary, G., Kavathekar, S. A., & Saxena, S. (1996). Preliminary report of psychiatric disorders in survivors of a severe earthquake. *American Journal of Psychiatry, 153,* 556–558.

Shear, M. K., McLaughlin, K. A., Ghesquiere, A., Gruber, M. J., Sampson, N. A., & Kessler, R. C. (2011). Complicated grief associated with Hurricane Katrina. *Depression and Anxiety, 28,* 648–657.

Strauss, A., & Corbin, J. (1998). *Basics of qualitative research: Techniques and procedures for developing grounded theory*. Thousand Oaks: Sage.

Chapter 14
Families and Faith-based Communities After a Disaster: Successes and Failures in the Wakes of Hurricanes Katrina and Rita

Loren D. Marks, Trevan G. Hatch, Yaxin Lu and Katie E. Cherry

Introduction

"Religion" is a term of such staggering breadth that it is typically necessary to divide it into separate dimensions when conducting social science research. Three dimensions of religion, as outlined by Marks (2005), include: (a) *spiritual beliefs* (personal, internal beliefs, framings, meanings, and perspectives), (b) *religious practices* (e.g., outward, observable expressions of faith such as prayer, scripture study, rituals, traditions, or less overtly sacred practice or abstinence that is religiously grounded), and (c) *faith communities* (support, involvement, and relationships grounded in one's congregation or religious group; pp. 175–176). With reference to the latter dimension, which serves as the focus of the present chapter, Krause (2012) has made the point that church attendance provides opportunity for older adults to share what they have learned in life with other members whom they believe value such experiences, which in turn enhances older persons' sense of self-worth and feelings of belonging. Most would agree that faith communities can be influential for people

K. E. Cherry (✉)
Department of Psychology, Louisiana State University, 236 Audubon Hall, Baton Rouge, LA 70803-5501, USA
e-mail: pskatie@lsu.edu

L. D. Marks
School of Family Life, Brigham Young University, 2092C Joseph F. Smith Building, Provo, Utah 84602, USA
e-mail: loren_marks@byu.edu

T. G. Hatch
School of Social Work, Louisiana State University, 335 Long Fieldhouse, Baton Rouge, LA 70803-5501, USA
e-mail: thatch8@lsu.edu

Y. Lu
Louisiana Department of Education, 1201 North Third Street, Baton Rouge, LA 70802, USA
e-mail: Yaxinlu3@gmail.com

K. E. Cherry (ed.), *Traumatic Stress and Long-Term Recovery*,
DOI 10.1007/978-3-319-18866-9_14

of all ages; however, a cautionary note is in order because this influence can be positive, negative, or both (Dollahite, Marks, & Goodman, 2004; Marks, 2006a, b).

In this chapter, we examine the role of faith-based communities for individuals and families coping with the 2005 Hurricanes Katrina and Rita. In particular, we explore *whether* faith communities were perceived as helpful by directly affected survivors coping with the aftermath of these hurricanes—or whether these organizations contributed to their frustrations and misery. In addition to examining this two-pronged question, we also address the deeper issues of *why* and *how* faith communities helped (or harmed) coastal residents of south Louisiana whose lives were forever changed by the 2005 storms. We begin by highlighting select results from the research literature on faith community to contextualize our findings.

A Brief Overview of Research Findings on Faith Community

Despite a US tendency to exaggerate religious participation, statistics indicate that religious involvement is an important part of life for many Americans (Burr, Marks, & Day, 2012). Although most married couples in America report a religious affiliation, there is significant variation in *actual levels of attendance* among persons who claim a faith affiliation (Burr et al., 2012). Around 60% report that religion is important or very important to them (McCullough, Hoyt, Larson, Koenig, & Thoresen, 2000), but Taylor (2003) found that only 36% attend a religious service once a month or more.

An expanding body of medical and social science research on *faith community* has yielded several recurring findings that are of relevance (Koenig, King, & Carson, 2012; Koenig, McCullough, & Larson, 2001; Marks, Dollahite, & Freeman, 2011). These six findings relate to the social and psychological issues that are focal points in the present study:

1. Faith community provides social and instrumental support for those who are actively involved (Koenig, 2002; Marks et al., 2011; Taylor, Chatters, & Levin, 2004).
2. Koenig et al. (2001) found nearly 100 studies suggesting that religion may be a deterrent to alcohol or drug abuse across the life span (i.e., Laird, Marks, & Marrero, 2011).
3. For those who develop alcohol and substance abuse addictions, evidence indicates "more successful rehabilitation among the more religious" (Koenig et al., 2001, pp. 179–180).
4. Actively involved religious persons have significantly lower cancer rates than those who do not attend regularly (Enstrom, 1998; Koenig et al., 2001; Marks, 2005).
5. In their comprehensive review of the literature, Koenig et al. (2001) found that 79 of 100 studies indicated "at least one positive correlation between religious involvement and greater happiness, life satisfaction, morale, or positive affect"

with 20 studies yielding complex, mixed, or no relationship findings, while only one study reported a negative correlation (p. 101).

6. Hummer, Rogers, Nam, and Ellison (1999) found a 7.6-year increase in life expectancy among persons who attend worship services more than once a week compared with nonattenders. African Americans who reportedly attended church services more than once a week *lived nearly 14 years longer* than African Americans who reportedly never attended (80.1 vs. 66.4 years; see also, Marks, Nesteruk, Swanson, Garrison, & Davis, 2005).

In summary, these six findings related to faith community indicate correlational relationships between regular worship service attendance and benefits including: (a) higher levels of social and instrumental support, (b) lower rates of alcohol or drug abuse, (c) greater success in overcoming addiction, (d) significantly lower cancer rates, (e) greater happiness and life satisfaction, and (f) significant increases in longevity. While these and other similar findings have been obtained, relatively little is known regarding *why* these associations exist (Marks et al., 2005). On the heels of these positive correlates of faith community involvement, however, we note an important counterpoint that will reemerge as a central theme in the section "Findings". This point of concern is drawn from qualitative research that indicates that when a faith community or congregation to which an individual or family is closely tied *lets them down or fails them* "it [is] both disappointing and hurtful in ways that…elicit deeper frustration and pain than failures by secular agencies and institutions" (Marks & Dollahite, 2001, p. 636).

Method

The sample, interview procedures, and team-based qualitative analyses are described in Chap. 12 (this volume). Here, we focus on participants' responses to the following question: *In times of trouble, people may turn to a faith community to help them cope with life stresses. Has a church or faith community helped you cope with Hurricanes Katrina and Rita, and, if so, in what ways?* They were encouraged to share illustrative personal stories and experiences, consistent with a narrative approach to qualitative methods (Josselson & Lieblich, 1993).

Findings

Our primary aim is to present our participants' voices and convey their experiences and observations with as much fidelity as possible. In keeping with this goal, our interpretation and explanations are brief. Four "core" themes related to faith community are as follows:

1. "The Hunger for Faith Community": In this theme, we see the pressing and almost urgent need for faith community *some* participants reported after the storms.

2. "My Church Family Kept Me Going": This theme illustrates how and why faith community was an important coping resource for many participants and their families.
3. "I Felt Like My Church Abandoned Me": This theme focuses on the deep and almost palpable pain reported by some who felt that their own faith communities let them and their families down in their hour of greatest need.
4. Helping Others: "Am I My Brother's Keeper?" This theme reflects the reported impact of receiving personal and familial help and assistance from a faith community to which the beneficiaries have no ties.

Theme 1: The Hunger for Faith Community

For many of the participants we interviewed, faith community was important because it promoted a sense of "peace" and "calm" in their lives. One explained:

> **212**[1] (69-year-old female): [Church] gives you an inner *peace*. I think I had told you, I'm not the holiest person in the world, but when I'm in my church, for some reason, a *calm* comes over me.

For the group we highlight next, however, faith community was more than just a calming spiritual and psychological experience, it was vital. The need to worship with others was so pronounced for some that they literally *created* or joined small, faith makeshift communities—in some cases, even under heavily damaged or primitive conditions (e.g., no electricity or running water). One married couple, for example, rallied the residents of an indirectly affected senior care facility that had become a home for her displaced and frail elderly relative for a weekly Sunday school.

> **262** (67-year-old female; Wife): [After Katrina]…we had a Sunday school, bible study on a Sunday morning. We had quite a few people that [would come]. Got to be like a little family.
>
> **263** (73-year-old male; Husband): All the residents of Jenny's Place[2]…
>
> **262** (Wife): [Well], all of the ones that wanted to come…. Oh it was a blessing…
>
> **Interviewer**: I bet they really enjoyed it.
>
> **262** (Wife): [I mean it was a blessing] for *us*…. Because you know, it allowed us to stay connected…
>
> **263** (Husband): Yeah.

---

[1] The designation of participants by ID number instead of by pseudonym is unusual in qualitative work. In part, this approach has been adopted because of the very large ($N=125$) and varied nature of the sample (by qualitative standards). The ID numbers also indicate group membership in a larger scale project (see Chap. 12, this volume).

[2] Some names of places and other identifying markers are pseudonyms to protect participants' anonymity.

> **262** (Wife): [It helped us]...with our faith, and not to become disconnected.... You know... when you teach, [that] is when you learn.... Every time you teach a lesson, you learn something yourself....And *they* seemed to enjoy it because they kept coming back.

Another participant similarly talked about the spontaneous interdenominational community that united at her neighbor's house in the weeks following Katrina. As she explained,

> **207** (67-year-old female): So, you know, we were all [a] different religion, if you want to talk about religion. But we would get together by Ralph's [he's my neighbor], and we would have a little church service and we'd sing and we'd have a meal and people lingered on for two hours or so afterwards, just talking and sharing and that really, really helped us to cope with a lot things. You know, we talked about *everything*. We talked about the politicians, we talked about the flood, we talked about where our houses [were, in terms of damage], we talked about if we had windows [left in them]... We talked about [everything]. [Eventually], from there, we went to the pastor's house, and he started having [a service] in his garage by his house.

Ralph, referenced in the previous quote, was also interviewed and recalled:

> **220** (63-year-old male): [For months after Katrina with few churches available], we had church services right underneath my carport back here.... And, when it got cold, we had them inside the shed. [We have] our woodstove in there.... We'd crank that woodstove up and we'd have it in there. And.... We had as many as 80...people back there.... You had people from Delacroix, Yscloskey, Shell Beach, from right here in this neighborhood all back there, all together. And, it was very simple. We tried to make the Gospel [real]...there wasn't nothing preached so high that nobody couldn't understand it. You know? There wasn't no collections taken, wasn't no money changing hands. It was strictly people coming together, enjoying each other, and enjoying the word of God. And, I wish it would have never left right there, really, to tell you the truth.

In the experience shared and narrated by this man, the reader almost feels the warmth of the stove and the literal and social warmth of individuals gathering for the unified blessing of believing and belonging—juxtaposed against the backdrop of a community in ruins. We have observed elsewhere that as human beings, we "long for something to *believe in*," that we "long for something to *belong to*," and that many persons strive to "satiate both of these craved, primary longings through [the] sacred" (Marks, Dollahite, & Barker, 2012, p. 186). For some participants, their faith community, in whatever form they could find it or create it, seemed to meet the dual needs of hope and connection during an almost incomprehensibly dark time.

In the preceding narratives, it is difficult to discern whether: (a) the need for strengthened faith and an assurance of the sacred was of fundamental importance or (b) whether the relationships, the connection, and the "sharing" were most salient in the coping efforts of the individuals, married couples, and families involved. Clearly, however, both were taking place.

The creative energy evidenced in the spontaneous faith communities is striking and fascinating, but these communities should not be overextended or portrayed as a primary emergent theme from our data. The spontaneous communities sketched out here offer but one expression (albeit a vibrantly colorful one) of the hunger and scramble for faith community in the aftermath of the hurricanes. Qualitative analyses yielded additional examples of satisfying this hunger through more traditional paths—although those paths were disrupted in most cases. The narratives presented next capture several participants' longing for some sense of their pre-Katrina/Rita "church family" and their efforts to restore and reestablish their faith communities in varying ways. As this participant reminded us:

> **203** (52-year-old female): Okay, I'm going to start by saying.... There *wasn't* any church community here to come to shortly after, so as far as here in St. Bernard, just like everything else, it got devastated, too. So there wasn't one to turn to here.

Even so, her desire to worship with others was sufficient that she did the best she could after evacuating and while being displaced for several months. She went on to explain,

> **203**: When I was moving around from place to place, and I wasn't familiar with the areas I was living in or staying in, even if it was for a couple of weeks, what I did was if I...the nearest church or one that I spotted on my way would be where I would go on Sunday, regardless of denomination. So after, as I moved from place to place, I went to a Methodist church, a Baptist church, a Unitarian church, a Episcopalian church.... If I could find a church, then I went to it....

Several other participants discussed their post-evacuation solutions to finding a new faith community as well. Two other participants explained:

> **238** (67-year-old male): As far as our church and that, yes because we (our family) always would try to stay as active as we can in our church. Even when we didn't have a church [because of the flood], we made our mass, no matter where it was. Even if we had to travel half an hour, 45 min, it didn't matter, we were going to mass [somewhere].

> **131** (56-year-old male): It was amazing because for a long time, people came from Baton Rouge, and Lafayette, and really all over Louisiana, and Mississippi, on Sunday morning to come to church [together].... [Y]ou don't really realize how much of a center of community is at the church, until something like [Katrina] happens. I never really realized it before. You'd see everybody in the church. You know, "Hey, how are you doing? How's your momma doing?" and all that kind of stuff. But you didn't really realize how strong those bonds were, I guess, until something like that happened.... [I] saw those people driving for two or three hours to get there, to go to a 1-hour mass.

Another evacuee strived to find remnants of her faith community in Slidell, LA (about an hour from New Orleans). She said,

> **204** (62-year-old female): [What helped me cope] was going to mass even though I was going in Slidell and [then] seeing the familiar faces of both the priests [who had also relocated] and being fed by their dynamic homilies.... They could just kind of knock your socks off...that really helped me.... [It also helped a lot to see some of] the [old church] friends that I was able to reconnect with.

We are reminded by this participant's recollections that while faith community worship is primarily sacred for some and primarily social for others, for many it serves *both* of these important functions (Dollahite, Marks, & Olson, 2002).

The previous three narratives remind us of the disruption of faith communities caused by evacuation and relocation of both congregants and clergy. For those who later returned (as opposed to permanently relocating elsewhere), some additional challenges remained. One woman recalled that, for her family and congregation,

> **214** (56-year-old female): [We had flood] water in the Church, about...three feet or so. So, we had Mass under a tent, which belonged to our congregation from here. You know,

> they went around salvaging what they could from different places. And…[we] had donated chairs…. I don't know where they came from, they were all different chairs. And, then when the Church was finally cleaned out, we went into the Church…of course there was no air conditioning, no whatever, and we had to make do with what [we] had.

The same participant (214) explained elsewhere that when she and her family

> …got back home, which was several weeks after…Katrina, we didn't have a Church. Church was…. Our Church building was damaged and would have to be repaired. And, our faith community, the Catholic community in St. Bernard, started with one Church and everybody went to the one Church, before any others could open. So we started with the one church and the one pastor and, you know, everybody from…which was once seven different parishes or churches going to the same place. So I think, you know, it's like everybody had been through the same thing, you know? And, I think that was a help with coping once you went to a place where everybody had been through the same thing and is going through the same thing….

Two other participants said, with respect to both their literal families and their "church families":

> **251** (71-year-old female): What we worried about coming back, [was that] we wouldn't have our religion, [that] we wouldn't have nothing…. When we first…[back] we didn't have [pews], but they had [borrowed] chairs…as a matter of fact, I think in the beginning we were sitting outside…. But we didn't care. We sat on the floor, we had to…but [it still] really it made your Sunday….

> **260** (64-year-old female): [After the hurricanes, we] had to rebuild Our Lady of Prompt Succor, our church which was my parish. [That was the church] where I was married. My children [were] baptized there, [and] they went to school from kindergarten to eighth grade there. And so we had a hand in [rebuilding our church]. So when you have a real role, it's a real ownership, and so that helped [us to be able to help to] put the church back together.

Another narrative supporting "The Hunger for Faith Community" shows a particularly determined participant who refused to let her faith community die:

> **228** (52-year-old female): We kept our [Our Lady of] Lourdes faith community together, even though we weren't a "church" [because our building was damaged and closed for a while]…. *The people were church.* We kept that *alive.* We kept in touch…. I had everybody's email [on a] distribution list. I kept them abreast of what was going on. [We] rallied in the troops for the rosaries at church, outside of church, [we'd even meet on] the levee walks. Everybody got the emails. "Okay, we're doing the [meeting at the] levee."… So we were church. We kept the same core people together and we knew we were going to [eventually re-] open our church. *And we did.* (Note: Our Lady of Lourdes reopened in November of 2009).

As previously illustrated, several participants and their families made pronounced (even remarkable) efforts to maintain, sustain, or even create faith communities after Katrina and Rita struck. Although most of our participants were Catholic and at least somewhat religious, the sample ranged widely in their reported faith affiliation and level of belief (see Cherry, Sampson, Nezat, Cacamo, Marks, & Galea, 2015). The following participant represents the atheist perspective of a few:

> **236** (76-year-old male): No, I don't believe, I don't believe [in God]. [Also], I don't like crowds [and I don't like church]. I have enough faith in my thoughts to overcome just about any problem that I find…. So religion has not been…[helpful].

For one or two other participants, having a faith community was not important, although they still held a belief in God and engaged in religious practices. One such participant (233) reported that in her home, "I probably read my Bible more after the storm and I probably prayed a lot more [but] my husband and I are not real fond of organized religion" *(49-year-old female)*.

To summarize, in Theme 1, "The Hunger for Faith Community," we see that while faith community was unimportant or only mildly important to a few of our participants, faith community was of profound importance to many other individuals, married couples, and families. Indeed, faith community was important enough to some that following the destruction of their traditional houses of worship, they employed a variety of alternatives including: (a) starting informal worship groups in their neighborhoods and homes, (b) finding new places to worship in whatever city or state they found themselves, and (c) involving themselves in restoration efforts for their buildings of worship after the storm. This first theme reflects the importance of faith community in the lives of many of our participants and their families. However, this theme offers only moderate insight regarding *why* they longed for a faith community. This issue is addressed in greater depth next.

Theme 2: "My Church Family Kept Me Going"

Both the religious and social force of faith community in the lives of many participants is evident in the narratives that follow, providing new insight into why participants may have longed for association with a faith community after the storms. The close-knit faith community ties of some were evidenced by reports of focused concern in the immediate aftermath of Katrina. One woman recalled,

> **203** (52-year-old female): [I remember] the frantic search online for people. [Trying to find out] who was missing and who wasn't. [It was awful] how long that went on after [Katrina hit], still not knowing who made it out, if everyone that you knew made it out, even if they weren't a close relative. [Especially], *you still were concerned [for] your fellow church community [members]*. And as the list of names of [those] who didn't make it came out… we lost quite a few, I'd say I knew at least a good five people from church that didn't evacuate and drowned.

For this participant, the first reported source of human concern, after "close" family, was "fellow church community" members. As the death tolls rose, and names of "church family" were added to the list, it is interesting to note that some participants also turned to their faith community, not only in terms of "religious coping" but also in terms of social support, a listening ear, and someone with whom to break bread. Another woman summarized:

> **223** (63-year-old female): I think just going to church has helped us…cope. Just, just going to church and being with our friends and all [our loved ones] at church. And after church on Saturday…evening…a group of us go out to eat [and visit together].

Other participants similarly discussed the impromptu social meetings after the formal worship service—meetings the survivors seemed to *need*—to grieve, to catch up, and to face the future:

143 (59-year-old female): It's not [just] that you're going to the building.... You could pray at *home*...[but] it's just being a part of the community, knowing that if something happens, [you]'ve got other people there...that would help or that you can turn to.... That's the whole point of going to church.

238 (67-year-old male): Yes, [the faith community] helped you cope with life's stresses. The best thing about [our church] to me is that you get to be...a community again [after all we have been through].... [I remember], even [after] mass left out, we'd all gather after mass to eat.... There was a time of community that everybody got together after the mass. Nobody hurried up and got in their own vehicle and left. No, we just...stood around and talked and, we'd have conversations with [our] people that you [see]...once a week... you've known them all your life. Just to have that sense of community.... It helps you cope.

The following participants had similar recollections following the storms. One man reported:

254 (59-year-old male): Has a church or faith community helped [us] cope with Hurricanes Katrina and Rita? I would say, "Yes." And the reason is: number one...we went to church the first mass at Prompt Succor the third weekend in October. And, that...mass then for the next [couple of months]...became the meeting place where you could network with people, you know? Because prior to that event, you [were] lucky [if] you found people because everybody's cell...phones didn't work; [and] people were living out of town. [Our church family was] scattered all over the place.... [The services starting back up at Prompt Succor gave us all] a chance to make contact with friends and people to get your life going again. So,...[when] the Church started, we had a place to go, [to reunite].... [And the] networking is a big plus that came out of that, being able to see the people and people networking, and then [the additional] moral support.

We pause here to highlight a couple of important points related to Theme 2 that these narratives are illustrating. First, a glance at the interview excerpts just reported does not produce a single mention of "God." There are many references to the divine in these data (displayed next). However, the power of faith community as a *social* force for many participants and their families was repeatedly emphasized in the interviews. Second, even without yet invoking divine or religious elements, the participants have offered several reasons, meanings, and explanations regarding *why* their faith communities helped them. These reasons "why" included (a) they "helped me cope," (b) they are my "church family," (c) "I needed the people," (d) they helped me "get [my] life going again," (e) "networking," and (f) "moral support." This list of reasons is rich, but it is not comprehensive. The next participant's response captures several of the previously mentioned reasons as well as additional novel benefits of faith community that warrant attention.

234 (59-year-old male): I would definitely say [our faith community] helped. And it helps because we get together with...our church families, and *we're able to confide in each other*. When we're going through these things, we almost think it's only happening to us, and then *we see what others went through*, what they're going through, and how they struggled.... Also, being able to do things at church gives me a sense that I'm helping out, that I'm doing something to give back. I don't know why I still get emotional about this.... *Being able to work within the church, and have the feeling that I'm giving back to the people who helped us; [that has] helped me*. I think that's a big part of a certain sense of healing. Being able to give back. Feeling...useful, just being able to do something for someone.... I think it's a [part of the] healing process.

In addition to finding close confidants and others who could truly empathize, this man explains that a great benefit provided by his church family has been the opportunity to "work within the church" and "give back"—and that for him this "giving back" has been an important part of the healing process. Similarly, a woman from our earlier but related work reported:

> *Helping [other] people, that [is what] helped me to cope*.... I took on so much other stuff helping other people [that] it kind of drowned out what I was going through and God fixed it. So while I was trying to fix somebody else['s situation], God was fixing *mine*. I...just continued to stay in prayer and helped those that needed help [and in the process, God helped me] (Silva, Marks, & Cherry, 2009, p. 236).

Like this individual, several of our participants emphasized both people *and* God as they explained their faith community...often in ways that blended aspects of the social and divine. The following two examples are illustrative:

> **227** (54-year-old male): [When you] have a community of people who love the Lord, then they're there to help one another. They're not just selfish thinking about their own needs or their own selves. They're more concerned. Even the Bible says, "Love your neighbor as yourself," and if you take these principles...to heart and begin to do what Jesus says, you'll find that...God's going to make sure your needs are provided [for when]...you can quit focusing on yourself and focus on someone else, ...God's going to bless you while you're focusing on somebody else, you know?

> **246** (77-year-old female): Just being in church is helpful. Just be in the presence of God's place.... I can sum up...why [I] come here [to church in this way. I can] be totally relaxed, and spend time with God. What church does is to provide us with community that I don't have otherwise. Because I don't have any family around me, [just church family].

In these two participants' responses, it is difficult to distinguish whether the primary motivations behind their faith community's involvement are rooted in a sense of connection with God or with "neighbors" and church family. Both influences appear salient. Indeed, almost no faith community references were solely related to God—the social dimension was nearly always implicitly (if not explicitly) emphasized, as captured next:

> **254** (59-year-old male): I'm a person who believes that if everybody went to the church of their choice on Sunday that you would, you could correlate any number of social problems in this country and watch them go down. I think the crime rate would drop. I think people would be naturally happier, and I think that you'd have a whole lot less to study [in the way of] psychological [problems].... If you go...to Church on Sunday, there's three or four hundred people in the Church that are all positive and like-minded, you know? And, you get to spend an hour with them, you get to reinforce that fact that: (a) You're not in it by yourself, and (b) There are actually positives out there, that you may not see [everyday].

> **227** (54-year-old male): I believe that Church is important. I believe that trusting in the Lord in times of trouble. The Church itself is there to help people, to encourage people, to point people to trust the Lord and to have faith in God. And I believe that the Church is... [something we should] be involved in.... Just like we have a personal relationship with the Lord, we should have friends and relations...who love the Lord. Because who we hang around with is who we become, and if we have people that are encouragers, people who want to help you and help each other...that helps you to cope. It helps you to have more faith because they're encouraging you to trust the Lord.

The seemingly stable and almost conversational tone of the previous excerpts may lull us into forgetting the carnage that was witnessed and confronted by those who experienced the storm directly in 2005. In this respect, the normalcy with which they speak may be indicative of remarkably successful coping in an otherwise tragic situation—a normalcy that some attributed in part to their faith community's stabilizing influence, as illustrated by this participant:

> **240** (49-year-old female): I think it's just the normalcy of going to church and praying, and it's just a normal thing. You got back to that "normal."

In many ways, however, "normal" was gone forever for participants and families in our study (see Chap. 12, this volume, for related discussion). Even those who coped well and found relative stability were, in some ways, forever changed by what they had experienced. Few faith community-related narratives captured this reality with more richness than those that reflected the efforts of some participants' clergy, who strived to offer solace and support during a time when they too had lost just about everything but their faith. The following illustrations, although brief, offer meaningful sketches regarding what select clergy meant to some of the participants:

> **258** (71-year-old female): [After Katrina], I'd go to church. That's all I did was go to church. And the pastor kept praying on me because I told him I was never going to be [able to pull it] back together, [but] he said, "Oh yes you are, sister, *you are*." I didn't think I was [but he helped me].

> **241** (71-year-old female): Pastor Warren.... I can call him anytime of the day. If I'm depressed.... He always tells me, "Turn it over to the Lord, leave it in God's hands." [He also says], "If you have any problems, you call me anytime of the day.".... And that's how I dealt with [Katrina].... When I was in the hospital for my knee surgery, he came up there and seen me, and prayed with me, and everything, before they took me to the operating room.

The affection and sense of relationship are evident in each of the previous excerpts. The next two narratives reflect a similar depth of gratitude for the clergy referenced.

> **203** (52-year-old female): I was fortunate enough when I lived in Slidell [after evacuating]...that my pastor from St. Mark was reassigned to the church parish that I lived in there. I mean, how much of a coincidence can you get? So immediately I started going there; and what would happen as people found out that Father Mark was there, people would start coming from all directions, and then of course that [church became] a big healing place because you were not only going there for your spiritual needs...but...the [former] St. Mark parishioners [that had evacuated] were coming in droves because somebody that they knew was there.... [Our] priest [was] there.

> **251** (71-year-old female): [After Katrina], our priest made a lot of services that would help us to get through it, [to] talk about it and stuff like that.... [The priest]...was really good with us, you know. I mean we stood along, almost every Sunday we [would] all talk about it, everybody'd talk about it. He'd talk about it. But I mean, he helped us cope with it, and [he would] explain why we [are] doing this and just bragging on how well we [were] doing when we came back [to rebuild], and how we [are] getting our parish back.... It was very encouraging.... [Coming together with him at the church] made everybody feel good because they realized that we were all in the same predicament.

Most of the narratives shared in connection with Theme 2, "My Church Family Kept Me Going," were from Catholics, which was the predominant religious affiliation in the sample (Cherry et al., 2015). The next theme, "I Felt Like My Church Abandoned Me," takes us in a very different direction than the two previous themes. Most of the narratives of frustration in the next theme relate to the Catholic Church (as would probably be expected, due to the predominantly Catholic composition of the sample). Our intent here is not to malign any church, including the Catholic Church.[3] However, we have an obligation as researchers to present with accuracy and fidelity the reports of our participants, including reports that were critical of their own faith communities. In Theme 3, we hear from an array of new participant voices—voices that seem to resound with frustration and hurt.

Theme 3: "I Felt Like My Church Abandoned Me"

In contrast to the previous narratives which document a faith community as a meaningful source of social support and a helpful temporal support for many of our participants and their families, others were deeply disappointed with their faith community's response (or lack of response) in the hurricane aftermath. Specifically, more than one fifth of the participants shared experiences or feelings that conveyed a *negative* attitude toward their faith community after the hurricanes. In fact, some participants gave up or changed their church affiliation.

As noted near the conclusion of Theme 2, some participants discussed with clergy who were "there" when their faith community needed them the most. The next excerpt portrays one priest who fled, and one who returned:

> **213** (64-year-old male): As I said before, it restores your belief in God…to know that your church was there for you. A lot of people thought that the Catholic Church wasn't there for them, but that's not so….Now, we had a priest in our area that kind of abandoned us, unfortunately. But the church…the *church* didn't abandon us, and they had people down here…. The former priest that was here [years ago], he came [back] down, and he comforted a lot of people. So it restored a lot as far as faith is concerned.

This man's perception was that one priest "kind of abandoned us," while another "came back down" to New Orleans to offer comfort. This participant seems to assume some level of personal choice for both of the priests he references. A few other participants placed blame, not on individual priests who served in the New Orleans area, but on the "archdiocese," meaning the higher church leadership. The following two criticisms are illustrative:

> **201** (56-year-old female): I know that the *Archdiocese* certainly had their issues, but all of our priests were pulled and were pretty much not allowed to come back…. I know other people who felt that they were let down because it took a very long time before there was a presence again with our Catholic churches.

[3] The authors have published several previous articles that present the Catholic faith very positively, based on participants' reports. Including one article focused on the strengths of Catholic families (Batson & Marks, 2008).

224 (51-year-old female): I [told you] how let down we all felt by the *Archdiocese* of New Orleans. You know, I could understand them not opening many churches because the[re] weren't enough people down here. I can understand that kind of situation where we were only able to re-open [Our Lady of] Prompt Succor in the beginning. Of course it was easier on me because that was the church I was attending at the time. But other people of course wanted *their* church to be the one to come back. But that was the only one that was… repaired.

The first Catholic Church in St. Bernard that was reopened for worship services after Katrina was Our Lady of Prompt Succor. For those, like the preceding participant, who attended that church before the hurricanes, Prompt Succor (meaning "timely help") was an apt name. For others whose "home" churches remained closed and, in some cases, were bulldozed into the ground, a sense of loss, abandonment, or even betrayal was evident. One participant reflected that she and her family felt that:

231 (50-year-old female): We were pretty much abandoned by the Catholic Church down here and they…they never gave you closure to your church connection, your spiritual connection, to your Church…. [The] Catholic Church did not solicit any input from the parishioners, as far as I know, about which church would reopen.

Another participant reported that from her perspective:

118 (53-year-old female): [The Catholic Church] is the one church that offered no help…. And not only that, they have closed many of the Catholic churches we have belonged to in St. Bernard Parish. So actually they tore them down. So here's the thing, you're raised Catholic, you were built in with the stress cope, things that help you cope with stress, but when the storm came, there was no help from the Catholic Church.

One father similarly shared:

236 (76-year-old male): We *built* that church. We paid for it, and they took it away. They took the money away and everything. The only thing the Catholic [Church] did for us was [open the] Prompt Succor [church] on the mass.

One of the cruelest consequences of the storms for our participants who were heavily invested in faith community was that those neighborhoods who suffered the most severe damage to homes were the same neighborhoods most likely to lose their (heavily damaged) neighborhood churches. Thus, those who arguably needed their *own* faith community, their *own* priest, their *own* familiar sacred building most profoundly were least likely to have access to them.

As the churches devastated by 16-feet (or more) of contaminated floodwater remained closed and were, in some cases, torn down, emotions surged among directly affected participants. Even years later, some hearts were still pained, as evidenced by the following excerpts:

244 (76-year-old female): I just ask God to help me, that's the only thing I can do. And I mean, if they had churches, maybe we'd go. But *they tear them down*, and they take the priests away. So, it's *their* fault; they should have left a couple of them open.

208 (66-year-old female): No, not really, [my faith community did not help]. I really…since St. Mark's got *torn down*, and I was into that community so much, I really haven't gotten to blend into the other community…. I don't feel at home….

226 (81-year-old male): This is what shocks me the most about the Catholic [Church]. They take the…for years they get everything they want, then when something goes wrong,

> they back out. Down here we had two buildings for the older people. It only had four feet of water in it. The Catholic Church took the money for the full buildings for the elder[ly] people, never fixed the buildings, *tore [them] down*, [and] took the money. Where's [all] the old people? Where's all that money they got from them people? And, that upsets me about the Catholic religion.

Another father and grandfather said of his family:

> **243** (78-year-old male): We were involved in the church and the school since…oh, I'd say the late fifties until the seventies…you know helping [with the] fundraisers, and all that stuff. The churches, [the] parishes [that] aren't making any money, they're closing them down. They're closing them down and they're building new churches other places, and they're the ones that tell you, "You should help the poor." Well, how come the rich parishes don't help the poor parishes? When the poor parishes aren't making money, they shut them down. That's what's been happening. All of the churches in my neighborhood, they shut them all down…. Instead of being about the Almighty, it's about the Almighty Dollar…. It's a shame to say it, but it's true.

Other Catholic participants were more moderate and measured in their criticism. One participant who was involved in the Catholic Church's response as a council member explained:

> **214** (56-year-old female):…[Look, our church] had to start from the ground up. And, I was on the council over there; they had actually picked a representative from each parish to be on the council [and we did what we could].

Another participant recalled:

> **215** (77-year-old female): [The Catholic Church] couldn't give us really anything but spiritual guidance. They didn't come help us and say, "What do you need here? What can we help you with? Can we help you find a good contractor?…Can we help you with your insurance company? Can we help you with FEMA (i.e., the Federal Emergency Management Agency)?" Okay? [But remember], *they were going through all of this themselves.*

The same participant later offered the following sketch of New Orleans at the time:

> **215**: When I came back here [after the flooding] everything was so disorganized…*the church was suffering the same way we all were.* The church lost everything too. Remember? The rectory, the church was flooded. Everything was flooded]. The church was in dire need of help itself. I mean as far as the community goes…basically, there was hardly any community. Everybody was in the same boat. Everybody…that came back was rebuilding their houses, rebuilding their lives. The church was trying to rebuild.

Several Catholic participants were less moderate, however, and reported their frustration and disappointment at what they perceived as a relative lack of outreach effort by their church in the immediate aftermath, as captured in the following interview excerpts:

> **124** (69-year-old female): After the hurricane, [our family], we were able to get in touch with our pastor…. I was crying and he said, "Baby, don't cry. We're going to help you." Well that was B.S. That was a bunch of…excuse me…I got very angry, because in one sermon…he said, you know, "White Dove[Church] is not FEMA," and it was like just putting a…stabbing me in the heart because I was raised in a church community that when… that's what the church was there for…to not only help people through spiritual things, but through physical things also. And I got angry…and it took so much out of me to be angry, and recently, this year, this year, five years, almost five years after Katrina, and this anger at this particular person.

216 (80-year-old male): I can't say nothing about the Catholic Church because they didn't do nothing…they didn't do hardly anything.

231 (50-year-old female): [During the relief efforts, the Catholic] Church was not visible like some of the volunteers or the other churches were….

201 (56-year-old female): Other faiths [responded] much quicker [than ours].

237 (52-year-old male): You see Catholic [based help groups] but not like you see other faiths.

Other participants were specific in their criticism of financial allocations by the Church and Catholic charities, including these two reports:

233 (49-year-old female): You know, the Catholic Church has wasted so much money. And then you [have] all these people after the storm that were looking for help. The Catholic Church said, "We only give our money overseas." I was like, "Ninety percent of the [people in this] parish are Catholic. Ninety percent of the parish have been supporting these churches for years and you only give the money *overseas*?"

208 (66-year-old female): I really…I thought when all the storm[s] took place, [that] Catholic Charities and things like that would come forth, but they never did. And I really put a lot of hope into that. Because I felt like, *that's my religion*; they should be there for me. But they weren't.

Earlier in this chapter, we noted that in previous qualitative work (with Latter-day Saint families) that when an individual or family's faith community failed them "it was both disappointing and hurtful in ways that seemed to elicit deeper frustration and pain than failures by secular agencies and institutions" (Marks & Dollahite, 2001, p. 636). Certainly, our participants, Catholic and non-Catholic, expressed abundant frustration with state and federal government. However, the pain expressed in connection with their church's failures seemed to be more profound, piercing, and emotional. Although no participant explicitly reported losing faith in God as a result of the hurricanes and ensuing struggles, a few Catholic participants did report that they lost faith in "their church" as portrayed in the two following excerpts:

240 (49-year-old female): Actually, I was going to the Catholic Church. Now I'm going to a Baptist church….

115 (48-year-old female): I used to be a practicing Catholic and I can tell you now that I am in a crisis of religion, not a crisis of faith. I am having a crisis of religion. The Catholic Church and I are not simpatico.

Another participant reflected on her family's experience:

231 (50-year-old female): [The Church's slow response] became depressing…. They eventually fixed the church, but *we never connected to any church again*…. So we have gone from being weekly church-going people to…[Well], we haven't even been to church on Christmas the past [several] years [since Katrina]…. So that has been a huge change…. Honestly. [My belief in the church was] interrupted and then disappointed. [I was hurt by]…my Catholic Church's response.

Note that even after expressing deep disappointment with the Church…and after admitting years of estrangement from the Church, this participant still concludes by calling the Church "*my* Catholic Church." With a few exceptions, the majority of the Catholic participants who criticized their church did not appear to be incensed or filled with vitriol—they instead came across as heartbroken or let down, but most of these individuals and families were not ready to entirely separate themselves from the Church.

Another participant conveyed a varied mixture of emotions throughout his interview. The next excerpt is actually pieced together from different portions of the interview, as hurt and disappointment seemed to surface over and over.

> **230** (49-year-old male): …Catholic Charities did not set anything [up] down here. We had Baptists; we had Methodists; we had Episcopal[ians]; we had Presbyterians; we had non-denominational groups…. [But the Catholic Church] used us. They took all of the insurance money that they received from all the churches down here and reallocated it to other areas. They were more interested in money than they were in actually helping their congregants… [their own] church members…. That's why I have lost my religious affiliation since the hurricane. I was born and raised Roman Catholic. I was an altar boy, believe it or not, until I was almost 16-years old at St. Rita's Church, which is right around the corner. That's where I went to school…. Oh yes, born and raised and infused in Catholic dogma…. But, no, they weren't here after the storm, and they…essentially *I had felt abandoned by my church.* So I have abandoned them…. I don't want to drag this on too long because that really sums it up really well for me.

Like several other participants, and as reflected in the title of Theme 3, this participant selects the word "abandoned" to summarize his feelings. Even so, note that like participant 231 in the preceding excerpt, this participant does not refer to "*The* church"; he chooses the personal possessive "*My* church."

It has been observed by the existential therapists Lantz and Frankl (1993), among others, that anger is often an expression of unresolved pain. It is difficult at best, and likely impossible, to convey the pain that our participants experienced on multiple levels (e.g., personal, familial, financial, and, yes, faith community). Indeed, it is worth remembering that the interviews captured in the chapter were conducted at least *5 years* after Katrina and Rita. The apparent pain several individuals are still wrestling with may be chronic, additive, or residual, but it does not appear to be "knee-jerk" angst. We suspect these are ideas and emotions that have been either sustained or developed across time.

We conclude this theme, "I Felt Like My Church Abandoned Me," by emphasizing that, with very few exceptions, local clergy were not criticized, nor were fellow parishioners or members of "church family" maligned. Our participants seemed to level their frustrations almost solely at institutional (archdiocesan) decisions. By contrast, there were some very positive reports of congregation-level outreach. We leave this theme with one such example from a participant who recalled attending a church with his family in Lafayette, LA, after evacuating New Orleans:

> **224** (51-year-old female): [Right after Katrina hit], we went to the church that was around U[niversity of] L[ouisiana]'s campus. I can't remember the name of it…[but] it was a Catholic Church. It was a larger church…[but] they were very understanding. And in fact, they ended up giving us some things. They ended up giving us a microwave. They [also] said they had some [more] things at the rectory if anyone would like to come see. And they gave us…a gift card to Wal-Mart. And I mean [their kindness]…*it gave me a different outlook….*

Rich qualitative data can provide us with "a different outlook." The present study offers selections from 125 different outlooks on a bona fide crisis that intertwined with each of the 125 person's lives. However, a crisis, according to the psychological theorist Erik Erikson, is not a disaster but a choice point…an opportunity for growth (see also Boss, 1999, 2002). For many of our participants, the crisis of Hurricanes Katrina and Rita provided an opportunity for growth and, perhaps ironically, a renewed and deepened faith in people. Our final theme captures these reports.

Theme 4: Helping Others: "Am I My Brother's Keeper?"

We anticipated that participants' responses would relate primarily to *their own* faith community in response to the question, "Has a faith community helped you cope with Hurricanes Katrina and Rita, and if so, in what way?" Our team-based analyses revealed, however, that the vast majority of the participants spontaneously discussed the helping hands offered by an array of "other" churches. Such reports even recurred among interviews with participants and families who were not religiously affiliated themselves. In addition, a few participants who were closely tied to their religion reported on how members of their denomination (but from other cities, or even other states) came to "their" personal faith community's assistance. As one woman explained:

> **214** (56-year-old female): We also had church groups come in from other Catholic churches all over the country. Well, actually, New York and New Jersey, they sent a few groups in to help us down in St. Bernard, as well as up at [Our Lady of] Prompt Succor [Church], when we were fixing [those two] church[es], they had groups come in. In fact, the[y] remain friends with the community; they [still] send people [down] every now and then.

The same woman and her husband added:

> **214** (56-year-old female) (wife): And, we have a lot of Protestant friends, too. We got quite a few that belong to other churches…. I think all the Churches helped [out in the community].

> **213** (64-year-old male) (husband): Another thing about [Katrina] is that religions [came] together.

Several participants offered similar reports of brotherhood and kindness across denomination. A few brief but illustrative examples include:

> **235** (43-year-old female): These Baptist people came out; they brought us food, clothes…. I mean it was unreal. Coming back home after the storm, other religions did [a great deal]…. There were religions with tents and stuff, giving water out to people, and there were just a lot of religions here…

> **201** (56-year-old female): [Katrina] just showed to me [that] Episcopalians or Baptists or whatever, were quite willing to come into a heavily Catholic community and help.

Some of the participants were zealous and emphatic in their praise of the outreach efforts by faith communities. One individual exclaimed:

> **213** (66-year-old male): [Did faith community help me?!] Oh, absolutely. [Churches and people] from everywhere. All denominations of Christians. All denominations. Anybody [that] needed any spiritual help from any denomination, they were there for them. And they brought things. Clothes, food, water, whatever they could bring and help clean up. Yards, cut [and clean up] branches [and] the trees. [There were] unbelievable things that they'd do. Everybody from Southern Baptists to Mormons.

Not every person and family was similarly helped by a faith community, however. A couple of our participants were less enthusiastic, like the following:

> **222** (66-year-old male): Now there were a lot of groups down here, but we never had any church group come to our house.

> **215** (77-year-old female): Of course, we used to go get some free meals, things like that, but to actually say anyone came and helped [us] physically or rebuilt [our] house or help[ed] [us] with finding anyone to rebuild [our] house, that didn't happen for me. Nobody helped me.

We previously saw in Theme 3 that some participants were disappointed in their *own* faith community's relief and/or response efforts. A much smaller number were dissatisfied with the efforts of *other* faith communities. Another example of this perspective is captured in the following participant's recollection:

> **230** (49-year-old male): [I remember there were] the church groups with the mops and bleach. They had come with 5-gallon [buckets with]...brushes and bleach and stuff like that. Some of [that stuff] came in handy, paper towels and stuff like that.... [Those church groups were] good hearted people [but]... you see, that's some of the dark humor.... Real dark humor. It was bizarre. It was like, "Okay, these people must need bleach. They must need bleach."

The juxtaposition of perspectives in the two previous groups of narratives provides a stark contrast. On the one hand we hear, "Anybody [that] needed any spiritual help from any denomination, they were there for them.... [There were] unbelievable things that they'd do. Everybody from Southern Baptists to Mormons." On the other hand we hear, "Nobody helped me," and "we never had any church group come to our house," and "[they brought us] bleach...that's some real dark humor." We are left wondering whether the wide range of perceptions is most closely linked to varied experience...or, perhaps, to individual perception.

While a wide array of faith communities reached out to the people of New Orleans during the immediate aftermath and longer-term relief efforts, our participants reported faith community outreach efforts from congregations originally based from Texas to Georgia that helped them cope as evacuees. Whether our New Orleans area participants and their families ultimately decided to permanently relocate *or* return and rebuild, they had to temporarily forge a life where they landed after emergency evacuation. The following narratives capture this reality and the role of faith communities in helping.

> **211** (55-year-old female): I think that the most help we got was from a church community was when we were in Alabama. We were in a hotel for about a week before we moved to Georgia, and it was honestly...it was amazing what these [Baptist] people did for us. Every day we never had to worry about food. They either brought in food, or they were taking us somewhere. They got clothes and they got a hold of Wal-Mart. Wal-Mart had come and taken the ages and sizes of all the children. They brought clothes and toiletries and stuff, and they were wonderful people. Yes, they did have a lot of churches. A lot of churches were involved. And...they were very understanding. I think they were a big help. They were a big help...[even though] our faith was [on]...the Catholic side.... But I mean as far as actually helping with different aspects of the hurricane, yes, there was a lot of community churches...and they...were very, very good people.

The preceding example, from Alabama, harmonizes with the following example from Lake Charles, LA, not far from the Texas/Louisiana border. This participant said of her family's experience:

> **221** (46-year-old female): When we were in Lake Charles, LA, [after evacuating] it was a faith-based…a faith-based organization that…that put this together. [T]hey were just taking in all the donations…we needed them right away….

Another example, from Atlanta, GA, similarly reflects the kindness and human outreach by faith communities far from New Orleans.

> **211** (55-year-old female): [When churches helped after the hurricanes] They weren't thinking [that it would last] *months* [in many cases]…. But…they were [a] big, big, big help. Especially when you're away from home. You don't know where to turn, where to go, you know? And then we went to Georgia, one of the things one of the churches helped us with was…they got…one of those little bitty transport [buses]…. And they took everybody [who had evacuated and needed to go to] Atlanta…. And they brought us and we registered for Red Cross and whatever we needed. Other churches had brought school supplies, and they had different stations [with] clothes…. They made sure all of those things were taken care of for you so that while you were waiting to be handled by the Red Cross or whatever that you were being taken care of [by the churches]…. I'll tell you…[I made it] a point to go to the table and say, "We thank you that you're here. You don't know how much difference you make by being here."

As we conclude Theme 4, Helping Others: "Am I My Brother's Keeper?" we return to a handful of narratives drawn from the home front in "heavily Catholic" New Orleans.

> **225** (68-year-old male): The churches got out, and they asked them to fill up a gallon bag with the things that we need…. The Baptist churches got together and they gave us, they collected food and they collected clothing and all, and toiletry items over there, the Red Cross gave us a gallon Ziploc bag. They had soap, toothbrush in there, toothpaste, a washcloth, and nail clippers and a comb and things like that that people donated…. So the churches, [including] the Baptist church, helped out tremendously. I'll never forget as long as I live, no matter where we went the Baptists were there to help the people. Food, clothing, whatever. We even gave a concert to them [out of thanks].

The next participant, without referencing personal denomination (if any), still emphasizes both work-related and financial assistance from one or two faith communities that are not noted by name, but were tremendously appreciated.

> **251** (71-year-old female): Oh yes. Definite[ly, faith community helped]…. [One church group] helped me to get some of my sheetrock [pulled out of my house]. They helped me, gave us money to go to Winn-Dixie [for groceries] and everything. So I find they helped [tremendously].

The following participant also shared recollections of kindness across denomination:

> **249** (51-year-old female): [There were] ones that were non-Catholic reaching out, feeding you when we didn't have a way to cook. I had a microwave—but they were companions, [they were] there for you and they were faithful. They were there almost every day…and very welcoming, very warm and there to help if you need[ed] it.

A final narrative emphasized the help provided by Catholic and other faith communities to the participant and her family during the monumental clean-up effort:

> **239** (77-year-old female): The Catholic Charities came and helped us out, and I think they gave us the strength to keep going, you know.... [There were] different churches from all over the country came down, and if it wouldn't have been for them, to help clean up the parish I don't know where we would be right now.

We reiterate this participant's explicit reflection, "If it wouldn't have been for [the churches]...I don't know where we would be right now." A recent Katrina-related article similarly posits:

> [A] central question related to the Katrina disaster that went largely unasked (much less addressed) by the state and national media was: *What went right?* A key response to this question was the immediate and comprehensive mobilization of south Louisiana's churches (Tausch et al., 2011, p. 243).

Based on some of our participants' interviews, the response of faith communities to the Katrina/Rita disaster was far from perfect. Outreach efforts missed some who were in need. Some faith community efforts were perceived as so slow and inadequate that a few participants and their families distanced themselves from their long-time denomination as a result. Even so, the overwhelming color and tone of our participants' reports seems to provide a textured picture of faith communities striving to answer the Biblical query, "Am I My Brother's Keeper?" in the affirmative. Particularly striking, perhaps, is the denominational blurring that took place as various churches reached out to members and nonmembers alike during times of profound need. We see this as a poignant but largely untold story of Katrina.

Conclusion

Our purpose in this chapter was to shed new light on faith communities as a coping resource in the aftermath of what has been described as the costliest natural disaster in US history. Qualitative analyses yielded four emergent themes pertaining to the role of faith-based communities in the immediate aftermath of the 2005 storms. Briefly, we have seen rather remarkable demonstrations of "The Hunger for Faith Community" (Theme 1)—including narratives that portrayed hurricane survivors literally gathering in sheds and garages to celebrate a unity of faith and relationship. We heard reports that, for some, "My Church Family Kept Me Going" (Theme 2). Considered together, Themes 1 and 2 are generally compatible with prior research which has shown that religiosity offsets the negative impact of major life stressors among older adults using quantitative methods (Krause & Tran, 1989; Krause, 1992). From this vantage point, faith community involvement in a post-disaster context offers a beacon of hope to those who have suddenly become homeless, having lost most, if not all material possessions in the storm.

In sharp contrast, "I Felt Like My Church Abandoned Me" (Theme 3) provided a startling counterpoint, illuminating the disappointment and seeming neglect by familiar faith-based institutions. Finally, and perhaps most significantly, "Helping Others: Am I My Brother's Keeper?" (Theme 4) brought to light the Herculean efforts of an array of faith communities that offered much to the survivors who were in need, without regard for denomination or belief. This theme is consistent with the well-documented outpouring of goods and services in the Katrina relief efforts orchestrated by most of the major denominations at local and national levels (Cain & Barthelemy, 2008; Cherry, Allen, & Galea, 2010; Phillips & Jenkins, 2010).

On a broader note, the themes presented here have implications for disaster preparedness and the coordination of relief efforts after a catastrophic disaster. Taken together, these four themes strongly suggest that faith-based institutions occupy both a helpful and harmful place in the psychological experience of trauma-exposed hurricane survivors. On the one hand, this dualistic (helpful/harmful) nature could be viewed as a threat to people's core beliefs and assumptions about their own faith traditions in times of great need. Alternatively, the complex nature of faith-based community presence (or absence) presents a unique opportunity for multidisciplinary collaborations to be formed among religious leaders, disaster relief personnel, and mental health professionals (see Putman et al., 2012; Smith et al., 2010, for related discussion). Collaborative efforts that build on church-affiliated social ties may foster *spiritual connectedness*, defined as "…the belief that there is a close bond among all people, regardless of whether they are religious or not" (Krause & Batista, 2009, p. 77). Spiritual connectedness, in turn, may facilitate the disaster relief efforts carried out by culturally diverse professionals from both the sacred and secular service realms for disaster survivors of all ages, an exciting possibility that awaits future research (see Chap. 19, this volume, for a related discussion). Given that older persons are often reluctant to seek social services compared to their younger counterparts (Cherry et al., 2010), faith-based communities may be key to effective resource linkage for the older segment of disaster-affected populations.

In conclusion, the abundant presentation of primary data with limited commentary has been intentional. As authors, we have kept our own voices somewhat checked in favor of the "insider experts" *who actually lived through and directly experienced the Katrina/Rita crisis* we have endeavored to study. Given this participant-centered path, it seems both consistent and wise to be brief in our concluding thoughts. As researchers on this project related to coping in the wake of one of the worst natural disasters in the US history, our aim is not to engage in attacks on any church (or other institution), nor is our intent to engage in apologetics. Our participants engaged in both of these exercises. Consequently, the chapter reflects both of these reported realities. The story of an aging sample coping with catastrophic disaster in the cultural center of New Orleans is not a simple one to tell.

From the revelry of Mardi Gras to the solemnity of Ash Wednesday, from the steeple of St. Louis Cathedral to the rebuilt doors of Our Lady of Lourdes in the outlying area of Violet—New Orleans is arguably the consummate French/Catholic community in the USA. Another pinnacle of French greatness, Victor Hugo, wrote not of a city but a man in need of aid. In his epic *Les Miserables*, the protagonist, Jean Valjean, stumbles to the door of a good bishop on the verge of starvation. The Bishop responds to Valjean's plea for help with the following:

> …This door does not ask a man who enters whether he has a name, but if he has a sorrow; you are suffering, you are hungry and thirsty, and so be welcome…. Why do I want to know your name? Besides, before you told it to me you had one which I knew.
> The man [Valjean] opened his eyes in amazement.
> Is that true? You know my name?
> "Yes," the Bishop answered, "you are *my brother*."[4]

It would seem that there are *still* those who know their brother's name.

Acknowledgments We are grateful to Sr. Mary Keefe and Fr. John Arnone of Our Lady of Lourdes Catholic Church in Violet, LA, and Gayle Buckley, Judy Chiappetta, and Catherine Serpas for their assistance with recruitment. We thank Susan McNeil of the St. Bernard Council on Aging and Sean Warner of the Gulf Coast Trust Bank in Chalmette, LA, for providing space for interviews. We thank Kelli Broome, Susan Brigman, Ashley Cacamo, Pamela Forest Nezat, and Mary Beth Tamor for their help with data collection and Robert Pressley, Penni Fontenot, Sarah Finney, Lauren Edwards, Allison Kennedy, Amy Goff, and Graham Belou for their assistance with transcriptions. We also thank Emily Allen, Savannah Ballard, Timothy Benedetto, Sarah Hebert, Trevor Johnson, Keri Kytola, and Bethany Pinkston for assistance with data coding and qualitative analyses.

This research was supported by grants from the Louisiana Board of Regents and the BP Gulf of Mexico Research Initiative, Office of Research and Economic Development, Louisiana State University. This support is gratefully acknowledged.

References

Batson, M., & Marks, L. D. (2008). Making the connection between prayer, faith, and forgiveness in Roman Catholic families. *The Qualitative Report, 13*, 394–415.

Boss, P. (1999). *Ambiguous loss*. Cambridge: Harvard University Press.

Boss, P. (2002). *Family stress management: A contextual approach*. Thousand Oaks: Sage.

Burr, W. R., Marks, L. D., & Day, R. (2012). *Sacred matters*. New York: Routledge.

Cain, D. S., & Barthelemy, J. (2008). Tangible and spiritual relief after the storm: The religious community responds to Katrina. *Journal of Social Service Research, 34*, 9–42.

Cherry, K. E., Allen, P. D., & Galea, S. (2010). Older adults and natural disasters: Lessons learned from Hurricanes Katrina and Rita. In P. Dass-Brailsford (Ed.), *Crisis and disaster counseling: Lessons learned from Hurricane Katrina and other disasters* (pp. 115–130). Thousand Oaks: Sage.

Cherry, K. E., Sampson, L., Nezat, P. F., Cacamo, A., Marks, L. D., & Galea, S. (2015). Long-term psychological outcomes in older adults after disaster: Relationships to religiosity and social support. *Aging & Mental Health, 19*(5), 430–443.

Dollahite, D. C., Marks, L. D., & Olson, M. M. (2002). Fathering, faith, and family therapy. *Journal of Family Psychotherapy, 13*, 263–294.

Dollahite, D. C., Marks, L. D., & Goodman, M. (2004). Religiosity and families. In M. J. Coleman & L. H. Ganong (Eds.), *The handbook of contemporary families* (pp. 411–431). Thousand Oaks: Sage.

Enstrom, J. E. (1998). Health practices and mortality rates among active California Mormons, 1980–1993. In J. T. Duke (Ed.), *Latter-day Saint social life: Social research on the LDS Church and its members* (pp. 461–471). Salt Lake City: Bookcraft.

Hugo, V. (1893). *Les miserables*. Boston: Little Brown.

[4] Hugo (1893) (trans.), vol. 1, p. 114, emphasis added.

Hummer, R., Rogers, R., Nam, C., & Ellison, C. G. (1999). Religious involvement and U. S. adult mortality. *Demography, 36*, 273–285.

Josselson, R., & Lieblich, A. (1993). *The narrative study of lives*. Newbury Park: Sage.

Koenig, H. G. (2002). Religion, congestive heart failure, and chronic pulmonary disease. *Journal of Religion and Health, 41*, 263–278.

Koenig, H. G., McCullough, M. E., & Larson, D. B. (Eds.) (2001). *Handbook of religion and health*. New York: Oxford University Press.

Koenig, H. G., King, D. E., & Carson, V. B. (Eds.) (2012). *Handbook of religion and health* (2nd ed.). New York: Oxford University Press.

Krause, N. (1992). Stress, religiosity, and psychological well-being among older blacks. *Journal of Aging and Health, 4*, 412–439.

Krause, N. (2012). Valuing the life experience of old adults and change in depressive symptoms: Exploring an overlooked benefit of involvement in religion. *Journal of Aging and Health, 24*, 227–249.

Krause, N., & Batista, E. (2009). Core religious beliefs and providing support to others in late life. *Mental Health, Religion, & Culture, 12*, 75–96.

Krause, N., & Tran, T. V. (1989). Stress and religious involvement among older Blacks. *Journal of Gerontology: Social Sciences, 44*, S4–S13.

Laird, R., Marks, L. D., & Marrero, M. (2011). Religiosity, self-control, and antisocial behavior: Religiosity as a promotive and protective factor. *Journal of Applied Developmental Psychology, 32*, 78–85.

Lantz, J. E., & Frankl, V. E. (1993). *Existential family therapy: Using the concepts of Viktor Frankl.* Northvale, NJ: Aronson, Inc.

Marks, L. D. (2005). Religion and bio-psycho-social health: A review and conceptual model. *Journal of Religion and Health, 44*, 173–186.

Marks, L. D. (2006a). Religion and family relational health: An overview and conceptual model. *Journal of Religion and Health, 45*, 603–618.

Marks, L. D. (2006b). Mental health, religious belief, and "the terrifying question." *Journal of Child and Family Studies, 15*, 133–139.

Marks, L. D., & Dollahite, D. C. (2001). Religion, relationships, and responsible fathering in Latter-day Saint families of children with special needs. *Journal of Social and Personal Relationships, 18*, 625–650.

Marks, L. D., Dollahite, D. C., & Freeman, J. J. (2011). Faith and prayer in family life. In T. W. Draper, A. J. Hawkins, & D. C. Dollahite (Eds.), *Strengthening our families* (2nd ed., pp. 185–195). Provo: BYU.

Marks, L. D., Dollahite, D. C., & Barker, K. (2012). Don't forget home. In J. Hoffman (Ed.), *Understanding religious ritual* (pp. 186–203). New York: Routledge.

McCullough, M. E., Hoyt, W. T., Larson, D. B., Koenig, H. G., & Thoresen, C. E. (2000). Religious involvement and mortality: A meta-analytic review. *Health Psychology, 19*, 211–222.

Marks, L. D., Nesteruk, O., Swanson, M., Garrison, M. E. B., & Davis, T. (2005). Religion and health among African Americans. *Research on Aging, 27*, 447–474.

Putman, K. M., Blair, R., Roberts, R., Ellington, J. F., Foy, D. W., Houston, J. B., & Pfefferbaum, B. (2012). Perspectives of faith-based relief providers on responding to the needs of evacuees following Hurricane Katrina. *Traumatology, 18*, 56–64.

Phillips, B., & Jenkins, P. (2010). The roles of faith-based organizations after Hurricane Katrina. In R. P. Kilmer, V. Gil-Rivas, R. G. Tedeschi, & L. G. Calhoun (Eds.), *Helping families and communities recover from disaster: Lessons learned from Hurricane Katrina and its aftermath* (pp. 215–238). Washington, D.C.: American Psychological Association.

Silva, J. L., Marks, L. D., & Cherry, K. E. (2009). The psychology behind helping and prosocial behaviors: An examination from intention to action in an adult population. In K. E. Cherry (Ed.), *Lifespan perspectives on natural disasters: Coping with Katrina, Rita and other storms* (pp. 219–240). New York: Springer.

Smith, R. P., Taylor, J., Larkin, G. L., North, C. S., Ryan, D., & Holmes, A. (2010). On reentering the chapel: Models for collaborations between psychiatrists, communities of faith, and faith-based providers after Hurricane Katrina. In G. H. Brenner, D. H. Bush, & J. Moses (Eds.), *Creating spiritual and psychological resilience* (pp. 125–132). New York: Rutledge.

Tausch, C., Marks, L. D., Silva Brown, J., Cherry, K. E., Frias, T., McWilliams, Z., et al. (2011). Religion and coping in the aftermath of Hurricanes Katrina and Rita: Qualitative themes from the Louisiana Healthy Aging Study. *Journal of Religion, Spirituality, and Aging, 23*, 236–253.

Taylor, H. (15 Oct 2003). The Harris Poll #59: While most Americans believe in God, only 36% attend a religious service once a month or more often. *Harris Interactive*. http://www.harrisinteractive.com/vault/Harris-Interactive-Poll-Research-While-Most-Americans-Believe-in-God-Only-36-pct-A-2003-10.pdf. Accessed 8 October 2014.

Taylor, R. J., Chatters, L. M., & Levin, J. (2004). *Religion in the lives of African Americans*. Thousand Oaks: Sage.

Chapter 15
Trauma and Ambiguous Loss: The Lingering Presence of the Physically Absent

Pauline Boss and Chikako Ishii

Introduction

We begin with three events from different parts of the world. Each, however, illustrates the same phenomenon, a loss that requires long-term resilience.

- On September 11, 2001, terrorists attacked the World Trade Center towers in New York City and the Pentagon near the nation's capital, using hijacked airliners as weapons. Since that day, the number of missing keeps changing as remains are still being identified. As of this writing, 2,753 are verified as dead in the World Trade Center attack, but 1,115 remain missing (Valenti, 2013).
- On March 11, 2011, it was reported that the death toll from the earthquake and tsunami in Japan was the highest ever recorded—in the hundreds, but government officials said, "It would almost certainly rise to more than 1,000" (Fackler, 2011). Sadly, the death toll as of this writing has reached 15,887, and the number of missing is 2612 across 22 prefectures—which are similar to states in the USA (National Police Agency of Japan, 2014).
- On March 8, 2014, Malaysia Airlines Flight 370 disappeared with 227 passengers, 2 infants, and 12 crew aboard ("Malaysia Airlines plane," 2014). As of this writing, their families still do not know where they are or if they are dead or alive. All have vanished without a trace.

P. Boss (✉)
Department of Family Social Science, College of Education and Human Development, University of Minnesota, 290 McNeal Hall, 1985 Buford Avenue, St. Paul, MN 55108, USA
e-mail: pboss@umn.edu

C. Ishii
TELL Counseling, 6-10-11 Minami Aoyama, Minato-ku, Tokyo 107-0062, Japan
e-mail: cishii@telljp.com

K. E. Cherry (ed.), *Traumatic Stress and Long-Term Recovery*,
DOI 10.1007/978-3-319-18866-9_15

The common phenomenon in each of these catastrophic events is called ambiguous loss (see Boss, 1999, 2006). It is a unique kind of loss where people disappear without proof of death—or life. Because the fate or whereabouts of the missing persons remains in doubt, sometimes for a lifetime, there is no possibility of closure or even resolution for this type of loss. The ongoing ambiguity and state of "not knowing" create a unique condition of helplessness and thus trauma for family members and friends left behind. It is important then to bear in mind that ambiguous loss and the impossibility of closure are conceptually and painfully linked.

With verified deaths of family members, however, there may also be trauma, especially if the death is untimely and off-time based on the expected human life cycle, for example, the death of an infant, child, or youth. But such phenomena are different from having a loved one swept away without a body to bury. Such unverified and unclear loss is additionally traumatic because it is inevitably long term and without possibility of closure. Because there may never even be resolution after such loss, the families' ongoing grief should be considered reasonable and understandable. Symptoms may mimic complicated grief, but even the healthiest people can show symptoms of depression and anxiety after an ambiguous loss. What scholars and professionals need to know to work effectively with families of the missing is that *it is the type of loss, not the type of grief, which is the core problem.*

The basic premise of the theory of ambiguous loss is that "not knowing" the whereabouts or fate of a family member is a stress beyond normal human expectations; thus an ambiguous loss is the most stressful of losses because there is no possibility of closure (for details, see Boss, 1987, 1999, 1988/2002, 2004, 2006, 2007; Boss & Dahl, 2014; Boss & Yeats, 2014). The culprit is the ambiguity surrounding the loss. Personal and family symptoms result from the stress of "not knowing" as relationships rupture from the uncanny context of loss more than from one's personal weakness. For even the strongest of individuals and families, ambiguous loss creates a painful, often lifelong mystery. Because it is more common than we think (Boss, 1999), we need to know more about this challenging type of loss and how to ease the stress of the many families facing ambiguous losses today.

Definition of Ambiguous Loss

Ambiguous loss is defined as a loss that remains unclear, unverified—yes, ambiguous. There is no proof of the missing person's whereabouts or status as dead or alive. As a result, perceptions of absence and presence are confused, relationships rupture, coping strategies are blocked, and grief is frozen. This overall immobilization increases feelings of helplessness. For this reason, ambiguous loss is one of the most traumatizing types of loss. Family members and friends are in a double bind; they hesitate to grieve and perform the usual funeral rituals after a death in the family, and at the same time, they cannot continue to act as if that person is alive or returning as they were. Unless changes are made in family roles and boundaries, they are sociologically, psychologically, and economically trapped in an indeterminate state of "not knowing" (Boss, 1999, 2006).

There are two types of ambiguous loss in the theoretical framework (see Table 15.1). In the first type, which is the primary focus of this chapter, a family member goes missing *physically* (Boss, 2004, 2006). Their loss may be a consequence of war, terrorism, captivity, kidnapping, airline explosion, tsunami, earthquake, and forced uprooting. The second type of ambiguous loss occurs when a loved one goes missing *psychologically*. Examples are dementia, depression, addiction, etc., all of which impair cognitive and emotional presence (for more information on this second type of ambiguous loss, we refer you to Boss, 2006, 2011, 2012; Boss, Caron, Horbal, & Mortimer, 1990; Boss & Kaplan, 2004).

It is important to note that both types of ambiguous loss can occur simultaneously in one person or one family. For example, in Fukushima, many families are not only experiencing type 1 ambiguous loss with physically missing loved ones, but due to relocation, they have also lost the psychological presence and support of longtime friends and neighbors who were also uprooted and relocated (see Chap. 5, this volume). Multiple ambiguous losses also occurred after 9/11 in New York. Some children with a parent lost in the rubble of the World Trade Center towers told us months later they felt as if they had lost both of their parents. We were puzzled as their mothers were sitting at the other end of the room. However, many of the mothers were so depressed that they apparently were no longer "there" for their children (Boss, Beaulieu, Wieling, Turner, & LaCruz, 2003). They were now psychologically absent because their husbands were physically missing. Both types of ambiguous loss were impacting the children.

Experiencing both types of ambiguous loss at the same time also impacts adults. For example, after 9/11, a woman we worked with had a physically missing husband and also a psychologically missing mother. That is, her mother suffered from Alzheimer's disease, a pathological condition characterized by severe deficits in memory and cognition that differ dramatically from normal aging (see Cherry &

Table 15.1 Two types of ambiguous loss. (For other examples, see Boss, 2006.)

Examples of *physical* ambiguous loss
Missing from earthquake and tsunami (3/11)
Missing from terrorist explosion (9/11)
Vanished without a trace (lost at sea, lost airplane)
Kidnapped by political or religious terrorists
Forced relocation, uprooting, and loss of home, land, animals, and community
Examples of *psychological* ambiguous loss
Depression, unresolved grief
Preoccupation with missing person
Addiction to drugs or alcohol, gambling
Obsession with computer games, Internet, TV, etc.
Dementia from Alzheimer's disease and other cognitive disorders
Chronic mental illness

Smith, 1998). Understandably, she felt doubly sad and confused. Such situations are likely to be of higher risk and require more attention and support.

Depending on cultural values and beliefs, many family members, however, manage to find a surprising resilience, which helps them to live well despite “not knowing.” For example, people may use religious beliefs or even dreams to create one or multiple endings to their mystery. They symbolically construct an ending to their story that brings them relief (Boss & Carnes, 2012; Robins, 2013, 2014).

The theory of ambiguous loss provides a useful lens, which focuses less on pathology and more on resilience. It is a stress-based model which aims at *prevention*—the prevention of further trauma and stress and subsequent medical symptoms with whomever we work—individuals, couples, individual families, or groups of families in a community.

To illustrate ambiguous loss, its effects, and the resilience that allows survivors to move forward in a new way, we will use primarily the March 11, 2011 (3/11) disaster, officially called “The East Japan Great Earthquake,” which brought a devastating tsunami to the East Japan region, the most serious in the Iwate, Miyagi, and Fukushima prefectures (see Chap. 5, this volume), as well as the September 11, 2001, terrorist attacks on the USA (9/11) in New York City and Washington, D.C. Both the Japanese (3/11) and the New York City (9/11) events, plus all too many ensuing events such as the lost Malaysia Airlines Flight 370, create a unique suffering comprised of complex grief and long-term sorrow for individuals, families, and even entire communities.

Because grief therapies are insufficient and often offensive to people experiencing ambiguous loss, this chapter also focuses on how to help and support them to increase their tolerance for ambiguity and thus gain the resilience and strength for the long journey ahead.

The Difference Between Ambiguous Loss and Death

Ambiguous loss differs from death because it has no clarity, finality, or proof of death. However, as with some kinds of death, for example, a child’s, ambiguous loss often leads to a complicated grief. With the missing, however, it is not due to the untimeliness of death, but due to the lack of facts surrounding the loss. Without proof of death, families must construe their own ending to their traumatic story.

With loss ongoing and without finality, the grief process is beyond normal human expectation and thus challenges a family’s ability to find meaning in their suffering. Without facts, they cannot make sense of the loss. We think of the families of passengers and crew on the missing Malaysia Airlines Flight 370 who may have to live a lifetime without knowing the fate and whereabouts of their loved ones.

When a loved one is lost physically without verification of death or a body to bury, such loss is in essence a “complicated loss” and thus leads to symptoms of complicated grief. Through no fault of family members, this type of unclear loss understandably causes open-ended and long-term grief. It may resemble “malingering” but because there is no possibility of closure or even resolution, we must note: If the loss remains ambiguous, the cause of chronic sorrow and lingering grief lies in the *type of loss* experienced and not in the pathology of the persons who are grieving (Boss, 1999, 2004, 2006).

The Difference Between Ambiguous Loss and Post-traumatic Disorder

Ambiguous loss is a traumatic loss and thus can lead to symptoms that are similar to those of post-traumatic stress disorder (PTSD): depression, anxiety, guilt, psychic numbing, flashbacks, and distressing dreams. There are differences, however, in how these symptoms are viewed and treated.

PTSD is viewed as an individual disorder. Based on the *Diagnostic and Statistical Manual of Mental Disorders* (5th ed.; DSM-5; American Psychiatric Association, 2013), it is medically defined, individually diagnosed, and individually treated. The family has not typically been involved. The therapeutic goal is to return the patient to health.

On the other hand, ambiguous loss is viewed as a relational disorder. It is a relational rupture that presumes a close relationship with the lost person. For this reason, relational interventions are most effective. For this trauma, family therapy and peer group meetings are recommended over individual therapy. The goal when treating ambiguous loss is to help family members and the family as a whole to find the resilience they need to live with long-term stress of ambiguity. That means empowering and remobilizing the family processes that involve decision making, day-to-day functioning, caring for one another, and finally, grieving what has been lost. While the treatment goal for PTSD has been recovery, the goal for ambiguous loss is resiliency (Boss, 2006).

The Difference Between Depression and the Normal Sadness of Grief

To work effectively with families of the missing, we must first know the difference between depression and sadness. Depression involves an intense grief that interferes with daily functioning (eating, sleeping, working, etc.) and often contains aspects of the individual's existing or preexisting conditions or disorders.

Symptoms of depression are a preoccupation with the lost person, difficulty finding meaning, putting life on hold, feelings of helplessness and hopelessness, and not accepting the loss. But family members with loved ones ambiguously lost also manifest these symptoms. Caution is required before a medical diagnosis of depression is warranted. Professionals may not see the sadness and sorrow of normal grieving because no visible death has occurred. Being sad when there is ambiguous loss is typical and should not be medicalized. While common treatment approaches to depression include talk therapy, often cognitive behavioral therapy (CBT) and medication, the treatment for the sadness of grief is human connection (Boss, 1999, 2006). Professional therapeutic guidance may or may not be required, but it should involve systemic work.

Cultural Beliefs that Influence Coping with Ambiguous Loss: The Example of 3/11

To understand and help families distressed by ambiguous loss, we begin by asking what their perceptions are about the situation: "What does this situation mean to you?" In Japan, for example, we begin by determining how people perceive the phenomenon of a tsunami (see Chap. 5, this volume). From the second author's perspective, many Japanese people think of a tsunami as unavoidable, but that they can make preparations to prevent or reduce disaster and loss.

There has been a phrase used in the tsunami-hit regions, "Tsunami, tendenko," literally meaning "At the time of tsunami, each person runs away separately." What this means is that in the event of a tsunami, the top priority is to save oneself. You have to be the first one to run to higher ground, so that people around you will also run. That is, by immediately running to save yourself, you inspire "tendenko" in others and in that way save others who might not see the urgency to escape to higher ground. (For more information, see Professor Toshitaka Katada's YouTube interview, Don Productions TV, 2013.) While "tendenko" begins individualistically, it is a strategy that benefits the collective. Paradoxically, running to save oneself helps to save one's family and community.

Today, there are even YouTube training sessions for students about "Tsunami, tendenko" because there have been so many sad stories of losing almost entire families in a tsunami. In 1993, for example, there was the case of the Kondo family in Hokkaido. Mrs. Kondo started to escape with her two children, but on the way to the hill, they made a detour to look for her mother. While looking for her mother, Mrs. Kondo and her children were swept away by the tsunami. In the meantime, her mother had already escaped up the hill and was safe. Mrs. Kondo's family, which had included three generations, was now only her mother. This kind of tragedy has been reported so many times, and that is why "Tsunami tendenko" has been emphasized.

As a result of historically losing entire families (or nearly so), citizens are now taught to trust each other and save themselves first. In this unique way, the individual acts alone to become responsible to save not only his or her own life but also the life of the family itself.

On March 11, 2011, students of the elementary school and middle school in Kamaishi followed "tendenko." They all ran up and away from the tsunami for 2 km, and thus 600 other lives were saved by such spontaneity. The adolescents and children saved their own lives while inspiring and helping others, young and elderly, to escape the rising water (NHK, 2013; Sashida, 2013). Because their schools were located next to the ocean, they had routine training sessions to be able to judge how far they should run and how to make their points clear to family members who did not take the situation that seriously (NHK, 2013). In this area, even the young children and adolescents who were back home actually persuaded their family members to follow their judgment.

With such training, the Japanese people—school children included—traditionally have had a sense of at least some mastery and control over this occasional but terrible event. However, after the behemoth tsunami of 3/11, people realize that it is even more challenging now to avoid disastrous outcomes from a tsunami. In 1896, the small town of Taro near Miyako in Iwate Prefecture experienced massive damage from a tsunami and lost 83 % of their population. In 1933, they experienced damage from another tsunami, losing 32 % of their population (Onishi & Ishiwatari, 2012). So in 1958, they started to build huge walls against future damage (Ito, 2011). When the tsunami of the Chilean earthquake hit this Japanese town of Taro in 1960, the walls saved the people (Wakefield, Ito, Toshio, Swanson, Revell, & Klein, 2013). As a result, they continued to build even higher and stronger walls until 1979, thinking that was the way to master and prevent disaster. Yet, in 2011, the tsunami waters on 3/11 breached even these higher walls. People now realized that disaster can occur despite preparation (Yoshimura, 2011). This increased their feelings of helplessness.

To increase such anxiety and worry for families even today, there is now more than a tsunami that can cause disaster for people living in the coastal areas. Ships and boats now carry chemicals and crude oils that can spill, a new threat bringing different kinds of damage in addition to a tsunami. Additionally and critically, the damaged Fukushima Daiichi Nuclear Power Plant was disabled by the 3/11 earthquake and tsunami and caused massive additional losses of homes, property, and communities due to radiation poisoning of ancestral farmlands. Indeed today, the prevention of loss and disaster and the preparation for coastal families is increasingly complex and challenging.

How do people experiencing ambiguous losses cope, not only from loved ones gone missing or deceased but also from their loss of home and community? People often talk directly to their dead relatives in a culture of ancestral worship (Ishii, 1996; Klass, 1996). While there is also support from the community and helpful people around them who are physically present, families of the missing as well as the dead continue to feel support from ancestors who are kept psychologically present. These families do not talk much about their missing or dead in their daily lives, but they do feel supported by talking to an ancestor no longer here physically, but nevertheless, psychologically present.

In Japan, the deceased are regarded as Buddha after 49 days, and the bereaved often talk individually to those dead persons at a home altar asking them to keep the bereaved family safe. This tradition of ancestral worship is kept among not only Buddhists but also non-Buddhists. Such psychological connection with a loved one is useful in Japan. The family members of the missing sometimes talk silently to those ancestors in front of a home altar so that the ancestors will keep their eyes on the missing to help them stay safe (J. Yoshino, personal communication, August 18, 2014).

In addition, there is financial support from the government. This support, however, may inadvertently block coping and increase family stress. In order to receive financial compensation for their loss, families must accept the fact that a body has not been found—and that their loved one is dead! Some family members do accept the second term, and turn in the official form, but others may disagree with that decision, causing family conflict. (We note that this dynamic was also found in families after New York's 9/11; see Boss, Beaulieu, Wieling, Turner, & LaCruz, 2003; and in the families of MIA pilots; see Boss, 1977, 1980).

To prevent permanent family rifts and alienation, our therapeutic task then is to meet with the family as a whole and explain that it is all right for them to disagree on how they perceive the loss. From research, we now know that each person grieves in his or her own way (Neimeyer, Harris, Winokuer, & Thornton, 2011), but we must also recognize that each family member may perceive the loss, especially an ambiguous loss, in his or her own way (Ishii & Setou, 2014). When loved ones vanish, with no facts available about their fates, it is no wonder that family members disagree about how to proceed. Without a body to bury, they have the added burden of needing to tolerate each other's interpretations of the loss. We may have to repeat these ideas for families many times because they often believe that everyone in a family has to feel the same way.

In addition, many people, because of discrimination, prejudice, stigma, poverty, war, or terrorism have little or no mastery or control, and thus need first to be empowered before they can find the resiliency they need to move forward with their lives (Robins, 2010; Une 2014). Across cultures and religions, the empowerment of people who live with ambiguous loss requires family and community support and professional education.

Religious and Secular Beliefs

In Japan, Buddhism is the dominant tradition when death occurs. While most Japanese people do not follow any one particular religion, most nevertheless follow the traditional rituals of Buddhism when a family member dies. Customs and traditions which are commonly observed are summarized by the second author: From the Obon tradition, serious attention is paid to the custom of visiting graves where people typically talk to the deceased family member. In addition, they maintain a role for the deceased by attending rites for them, which do not end with the funeral (for a fuller discussion, see Ishii, 1996, p. 225).

With a clear and validated death, Buddhist beliefs offer opportunities to meet together for the bereaved. Those rituals are not only a wake and a funeral right after death but also the anniversary ceremonies for family and relatives that take place at the 1st, 3rd, 7th, and 13th years. On a daily basis, there is a custom for family members to place food and drink in front of their home altar and talk in silence to the dead. They do this individually. In addition, communities have annual ceremonies or festivals during Obon in summer to remember those who died.

The problem is that Buddhism does not provide any of these rituals to the families of the missing (Y. Taniyama, personal communication, August 28, 2014). While Buddhist priests may help such families to feel calm about the dead, this practice of not allowing families of the missing to meet together for these traditional grief rituals requires rethinking. In New York City, after 9/11, there were similar restrictions at first. Some religions did not allow burial without a body, but after some discussion, church leaders reconsidered and ultimately allowed the burial of empty caskets or symbols representing the missing person. Especially for those who must live with the lifelong pain of a loved one gone missing, religious rituals of grief are often necessary to find some measure of peace. Presently in Japan, there are no ways to talk directly to a missing loved one in front of the home altar, but some family members, as they continue to talk to their deceased relatives, who are now turned into Buddha, ask them to take care of the missing person(s). This can provide a measure of comfort to the families of the missing.

For families who do not find solace from traditional religion, there are also secular beliefs. They may go to a medium (Takahashi, 2014; Yanagida & Suzuki, 2014) and ask about the missing person. The mediums are found in some regions and, in particular, in the coastal area where the 3/11 tsunami hit. The medium's answer may give the family some sense of relief, so this is widely done in certain regions in East Japan (Sato, 2014). Another experience, also nonreligious, is that one family member often talks to the missing person privately. One way is in a dream. That way, the surviving person feels relieved. But such dreams are not talked about openly. The experience of seeing the missing in dreams is kept private, very private. More generally among the Japanese, people do not talk about that experience with other family members, saying that is because they are worried what they saw in the dream might disappoint other family members (J. Yoshino, personal communication, August 18, 2014). When the dream gives some clue about the missing, for example, where the lost person is, how he or she is doing, or whether no more living, the dreamer may choose not to share this information with the family members. Typically, unless people know for sure that what they dreamt about will make everyone happy, they try not to talk about it. When the dreamer feels that he or she has a certain relationship with the missing person, they may not want to disclose this to other family members.

Resilience as the Tolerance for Ambiguity

Like a flexible cable bridge bending with the force of a big wind, human resilience is the ability to bend in response to a traumatic force that pummels for some time—and then regain one's stability. Resilience then is more than recovery—and more than "bouncing back." It implies growth in flexibility and strength rather than simply regaining one's status quo (Boss, 2006; see also Chap. 16, this volume).

When a family must live with ambiguous loss, resilience means specifically the ability to embrace the "not knowing." There is no end point to the uncertainty, so it becomes a constant and adaptive trait requiring flexibility, strength, and change. The upside is that people often grow stronger from that struggle. New human connections are made; new ways of being are discovered. Life goes on reasonably well despite ambiguous loss.

Because resiliency lies in one's ability to accept the lack of information and the "not knowing," this is challenging in a can-do culture and information age where certainty holds more value than uncertainty. Nevertheless, we see evidence of resilience in surprising places.

A Story of Resilience in a Miyagi High School

To set the stage for this story, we must know the cultural context in Japan high schools regarding the teacher–student hierarchy, which is strictly kept. This is very different compared to the USA, where students often view themselves as consumers who are entitled to personal access to their teacher as part of the educational experience they or their parents have paid for. In Japan, however, as in many other countries, teachers are revered and considered authorities who do not share their private lives with their students. Overall, the teacher–student relationship is more formal with a strict hierarchy. Nevertheless, after 3/11, the teacher in the following story saw a need for change in this relationship. He was resilient, so in the wake of disaster and loss, he could shift and change his traditional way of interacting with his students. The following is the second author's personal communication with that teacher whom we shall call Mr. K. (personal communication, November 9, 2013):

> Mr. K. is a highly respected schoolteacher, leader of his clan, and community leader in Miyagi. On March 11, 2011, often called 3/11 in Japan, he lost many family members and relatives: 19 dead and three still missing. His maternal grandfather's brother A. was washed away by the Tsunami with his wife B. and his daughter C. C. happened to be visiting her father on that terrible day. A.'s son, a fisherman, told his sister C. to flee to a higher place with his father A. who was weak. Then he headed his boat out to sea before the Tsunami's arrival. He was too late and was caught by the Tsunami and washed away in his boat, but he managed to keep popping into other less damaged boats, and finally got hooked on the branch of a tree. He survived. His father and sister, however, are still missing. His mother B.'s body was found far from their town. Mr. K. thought the Tsunami took her body and then the waves brought her back to another part of the affected area.
>
> He also told how his family survived after 3/11. Since his home is located in a tiny fishing village and is isolated by surrounding mountains and rivers, when the roads, bridges, and train truck were damaged, supplies could not arrive compared to other parts of the same city. For more than 100 days, traveling miles and miles, he had to find a way to get water for all his clan and the village people who stayed in houses which survived, every day. One of his nieces was only several months old, and there was neither baby milk supply nor Pampers. So he made every effort to go to other evacuation centers and see if they happen to keep those supplies. He also went around to many centers where the bodies were kept. He checked more than 1,000 bodies in a day while he searched for his missing aunt and finally found her. Her face and body was not identifiable, but her key matched her husband's.
>
> On a hilltop overlooking the ocean, there is a community memorial site where a statue of Kannon (Buddha) has been placed. Mr. K.'s family provided the land for this site. With a

good view of the damaged area, the statue has become the place for survivors to pray for their family and friends dead—and still missing.

On December 7, 2012, more than a year and a half after the Tsunami devastated the community, there was a minor earthquake after dark. Some students got very upset. Some cried. The Tsunami warning was given, but soon after lifted, and the students went home. On the following Monday, some students were still showing signs of trauma and stress.

Earlier, in April of 2012, nearly a year after the Tsunami of 3/11, a student who lost his father in the Tsunami overheard Mr. K. playing his guitar; the boy asked if he could have lessons and that occurred. The boy had been taking lessons for some time, seemingly stable again. Yet, three days after the minor earthquake in December 2012, Mr. K. found the boy crouching in a corner of a dark classroom after everyone left. When Mr. K. spoke to him, the student for the first time started to share his story about his experiences from 3/11—his missing father and his current family situation. (Many times, a mother who loses her husband goes back to her family of origin with her children. And later they find it difficult to live that way. This boy's family was no exception.) He told his teacher about his bad experiences. Surprisingly, Mr. K. told the student his own story about missing and dead family members. Culturally, it was unusual for a teacher to share a personal story with a student. But he did, and it made it seem all right to the boy for having been afraid and sad.

On the next day, Mr. K. had another guitar lesson with this student, so he asked him how he was doing. He told Mr. K. that he now felt close to Mr. K. because he was also suffering from losing family members. And he learned that it is okay to recall the parent who is missing. He also found out that it is important to remember the person who is gone.

Though the guitar lessons started with this student, Mr. K. invited some other boys to join. He was aware from a Tohoku newspaper that nobody at home or at school would talk about 3/11. Especially with children, Mr. K. had shifted those cultural rules.

The boy told his teacher, Mr. K., that he had never before talked about his missing father. He felt that it was not allowed to talk about this, even at home. Later, after their talking, the boy told his teacher that he had been seeing his father in dreams since early 2013 and that his father looked as if he supported his son's playing guitar. He liked this. The boy said that he does not see his father in dreams any more, but he feels somehow that his father approves and enjoys watching him playing the guitar.

This is a story of resiliency for several reasons: *First,* the teacher's wisdom and ability to set aside the usual teacher–student hierarchy by sharing personal stories allowed the student to see that he was not alone in his grief and loss. The teacher minimized the hierarchy, especially with students who were visibly suffering from loss, clear and ambiguous. By showing his own feelings and revealing his own losses, the students could see that even their esteemed teacher was grieving, and that it was permissible to talk about the pain. *Second,* while the community rules prescribed private grieving, once the teacher broke this rule by sharing his story, the students realized they could also. Breaking the silence was functional for moving forward with life after loss. Here, social support came in the form of a classroom and guitar lessons, all very functional for human connection. *Third,* the transformation to music, in this case guitar lessons, provided a serene and supportive setting for easing posttraumatic stress. It normalized the pain of loved ones gone missing with music as the calming balm. The control and orderliness of the notes balanced the chaos of the aftermath of 3/11. The teacher and fellow students became a musical psychological family for living well despite the pain of loss. *Finally,* this story shows us that resilience can be found in surprising places, in this case, in a schoolroom and in a wise teacher—and in a boy's dream of approval from his missing father. Perceptions matter, and in this case, the boy believed his father liked his guitar playing, and thus it can become satisfying to him, perhaps for the rest of his life. It becomes his special coping mechanism (Boss, 1992).

Assessment and Interventions: Finding the Resilience to Live Long Term with Ambiguous Loss

The basic theoretical premise for assessment and shaping treatment or intervention depends on one's training or discipline. From a *sociological perspective,* ambiguous loss is assessed structurally as it leads to boundary ambiguity (Boss, 1988/2002; Boss & Greenberg, 1984). That is, the clarity needed for boundary maintenance (in the sociological sense) is unattainable. Parenting roles are ignored, decisions are put on hold, daily tasks are undone, family members are ignored or cut off, and rituals and celebrations are canceled even though they are the glue of family life. To function, a family needs to know who is in and who is out of the system and with a missing member, the therapeutic challenge focuses on reshaping the family while not closing out the missing member.

From a *psychological perspective,* ambiguous loss is assessed more individually and relationally. Whether we meet with the community or one family, a couple or an individual, we look for feelings of hopelessness along with depression, and feelings of ambivalence that can lead to guilt, anxiety, and immobilization (Boss, 1999, 2006). While we treat the symptoms, it is essential to remember the social context of ambiguous loss in which the individual and family are now embedded. Their psychological symptoms are often less about personal or familial pathology than a result of living in an environment of ruptured relationships.

Individual Effects of Ambiguous Loss

The individual effects of ambiguous loss are often depression, anxiety, guilt, and feelings of hopelessness, helplessness, ambivalence, and anxious attachment. Grief is frozen, but there is a chronic sadness that is often diagnosed as a full-blown clinical depression. It is thus essential to differentiate between what we call normal sadness and a depression that needs medical treatment. (See also pp. 275–276 regarding sadness versus depression.) With an ambiguous loss, grief often lingers, sometimes for a lifetime; this is understandable and not pathological. Despite times of sadness, those people suffering from ambiguous loss function well in work and daily life, in their relationships, and in their social connections. On the other hand, the person who is depressed does not function well in these areas; he or she may become isolated and disabled in daily life or/and work.

Family and Couple Effects of Ambiguous Loss

Family or marital roles, rules, and rituals all need to be adjusted after ambiguous loss. We ask families: "What marital/family roles or tasks have you lost? What roles or tasks have you gained? Can you manage the change? Where do you need help?" Regarding family rules, we ask them who makes the decisions and plans for daily routines and for special occasions. We also ask if gender, race, age, class, or religion is affecting the ability to cope. We ask whether safety or economic security is an issue.

To assess family rituals, we ask what family and community celebrations, holiday events, and religious rituals they observed *before* their ambiguous loss. We also ascertain whether family members are adapting their usual rituals and celebrations *since* the ambiguous loss, as it is important that they continue. Finally, because community memorialization is so helpful to couples and families, we ask if there is such a place for them to go: "Does your community offer a place or symbol of remembrance to help you remember and honor your missing family member?" (See Robins, 2013; Saul, 2013.)

Six Guidelines for Strengthening Resilience in Families of the Missing

For the resiliency-based approach, we offer six research-based guidelines to help ease the lingering presence of stress and grief for the families suffering with the ambiguous loss. Brief descriptions are given for each of the six guidelines, but we encourage the reader to see Boss (2006) and its Japanese translation (Boss, 2015) or the German translation (Boss, 2008) for a deeper discussion of each guideline.

1. *Finding meaning:* What helps for finding meaning is to give the problem a name. We tell family members, individually as well as in groups: "What you are experiencing is ambiguous loss. It is one of the most difficult types of loss because there is no closure. It is not your fault."
   People cannot cope with a problem until they know what the problem is. Giving it a name (ambiguous loss) allows survivors to better understand this mysterious type of loss. Having a name eases their feelings of helplessness and blame (self or other) and allows the coping process to begin. Talking with others who are experiencing the same type of loss helps people learn the dialectic of *both–and* thinking. That is, they slowly learn to embrace the paradox of ambiguous loss: "She is probably dead, but maybe not," "He is gone, but still here sometimes in my thoughts and dreams." To find some measure of meaning in the meaninglessness of ambiguous loss, they give up on absolute thinking and accept the paradox. They learn to hold two opposing ideas in their minds at the same time.
2. *Adjusting mastery:* This guideline means helping individuals and families to adjust their sense of mastery and being in control when ambiguity persists.

Depending on family and community culture, the sense of mastery and control may need to be raised or lowered in order to find empowerment and safety after a family member disappears. What helps is to externalize the blame (the culprit is the ambiguity).

Because mastery is the opposite of helplessness, intervention guidelines are aimed at increasing the empowerment of disenfranchised, neglected, or abused family members so that they can begin to cope and adapt to their new situation. If, however, the survivors are already highly competent and mastery-oriented people, accustomed to solving all problems, we need to soften and temper their need for mastery in the face of ambiguous loss. Often, there are also gender differences regarding need for adjustment and empowerment. For the most part, however, a mastery orientation is a good thing (Boss, 2006, p. 98); as a consistent moderator of stress and trauma, it allows survivors to move forward with the tasks and relationships of everyday life. Finding some mastery and control in their lives, even after ambiguous loss, helps survivors feel less helpless.

To find mastery in the face of ambiguous loss, we recommend that families perform rituals; they are functional because they require actively doing something on behalf of the lost person. When the community also memorializes the missing, people know they are not alone, and they also have a place to go in lieu of a cemetery to honor and remember their lost person. For this reason alone, it is essential for families of the missing to be offered some type of ritual by the larger community. This recognition validates the loss and increases the survivor's sense of mastery in the face of utter helplessness.

If survivors continue to feel helpless and hopeless, we encourage them to begin mastering their *internal* selves through, depending on their culture and beliefs, meditation, prayer, mindfulness, physical activity, music (guitar playing as mentioned earlier), art, and dance, among others. Mastering a musical instrument or a drawing or simply being in prayer are ways many have lessened their sense of helplessness and thus gained mastery and resilience.

It is important to know, however, that not being allowed to be empowered or have a mastery orientation at all (e.g., discrimination, poverty, stigma, or imprisonment) can weaken that resiliency. For clinical work, this means empowering those family members whose voices have not been heard due to discrimination or confinement or intimidation and abuse. Women in patriarchal cultures, for example, whose husbands are kidnapped become neither wife nor widow, and thus are without status, agency, or power within what was their family. They are often abused. The intervention then is to increase their levels of mastery in order for them to survive. How do we do this when their families are at best, nonsupportive? These women are urged to gather together with other wives of missing husbands in a community group meeting where they are no longer isolated and thus can regain some measure of mastery over their own welfare (Robins, 2013). Their family of support becomes one of peers. While they may still live with their missing husband's family, they now have a psychological family that allows them to feel more in charge of their own destinies.

3. *Reconstructing identity:* This guideline concerns an identity that has been altered by having a relationship ruptured by ambiguous loss. To move forward, we counsel family members to practice performing new roles and reflect on who they are now that someone in the family is gone. We ask them to ask themselves: "Who am I now that a family member is missing? What new roles must I now perform to make up for the loss? Who is my family now? Have some people (nonrelatives) become like family to me now?"
   Over time, family members reflect on these questions as their identities change with age, with life experiences, and across the lifespan, as well as across the family life cycle. We ask family members: "Who are you now? Are you a widow or a widow waiting to happen? Are you still married?" It helps to redefine family and marital boundaries: who is in, who is out, and who plays what roles now. Staying connected with friends and making new social connections helps in this process of discovering identity after a loss. Being able to reconstruct identity after loss is a sign of flexibility and resilience.
4. *Normalizing ambivalence:* Recognize that family members might have some mixed emotions about the lost person. We suggest they talk with others (peer or professional) about their mixed emotions (love/hate, anger/sorrow) regarding the missing person. The negative emotions often cause unnecessary guilt and anxiety, but it is typical to "wish it was over," that a body would be found to bring some sense of closure to the tension. Once it is recognized that the ambivalence is the result of the ambiguity, and thus sociological and not psychiatric, then the tension of mixed emotions is more easily normalized and lowered to a manageable level. We normalize anger and guilt, but not harmful actions such as harming self or others by seeking retribution in cases where there may be a clear perpetrator.
5. *Revising attachment:* This requires the *both–and* approach of both letting go and remembering the lost person. We work with family members to recognize that their loved one is both here and gone and to grieve what was lost but also celebrate what they still have. We help them to join recreational or support groups and find social activities to develop new attachments so they do not stay isolated. No one they love is fully present all the time; nor are they fully absent, even after disappearance or death. They do not have to close them out of their lives. We support them to let go of the idea of closure and, instead, remember and honor them while also moving forward with life in a new way.
6. *Discovering new hope:* We remind readers that the six guidelines are not linear; thus discovering hope is not necessarily a last step. We see guidelines as process more than steps to be taken in a particular order. Families with missing loved ones often discover new hope in bits and pieces along the way of dealing with the other guidelines. Hope is tied to meaning and meaning to hope but mastery, identity, ambivalence, and attachment are essential components on the journey to discover both meaning and hope. It helps to become more comfortable with ambiguity, which for some is viewed as a type of spirituality; to at times laugh at the absurdity of ambiguous loss; to redefine justice because sometimes life is unfair and illogical; and with others, to imagine new options for a now altered

life. One can be both sad about the loss of a parent, for example, and also searching to find new connections and social support. The Japanese school boy whose father was lost in the 3/11 tsunami asked his teacher, Mr. K., for guitar lessons; later on, other boys joined in so that this group became a kind of psychological family, with the teacher being a kind of psychological father. Such human connection allows for the discovery of new meaning and hope and thus the ability of survivors to move forward despite their terrible losses.

The Need for Professional Self-Reflection

From our decades of experience working with families of the missing, we recognize that we cannot bring the families we work with further than we ourselves can go in tolerating ambiguity. Before we end this chapter, we emphasize that not just survivors, but those of us who work with them, must also consider the six guidelines just presented. We need to be clear about who we are as we work with families of the missing: "Who am I as I do this work? Is my family of origin relevant in how I respond to this work? What is my level of tolerance for ambiguity? Do I feel helpless if I cannot find a solution for the people I am trying to help?"

We therefore regularly reflect on our own losses, our meaning of them, our mastery, identity, ambivalence, attachment, and hope in spite of them. If we are to be effective in understanding and helping families experiencing ambiguous loss, we must first recognize and reflect on our own. They may not be as extreme as those we described in this chapter, but they can, nevertheless, be stressful and long term. We can learn from them how to work with the more extreme losses.

But first, we as scholars and professionals must increase our own tolerance for ambiguity, not an easy task for those of us trained to find answers, cure pain, solve problems, and fix what has been ruptured. Learning to live with an unanswered question is a new challenge.

Summary

Ambiguous loss is one of the most painful kinds of losses because there is no possibility of resolution or closure in the classic sense of resolution or completion in the fullness of time. Grief often continues for a lifetime, even across generations as with slavery, the World War II Holocaust (see Chap. 23, this volume), and likely with the more recent ambiguous losses from New York's 9/11 and East Japan's 3/11. The challenge then for researchers and practitioners is to discover ways to help people live well despite such irresolvable loss. Resilience in this case means increasing one's tolerance for ambiguity. Individuals and families learn to hold the ambiguity and become less distressed by the lack of closure.

What we have learned thus far is that the theory of ambiguous loss is a useful theory for easing the stress of "not knowing" where a loved one is or whether they are dead or alive (Boss, 2006; Robins, forthcoming special issue of *Journal of Family Theory & Review,* 2016). *First,* the theory helps researchers, practitioners, and laypersons to better understand the complexities of ambiguous loss and its effects—individually, relationally, and systemically. *Second,* while further testing in progress, globally, research thus far indicates that despite the lack of knowing where a loved one is, the theory of ambiguous loss is useful in Eastern as well as Western cultures (Robins, 2010, 2013). *Third,* ambiguous loss theory enables practitioners to help people move forward with their lives despite the pain of ambiguous loss by holding the two opposing ideas of absence and presence in their minds at the same time. Resilience increases with acceptance of paradox: "My loved one is probably dead—and maybe not. She or he is physically gone and yet, psychologically still here." *Fourth,* having the name for a pain—in this case, ambiguous loss—allows people to begin the essential processes of coping and grieving even without a validated death.

Finally, applying the six guidelines for resilience, in any order, helps survivors live reasonably good lives despite ambiguous loss. They find that holding two opposing ideas simultaneously is an effective way to cope with the long-term stress of "not knowing." Thinking of a missing person as both here and gone may be as close to the truth as they can ever get. By accepting this dialectic, people are more able to find meaning and thus resilience to live reasonably good lives despite their loved one's disappearance. This is the good news.

References

American Psychiatric Association. (2013). *Diagnostic and statistical manual of mental disorders* (5th ed.). Washington, DC: American Psychiatric Association.

Boss, P. (1977). A clarification of the concept of psychological father presence in families experiencing ambiguity of boundary. *Journal of Marriage & the Family, 39*(1), 141–151.

Boss, P. (1980). The relationship of psychological father presence, wife's personal qualities, and wife/family dysfunction in families of missing fathers. *Journal of Marriage & the Family, 42*(3), 541–549.

Boss, P. (1987). Family stress: Perception and context. In M. Sussman & S. Steinmetz (Eds.), *Handbook of marriage and family* (pp. 695–723). New York: Plenum.

Boss, P. (1992). Primacy of perception in family stress theory and measurement. *Journal of Family Psychology, 6*(2), 113–119.

Boss, P. (1999). *Ambiguous loss: Learning to live with unresolved grief.* Cambridge: Harvard University Press.

Boss, P. (1988/2002). *Family stress management: A contextual approach* (1st & 2nd eds.). Thousand Oaks: Sage.

Boss, P. (2004). Ambiguous loss research, theory, and practice: Reflections after 9/11. *Journal of Marriage & Family, 66*(3), 551–566.

Boss, P. (2006). *Loss, trauma, and resilience: Therapeutic work with ambiguous loss.* New York: Norton.

Boss, P. (2007). Ambiguous loss theory: Challenges for scholars and practitioners [Special issue.] *Family Relations, 56*(2), 105–111.
Boss, P. (2008). *Verlust, trauma, und resilience* [Loss, trauma, and resilience]. (A. Hildenbrand, trans.). Stuttgart: Klett-Cotta.
Boss, P. (2011). *Loving someone who has dementia: How to find hope while coping with stress and grief.* San Francisco: Jossey-Bass.
Boss, P. (2012). The ambiguous loss of dementia: A relational view of complicated grief in caregivers. In M. O'Reilly-Landry (Ed.), *A psychodynamic understanding of modern medicine: Placing the person at the center of care* (pp. 183–193). London: Radcliffe.
Boss, P. (2015). *Aimaina sooshitsu to torauma karano kaifuku: Kazoku to komyuniti no rejiriensu* [Loss, trauma, and resilience: Therapeutic work with ambiguous loss]. (S. Nakajima & C. Ishii, trans.). Tokyo: Seishin Shobo.
Boss, P., & Carnes, D. (2012). The myth of closure. *Family Process, 51*(4), 456–460.
Boss, P., & Dahl, C. M. (2014). Family therapy for the unresolved grief of ambiguous loss. In D. W. Kissane & F. Parnes (Eds.), *Bereavement care for families* (pp. 171–182). New York: Routledge.
Boss, P., & Greenberg, J. (1984). Family boundary ambiguity: A new variable in family stress theory. *Family Process, 23*(4), 535–546.
Boss, P., & Kaplan, L. (2004). Ambiguous loss and ambivalence when a parent has dementia. In K. Pillemer & K. Luescher (Eds.), *Intergenerational ambivalences: New perspectives on parent-child relations in later life* (pp. 207–224). Oxford: Elsevier.
Boss, P., & Yeats, J. R. (2014). Ambiguous loss: A complicated type of grief when loved ones disappear. *Bereavement Care, 33*(2), 63–69.
Boss, P., Caron, W., Horbal, J., & Mortimer, J. (1990). Predictors of depression in caregivers of dementia patients: Boundary ambiguity and mastery. *Family Process, 29,* 245–254.
Boss, P., Beaulieu, L., Wieling, E., Turner, W., & LaCruz, S. (2003). Healing loss, ambiguity, and trauma: A community-based intervention with families of union workers missing after the 9/11 attack in New York City. *Journal of Marital & Family Therapy, 29*(4), 455–467.
Cherry, K. E., & Smith, A. D. (1998). Normal memory aging. In M. Hersen & V. B. Van Hasselt (Eds.), *Handbook of clinical geropsychology* (pp. 87–110). New York: Plenum.
Don Productions TV. (20 July 2013). *Wisdom to survive a tsunami. Professor Toshitaka Katada interview*. [Video file]. https://www.youtube.com/watch?v=dbnz0FZU73Q. Accessed 25 June 2015.
Fackler, D. (11 March 2011). Powerful quake and tsunami devastate Northern Japan. *The New York Times*. http://www.nytimes.com/2011/03/12/world/asia/12japan.html?pagewanted=all&_r=1&. Accessed 25 June 2015.
Ishii, C. (1996). The language of grief in today's Japan. *Theologia-Diakonia, 30,* 225–236.
Ishii, C., & Setou, N. (2014). Kazoku ryohoni motoduku "aimaina soshitsu" eno shien: Fukushimani okeru shiensha shienno keiken kara [Support for "ambiguous loss" based on family therapy: Through our experience of helping aid workers in Fukushima]. *Japanese Journal of Family Therapy, 31*(1), 101–105.
Ito, S. (26 March 2011). Japan's tsunami defences brutally exposed. *Asiaone*. http://news.asiaone.com/News/Latest%2BNews/Asia/Story/A1Story20110326-270285.html. Accessed 25 June 2015.
Klass, D. (1996). Grief in an Eastern culture: Japanese ancestor worship. In D. Klass, P. R. Silverman, & S. L. Nickman (Eds.), *Continuing bonds: New understandings of grief* (pp. 59–72). New York: Taylor & Francis.
Malaysia Airlines plane, flight MH370, goes missing (7 March 2014). *Huffington Post*. http://www.huffingtonpost.com/2014/03/07/malaysian-airlines-plane-_n_4922705.html. Accessed 25 June 2015.
National Police Agency of Japan. (10 July 2014). *Damage situation and police countermeasures associated with 2011 Tohoku District—off the Pacific Ocean Earthquake*. https://www.npa.go.jp/archive/keibi/biki/higaijokyo_e.pdf. Accessed 25 June 2015.

Neimeyer, R. A., Harris, D. L., Winokuer, H., & Thornton, G. F. (Eds.). (2011). *Grief and bereavement in contemporary society*. New York: Routledge.

NHK (Producer). (2013). *Kamaishi no kiseki: Kodomo ga kataru 3.11* [Kamaishi Miracle: 3.11.: Children talk about what they experienced on 3.11] [DVD]. Japan: Producer.

Onishi, T., & Ishiwatari, M. (2012). *Urban planning, land use regulation & relocation*. Washington, DC: World Bank Group. http://wbi.worldbank.org/wbi/Data/wbi/wbicms/files/drupal-acquia/wbi/drm_kn2-7.pdf. Accessed 26 June 2015.

Robins, S. (2010). Ambiguous loss in a non-Western context: Families of the disappeared in post-conflict Nepal. *Family Relations, 59*, 253–268.

Robins, S. (2013). *Families of the missing: A test for contemporary approaches to transitional justice*. New York/London: Routledge Glasshouse.

Robins, S. (2014). Constructing meaning from disappearance: Local memorialisation of the missing in Nepal. *International Journal of Conflict and Violence, 8*(1). http://www.ijcv.org/earlyview/342.pdf. Accessed 25 June 2015.

Robins, S. (2016). Discursive approaches to ambiguous loss: Theorizing community-based therapy after enforced disappearance. *Journal of Family Theory & Review*. (Manuscript in preparation).

Saul, J. (2013). *Collective trauma, collective healing: Promoting community resilience in the aftermath of disaster*. New York: Routledge.

Sashida, K. (2013). *Tsunami tendenko: Hashire, ue ni!* [At the time of Tsunami, run high upward]. Tokyo: Popura-sha.

Sato, K. (2014). Nihonno shamanisumu to shisha tono koryu [Shamans possessed by the spirits of the dead in Japanese shamanism]. *Annual of The Institute of Thanatology, Toyo Eiwa University, 10*, 91–110.

Takahashi, H. (2014). Darega hanashio kikunoka: Hisaichini okeru reino hanashi to shukyosha [Who listens to their stories?: How religious professionals are dealing with occult phenomena in the Great East Japan Earthquake Disaster area]. *Annual of The Institute of Thanatology, Toyo Eiwa University, 10*, 237–254.

Une, T. (2014). Machi wa hosupisu ni narenaika: Hisaichi de kea ni tazusawatte mietekita koto [Can a town be a hospice?: What we discovered from providing psychologist and spiritual care in the earthquake disaster area]. *Annual of The Institute of Thanatology, Toyo Eiwa University, 10*, 255–271.

Valenti, J. (16 Sept 2013). Victim of 9/11 attacks on WTC identified. *Newsday*. http://www.newsday.com/news/new-york/victim-of-9-11-attacks-on-wtc-identified-1.6082613. Accessed 25 June 2015.

Wakefield, J., Ito, K., Toshio, A., Swanson, K., Revell, M., & Klein, P. (2013). National identity case study: How do disasters affect the construction of place identity? In Solem, M., Klein, P., Muñiz-Solari, O., & Ray, W., (Eds)., *AAG center for global geography education*. http://www.aag.org/cgge. Accessed 29 June 2015.

Yanagida, K., & Suzuki, I. (Aug 2014). Hitowa naze "yurei" o mirunoka [Why people see "ghosts"?]. *Bungei Shunju*, 338–345.

Yoshimura, H. (21 March 2011). City's concrete 'protector' fails to stop killer tsunami. *The Asahi Shimbun*. http://ajw.asahi.com/article/0311disaster/quake_tsunami/AJ201103213218. Accessed 26 June 2015.

Part III
Healing after Trauma: Resilience and Long-Term Recovery

Chapter 16
Aging with Trauma Across the Lifetime and Experiencing Trauma in Old Age: Vulnerability and Resilience Intertwined

Yuval Palgi, Amit Shrira and Dov Shmotkin

Introduction

During their lifetime, most people are exposed to at least a few occurrences of traumatic, or potentially traumatic, events (Breslau et al., 1998; Norris, 1992; Shmotkin & Litwin, 2009). According to criterion A of the Diagnostic and Statistical Manual (DSM, 5th edition; American Psychiatric Association, 2013), a traumatic event may occur when the individual is exposed to, witnesses, or learns about actual or threatened death, serious injury, or sexual violence. These events may occur directly to the person himself/herself or to others. Adverse conditions that do not ostensibly meet the DSM criterion A (e.g., experiencing severe economic deprivation, providing long-term care to a severely disabled family member) may be potentially traumatizing if they pervasively and chronically disrupt one's ability to meet essential needs and goals (Bonanno, Westphal, & Mancini, 2011). In most cases, these exposures do not lead to a justifiable diagnosis of posttraumatic stress disorder (PTSD; Breslau, Peterson, Poisson, Schultz, & Lucia, 2004; Kessler, Sonnega, Bromet, Hughes, & Nelson, 1995). However, for many, such exposures bear long-lasting consequences on physical and mental health, as evident in later life (Keinan, Shrira, & Shmotkin, 2012; Krause, 2009). Nevertheless, alongside its deleterious consequences, traumatic experiences may also be associated with resilience (Seery, Holman, & Silver, 2010; Shmotkin, 2003; Shrira, Palgi, Ben-Ezra, & Shmotkin, 2011b). The body of

Y. Palgi (✉)
Department of Gerontology and the Center for Research and Study of Aging, University of Haifa, 199 Aba Khoushy Ave., Mount Carmel, Haifa, 3498838, Israel
e-mail: ypalgi@research.haifa.ac.il

A. Shrira
Interdisciplinary Department of Social Sciences, Bar-Ilan University, Ramat Gan, 52900, Israel
e-mail: amit.shrira@biu.ac.il

D. Shmotkin
School of Psychological Sciences and the Herczeg Institute on Aging, Tel Aviv University, Tel Aviv 69978, Israel
e-mail: shmotkin@post.tau.ac.il

K. E. Cherry (ed.), *Traumatic Stress and Long-Term Recovery*,
DOI 10.1007/978-3-319-18866-9_16

literature on these topics often interchanges, or even confuses, related experiences or events such as trauma, traumatic stress, potential trauma, and adversity. Therefore, for the sake of clarity, we opted to use in this chapter the term "trauma" in its broad sense, denoting a presumably forceful experience or event that one perceives as an overwhelming threat to one's life or to one's physical and mental integrity.

For many years, the psychiatric literature paid little attention to the consequences of early-life, as well as late-life, traumatic experiences in older adults' lives. Also, it was common to overlook real differences of manifest traumatic symptoms existing in younger versus older age (Thorp & Blazer, 2012). For example, certain symptoms accounting for PTSD according to the DSM-5 (e.g., inability to remember an important aspect of a traumatic event, diminished interest in significant activities, sleep disturbance, and problems with concentration; American Psychiatric Association, 2013) may overlap in old age with aging-related symptoms. Possibly, this insufficient sensitivity to the impact of age indicated that developmental trajectories of traumatic reactions among adults were not taken into account (Scott, Poulin, & Silver, 2013). It seems that the perception of trauma in old age is typically "age centric" because it is shaped from a young adult perspective.

Due to the demographically expanding segment of older individuals in the population, it becomes even more imperative to better understand what characterizes traumatic and posttraumatic reactions in old age (Shenk, Ramos, Kalaw, & Tufan, 2009). Moreover, it is questioned whether the fusion of traumatic experiences and aging processes can be explained in terms of positive human adaptation. Presenting the *pursuit of happiness in a hostile world* model (Shmotkin, 2005, 2011), we aim, in this chapter, to address the interrelated roles of vulnerability and resilience among individuals who age while still bearing past experiences of trauma, or otherwise facing trauma that typically occurs in old age.

How Is Trauma Across the Lifetime Manifested in Old Age?

The literature presents two differing perspectives concerning the manifestation of lifetime trauma in old age. The first is the psychiatric–epidemiological perspective, which seeks differences between younger and older adults mainly in the *levels* (i.e., severity) of PTSD symptoms. Following this perspective, it was suggested that older adults presented similar levels of symptoms as those reported among younger adults (Bleich, Gelkopf, Melamed, & Solomon, 2005). However, in a longitudinal study, Yehuda (2009) found that posttraumatic symptoms decreased with age among older adults who endorsed PTSD, with the greatest decline revealed in intrusive thoughts and the survivor's guilt (Averill & Back, 2000; Lapp, Agbokou, & Ferreri, 2011).

The second perspective is psychological–developmental, claiming that developmental processes along the life span shape the nature of the trauma in late life. According to this perspective, posttraumatic reactions join to aging processes in creating certain modes by which traumatized people survive to old age. In this vein,

Shmotkin, Shrira, and Palgi (2011) delineated three cardinal modes: dementia-molded survival, embattled survival, and robust survival.

Dementia-molded survival refers to older adults with cognitive dysfunction due to dementia. For these persons, the dementia seems to reshape their traumatic memories while, in turn, the traumatic memories are presumably operative in the development and manifestations of dementia (Burnes & Burnette, 2013). As traumatic remnants are mostly embodied in memory, two trajectories regarding this mode are available. In the first one, dementia-related deterioration of memory blurs, and consequently relieves, the long-lasting, agonizing experience of trauma (Kensinger, 2006). In the second trajectory, the traumatic stress is intensified by dementia because common regulatory mechanisms are undermined, and formerly controlled traumatic memories are thus disinhibited (Butters & Delis, 1995; Cook, Ruzek, & Cassidy, 2003).

The mode of *embattled survival* refers to cognitively intact older adults, for whom traumatic events that occurred during their lives have an accumulating detrimental effect on their late-life adaptation (Kraaij & De Wilde, 2001). For these older adults, the lingering trauma may induce accelerating aging processes that intensify physical and mental frailty (Shrira, 2012, 2014; Shrira & Litwin, 2014). Lingering trauma, in this mode, may appear as a chronic condition (Averill & Beck, 2000), possibly in the form of PTSD.

Robust survival refers to older adults who exhibit good adaptation relative to their age, despite their past trauma. This mode is compatible with evidence that older persons do not differ from, or are even more resilient than, younger adults in their reactions to trauma (Bleich et al., 2005), and show relatively low symptom levels even after high trauma exposure (Schnurr, Spiro, Vielhauer, Findler, & Hamblen, 2002). This potential inoculation in old age can be explained by the maturity and experience that come with age (Hyer & Sacks, 2008), as well as by the underestimated reserves of resilience that traumatized people can sustain in old age (Ryff, Friedman, Morozink, & Tsenkova, 2012).

To sum, whereas the psychiatric–epidemiological perspective focuses mainly on age-related changes in levels of symptoms, the psychological–developmental perspective dwells on presumable processes operating behind the symptoms along the course of time. In fact, review studies on older adults found inconclusive results regarding the long-lasting effect of trauma (Böttche, Kuwert, & Knaevelsrud, 2012; Shenk et al., 2009). In the chapter, we further pursue the psychological–developmental perspective in order to examine the mechanisms that mingle issues of trauma and aging.

Aging Trauma Versus Trauma in Old Age

We define *aging trauma* as *a distal traumatic experience or event that happened at an earlier point in the life span, but is still activated in one's aging process*. On the other hand, *trauma in old age* is *a proximal traumatic experience or event that happened when one was already old and often in the context of aging-related contingencies* (Martin, da Rosa, & Poon, 2011). These two types of experiences present different, but not mutually exclusive, trajectories of trauma.

Aging trauma may exacerbate, or otherwise inoculate, one's adaptation to aging. Often, it incorporates a number of events that involve life course chains of adversity (e.g., poverty, engaging in skirmishes, drug abuse, problems with the law, early marriage, occupational instability, divorce, social isolation), which placed a person at a greater risk to further deterioration in old age (Pearlin, Schieman, Fazio, & Meersman, 2005). This cumulative effect may be exponential when a primary event leads to a secondary event. Moreover, the fact that the primary experience has been intensified challenges the individual's ability to adjust to stress, especially in old age when adaptation mechanisms may be less flexible. The *cumulative inequality theory* (Ferraro & Shippee, 2009) takes a life-span perspective that might be relevant to understanding aging trauma. This theory proposes that social systems (class, race, income), as well as personal exposure to risk, generate inequality between individuals that accumulates across the life span. Hence, trauma occurring at young age, besides taxing one's functioning at the time, may also create ruptures in abilities and resources that perpetuate inequality of functioning levels up to the particularly demanding period of old age. In contrast, other findings showed that aging trauma may enhance better preparedness for the challenges of aging. Thus, research showed that aging Holocaust survivors showed general resilience in their adaptation and only specific vulnerabilities in part of their functioning (Amir & Lev-Wiesel, 2003; Barel, Van IJzendoorn, Sagi-Schwartz, & Bakermans-Kranenburg, 2010; Shmotkin & Lomranz, 1998; Shmotkin, Blumstein, & Modan, 2003; Shrira, Palgi, Ben-Ezra, & Shmotkin, 2011a).

Aging trauma is often reprocessed through the task of *life review* whereby older adults integrate their past experiences in a coherent way (Butler, 1963; Erikson, 1998). This task provides another opportunity to narrate, and thus transform and integrate, the past trauma into one's identity-defined life story (Maercker, 2002; Pals & McAdams, 2004). The idea of treating present traumatic symptoms by retelling and reconstructing past events is well documented in the trauma literature (see, e.g., Palgi & Ben-Ezra, 2010; Palgi, Palgi, Ben-Ezra, & Shrira, 2014). Indeed, older individuals are better off if they are able to contrast their past suffering with their present well-being and formulate a life story where the trauma is demarcated and controlled (see Chap. 23, this volume). These mechanisms appear empirically intricate. Thus, while Holocaust survivors were found to be less able than controls to separate between their most miserable period in the past and their present life satisfaction, there were still survivors who were able to better separate between suffering in other periods and their present life satisfaction (Shrira & Shmotkin, 2008). Also, Holocaust survivors were found to maintain a higher subjective well-being (SWB) if they could deflate their emotional investment in the Holocaust period of their life while strengthening their emotional investment in non-Holocaust periods (Cohen & Shmotkin, 2007).

Furthermore, one's time perspective can either help or hinder coping with the challenges of aging. For example, it was found that the best-functioning participants in very advanced age were those whose time trajectory appeared stable, meaning that they could make their past experiences and future expectations correspond with their present experience (Palgi & Shmotkin, 2010). Traumatized older adults, however, may find it hard to do this integration. Separating the survivors into those who conceived the Holocaust *as past* and those who conceived the Holocaust *as present,* showed that those in the former category were able to draw an effective line between the traumatic past and their present, thus allowing themselves to move forward (Shmotkin & Barilan, 2002).

Summing together the previously mentioned studies suggests that aging trauma, by its nature, keeps the traumatic remnants of the past active through interaction with one's aging processes in ways that either ameliorate or aggravate the lingering endurance of the trauma during late life.

Unlike aging trauma, *trauma in old age* represents a usually proximal traumatic experience or event that occurs after one's aging processes have evolved. Naturally, the typical declines of old age may restrict the vigor and scope with which older adults encounter newly experienced traumas (Bei et al., 2013),. In this case, aging-related phenomena may serve as moderators of the occurrence. For example, it was found that among American older adults, exposure to Hurricane Sandy (which hit the US East Coast in 2012) was associated with PTSD symptoms to a higher degree for those who reported stronger fear of aging (Palgi, Shrira, Goodwin, Hamama-Raz, & Ben-Ezra, 2014).

Yet, not in line with lay notions, older adults largely exhibit a better emotional regulation and a stronger bias for positivity (Mather & Carstensen, 2005). This old-age resilience is further supported by the tendency of older adults to retain positive, meaningful social interactions (Carstensen, Isaacowitz, & Charles, 1999). Hence, despite the expectation to see much frailty in old age, older adults may appear surprisingly potent in front of exposure to current traumas (Böttche et al., 2012). In this vein, post-disaster psychopathology is generally lower among older adults (Norris, Kaniasty, Conrad, Inman, & Murphy, 2002; Shrira, Palgi, Hamama-Raz, Goodwin & Ben-Ezra, 2014).

Studies that examined the effect of *age* at the time of the exposure to trauma found that older adults who experienced their most distressing traumatic event during childhood exhibited higher symptoms of PTSD and lower subjective happiness compared with those who experienced their most distressing event after the transition to adulthood (Ogle, Rubin, Berntsen, & Siegler, 2013; Ogle, Rubin, & Siegler, 2014). However, some studies indicated that traumatic events that occurred at young adulthood and midlife, compared to other life periods, were stronger predictors of negative posttraumatic outcomes in old age (Dulin & Passmore, 2010; Krause, 2005). Another study showed that events experienced after 50 years of age are most detrimental for late-life mental health (Shrira, Shmotkin, & Litwin, 2012). The aforementioned findings, which present examples of aging trauma in our current term, point to the importance of *timing* in traumatization, and yet they are not conclusive. Even less is known about the timing effect of trauma during old age (Palgi, Gelkopf, & Berger, 2015), as the temporal boundary between aging trauma and trauma in old age may in some cases be blurred because aging itself is socially constructed, with no clear start point that is immanently felt by individuals.

Overall, our proposed distinction between aging trauma and trauma in old age may facilitate a closer inspection of the dynamics underlying each kind of experience. In the case of aging trauma, the various aging processes have to accommodate one's handling of the lingering traumatic narrative, whereas in the case of trauma in old age, the relatively recent traumatic narrative often appears assimilated within one's aging processes. While overlaps of the two kinds of trauma are evident, the suggested difference between the two becomes clearer in view of the typical themes associated with each. Aging trauma often relates to events such as childhood deprivations, sexual abuse, wars and violent conflicts, car and occupational accidents, or breakup of marriage and close relationships (see Chap. 9, this volume for discussion of early childhood adversity). In comparison, trauma in old age typically relates to late-life events such as bereavement and widowhood, major debilitating and life-threatening diseases, caregiving, and dependency due to loss of vital functions.

Resilience Versus Vulnerability: Which One Prevails?

As implied in the previous discussion, the gerontological literature dealing with the contradiction of vulnerability versus resilience in coping with trauma suggests two competing hypotheses. The *vulnerability hypothesis* (Shrira et al., 2014; Solomon & Ginzburg, 1998) argues that older adults constitute an at-risk group with regard to the impact of trauma due to the age-related decline in functioning and the depletion of physical, social, and financial resources. In contrast, the *inoculation hypothesis* (Eysenck, 1983; Lapp et al., 2011) argues that older adults are less vulnerable to trauma than younger counterparts due to a better emotional regulation, higher maturity, and longer life experience (Hyer & Sacks, 2008; Urry & Gross, 2010).

Nevertheless, these two hypotheses are not mutually exclusive and sometimes complement each other. One kind of resilience is *posttraumatic growth,* referring to a positive psychological change that occurs as a result of a struggle with the consequences of a traumatic exposure. Such change is manifested by a new meaning in one's perspective on life, enhanced personal strength, and better relations to others (Tedeschi & Calhoun, 2004; see Chap. 17, this volume, for a related discussion). However, studies have suggested a paradoxical "double-edge sword" association between higher posttraumatic stress and higher posttraumatic growth (Boals & Schuettler, 2011). The intricate links between vulnerability and resilience were also exposed in studies of massive trauma such as the Holocaust, showing that it is nearly impossible to disentangle resilience and vulnerability within the individual survivors (Shmotkin, 2003; Shmotkin, Shrira, Goldberg, & Palgi, 2011). However, research sheds light on specific moderating variables that may determine whether resilience or vulnerability prevails. Certain variables of this kind are mentioned next.

In line with the aforementioned inoculation hypothesis, *prior exposure* strengthens resilience in face of current trauma. For example, a recent study showed that older adults, who reported to have experienced lower levels of traumatic events, found it harder to cope with first-time exposure to rocket attacks at the south of Israel, compared to those who had previously experienced higher levels of traumatic events (Palgi et al., 2015). Similarly, American older adults who had had a low level of exposure to the World Trade Center terrorist attacks on September 11, 2001, reported higher PTSD symptoms following Hurricane Sandy that occurred 11 years later (Shrira et al., 2014). While these studies suggest that older adults tend to rely on successful coping with previous traumatic experiences when confronting a new potential trauma, younger adults, on the other hand, may use other resources that are more easily available to them, such as broader social support and greater flexibility in response to stressors.

Another moderating variable that may explain the relative prevalence of resilience versus vulnerability is the *quantitative aspect of the trauma*. Thus, findings showed that the accumulation (i.e., the number) of lifetime adversities is associated with decline, as well as with continuous impairment, in major markers of physical, cognitive, and psychological health at the second half of life (Shrira, 2012, 2014; Shrira & Litwin, 2014). On the other hand, the mere exposure to a single traumatic event, even if extreme in its nature, may still leave easier ways to mobilize coping mechanisms and focus them on the particular experience (Averill & Beck, 2000; Böttche et al., 2012; Lapp et al., 2011). These findings are in line with the dose–response model, which posits that the extent of repeated exposures to a traumatic event has a specific impact on the trauma's sequelae (March, 1993). Notably, this experiential dose of cumulative life adversity is not necessarily linear in its effect on functioning outcomes (i.e., the highest dose of exposure may not generate the strongest impact), and it may be associated not only with a stronger distress (as usually expected) but also with eventually enhanced well-being (Keinan et al., 2012).

Still another moderating variable relating to the prevalence of resilience versus vulnerability is the *durational aspect of the trauma*. Whereas individuals can recover from prolonged exposure to trauma occurring in young age (Brom, Durst, & Aghassy, 2002; Shrira et al., 2011a), prolonged exposure to trauma occurring in old age tends to prove more deleterious due to lower flexibility and plasticity of the nervous system and the behavioral repertoire in late life (Charles, 2010; Charles & Piazza, 2009). Research has shown that prolonged chronic stressors are associated with increased morbidity and mortality (Troxel, Matthews, Bromberger, & Sutton-Tyrrell, 2003). These findings are in line with the *allostatic load theory,* which postulates that frequent activation of the body's stress response, while essential for managing acute threats, can damage the body in the long run (McEwen, 1998; see Chap. 9, this volume, for related discussion). Furthermore, several studies conducted among Israelis exposed to prolonged missile attacks for years found age to be positively associated with PTSD symptoms (Dekel & Nuttman-Shwartz, 2009; Gelkopf, Berger, Bleich, & Silver, 2012).

Mechanisms That Help Older Adults Deal with Trauma

It is curious to identify the coping mechanisms that older adults use in order to adjust to aging trauma, or trauma in old age, while handling the common burdens of aging. In fact, we have presented here certain mechanisms stemming from larger adaptational strategies that become particularly vital for sustaining the mental health of older people. The aforementioned strategies include the formulation of one's life story, the adoption of a time perspective on one's life course, and the emotional regulation that improves with age. Next, we address several more mechanisms of particular relevance.

Selection, Optimization, and Compensation Baltes (1997) maintained that in old age, the incomplete segment in the architecture of human development is getting larger, as optimal functioning is doomed to disruption by irreparable biological dysfunctions. Nevertheless, psychological mechanisms such as selection, optimization, and compensation may attenuate this process. Moreover, these mechanisms are not overwhelmed by physical deterioration and may even gain power among older adults who were exposed to traumatic events. In a later conceptual development, the *socioemotional selectivity theory* (Carstensen et al., 1999) claims that, in the face of shorter time horizons, people optimize their priorities regarding their emotional goals. While young adults invest their efforts in knowledge-related goals, older adults adopt goals related to emotional regulation (Carstensen et al., 1999). Thus, older adults focus more on positive emotional experiences and less on negative ones (Charles, Mather, & Carstensen, 2003), and select particularly positive and meaningful social interactions (Carstensen, 1995; Carstensen et al., 1999). This positivity bias of older adults (Mather & Carstensen, 2005) can attenuate, to some degree, the negative consequences of trauma, provided that the trauma does not disrupt irrevocably one's primary adaptational resources, notably the supportive social networks (Isaacowitz, Smith, & Carstensen, 2003).

Wisdom According to Baltes and Staudinger (2000), wisdom is defined as a person's expertise in the fundamental pragmatics of life. That is, wisdom entails abilities of retaining knowledge and exercising judgment about the essence of the human condition, as well as conceived ways as to how people might best plan, manage, and understand the lives they lead within the context of whatever values they hold important. Wisdom does not refer to intellectual or acquired academic knowledge, but rather to insight into human nature and the ability to resolve life complexities through practical experiences and personal reflections. Unlike cognitive functioning that decreases with age, wisdom is appropriate for aging-related developmental tasks as it frequently remains intact in old age.

Wisdom has been shown to be related to stress and posttraumatic growth (Webster & Deng, in press). Similarly, Linley (2003) has suggested that adaptation to traumatic exposure requires recognition and management of uncertainty, integration of affect and cognition, and the awareness and acceptance of human limitations. Arguably, adaptation to traumatic exposure also requires an effortful reconstruction of world assumptions, such as living in a benevolent and predictable world, which are often utterly shattered by trauma (Janoff-Bulman, 1992; Webster & Deng, in press). Older adults may be particularly in need of integrating and stitching together non-cohesive parts of their perceptions regarding human nature and themselves. One manifestation of wisdom in old age is understanding the dialectical nature of the world after experiencing trauma. This ability to withstand contradictions and paradoxes in life is explicated in the *aintegration theory* (Lomranz, 2005). Following this conception, wisdom among older adults facilitates adjustment to trauma by the ability to reconcile with unbridgeable parts of the self, such as a devastating trauma and everyday life.

Maturity Older adults may benefit from their maturity of personality and lifelong experience. Maturity is attained from innate and psychological growth propensities that tend to promote one's positive developmental changes over time (Sheldon & Kasser, 2001). It was suggested that maturity is gained by succeeding in completing age-related developmental tasks (Erikson, 1998). Lifelong personality processes indicate that older individuals may be more psychologically mature, and that this maturation mediates the relationship between age and well-being (Sheldon & Kasser, 2001). Young–old individuals, for example, have shown better emotional functioning after exposure to earthquake compared to midlife participants. However, this age difference was also presented prior to the earthquake (Knight, Gatz, Heller, & Bengston, 2000). Therefore, it is possible that the effect of maturity may sometimes interweave with inoculation effect related to exposure to past traumatic events (Shrira et al., 2014).

Maturity may improve one's coping with trauma in old age as maturity provides older adults with several advantages. First, maturity stems from experience. Most older adults experienced in their lifetime successful coping with harsh challenges that strengthened their sense of resilience (Shenk et al., 2009), optimized the buffering effect of these successes for emotionally hard times (Blazer & Hybels, 2005), and provided useful lessons concerning how to tackle traumatic events at hand (Hyer & Sacks, 2008). Apart from relying on beneficial experience, maturity overlaps the notion of wisdom in the ability to acknowledge the complexities of life as well as facilitates a positive outlook of hope and happiness (King & Hicks, 2007; see also Chap. 17, this volume). As suggested previously, all these features constitute assets of coping with trauma.

Proposing a Unifying Model: The Pursuit of Happiness in a Hostile World

So far, our review has detailed multiple pieces of knowledge on trauma in older adults, but it still needs a unifying conceptual framework to put these pieces in. Next, we present a broadened version of the *pursuit of happiness in a hostile world* model, proposed earlier by Shmotkin (2005, 2011; Shmotkin & Shrira, 2012, 2013).

By this model, we seek to further understand resilience and vulnerability trajectories regarding the experience of trauma by older adults. We suggest that getting older elevates the salience of self-beliefs concerning actual or potential threats to one's life or, more broadly, to one's physical and mental integrity. These threats may include war, natural disasters, accidents, critical illness, loss of functional independence, bereavement and separation of loved ones, breakup of close relationships, violence and crime, and imminent death. Nourished by further representations of traumatic catastrophes, these perceived threats collectively form an image of adversity termed by Shmotkin (2005) as the *hostile-world scenario* (HWS). When activated adaptively, the HWS helps the individual to keep vigilant and prudent in the struggle to remain safe and well. Thus, the HWS usually functions as a system that scans and appraises any potentiality of a negative condition, or an even worse condition when a negative one already prevails. Nevertheless, under certain situations, an excessive activation of the HWS may generate a disturbing sense of precarious living in a disastrous world. Along with aging, the activation of this scenario is expected to increase in various ways. First, real threats that characterize old age (e.g., disease, death of spouse and close friends, elder abuse) may come up. Second, the aforementioned, life review process may sensitize unresolved traumas of the past. Finally, cognitive impairment processes may intensify traumatic emotional memories, both distal and proximal, due to increasing neurological deficits in the functions of emotional inhibition and regulation (Budson et al., 2004).

According to the presented model, the HWS is complementary to, and interactive with, positively oriented systems that provide individuals with a favorable psychological environment (Shmotkin & Shrira, 2012; Shrira et al., 2011b). Such positive systems notably include SWB (people's evaluations of the satisfaction and pleasantness in their life) and *meaning in life* (MIL; people's conceptions that they lead a life corresponding to their values and potentials). Humans are geared to seek both SWB (Diener, Lucas, & Scollon, 2006) and MIL (Frankl, 1963). Evidently, the various strategies and mechanisms discussed earlier as essential for coping with trauma (e.g., regulating the dominance of positive over negative emotions, establishing a life story and the temporal perspective of one's life, exercising optimization and wisdom) are closely interwoven with derivatives of both SWB and MIL.

By employing the counteracting, or ameliorating, effects of SWB and MIL over the HWS, older adults largely succeed in living normal lives at a period of overall functional decline. This achievement is made possible due to the dynamic and agentic features of the systems explicated in our guiding model (Busseri & Sadava, 2013). Thus, the model proclaims that one's HWS and the favorable psychological environment (the latter being induced by SWB and MIL) can attenuate each other according to the adaptational demands of the situation (Palgi, 2013; Shmotkin & Shrira, 2013). This reciprocal relationship resolves the unsettling contradiction between the intimidating and merciless world represented by the HWS on the one hand, and people's efforts to sustain generally happy and meaningful lives on the other hand. Moreover, SWB and MIL work as complementary systems (amplifying each other) and compensatory systems (replacing each other). Thus, SWB can make a traumatic experience more manageable by letting individuals evaluate their lives as basically favorable, whereas MIL can make a traumatic experience more interpretable by letting individuals conceive their lives in comprehensible terms. In other words, SWB *regulates* the HWS, whereas MIL *reconstructs* it (Shmotkin & Shrira, 2012). As revealed in different studies, these two functions may substitute for each other in case of need. For example, when either SWB or MIL is low, the other one takes a stronger role in moderating the deleterious effect of cumulative adversity on one's functioning (Shrira et al., 2011b).

Despite the basically adaptive function of the HWS in monitoring potential adversity, this system may also turn to amplify negative dispositions (e.g., neuroticism, pessimism, depression) and act as a hub for unresolved negative conditions (e.g., disability, irresistible pain, devastating loss). The presented model should then account for the failure of the positive regulatory systems to repair the self-intensification of the HWS. In this way, an irreparable damage in various functioning domains may be caused by prolonged experiences of aging trauma (Shrira, 2012, 2014; Shrira & Litwin, 2014) as well as trauma in old age (Dekel & Nuttman-Shwartz, 2009; Gelkopf et al., 2012).

The *pursuit of happiness in a hostile world* model presents certain unique formulations that offer more insight into the study areas of aging and trauma. These include the conception of SWB and MIL as agentic forces rather than mere outcomes of other psychological processes, the adaptive role of perceived adversity as embodied in one's cohesive image of the HWS, and the dynamic interrelations between opposing systems, as in the simultaneous activation (or, rather, the mutual inhibition) of SWB and the HWS (for fuller details, see Shmotkin, 2011; Shmotkin & Shrira, 2012, 2013). As these particular formulations focus on adaptation in the face of challenge, the presented model is basically congruent with other theoretical models that address well-being and adversity in an adaptational framework. For example, according to the model of *strength and vulnerability integration* (SAVI; Charles, 2010; Charles & Piazza, 2009), age-related appraisals, behaviors, and attentional strategies increase the individual's strength to regulate life experiences. Such strategies may become more efficient with age and often allow individuals to circumvent or minimize negative experiences. Well-being also has a crucial role in the *broaden-and-build theory* (Fredrickson, 2001, 2013), which posits that under traumatic conditions, experiences of positive emotions may broaden one's momentary thought–action repertoires, and thus serve to build enduring personal resources. Each of these models depicts coping with trauma in terms of processes that underlie a larger view of psychological adaptation.

Conclusion

We reviewed in this chapter several main issues regarding trauma among older adults and suggested a model for better understanding the dialectical appearances of resilience versus vulnerability vis-à-vis life adversity. Briefly, the model (Shmotkin, 2005) dwells on a dynamic interplay between a favorable psychological environment and the HWS. Concepts like *aging trauma* and *trauma in old age* extend this model by complicating the pursuit of happiness among older adults with hostile contingencies stemming from two sources: lingering disruptive remnants of one's past along with disruptive experiences that are newly imposed on one's declining functions at the present. Findings reviewed in this chapter may instruct clinicians and practitioners how to identify certain developmental processes that may enlarge, rather than restrict, the options of older adults for coping with trauma and adversity in later life.

References

American Psychiatric Association. (2013). *Diagnostic and statistical manual of mental disorders* (5th ed.). Arlington: American Psychiatric Publishing.

Amir, M., & Lev-Wiesel, R. (2003). Time does not heal all wounds: Quality of life and psychological distress of people who survived the Holocaust as children 55 years later. *Journal of Traumatic Stress, 16,* 295–299.

Averill, P. M., & Beck, J. G. (2000). Posttraumatic stress disorder in older adults: A conceptual review. *Journal of Anxiety Disorders, 14,* 133–156.

Baltes, P. B. (1997). On the incomplete architecture of human ontogeny: Selection, optimization, and compensation as foundation of developmental theory. *American Psychologist, 52,* 366–380.

Baltes, P. B., & Staudinger, U. M. (2000). Wisdom: A metaheuristic (pragmatic) to orchestrate mind and virtue toward excellence. *American Psychologist, 55,* 122–136.

Barel, E., Van IJzendoorn, M. H., Sagi-Schwartz, A., & Bakermans-Kranenburg, M. J. (2010). Surviving the Holocaust: A meta-analysis of the long-term sequelae of a genocide. *Psychological Bulletin, 136,* 677–698.

Bei, B., Bryant, C., Gilson, K. M., Koh, J., Gibson, P., Komiti, A., et al. (2013). A prospective study of the impact of floods on the mental and physical health of older adults. *Aging and Mental Health, 17,* 992–1002.

Blazer, D., & Hybels, C. (2005). Origins of depression in later life. *Psychological Medicine, 35,* 1241–1252.

Bleich, A., Gelkopf, M., Melamed, Y., & Solomon, Z. (2005). Emotional impact of exposure to terrorism among young-old and old-old Israeli citizens. *American Journal of Geriatric Psychiatry, 13,* 705–712.

Boals, A., & Schuettler, D. (2011). A double-edged sword: Event centrality, PTSD and posttraumatic growth. *Applied Cognitive Psychology, 25,* 817–822.

Bonanno, G. A., Westphal, M., & Mancini, A. D. (2011). Resilience to loss and potential trauma. *Annual Review of Clinical Psychology, 7,* 511–535.

Böttche, M., Kuwert, P., & Knaevelsrud, C. (2012). Posttraumatic stress disorder in older adults: An overview of characteristics and treatment approaches. *International Journal of Geriatric Psychiatry, 27,* 230–239.

Breslau, N., Kessler, R.C., Chilcoat, H. D., Schultz, L. R., Davis G. C., & Andreski, P. (1998). Trauma and posttraumatic stress disorder in the community: The 1996 Detroit area Survey of trauma. *Archives of General Psychiatry, 55,* 626–632.

Breslau, N., Peterson, E. L., Poisson, L. M., Schultz, L. R., & Lucia, V. C. (2004). Estimating post-traumatic stress disorder in the community: Lifetime perspective and the impact of typical traumatic events. *Psychological Medicine, 34,* 889–898.

Brom, D., Durst, N., & Aghassy, G. (2002). The phenomenology of posttraumatic distress in older adult Holocaust survivors. *Journal of Clinical Geropsychology, 8,* 189–201.

Budson, A. E., Simons, J. S., Sullivan, A. L., Beier, J. S., Solomon, P. R., Scinto, L. F., et al. (2004). Memory and emotions for the September 11, 2001, terrorist attack in patients with Alzheimer's

disease, patients with mild cognitive impairment, and healthy older adults. *Neuropsychology, 18,* 315–327.
Burnes, D. P., & Burnette, D. (2013). Broadening the etiological discourse on Alzheimer's disease to include trauma and posttraumatic stress disorder as psychosocial risk factors. *Journal of Aging Studies, 27,* 218–224.
Busseri, M. A., & Sadava, S. W. (2013). Subjective well-being as a dynamic and agentic system: Evidence from a longitudinal study. *Journal of Happiness Studies, 14,* 1085–1112.
Butler, R. N. (1963). The life review: An interpretation of reminiscence in the aged. *Psychiatry, 26,* 65–76.
Butters, N., & Delis, D. C. (1995). Clinical assessment of memory disorders in amnesia and dementia. *Annual Review of Psychology, 46,* 493–523.
Carstensen, L. L. (1995). Evidence for a life-span theory of socioemotional selectivity. *Current Directions in Psychological Science, 4,* 151–156.
Carstensen, L. L., Isaacowitz, D. M., & Charles, S. T. (1999) Taking time seriously: A theory of socioemotional selectivity. *American Psychologist, 54,* 165–181.
Charles, S. T. (2010). Strength and vulnerability integration: A model of emotional well-being across adulthood. *Psychological Bulletin, 136,* 1068–1091.
Charles, S. T., & Piazza, J. R. (2009). Age differences in affective well-being: Context matters. *Social and Personality Psychology Compass, 3,* 711–724.
Charles, S. T., Mather, M., & Carstensen, L. L. (2003). Aging and emotional memory: The forgettable nature of negative images for older adults. *Journal of Experimental Psychology: General, 132,* 310–324.
Cohen, K., & Shmotkin, D. (2007). Emotional ratings of anchor periods in life and their relation to subjective well-being among Holocaust survivors. *Personality and Individual Differences, 43,* 495–506.
Cook, J. M., Ruzek, J. I., & Cassidy, E. (2003). Possible association of posttraumatic stress disorder with cognitive impairment among older adults. *Psychiatric Services, 54,* 1223–1225.
Dekel, R., & Nuttman-Shwartz, O. (2009). Posttraumatic stress and growth: The contribution of cognitive appraisal and sense of belonging to the country. *Health and Social Work, 34,* 87–96.
Diener, E., Lucas, R. E., & Scollon, C. N. (2006). Beyond the hedonic treadmill: Revising the adaptation theory of well-being. *American Psychologist, 61,* 305–314.
Dulin, P. L., & Passmore, T. (2010). Avoidance of potentially traumatic stimuli mediates the relationship between accumulated lifetime trauma and late-life depression and anxiety. *Journal of Traumatic Stress, 23,* 296–299.
Erikson, E. H. (1998). *The life cycle completed: Extended version with new chapters on the ninth stage by Joan M. Erikson.* New York: Norton.
Eysenck, H. J. (1983). Stress, disease, and personality: The inoculation effect. In C. L. Cooper (Ed.), *Stress research* (pp. 121–146). New York: Wiley.
Ferraro, K. F., & Shippee, T. P. (2009). Aging and cumulative inequality: How does inequality get under the skin? *The Gerontologist, 49,* 333–343.
Frankl, V. E. (1963). *Man's search for meaning: An introduction to logotherapy.* New York: Washington Square Press.
Fredrickson, B. L. (2001). The role of positive emotions in positive psychology: The broaden-and-build theory of positive emotions. *American Psychologist, 56,* 218–226.
Fredrickson, B. L. (2013). Updated thinking on positivity ratios. *American Psychologist, 68,* 814–822.
Gelkopf, M., Berger, R., Bleich, A., & Silver, R. C. (2012). Protective factors and predictors of vulnerability to chronic stress: A comparative study of 4 communities after 7 years of continuous rocket fire. *Social Science and Medicine, 74,* 757–766.
Hyer, L., & Sacks, A. (2008). PTSD (post-traumatic stress disorders) in later life. In D. Gallagher-Thompson, A. M. Steffen, & L.W. Thompson (Eds.), *Handbook of behavioral and cognitive therapies with older adults* (pp. 278–294). New York: Springer.
Isaacowitz, D. M., Smith, T. B., & Carstensen, L. L. (2003). Socioemotional selectivity and mental health among trauma survivors in old age. *Ageing International, 28,* 181–199.

Janoff-Bulman, R. (1992). *Shattered assumptions: Towards a new psychology of trauma*. New York: Free Press.

Keinan, G., Shrira, A., & Shmotkin, D. (2012). The association between cumulative adversity and mental health: Considering dose and primary focus of adversity. *Quality of Life Research, 21*, 1149–1158.

Kensinger, E. A. (2006). Remembering emotional information: Effects of aging and Alzheimer's disease. In E. M. Welsh (Ed.), *Frontiers in Alzheimer's disease research* (pp. 213–226). Hauppauge: Nova Science.

Kessler, R. C., Sonnega, A., Bromet, E., Hughes, M., & Nelson, C. B. (1995). Posttraumatic stress disorder in the National Comorbidity Survey. *Archives of General Psychiatry, 52*, 1048–1060.

King, L. A., & Hicks, J. A. (2007). Whatever happened to "what might have been"? Regrets, happiness, and maturity. *American Psychologist, 62*, 625–636.

Knight, B. G., Gatz, M., Heller, K., & Bengtson, V. L. (2000). Age and emotional response to the Northridge earthquake: A longitudinal analysis. *Psychology and Aging, 15*, 627–634.

Kraaij, V., & DeWilde, E. J. (2001). Negative life events and depressive symptoms in the elderly: A life span perspective. *Aging and Mental Health, 5*, 84–91.

Krause, N. (2005). Traumatic events and meaning in life: Exploring variations in three age cohorts. *Ageing and Society, 25*, 501–524.

Krause, N. (2009). Lifetime trauma, prayer, and psychological distress in late life. *International Journal for the Psychology of Religion, 19*, 55–72.

Lapp, L. K., Agbokou, C., & Ferreri, F. (2011). PTSD in the elderly: The interaction between trauma and aging. *International Psychogeriatrics, 23*, 858–868.

Linley, P. A. (2003). Positive adaptation to trauma: Wisdom as both process and outcome. *Journal of Traumatic Stress, 16*, 601–610.

Lomranz, J. (2005). Amplified comment: The triangular relationships between the Holocaust, aging, and narrative gerontology. *The International Journal of Aging and Human Development, 60*, 255–267.

Maercker, A. (2002). Life-review technique in the treatment of PTSD in elderly patients: Rationale and three single case studies. *Journal of Clinical Geropsychology, 8*, 239–249.

March, J. S. (1993). What constitutes a stressor? The "Criterion A" issue. In J. R. T. Davidson & E. B. Foa (Eds.), *Posttraumatic stress disorder, DSM-IV and beyond* (pp. 37–54). Washington, DC: American Psychiatric Association Press.

Martin, P., da Rosa, G., & Poon, L. W. (2011). The impact of life events on the oldest old. In L. W. Poon & J. Cohen-Mansfield (Eds.), *Understanding well-being in the oldest old* (pp. 96–110). Cambridge: Cambridge University Press.

Mather, M., & Carstensen, L. L. (2005). Aging and motivated cognition: The positivity effect in attention and memory. *Trends in Cognitive Sciences, 9*, 496–502.

McEwen, B. S. (1998). Protective and damaging effects of stress mediators. *New England Journal of Medicine, 338*, 171–179.

Norris, F. H. (1992). Epidemiology of trauma: Frequency and impact of different potentially traumatic events on different demographic groups. *Journal of Consulting and Clinical Psychology, 60*, 409–418.

Norris, F. H., Kaniasty, K., Conrad, M. L., Inman, G. L., & Murphy, A. D. (2002). Placing age differences in cultural context: A comparison of the effects of age on PTSD after disaster in the United States, Mexico, and Poland. *Journal of Clinical Geropsychology, 8*, 153–173.

Ogle, C. M., Rubin, D. C., Berntsen, D., & Siegler, I. C. (2013). The frequency and impact of exposure to potentially traumatic events over the life course. *Clinical Psychological Science, 1*, 426–434.

Ogle, C. M., Rubin, D. C., & Siegler, I. C. (2014). Cumulative exposure to traumatic events in older adults. *Aging and Mental Health, 18*, 316–325.

Palgi, S., Palgi, Y., Ben-Ezra, M., & Shrira, A. (2014). I will fear no evil, for I am with me: Mentalization-oriented intervention with PTSD patients—A case study. *Journal of Contemporary Psychotherapy, 43*, 1–10.

Palgi, Y. (2013). Ongoing cumulative chronic stressors as predictors of well-being in the second half of life. *Journal of Happiness Studies, 14,* 1127–1144.

Palgi, Y., & Ben-Ezra, M. (2010). "Back to the future": Narrative treatment for post-traumatic, acute stress disorder in the case of paramedic Mr. G. *Pragmatic Case Studies in Psychotherapy, 6,* 1–26.

Palgi, Y., & Shmotkin, D. (2010). The predicament of time near the end of life: Time perspective trajectories of life satisfaction among the old-old. *Aging and Mental Health, 14,* 577–586.

Palgi, Y., Shrira, A., Goodwin, R., Hamama-Raz, Y., & Ben-Ezra, M. (2014). Fear of aging moderates PTSD symptoms among older adults exposed to Hurricane Sandy. *American Journal of Geriatric Psychiatry, 22,* 741.

Palgi, Y., Gelkopf, M., & Berger, R. (2015). The inoculating role of previous exposure to potentially traumatic life events on coping with prolonged exposure to rocket attacks: A lifespan perspective. *Psychiatry Research, 227,* 296–301.

Pals, J. L., & McAdams, D. P. (2004). The transformed self: A narrative understanding of posttraumatic growth. *Psychological Inquiry, 15,* 65–69.

Pearlin, L. I., Schieman, S., Fazio, E. M., & Meersman, S. C. (2005). Stress, health, and the life course: Some conceptual specifications. *Journal of Health and Social Behavior, 46,* 205–219.

Ryff, C. D., Friedman, E. M., Morozink, J. A., & Tsenkova, V. (2012). Psychological resilience in adulthood and later life: Implications for health. *Annual Review of Gerontology and Geriatrics, 32,* 73–92.

Schnurr, P. P., Spiro, A., Vielhauer, M. J., Findler, M. N., & Hamblen, J. L. (2002).Trauma in the lives of older men: Findings from the Normative Aging Study. *Journal of Clinical Geropsychology, 8,* 175–187.

Scott, S. B., Poulin, M. J., & Silver, R. C. (2013). A life span perspective on terrorism: Age differences in trajectories of response to 9/11. *Developmental Psychology, 49,* 986–998.

Seery, M. D., Holman, E. A., & Silver, R. C. (2010). Whatever does not kill us: Cumulative lifetime adversity, vulnerability, and resilience. *Journal of Personality and Social Psychology, 99,* 1025–1041.

Sheldon, K. M., & Kasser, T. (2001). Getting older, getting better? Personal strivings and psychological maturity across the life span. *Developmental Psychology, 37,* 491–501.

Shenk, D., Ramos, B., Kalaw, K. J., & Tufan, I. (2009). History, memory, and disasters among older adults: A life course perspective. *Traumatology, 15,* 35–43.

Shmotkin, D. (2003). Vulnerability and resilience intertwined: A review of research on Holocaust survivors. In R. Jacoby & G. Keinan (Eds.), *Between stress and hope: From a disease-centered to a health-centered perspective* (pp. 213–233). Westport: Praeger.

Shmotkin, D. (2005). Happiness in face of adversity: Reformulating the dynamic and modular bases of subjective well-being. *Review of General Psychology, 9,* 291–325.

Shmotkin, D. (2011). The pursuit of happiness: Alternative conceptions of subjective well-being. In L. W. Poon & J. Cohen-Mansfield (Eds.), *Understanding well-being in the oldest old* (pp. 27–45). New York: Cambridge University Press.

Shmotkin, D., & Barilan, Y. M. (2002). Expressions of Holocaust experience and their relationship to mental symptoms and physical morbidity among Holocaust survivor patients. *Journal of Behavioral Medicine, 25,* 115–134.

Shmotkin, D., & Litwin, H. (2009). Cumulative adversity and depressive symptoms among older adults in Israel: The differential roles of self-oriented versus other-oriented events of potential trauma. *Social Psychiatry and Psychiatric Epidemiology, 44,* 989–997.

Shmotkin, D., & Lomranz, J. (1998). Subjective well-being among Holocaust survivors: An examination of overlooked differentiations. *Journal of Personality and Social Psychology, 75,* 141–155.

Shmotkin, D., & Shrira, A. (2012). On the distinction between subjective well-being and meaning in life: Regulatory versus reconstructive functions in the face of a hostile world. In P. T. P. Wong (Ed.), *The human quest for meaning: Theories, research, and applications* (2nd ed., pp. 143–163). New York: Routledge.

Shmotkin, D., & Shrira, A. (2013). Subjective well-being and meaning in life in a hostile world: Proposing a configurative perspective. In J. A. Hicks & C. Routledge (Eds.), *The experience of*

meaning in life: Classical perspectives, emerging themes, and controversies (pp. 77–86). New York: Springer.
Shmotkin, D., Blumstein, T., & Modan, B. (2003). Tracing long-term effects of early trauma: A broad-scope view of Holocaust survivors in late life. *Journal of Consulting and Clinical Psychology, 71,* 223–234.
Shmotkin, D., Shrira, A., Goldberg, S. C., & Palgi, Y. (2011). Resilience and vulnerability among aging Holocaust survivors and their families: An intergenerational overview. *Journal of Intergenerational Relationships, 9,* 7–21.
Shmotkin, D., Shrira, A., & Palgi, Y. (2011). Does trauma linger into old-old age: Using the Holocaust experience as a paradigm. In L. W. Poon & J. Cohen-Mansfield (Eds.), *Understanding well-being in the oldest old* (pp. 81–95). New York: Cambridge University Press.
Shrira, A. (2012). The effect of lifetime cumulative adversity on change and chronicity in depressive symptoms and quality of life in older adults. *International Psychogeriatrics, 24,* 1988–1997.
Shrira, A. (2014). Greater age-related decline in markers of physical, mental and cognitive health among Israeli older adults exposed to lifetime cumulative adversity. *Aging and Mental Health, 18,* 610–618.
Shrira, A., & Litwin, H. (2014). The effect of lifetime cumulative adversity and depressive symptoms on functional status. *Journal of Gerontology: Psychological Sciences and Social Sciences, 69,* 953–965.
Shrira, A., Palgi, Y., Ben-Ezra, M., & Shmotkin, D. (2011a). Functioning and mortality of Holocaust survivors: Physical resilience and psychosocial vulnerabilities. *Journal of Loss and Trauma, 16,* 67–83.
Shrira, A., Palgi, Y., Ben-Ezra, M., & Shmotkin, D. (2011b). How subjective well-being and meaning in life interact in the hostile world? *The Journal of Positive Psychology, 6,* 273–285.
Shrira, A., & Shmotkin, D. (2008). Can the past keep life pleasant even for old-old trauma survivors? *Aging and Mental Health, 12,* 807–819.
Shrira, A., Shmotkin, D., & Litwin, H. (2012). Potentially traumatic events at different points in the life span and mental health: Findings from SHARE-Israel. *American Journal of Orthopsychiatry, 82,* 251–259.
Shrira, A., Palgi, Y., Hamama-Raz, Y., Goodwin, R., & Ben-Ezra, M. (2014). Previous exposure to the World Trade Center terrorist attack and posttraumatic symptoms among older adults following Hurricane Sandy. *Psychiatry: Interpersonal and Biological Processes, 77,* 374–385.
Solomon, Z., & Ginzburg, K. (1998). War trauma and the aged: An Israeli perspective. In J. Lomranz (Ed.), *Handbook of aging and mental health: An integrative approach* (pp. 135–152). New York: Plenum.
Tedeschi, R. G., & Calhoun, L. G. (2004). Posttraumatic growth: Conceptual foundations and empirical evidence. *Psychological Inquiry, 15,* 1–18.
Thorp, S. R., & Blazer, D. G. (2012). Time does not heal all wounds: Trauma, stress, and resilience among older adults. *American Journal of Geriatric Psychiatry, 20,* 375–379.
Troxel, W. M., Matthews, K. A., Bromberger, J. T., & Sutton-Tyrrell, K. (2003). Chronic stress burden, discrimination, and subclinical carotid artery disease in African American and Caucasian women. *Health Psychology, 22,* 300–309.
Urry, H. L., & Gross, J. J. (2010). Emotion regulation in older age. *Current Directions in Psychological Science, 19,* 352–357.
Webster, J. D., & Deng, X. C. (in press). Paths from trauma to intrapersonal strength: Worldview, posttraumatic growth, and wisdom. *Journal of Loss and Trauma, 20,* 253–266.
Yehuda, R. (2009). Status of glucocorticoid alterations in post-traumatic stress disorder. *Annals of the New York Academy of Sciences, 1179,* 56–69.

Chapter 17
Lost Possible Selves and Personality Development

Laura A. King and Gerald L. Mitchell

Introduction

"What do you want to be when you grow up?" is a question that is frequently posed to children. With age, our answers to the question of "what we want to be" may be far removed from childhood dreams of becoming a firefighter, an astronaut, an artist, or a garbage collector. And certainly, we are less likely to be asked what we want to be when we grow up when we are, after all, grown-ups. Yet, in a sense, adults answer this question every day as we seek our life goals, striving to become the persons we hoped to be.

Personal goals are a key aspect of psychological well-being (e.g., Emmons, 1986, Sheldon & Hoon, 2007). Having, valuing, and making progress on personal goals are associated with psychological well-being (King, 2008a). Goals are the way we experience a sense of purpose, a key aspect of the experience of meaning in life (Heintzelman & King, 2013). Personal goals play an important role in a larger framework of self-regulation providing life with organizing principles, with beginnings, middles, and ends, so that experiences make sense (King, 2008b). Goals lend coherence to affective experience: We feel good or bad depending on how we are progressing in our valued motivational pursuits (Carver & Scheier, 2008). Striving toward personal goals attaches us to larger motivational concerns, allowing us to enact the behaviors that will meet our broader needs (Sheldon & Kasser, 2001). Goal pursuit might also play a role in personality development. An unreliable teenager might set a goal to become a more conscientious young adult. An adult who is hostile might set a goal to become more compassionate. Success at these goals would seem to imply that a person has matured: That the pursuit of a personal goal has contributed to development (see Hudson & Fraley, in press).

L. A. King (✉) · G. L. Mitchell
Department of Psychology, University of Missouri, McAlester Hall, Columbia, MO 65211, USA
e-mail: Kingla@missouri.edu

G. L. Mitchell
e-mail: glmf4d@mail.missouri.edu

K. E. Cherry (ed.), *Traumatic Stress and Long-Term Recovery,*
DOI 10.1007/978-3-319-18866-9_17

Nevertheless, for all its beneficial associations, goal pursuit is not without its downsides (King & Burton, 2003). There are numerous places where such pursuit can go awry. The selection of a goal may be poorly suited to one's abilities, skills, and opportunities. Beliefs about what future experiences will bring fulfillment can be inaccurate (Wilson & Gilbert, 2005). In addition, most of the time, people pursue multiple goals (Vancouver, Weinhardt, & Schmidt, 2010) and this multiplicity can engender conflict and stress (Boudreaux & Ozer, 2013; Emmons & King, 1988). Devoting resources to a particular goal may mean neglecting others. This prioritizing can be based on inaccurate perceptions of one's abilities, leading to poorer performance outcomes (Vancouver, Gullekson, Morse, & Warren, 2014). Furthermore, caring about a goal means monitoring progress and potentially experiencing negative emotions, when progress is lower than anticipated, and disappointment, in the face of failure (Pomerantz, Saxon, & Oishi, 2000). Pursuing a long-term life dream can involve delaying gratification, putting off immediate pleasures, to regulate behavior toward a distal desired end. Although such capacities are a hallmark of effective self-regulation (King & Trent, 2012), if those distal futures are never realized, sacrifices (or sunken costs) may be a source of considerable distress. Finally, not all goal-relevant outcomes are in the control of the person pursuing a goal. Life events may render goals unavailable, no matter our efforts. Traumatic life experiences can not only simply disrupt the pursuit of valued goals but also draw the very value of those goals into question, destroying a person's sense of meaning (Calhoun & Tedeschi, 1999; Janoff-Bulman, 1992). Having a life dream rendered impossible by life events leaves a person open to the experience of regret: Facing the awful truth that one's considerable efforts have been wasted time (King & Hicks, 2007). Mentally extrapolating our lives into future means attaching ourselves to a potentially precarious fiction: When we set a goal, we place a bet on the future and invest our present lives in the pursuit of that future. That investment, in turn, defines a degree of vulnerability if a goal cannot be attained.

Disengaging from cherished goals can be challenging and people seem more likely to redouble their efforts in the face of failure, rather than moving on (Brunstein & Gollwitzer, 1996; Emmons, Colby, & Kaiser, 1998). The capacity to disengage from unavailable goals predicts subsequent well-being (Wrosch, Amir, & Miller, 2011) and a well-regulated system would seem to be one that responds to failures by flexibly divesting from lost causes (Wrosch, Bauer, & Scheier, 2005) and investing in new goals that promise fulfillment. This optimal process speaks to remarkable human strengths, including the capacity to acknowledge failure and to courageously invest once again in the future, even when the risks of such investment have been borne out by experience. Contemplating this optimal process conjures images of the person, phoenix-like, rising up from the ashes of dashed life dreams to reinstate a sense of purpose.

Although such strengths are often (and justifiably) celebrated when they are demonstrated, we suggest that there may be value in attending to not only "the rising up" but "the ashes": That there may be value in digging into those dying embers to acknowledge and contemplate the hopes and dreams one once pursued. When life circumstances prevent the person from seeing their life goals to fruition, those lost futures are not merely a source of regret. Even as they can be thought of as implying a crisis, experiences that disrupt goal pursuit may also be opportunities to develop. The stance that a person takes toward lost motivational pursuits, the people they wished to be but no longer can, can serve both as an indicator of psychological maturity and as a portent of the maturational process (King & Hicks, 2007). Placing unattainable goals in a developmental context provides a window to the processes by which traumatic experiences can spur personality development.

In this chapter, we explore the ways that goals, life dreams, or *possible selves* that are disrupted by life experiences might play a role in personality development. To begin, we first step away from the context of goals to review, briefly, the concepts of posttraumatic growth (PTG) and personality development (from a trait perspective). We suggest although both of these approaches capture something about how life experiences can influence development, they each fall short in terms of uncovering the process of that development. Then, we describe an alternative approach to personality development, ego development, that is well suited to revealing that process. We show how narrative features suggesting accommodation provide a means of tracking active personality development. Then, we return to the potential place of goals in personality development, considering specifically how accommodation is demonstrated in narrative descriptions of lost goals or lost possible selves. Finally, we draw links from this research on rather dramatic life changes to everyday life and the types of goal changes that are required, perhaps, of all adults as they consider and reconsider what they want to be when they grow up.

PTG and Personality Development

Can negative life experiences be sources of personality development? The potential for stressful experiences to lead to positive changes has long been recognized. This idea is perhaps best reflected in accumulated evidence for stress-related or PTG. However, research on this intuitively appealing idea has limits which are largely absent from research on personality development from the trait approach. These two approaches to the potential for life events to contribute to adult personality development, though different, offer complementary approaches to the process by which having experienced a negative or traumatic experience a person is, in fact, better for it. Here, we review each of these literatures, highlighting their strengths and limitations. We then review an alternative approach to personality development in adulthood that allows for an examination of the role of the active developer in his or her development through challenging life experiences.

Posttraumatic Growth

Tedeschi and McNally (2011) defined PTG as positive personal change as a result of struggling with a trauma. Research demonstrates that individuals who have experienced a range of different negative life experiences report having grown as a result of these (e.g., Karanci & Acarturk, 2005; Klosky, et al., 2014; Lowe, Manove, & Rhodes, 2013; Morris, Shakespeare-Finsh, Reick, & Newberry, 2005). PTG is typically measured using self-report scales on which individuals rate the extent to which a traumatic events has led to positive changes in various domains. For instance, individuals might rate the extent to which a traumatic experience has led them to deeper relationships with others, a greater appreciation for each day, a better sense of life priorities, or a stronger sense of their own capacities to handle life difficulties (e.g., Park, Chmielewski & Blank, 2010; Park, Cohen, & Murch, 1996; Tedeschi & Calhoun, 1996). Research using such self-reports suggests that PTG is not uncommon, with between 30 and 70 % of survivors of various traumatic experiences reporting PTG (Joseph, Murphy & Regel, 2012). Reports of PTG following traumatic experiences are strongly related to psychological, social, and spiritual well-being (though not typically physical health; e.g., Joseph et al., 2012; Helgeson, Reynolds, & Tomich, 2006; Park et al., 1996, 2010; Triplett, Tedeschi, Cann, Calhoun, & Reeve, 2012).

Interestingly, PTG is not simply associated with a kind of Pollyannaish, naive thinking style. Self-reported PTG is related to appraisals of events as more severe, threatening, and stressful as well as heightened intrusive thoughts about the trauma (Helgeson et al., 2006). The relationship of intrusive thoughts on well-being is moderated by the perception of PTG: In a sample of younger adult cancer survivors, those who report high levels of PTG, intrusive thoughts were associated with *higher* well-being (Park et al., 2010). These results suggest that the subjective sense of PTG may transform even negative experiences into ones that support well-being. Thus, self-reported PTG captures quite well the subjective feeling that one has been changed for the better by a traumatic experience. Moreover, this subjective feeling is linked to subsequent adjustment in a way that suggests it is important to functioning.

Importantly, however, it is far from clear that individuals who report growing from traumatic life experiences have actually changed in an objective way. Conclusions about subjective reports of PTG may always be open to a variety of alternative explanations, including social desirability, positive illusions, and cognitive dissonance (Coyne & Tennen, 2010; Tennen & Affleck 2009; Bonanno, 2004). Certainly, *feeling* like one has grown through life events is a strong predictor of subsequent well-being. We might think of PTG as involving a healthy coping style (i.e., positive reappraisal or benefit-finding) but it is not clear that reports of PTG reflect the "actual" change (King & Trent, 2012). Claims about developing through life experiences require longitudinal research that tracks variables beyond the subjective feeling of having been changed for the better by experience. Researchers in personality psychology have begun to address this issue using the trait approach.

Adult Personality Development: The Trait Approach

When we think of the characteristics that make a person "mature," we might think of personality descriptors like stable, responsible, or compassionate. Trait psychologists have examined how personality traits (typically focusing on the Big 5: neuroticism, extraversion, openness to experience, agreeableness, and conscientiousness) change over the course of life, and this research largely lends empirical support to intuitive ideas about what it means to be mature. Meta-analyses of longitudinal studies show normative age-related changes in personality traits that look very much like maturation. Specifically, research shows that, particularly from adolescence through young adulthood, people are likely to become less neurotic, more conscientious, and more agreeable (e.g., Roberts, Walton, & Veichtbauer, 2006; Specht, Egloff, & Schmakle, 2011; Vaidya, Gray, Haig, Mroczek, & Watson, 2008). Such changes seem to indicate something like development, a movement toward a more "mature" (i.e., more emotionally regulated, more responsible, and more kind) level of personality functioning. The mechanisms of these changes (in keeping with their timing) have been suggested to be the additional demands and social roles that require young adults to cultivate conscientiousness and agreeableness (Lodi-Smith & Roberts, 2007). That these changes occur, at all, is notable. Traits might be the least likely aspects of a person to change through life, given that by definition traits are thought to represent enduring and stable behavioral tendencies (e.g., Allemand, Steiger, & Hill, 2013).

These trait changes are understood as loosely age related in a broad way and comparatively little research has examined whether *specific life experiences* are associated with personality development. A small but growing number of large longitudinal studies have allowed for an examination of the ways traits relate to life events over time. These studies identify two types of processes. First, they examine whether personality traits predict specific life events (a process called *selection*). Generally speaking they do, with studies showing, for instance, that extroverts are more likely to experience positive life events, while neuroticism is associated with experiencing more negative life events (Magnus, Diener, Fujita, & Pavot, 1993).

A second process, one that is more relevant to our purposes, refers to how events shape personality traits and predict trait change (a process called *socialization*). Some research supports the idea that experiences can influence later changes in personality. For example, the type of training college-aged students receive can predict personality changes over time (e.g., increases in conscientiousness; Lüdtke, Roberts, Trautwein, & Nagy, 2011). In addition, longitudinal research shows that success in the domains of career and romantic relationships can predict increases in extraversion and decreases in neuroticism over time (Scollon & Diener, 2006). More recently, one study showed that, compared to a control group, individuals who experienced military training failed to show the normative increase in agreeableness that was found in a control sample across 8 years (Jackson, Thoemmes, Jonkmann, Lüdtke, & Trautwein, 2012). Other research suggests that the experience of negative events predicts higher levels of neuroticism, and the experience of positive events predicts increases in extraversion and conscientiousness (Sutin, Costa, Wethington, & Eaton, 2010). Such patterns indicate that *negative* events, per se, might not be particularly likely to lead to personality development.

A strength of the trait approach is that it features the kind of longitudinal assessments required to make claims about "actual" change. Further, this research does not rely on subjective reports of change. Nevertheless, in comparison to research on

PTG, what is missing from the trait approach to development is a strong sense of the active developer and the process of change itself. That is, this approach does not seem to fully capture the importance of who the person is and his or her perceptions of experiences as playing an important role in the developmental trait change. A few studies do implicate the active developer and these perceptions. For example, in a study on a sample of the general population of Germany, individuals with higher life satisfaction showed more positive change in emotional stability, agreeableness, and conscientiousness during major life role transitions (Specht, Egloff, & Schmukle, 2013). These results suggest that coming from a position of psychological strength can spur developmental changes during potentially difficult times.

In addition, one longitudinal study examined how subjective feelings about a stressful life event in the trajectory of trait change over time (Sutin et al., 2010). In this study, longitudinal trait measurements were buttressed with an interview in which participants were asked to describe a stressful life event. Appraisals of these events as involving "learning a lesson" were measured in the interviews. The results showed that appraising stressful events as providing lessons predicted trait change (including increases in extraversion and conscientiousness and lowered neuroticism) over time (Sutin et al., 2010). This research suggests that how people think about stressful experiences can influence whether an event is associated with subsequent indications of higher (or lower) levels of maturity.

Comparing PTG and research on personality development from the trait perspective reveals a bit of a disconnect. PTG would seem to do a very good job of capturing the person's subjective feelings of change and some of PTG may be reflected in trait change. For instance, feeling that one has become more compassionate as a result of a traumatic experience might be reflected in higher levels of agreeableness. Learning to "not sweat the small stuff" might be reflected in decreases in neuroticism. Yet, other aspects of PTG may be irrelevant to traits, such as the sense that one has gained an appreciation of everyday life. Consider that a neurotic person might remain neurotic through challenging life experiences and an extravert might remain highly extraverted, but each of these individuals might change in a different way or on a different level: They might have come to experience themselves and the world in a way that is transformed by experience, qualitatively if not quantitatively. A person can show a great deal of stability at the trait level and yet feel that they have grown in ways that are missed by a trait approach. At the same time, there is no question that a person's subjective report of "growing" requires less subjective verification. Moreover, neither PTG nor the trait approach to development allow for a sense of how development occurs, the underlying process of change itself. We turn next to a different perspective on personality development that addresses these missing pieces.

An Alternative Approach: Ego Development

Although the trait approach is the dominant approach in contemporary personality psychology, it is not the only way to understand the person. Jane Loevinger (1976) used the term ego to refer to an individual's frame of reference in approaching the self and world. For Loevinger, the ego is "the striving to master, to integrate, and make sense of experience" (Loevinger, 1976, p. 59). The developmental level of the ego then would dictate what a person sees in the world and the sense the person makes of what he or she sees.

Ego development refers to the level of complexity with which one experiences oneself and the world (King & Hicks, 2007; Loevinger, 1976). At its lowest levels, the ego is dominated by impulses and thinking is simplistic. With development, the ego comes to see the world from an increasingly complex frame of reference, recognizing conflicts, the contextual nature of experience, and the relativity that characterizes many human decisions. High levels of ego development imply greater tolerance for ambivalence and a preoccupation with issues of identity and respect for the subjectivity of others (Pfaffenberger, Marko, & Combs, 2011).

Unlike PTG and traits, ego development is not proposed to be available to self-report. Rather, the complexity and sophistication of one's frame of reference is measured using the Sentence Completion Test (SCT; Hy & Loevinger, 1996). On this measure, participants are asked to complete sentence stems (e.g., "What gets me into trouble is…") and responses are scored by raters trained using standard guidelines. Low-level responses generally involve impulses, conventions, and rules. High-level responses include taking multiple perspectives, considering various possibilities, and conditional relationships. Although time-consuming, this measure has been shown to track changes in personality and cognitive complexity over time (e.g., Helson & Roberts, 1994).

Ego development (as measured by the SCT) relates to openness to experience increased compassion, intellectuality, tolerance (Helson & Roberts, 1994; Helson & Wink, 1987) as well as empathy and the capacity for interpersonal connectedness (Carlozzi, Gaa, & Liberman, 1983; Pals & John, 1998). Interestingly, ego development is *not* related to self-reports of personal growth through difficult experiences, and it is generally independent of psychological well-being (King, Scollon, Ramsey, & Williams, 2000). Ego development is not about feeling like one has grown. Rather, it appears to tap into a way of interpreting the world, about how one *is* rather than how one *feels* (King, 2011).

Ego development, though a rather unusual and somewhat difficult construct, is especially useful for tracking the process of personality development through difficult life experiences because Loevinger explicitly acknowledged that ego development *relies* on such experiences. Ego development is not normative age-related change. It has no such inevitability. Rather, Loevinger (1976) stated that only when the environment fails to meet the person's expectations can development occur. She described *pacers* as experiences that facilitate development by challenging a person to ever more sophisticated ways of experiencing the self and world. Loevinger (1976) conceived the ego as a buffer that determines how we experience the world around us. Experiences come through that buffer, perhaps beveling it in different ways, honing its relationship to the world and the self. This idea resonates very well with the notion that in adulthood personality development is driven by the need to accommodate life changes, as we now consider.

Process: Accommodation in Adulthood Drawing on Piaget's concepts of developmental processes, Block (1982) proposed that life experiences can play a role in adult personality development through assimilation and accommodation. As described by Piaget, assimilation involves using existing schemas to make sense out of the current environment. When these existing frames of reference are not up to the challenge of making sense of new experience, schemas are changed, revised, or invented. This is the process of accommodation. In adulthood, stressful or traumatic life experiences may call for accommodative change, revising one's sources of meaning, one's values, or philosophy of life.

Accommodation is the presumed mechanism underlying changes in ego development over time. Research has shown that experiencing a broad range of life events predicts ego development cross-sectionally and longitudinally (e.g., Helson, 1992; Helson & Roberts, 1994). This research suggests that the experience of difficult times (i.e., pacers) is associated with enhanced ego development. Studies linking difficult times to ego development, however, only assume accommodation has occurred in response to those life difficulties. Is there a way to measure the process of accommodation, making explicit the revising of meaning structures that is thought to precipitate these changes? One way researchers have sought to do this is by examining the stories people tell about difficult life experiences. These stories have been used as a window into the action of accommodation.

Narratives, Accommodative Processing, and Ego Development The life story approach to personality holds that the narrative we create about our lives provides a key source of identity (McAdams & McLean, 2013). The stories we create about life experiences are instantiations of meaning making and of how we have made sense of these important, sometimes crucial, life experiences. As the ego is proposed to be the author that makes sense of experience, King et al. (2000) proposed that stories of major life events might provide a way to examine the accommodative process itself. Research on narrative constructions of life transitions has examined this proposal.

For example, in one prospective study, parents of children with Down syndrome (DS) were asked to write a narrative account of finding out that they would be parenting a child with DS (King et al., 2000). Parents also completed measures of psychological well-being and the SCT as a measure of ego development. They were contacted 2 years later to complete the well-being and ego development measures a second time. The stories they provided were reliably coded for narrative features that tapped two dimensions, closure, and accommodation. We describe each of these dimensions and their correlates below.

Closure Closure included dimensions indicating narrative coherence including foreshadowing, positive affective tone, resolution, and happy endings. Excerpts of stories rated high in closure include the following (from King et al., 2000, p. 523).

> …We knew that our daughter was going to get a very loving supportive family who would make sure she achieved everything possible for her.

> I knew everything would be all right. He was first and foremost our baby boy and DS was one characteristic of Jamie. He is as much or more of a blessing to our family as any child could be.
>
> I know my daughter is quite special. It's as if she's part of another race or from another planet. She's definitely wired differently. And I think those wires are hooked directly to God. She's the closest I've come to an angel on Earth.

Excerpts from stories low on closure include (from King et al., 2000, p. 519):

> Images of adults with DS flooded my mind. They were not pretty images. I was afraid he would die from the surgery and more afraid that he wouldn't.
>
> Finding out was devastating. I was depressed, didn't want him. When I told my mother, she fainted. My other child became so upset due to the circumstances that she vomited. It was simply devastating.
>
> We were given an Exceptional Parents magazine. On the way home from the blood test, I found a picture of a crib with a lid on it, like a cage. I remember wondering, what do we have? What are we faced with? I also remember thinking that now we'll never be normal.

Results for closure were limited to concurrent measures. Specifically, those parents whose stories were highly coherent and conveyed a strong sense of closure were more likely to report higher concurrent well-being. No prospective relationships emerged, suggesting that it may be that those who are high on well-being tell more coherent stories about their experiences.

Accommodation Accommodation referred to features including how active the narrator was in the story, how much the person fully explored the experience, and the degree to which the person experienced a paradigmatic shift because of the event. These processes are, perhaps, less transparent than the coding for closure and so we share here an excerpt of the instructions for paradigmatic shift (King et al., 2000, p. 520):

> …the new experience requires a revision of structures—an essential change in response to the environment. For our sample, this concept serves as an analogy for qualitative change in how the person sees the world and him or herself. Accommodative change means that the person has been forced to change, centrally and qualitatively, his or her views of the self and world.

To get a sense of the richness with which accommodative processing is conveyed in narratives, consider the following examples, each of which received a high score in the content analyses:

> I was surprised how much I totally suppressed the information. Total denial for 3 weeks…. I was shocked at my own inability to deal with such an unexpected event. I cried a lot. The pain was so deep. I felt cheated—I could hardly function. I was so absorbed with my own fears. But I did regroup. I did grow. And I did learn to accept the situation. That opened the door for me to bond and love my child. But it took time. (King et al., 2000, p. 522)
>
> I cried some and experienced waves of "unknown" embracing me…. I knew little about DS—it was an abstraction. Any handicap fell into the category of a childhood memory of seeing "waterheads," as I was told or remember, out on a shopping trip getting into a bus. My daughter was flesh and blood and a good nurser, and that was the reality I remember dealing with. I thought very little about her future, but I knew I would bow to no predictions. Irrational thoughts came to me at times but did not consume much thinking time: "I must have DS too, it just hasn't been discovered yet" or "This child must be a consequence for wrong decisions in the past." (King, 2001, p. 60)

> It was long enough ago that the word was Mongoloid. I was alone, and it was late at night when the doctor told me. Of course, my mind clicked in to an offensive mode of denial—bad dream, etc. I chose not to call my husband…. Instead—I laugh at this now because I was 33—I called my parents. I think I wanted them to fix things—they had been pretty good at that in the past…. Then I realized that I was mourning as if my child had died, yet I still had a nice fat baby in the nursery. I rang for him to be brought to me expecting him to be a monster instead of the cute thing I saw in the delivery room. I tore all of his clothes off of him and just looked at him. He was beautiful. The doctor recommended immediately institutionalizing him and said it would be best if I never saw my son…. It took a day of being a totally hysterical mother before they would let me see or hold my son. The moment I held him, I knew he would stay with me. (King 2001, p. 65)

Clearly, narratives high in accommodative processing were highly vivid and often included (as the examples above show) a tendency to comment on one's own coping processes. Finally, they were also likely to show an intriguing tendency to focus on the physical reality of the child (King & Hicks, 2007). Importantly, although narratives including accommodative processing were, on average, longer than those low in this quality, they were not more negative or more traumatic.

Was accommodative narrative processing related to well-being and ego development? The results showed that this aspect of the narratives was generally unrelated to measures of well-being. However, accommodative processing was related to reports of concurrent stress-related growth. Moreover, accommodative processing prospectively predicted self-reported stress-related growth over 2 years (King et al., 2000). Interestingly, self-reported growth through the experience of parenting a child with DS was highest at 2 years for those whose stories were characterized by high levels of both accommodation and closure. This pattern suggests that the subjective sense of personal growth may require not only working through a potentially traumatic event but also finding a sense of positive resolution around that event.

Narrative accommodation was also associated with ego development concurrently. Furthermore, accommodative processing predicted gains in ego development over 2 years, particularly for parents who had "room to grow": Accommodation that is actively grappling with experience, letting go of previous meaning structures, and exploring new ones, at time 1 was especially associated with ego development among parents who were relatively lower on ego development at that time (King et al., 2000). These results suggest, first, that accommodative processing appears to be a characteristic of the mature ego. Second, they suggest that actively accommodating difficult experiences can facilitate ego development over time.

Similar patterns of results for closure and accommodation have been found in other samples (e.g., Lilgendahl, Helson, & John, 2013; Pals, 2006): Closure generally is associated with subjective well-being while accommodation is associated with ego development. And these two outcomes appear to be independent of each other. Such patterns have led to the suggestion that there are two narrative pathways that are associated with two different aspects of maturity (King, 2001; King & Hicks, 2007; Pals, 2006). Importantly, these two pathways are orthogonal. Accommodating a life transition does not imply a lack of closure. Individuals who fully explore potentially traumatic life experiences are not, by necessity, "sadder but wiser."

In sum, narratives of important life experiences are a context in which accommodative processing can be measured and such processing is associated with ego development both concurrently and prospectively. Might narratives about goals serve as a similar venue to capture accommodation and track its association with personality development? We address this question next.

Narrating the Future: Possible Selves and Ego Development

Examining accommodation in the context of goals requires that we consider something beyond a straightforward "to-do list." The construct of possible selves is especially useful in this regard. Possible selves are personalized representations of goals (Markus & Nurius, 1986). They involve images of the self in the future in a host of various roles. Possible selves link goals to broader identity concerns (Oyserman & James, 2011). Features of possible selves (e.g., their content and salience in a person's mental life) have been shown to predict important outcomes such as effort and performance in the academic domain (e.g., Oyserman, Bybee, & Terry, 2006). Possible selves provide a richer context in which to examine the process of accommodation. Because possible selves refer to the host of possible people a person may consider becoming, they allow for an examination of not only who one wishes to be, but who one *used to* wish to be, *the lost possible self*.

King and Raspin (2004, p. 607) defined lost possible future selves as representations of the self in the future, which might have once held the promise of positive affect, but which are no longer a part of a person's life. These possible selves represent the ashes referred to previously: The remnants of who one wished to be in another time, "what might have been" if circumstances had been different (King & Hicks, 2007).

Lost possible selves would seem to be an excellent context in which to measure the processes of personality development through life-changing events. Given the difficulty of letting go of previously cherished goals and the likelihood that these goals might be threatening sources of regret, the degree to which a person is able to elaborate on these goals would seem to be a good indicator of psychological complexity (or ego development). We might expect the developed ego to look upon these goals as legitimately good ones, even if they are no longer available to the self. Although a person's current best possible self is a likely source of well-being, we might expect that the capacity to elaborate on a lost possible self would be especially strongly related to ego development, concurrently and over time.

In order to examine these predictions, two samples of community adults who had experienced such events were recruited. These included women who had experienced divorce after more than 20 years of marriage (King & Raspin, 2004) and gay men and lesbian women (King & Smith, 2004). Although these samples clearly differ in many ways, they each can be seen as having once likely espoused a very different future than the one they were currently pursuing. While the divorced women almost assuredly had imagined their lives in the future with their ex-husbands during their long marriages, the gay and lesbian sample provided a somewhat different possibility. Although most of these participants had imagined that they would "grow up" to be straight (heterosexual), some did not. Nevertheless all of these participants certainly lived in a context in which a different path, a "straight possible self" was the norm.

Each sample was asked to write narrative descriptions of two possible selves and complete measures of psychological well-being and ego development. As with the parents of children with DS, they completed the well-being and ego development measures again, 2 years later.

The first possible self-narrative collected from these samples was their current best possible self. Instructions were:

> We would like you to consider the life you imagine for yourself currently, and in the future. What sorts of things do you hope for and dream about? Imagine that your life has gone as well as it possibly could have. You have worked hard and achieved your goals. Think of this as your "best possible life" or your "happily ever after."

The second narrative was their lost (or for the gay participants "straight") possible self. The instructions for the lost possible selves were variations on the following:

> We would like you to consider your future as you imagined it before [the life changing event]. Try to remember how you imagined your future to be. What sorts of things did you hope for and dream about for your life? Think of this as your "best possible life" or your happily ever after, if you had not experienced [the event].

Two characteristics of these possible selves were examined, their salience and their level of elaboration. Salience was measured using self-report. Immediately after writing each narrative, participants made rating of the salience of that possible self in their current mental life (e.g., "How easy was it for you to bring this description to mind? How vivid was the image for you?"). Elaboration measures were provided by content analyses. A team of coders reliably coded the narratives for their levels of detail, vividness, and richness. The level of elaboration of the lost possible self was the key measure of accommodation.

To appreciate the difference between high and low elaboration, consider the following examples. First, the following is a relatively elaborate lost possible self provided by a woman who experienced divorce after over 20 years of marriage:

> I think I was raised to be a wife and mother. I thought if I followed all the "rules," we would live happily ever after…. Living in a small town in a modest home, being a housewife in retirement years—it was sort of like the television show Mayberry RFD. I wanted to be "Aunt Bea," but with a contented husband who let me be myself—like "Andy." Life would be simple, easy and sweet. (King, 2001, p. 65)

In contrast, a low-elaboration lost possible self from a divorced women is:

> I am a realist and never expect anything from life. (King & Raspin, 2004, p. 616)

Similarly, an example of a highly elaborate straight possible self from a gay man:

> As I was growing up, I envisioned my life to be like the lives of those I admired. Those lives were something to aspire to. I grew up in a small town…. My parents and their friends were

> involved in volunteer work, owned businesses, and were active in community politics. My dream was to be a veterinarian. I imagined that I was married (as that is what is supposed to happen). I dreamed that my wife would be the manager of the pet store we both owned.... We would be active in the community. Small towns can be so much fun.... I would be well-known as someone who is a good person and down to earth.... The business would be successful and eventually passed down to our children. (King, 2001, p. 63)

Finally, an example of a straight possible self rated low on elaboration, from a gay man:

> As I am considered a handsome man, I imagine I would probably have a beautiful blonde wife to contrast to my own dark features. I probably would have concentrated more on education and not so much on partying. Therefore I'd have an executive type position, tidy house in the suburbs, and two kids. (King & Smith, 2004, p. 981)

How did current and lost possible selves relate to well-being and ego development? Although the results for each sample differed in some ways (see King & Raspin, 2004 and King & Smith, 2004, for the divorced women and gay samples, respectively), similar patterns emerged across these different groups. These patterns resonate with those identified for narratives more generally. That is, there were clear differences in the predictors of well-being and predictors of ego development. First, well-being was most strongly associated with the salience ratings for the possible selves. Specifically, endorsing a highly salient current best possible self was strongly related to concurrent well-being. In contrast, the salience of the lost (or straight) possible self was negatively related to well-being and positively related to regret. Thinking about an image of the self in a previously desired but unavailable future was associated with distress. In addition, in both samples, ego development was associated with elaborating on the lost (or straight) possible self. As predicted, the capacity to elaborate on "what might have been" predicted ego development concurrently and prospectively.

Closing Thoughts: Of Phoenixes and Their Ashes

The studies reviewed here were conducted in the hopes of uncovering a place for lost possible selves in personality development. The samples were chosen specifically because they had experienced potentially life-changing events, events that challenged identity and meaning and required a revision of the life story. The choice of ego development as the outcome of interest was, of course, no accident. This aspect of maturity was thought to be ideal for studying individuals who, because of life experience, might endorse lower levels of well-being but might, nevertheless, provide an opportunity to show that negative experiences can play a role in maturity (King & Hicks, 2007). What are the implications of these studies on these potentially exceptional samples for everyday life and everyday development?

Certainly, to the extent that goals are a common aspect of everyday life, all adults are likely to weather the experience of failure and disappointment. Although it may be tempting to simply avoid contemplating these losses, an examination of who we wanted to be may have its benefits: It may not be a pathway to ever increasing happiness but it might be an important step toward wisdom and perhaps acceptance of life-changing events (see Chap. 21, this volume).

These studies have another fascinating lesson for adulthood more generally. As we have noted throughout this chapter, the outcomes of well-being and ego development were independent of each other and were predicted by distinct narrative features. This independence suggests an important lesson about the "trade-offs" of adulthood. Specifically, they suggest that no trade-off is necessary. Happiness and complexity, these two sides of maturity, were never negatively correlated. In the long run, joy is not compromised by wisdom.

Among the participants in these studies there were certainly phoenixes who rose above the ashes of their previous hopes and dreams to construct amazing future selves toward which to strive. Some of these beautiful birds left the ashes of their previous lives behind with nary a thought. Others rose from those ashes, to be sure, but, prior to taking flight, they paused to allow themselves to be changed by their losses. Their eventual flight was no less joyful but perhaps it was made a bit richer by their willingness to contemplate what might have been, even as they perched to soar again toward who they hoped to become.

References

Allemand, M., Steiger, A. E., & Hill, P. L. (2013). Stability of personality traits in adulthood: Mechanisms and implications. *GeroPsych: The Journal of Gerontopsychology and Geriatric Psychiatry, 26,* 5–13.

Block, J. (1982). Assimilation, accommodation, and the dynamics of personality development. *Child Development, 53,* 281–295.

Bonanno, G. A. (2004). Loss, trauma, and human resilience: Have we underestimated the human capacity to thrive after extremely aversive events? *American Psychologist, 59,* 20–28.

Boudreaux, M. J., & Ozer, D. J. (2013). Goal conflict, goal striving, and psychological well-being. *Motivation and Emotion, 37,* 433–443.

Brunstein, J. C., & Gollwitzer, P. M. (1996). Effects of failure on subsequent performance: The importance of self-defining goals. *Journal of Personality and Social Psychology, 70,* 395–407.

Calhoun, L. G., & Tedeschi, R. G. (1999). *Facilitating posttraumatic growth: A clinician's guide.* Mahwah: Erlbaum.

Carlozzi, A. F., Gaa, J. P., & Liberman, D. B. (1983). Empathy and ego development. *Journal of Counseling Psychology, 30,* 113–116.

Carver, C. S., & Scheier, M. F. (2008). Feedback processes in the simultaneous regulation of action and affect. In W. Gardner & J. Shah (Eds.), *Handbook of motivation science* (pp. 308–324). New York City: Guilford.

Coyne, J. C., & Tennen, H. (2010). Positive psychology in cancer care: Bad science, exaggerated claims, and unproven medicine. *Annals of Behavioral Medicine, 39,* 16–26.

Emmons, R. A. (1986). Personal strivings: An approach to personality and subjective well-being. *Journal of Personality and Social Psychology, 51,* 1058–1068.

Emmons, R. A., & King, L. A. (1988). Conflict among personal strivings: Immediate and long term implications for psychological and physical well-being. *Journal of Personality and Social Psychology, 48,* 1040–1048.

Emmons, R. A., Colby, P. M., & Kaiser, H. A. (1998). When losses lead to gains: Personal goals and the recovery of meaning. In P. T. P. Wong & P. S. Fry (Eds.). *The human quest for meaning: A handbook of psychological research and clinical applications* (pp. 163–178). Mahwah: Erlbaum.

Heintzelman, S. J., & King, L. A. (2013). On knowing more than we can tell: Intuition and the human experience of meaning. *Journal of Positive Psychology, 8,* 471–482.

Helgeson, V. S., Reynolds, K. A., & Tomich, P. L. (2006). A meta-analytic review of benefit finding and growth. *Journal of Consulting and Clinical Psychology, 74,* 797–816.

Helson, R. (1992). Women's difficult times and rewriting the life story. *Psychology of Women Quarterly, 16,* 331–347.

Helson, R., & Roberts, B. W. (1994). Ego development and personality change in adulthood. *Journal of Personality and Social Psychology, 66,* 911–920.

Helson, R., & Wink, P. (1987). Two conceptions of maturity examined in the findings of a longitudinal study. *Journal of Personality and Social Psychology, 53,* 531–541.

Hudson, N.W., & Fraley, R. C. (in press). Volitional personality trait change: Can people choose to change their personality traits? *Journal of Personality and Social Psychology.*

Hy, L. X., & Loevinger, J. (1996). *Measuring ego development* (*2nd Ed*). Mahwah: Erlbaum.

Jackson, J. J., Thoemmes, F., Jonkmann, K., Lüdtke, O., & Trautwein, U. (2012). Military training and personality trait development: Does the military make the man, or does the man make the military? *Psychological Science, 23,* 270–277.

Janoff-Bulman, R. (1992). *Shattered assumptions.* New York: Free Press.

Joseph, S., Murphy, D., & Regel, S. (2012). An affective-cognitive processing model of post-traumatic growth. *Clinical Psychology and Psychotherapy, 19,* 315–325.

Karanci, N. A., & Acarturk, C. (2005). Post-traumatic growth among Marmara earthquake survivors involved in disaster preparedness as volunteers. *Traumatology, 11,* 307–323.

King, L. A. (2001). The hard road to the good life: The happy, mature person. *The Journal of Humanistic Psychology, 41,* 51–72.

King, L. A. (2008a). Personal goals and life dreams: Positive psychology and motivation in daily life. In W. Gardner & J. Shah (Eds.), *Handbook of motivation science.* (pp. 518–532). New York City: Guilford.

King, L. A. (2008b). Interventions for enhancing SWB: The pursuit of happiness. In R. J. Larsen & M. Eid (Eds.), *The science of subjective well-being* (pp. 431–448). New York: Guilford.

King, L. A. (2011). The challenge of ego development: Intentional vs. active development. In A. H. Pfaffenberger, P. W. Marko & A. Combs, (Eds.), *The Postconventional Personality* (pp. 163–174). Albany: SUNY Press.

King, L. A., & Burton, C. M. (2003). The hazards of goal pursuit. In E. Chang & L. Sanna (Eds.), *Personality, strategy, and adjustment: Beyond virtues and vices* (pp. 53–69). Washington, D.C.: American Psychological Association.

King, L. A., & Hicks, J. A. (2007). Whatever happened to "what might have been"? Regret, happiness, and maturity. *American Psychologist, 62,* 625–636.

King, L. A., & Raspin, C. (2004). Lost and found possible selves, well-being and ego development in divorced women. *Journal of Personality, 72,* 603–631.

King, L. A., & Smith, N. G. (2004). Gay and straight possible selves: Goals, identity, subjective well -being, and personality development. *Journal of Personality, 72,* 967–994.

King, L. A., & Trent, J. (2012). Personality strengths. In H. Tennen & J. M. Suls (Eds.) *Handbook of psychology, 2nd edition, Vol. 5: Personality and social psychology* (pp. 197–222). New York: Wiley.

King, L. A., Scollon, C. K., Ramsey, C. M., & Williams, T. (2000). Stories of life transition: Happy endings, subjective well-being, and ego development in parents of children with Down Syndrome. *Journal of Research in Personality, 34,* 509–536.

Klosky, J. L., Krull, K. R., Kawashima, T., Leisenring, W., Randolph, M. E., Zebrack, B., et al. (2104). Relations between posttraumatic stress and posttraumatic growth in long-term survivors of childhood cancer: A report from the childhood cancer survivor study. *Health Psychology, 33,* 878–882.

Lilgendahl, J. P., Helson, R., & John, O. P. (2013). Does ego development increase during midlife? The effects of openness and accommodative processing of difficult events. *Journal of Personality, 81,* 403–416.
Lodi-Smith, J., & Roberts, B. W. (2007). Social investment and personality: A meta-analysis of the relationship of personality traits to investment in work, family, religion, and volunteerism. *Personality and Social Psychology Review, 11,* 68–86.
Loevinger, J. (1976). *Ego development: Conceptions and theories.* San Francisco: Jossey-Bass.
Lowe, S. R., Manove, E. E., & Rhodes, J. E. (2013). Posttraumatic stress and posttraumatic growth among low-income mothers who survived Hurricane Katrina. *Journal of Consulting and Clinical Psychology, 81,* 877–889
Lüdtke, O., Roberts, B. W., Trautwein, U., & Nagy, G. (2011). A random walk down university avenue: Life paths, life events and personality trait change at the transition to university life. *Journal of Personality and Social Psychology, 101,* 620–637.
Magnus, K., Diener, E., Fujita, F., & Pavot, W. (1993). Extraversion and neuroticism as predictors of objective life events: A longitudinal analysis. *Journal of Personality and Social Psychology, 65,* 1046–1053.
Markus, H., & Nurius, P. (1986). Possible selves. *American Psychologist, 41,* 954–969.
McAdams, D. P., & McLean, K. C. (2013). Narrative identity. *Current Directions in Psychological Science, 22,* 233–238.
Morris, B. A., Shakespeare-Finch, J., Rieck, M., & Newberry, J. (2005). Multidimensional nature of posttraumatic growth in an Australian population. *Journal of Traumatic Stress, 18,* 575–585.
Oyserman, D., & James, L. (2011). Possible identities. In S.J. Schwartz, K. Luyckx, & V.L. Vignoles (Eds.), *Handbook of identity theory and research (Vols 1 and 2)* (pp. 117–145). New York: Springer.
Oyserman, D., Bybee, D., & Terry, K. (2006). Possible selves and academic outcomes: How and when possible selves impel action. *Journal of Personality and Social Psychology, 91,* 188–204.
Pals, J. L. (2006). Narrative identity processing of difficult life experiences: Pathways of personality development and positive self-transformation in adulthood. *Journal of Personality, 74,* 1079–1110.
Pals, J. L., & John, O. P. (1998). How are dimensions of adult personality related to ego development? An application of the typological approach. In P. M. Westenberg, A. Blasi, & L. D. Cohn (Eds.), *Personality development: Theoretical, empirical, and clinical investigations of Loevinger's conception of ego development* (pp. 113–131). Mahwah: Erlbaum.
Park, C. L., Cohen, L. H., & Murch, R. L. (1996). Assessment and prediction of stress-related growth. *Journal of Personality, 64,* 71–105.
Park, C. L., Chmielewski, J., & Blank, T. O. (2010). Post-traumatic growth: Finding positive meaning in cancer survivorship moderates the impact of intrusive thoughts on adjustment in younger adults. *Psycho-oncology, 19,* 1139–1147.
Pfaffenberger, A. H., Marko, P. W., & Combs, A. (Eds.) (2011). *The postconventional personality.* Albany: SUNY Press.
Pomerantz, E. M., Saxon, J. L., & Oishi, S. (2000). The psychological trade-offs of goal investment. *Journal of Personality and Social Psychology, 79,* 617–630.
Roberts, B. W., Walton, K. E., & Veichtbauer, W. (2006). Patterns of mean-level change in personality traits across the life course. *Psychological Bulletin, 132,* 1–25
Scollon, C. N., & Diener, E. (2006). Love, work, and changes in extraversion and neuroticism over time. *Journal of Personality and Social Psychology, 91,* 1152–1165.
Sheldon, K. M., & Hoon, T.H. (2007). The multiple determination of well-being: Independent effects of positive traits, needs, goals, selves, social supports, and cultural contexts. *Journal of Happiness Studies, 8,* 565–592.
Sheldon, K. M., & Kasser, T. (2001). Goals, congruence, and positive well-being: New empirical support for humanistic theories. *Journal of Humanistic Psychology, 41,* 30–50.
Specht, J., Egloff, B., & Schmukle, S.C. (2011). Stability and change in personality across the life course: The impact of age and major life events on mean-level and rank-order stability of the Big Five. *Journal of Personality and Social Psychology, 101,* 862–882.

Specht, J., Egloff, B., & Schmukle, S. C. (2013). Examining mechanisms of personality maturation: The impact of life satisfaction on the development of the Big Five personality traits. *Social Psychological and Personality Science, 4,* 181–189.

Sutin, A.R., Costa, P.T., Wethington, E., & Eaton, W. (2010). Turning points and lessons learned: Stressful life events and personality trait development across middle adulthood. *Psychology and Aging, 73,* 524–533.

Tedeschi, R. G., & Calhoun, L.G. (1996). The posttraumatic growth inventory: Measuring the positive legacy of trauma. *Journal of Traumatic Stress, 9,* 455–471.

Tedeschi, R. G., & McNally, R. J. (2011). Can we facilitate posttraumatic growth in combat veterans? *American Psychologist, 66,* 19–24.

Tennen, H., & Affleck, G. (2009). Assessing positive life change: In search of meticulous methods. In C. L. Park, S. C. Lechner, M. H. Antoni, A. L. Stanton, & Annette L. (Eds.), *Medical illness and positive life change: Can crisis lead to personal transformation?* (pp. 31–49, 261). Washington, D.C.: American Psychological Association.

Triplett, K. N., Tedeschi, R. G., Cann, A., Calhoun, L. G., & Reeve, C. L. (2012). Posttraumatic growth, meaning in life, and life satisfaction in response to trauma. *Psychological Trauma: Theory, Research, Practice, and Policy, 4,* 400–410.

Vaidya, J. G., Gray, E. K., Haig, J., Mroczek, D. K., & Watson, D. (2008). Differential stability and individual growth trajectories of Big Five and affective traits during young adulthood. *Journal of Personality, 76,* 267–304.

Vancouver, J. B., Weinhardt, J. M., & Schmidt, A.M. (2010). A formal, computational theory of multiple-goal pursuit: Integrating goal-choice and goal-striving processes. *Journal of Applied Psychology, 95,* 985–1008.

Vancouver, J. B., Gullekson, N. L., Morse, B. J., & Warren, M. A. (2014). Finding a between-person negative effect of self-efficacy on performance: Not just a within-person effect anymore. *Human Performance, 27,* 243–261.

Wilson, T. D., & Gilbert, D. T. (2005). Affective forecasting: Knowing what to want. *Current Directions in Psychological Science, 14,* 131–134.

Wrosch, C., Bauer, I., & Scheier, M. F. (2005). Regret and quality of life across the adult life span: The influence of disengagement and available future goals. *Psychology and Aging, 20,* 657–670.

Wrosch, C., Amir, E., & Miller, G. (2011). Goal adjustment capacities, coping, and subjective well-being: The sample case of caregiving for a family member with mental illness. *Journal of Personality and Social Psychology, 100,* 934–946.

Chapter 18
Younger and Older Coastal Fishers Face Catastrophic Loss after Hurricane Katrina

Katie E. Cherry, Loren D. Marks, Rachel Adamek and Bethany A. Lyon

Introduction

Natural disasters bring catastrophic destruction and traumatic stress. The psychosocial consequences of disasters include losses of material goods, property, and disruptions to social networks and lifestyle. Threats to mental health for survivors are an important public health consideration and may include post-traumatic stress disorder (PTSD), anxiety, and depression. These challenges, among others, are well documented in the disaster science literature in the first 2 years after a disaster (Cherry, 2009; Cherry, Galea, & Silva, 2008; Neria, Galea, & Norris, 2009). Comparatively less is known about long-term consequences for temporarily and permanently displaced residents of devastated communities more than 2 years after disaster (see Chaps. 10, 12, and 13, this volume).

The environmental consequences of hurricanes are of particular concern to commercial fishers for whom the water is a way of life. Coastal erosion and the progressive loss of barrier islands and marshland which have historically buffered the forceful impact of hurricanes are worrisome prospects. Louisiana's fishers produce a sizeable percentage of seafood worldwide and are recognized as the largest provider of seafood within the continental USA (Lee & Blanchard, 2012). Despite their

K. E. Cherry (✉) · R. Adamek · B. A. Lyon
Department of Psychology, Louisiana State University, 236 Audubon Hall,
Baton Rouge, LA 70803-5501, USA
e-mail: pskatie@lsu.edu

R. Adamek
e-mail: rachel54a@gmail.com

B. A. Lyon
e-mail: blyon2@tigers.lsu.edu

L. D. Marks
School of Family Life, Brigham Young University, 2092C Joseph F. Smith Building,
Provo, Utah 84602, USA
e-mail: loren_marks@byu.edu

K. E. Cherry (ed.), *Traumatic Stress and Long-Term Recovery*,
DOI 10.1007/978-3-319-18866-9_18

centrality to the seafood industry, relatively little research has addressed the impact of natural disasters on the US Gulf Coast commercial fishers, representing a serious gap in the disaster science literature. Because fishers' livelihood is dependent upon natural resources, one might expect greater risk for adverse psychological reactions after disaster compared to the general population. On the contrary, fishers' historical presence and longevity in hurricane-prone coastal regions imply a culture of resilience which may reduce vulnerability when treacherous hurricanes strike. Insights gained from commercial fishers and their families in the years after Katrina may shed new light on factors that lessen risk and promote resilience in the wake of catastrophic disaster.

On August 29, 2005, Hurricane Katrina made landfall in the US Gulf Coast region which includes (west to east) Texas, Louisiana, Mississippi, Alabama, and Florida. Katrina's swath of catastrophic destruction (declared a federal disaster area) was unusually wide, spanning an estimated 90,000 square miles, similar in size to Great Britain (Weisler, Barbee, & Townsend, 2006). Many fishers in the present study had sheltered in place on boats secured in the Violet Canal and other ostensibly safe locations within the levee protection system. Large fishing vessels that did not sink in the storm became a collection point for storm victims rescued from roof tops or pulled from the flooding which followed the levee breaches in Katrina's immediate aftermath. An early coroner's report (September, 2005) offered a snapshot of the loss of human life, estimating that over a 1000 bodies were recovered from Katrina's floodwaters in New Orleans in the first weeks after the storm (Cataldie, 2007). Considered the most devastating and costly hurricane to hit the USA, Katrina's estimated death toll overall stands at 1,800 and over 125 billion US dollars in damages (Graumann et al., 2006). On September 24, 2005, less than a month after Katrina, Hurricane Rita crashed into the western side of Louisiana and southeast Texas. Rita, also a category 3 hurricane at landfall, directly caused seven fatalities and property damage reaching an estimated 11.3 billion US dollars (National Hurricane Center, 2007). For specifics on the 2005 hurricanes, see Cherry (2009), Kessler, Galea, Gruber, Sampson, Petukhova, and Wang (2009), and Kilmer, Gil-Rivas, Tedeschi, and Calhoun (2010).

In this chapter, we focus on the commercial fishers of St. Bernard and Plaquemine Parishes. The rich cultural heritage of coastal fishers—lifestyles and traditions—and their intergenerational knowledge of hurricanes acquired over centuries of living in the bayous and natural waterways of south Louisiana warrant careful consideration. A glimpse of the history and cultural milieu that characterizes these south Louisiana fishing communities is given next.

Historic Overview: Two Fishing Communities, Cultural Heritage, and Hurricanes

Located approximately 5 miles southeast of the city of New Orleans, St. Bernard is a suburban community with an estimated pre-Katrina population of 68,000. The population of St. Bernard is smaller today with current estimates at 43,482

(US Census Bureau, 2013). Perhaps best known for its world-class seafood, St. Bernard is largely a fishing community and home to multigeneration families of fishers who have caught shrimp with nets on wooden boats ("double riggers") built with their own hands for over a century. A warm and personable community, St. Bernard also has a unique intergenerational aspect, where suburban families have grown up together as neighbors and friends for decades.

The longevity of fishing communities in St. Bernard is noteworthy, with a rich cultural heritage traced back to the 1780s when the first Isleños settlers from the Canary Islands came to south Louisiana. Spanish remains a predominant language spoken among some families of Isleños descent today (Coles, 2012). St. Bernard is also home to the Los Isleños Museum, which contains a treasure trove of Isleños' culture and folklore. Encapsulated in a quaint and historic wooden building (rebuilt in the years after Katrina) are ornate costumes and replicas of wooden fishing boats. Among the items on display are fascinating, although decidedly different home remedies for the treatment of a variety of maladies (Robin, 2000). The Isleño Fiesta, an annual festival sponsored by the Los Isleños Heritage and Cultural Society to celebrate Isleños' ways of life is held on the museum grounds in March (Los Isleños Learn, 2014).

Plaquemines Parish is another south Louisiana coastal community with a unique cultural heritage and is home to a multigenerational Croatian fishing community. As documented in *Yugoslavs in Louisiana* (Vujnovich, 1974), the first Croatian settlers came to south Louisiana in the 1800s and lived in camps on the bayous in Plaquemines, Jefferson, and Lafourche Parishes. Croatian men immigrated to south Louisiana and made their livelihood by oyster fishing, leaving their families, wives, and children in the old country. In the middle to late 1800s, the United Slavonian Benevolent Society (USBA) was formed. The USBA established tombs—one in Buras and one in the city of New Orleans—to allow proper burial for Croatian immigrants who died here (Ware, 1996).

Oyster farming is an important agricultural component in Plaquemines Parish, where residents have fished oysters on flat boats ("luggers") since the days of wooden rakes and backbreaking labor in the hot sun. Modern methods and mechanized dredging techniques are used to fish oysters today. In the 1950s, the Louisiana Oyster Dealers and Growers Association was formed to collectively lobby and promote the development of the oyster industry (Ware, 1996). Today, oyster farming remains a significant industry in Plaquemines Parish among other coastal parishes in south Louisiana, although the 2010 British Petroleum (BP) Deepwater Horizon Oil Spill has severely threatened this industry, as discussed in Chap. 4 (this volume).

In addition to the Croatian community and oyster farming, Plaquemines Parish is significant as the site where Hurricane Katrina made landfall. Packing 150 mph winds, the eye of Hurricane Katrina covered a 30–50-mile swath, from Buras to Pointe a la Hache (see Fig. 18.1). The levee surrounding this part of south Louisiana was not breached; it was overtopped, bringing a devastating 30–40 ft of water into south Plaquemines. With unrelenting force, this water punched a hole on the other side, a levee breach from the inside out, leaving a gaping 150-ft hole straight into

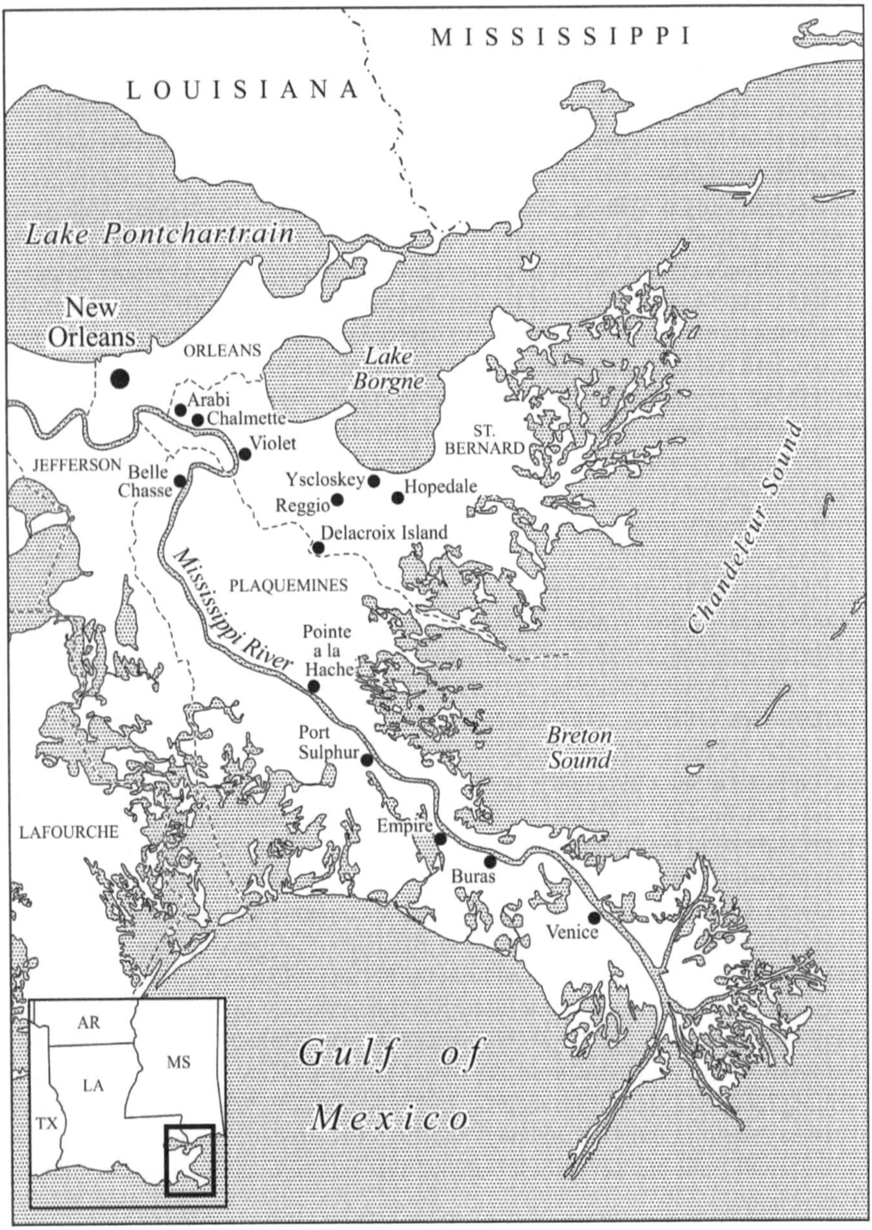

Fig. 18.1 St. Bernard and Plaquemines Parishes in South Louisiana. (Courtesy of Mary Lee Eggart, Cartographer, 2014)

the Gulf of Mexico. As the first author has been told by a resident of Buras who witnessed Katrina's aftermath, the flooded towns in south Plaquemines experienced a tide, bringing all manner of sea life from the Gulf directly into people's front yards.

Lifelong residents of the US Gulf Coast are well acquainted with the threat and environmental realities of severe weather. The Atlantic hurricane season begins on June 1 and concludes on November 30 (National Hurricane Center, 2015). Year after year, hurricane season comes and goes, sometimes with great activity churning in the Gulf of Mexico and other times with less activity and relative calm. Storm preparations and anticipation are fundamental to coastal residents. They either evacuate, leaving the area for a few days until the storm has passed, or they *hunker down* and ride out the storm as coastal residents have done for centuries. For commercial fishers, the large shrimping and oyster boats are moved to secure locations within the levee protection system or taken to distant ports well beyond the anticipated reach of a potentially deadly hurricane. No one would have imagined these austere and commanding sea vessels would become a safe haven for hundreds of storm-ravaged strangers rescued by first responders and brave citizens in the last days of August 2005.

For younger and older coastal residents alike, storms associated with flooding and significant property damage stand out in memory, serving as a reference point against which future storms are compared. Older coastal residents talk about hurricanes that destroyed homes before storms were named. For example, the unnamed storm of 1947 demolished homes in Yscloskey, Hopedale, and Delacroix Island (see Fig. 18.1). Less than a decade later, Hurricane Flossy struck the central Gulf Coast on September 24, 1956, as a category 1 storm that directly caused 15 deaths (Dunn, Davis, & Moore, 1956). Middle-aged and older coastal residents spoke of Hurricane Betsy on September 9, 1965, with flooding in New Orleans and portions of St. Bernard. At 90 years of age, one lifelong coastal resident spoke of losing homes in three different hurricanes, Flossy, Betsy, and Katrina. As she described it, rebuilding homes and reestablishing routines of everyday living were part of life, something one does without hesitation or complaint. Listening to very old adults describe losing everything and rebuilding multiple times without litany, self-pity, or blame, one gets the sense that *resilience* (referring to the tendency to bounce back from negative life events) is a developmental characteristic acquired over time through experience and repeated exposure to adversity.

To summarize, we explore Katrina's impact on commercial fishers and their family members who depend on natural resources for their livelihood in this chapter. The contrast between younger (less than 55 years of age) and older (55+ years) fishers is of particular interest. One might reasonably assume that distal variables such as cultural heritage and tradition may hold greater meaning among older fishers. Older fishers who have lived in hurricane-prone coastal regions for over a half-century have likely developed hurricane preparedness techniques and methods of coping, possibly passed down through fishing families for generations. These personal characteristics among seasoned fishers may contribute to individual and family resilience and the recovery and revitalization of communities when deadly and destructive hurricanes strike.

Method

Participants and Procedure

The sample was comprised of 64 fishers and their family members. All had experienced catastrophic losses in the 2005 hurricanes (Cherry et al., 2015; Chap. 4, this volume). To examine age-related differences in coping responses, the sample was split at the median age to form groups of younger (M=43.2, SD=10.9 years; age range: 21–54 years) and older adults (M=66.5, SD=10.5 years; age range: 55–90 years). In this chapter, we focus on fishers' responses to the following open-ended questions:

1. *In times of trouble, people often turn to their religion and spiritual beliefs to help them cope with life stresses. Have your religious beliefs and practices helped you cope with Hurricanes Katrina and Rita? If so, in what way?*
2. *In times of trouble, people may turn to a faith community to help them cope with life stresses. Has a church or faith community helped you cope with Hurricanes Katrina and Rita? If so, in what way?*
3. *They say every cloud has a silver lining, and even the most awful events can have positive outcomes. Do you think there are any positive outcomes that can come from Hurricanes Katrina and Rita? If so, what are they?*

Of the 64 persons in the sample, four couples responded jointly to the open-ended questions, and one participant declined for a total of 59 responses which were digitally recorded and transcribed verbatim. For each transcription, two separate data audits were performed by different graduate research assistants to ensure accuracy of these narrative data.

Analyses and Coding

Narrative data were content analyzed in a manner consistent with grounded theory methodology (Strauss & Corbin, 1998). Two student teams (each comprised of four coders and one team leader) met weekly during the 2014 spring semester to carry out the open-coding process (see Chap. 12, this volume, for a description). One team coded younger fishers' responses, and the other team coded older fishers' responses. Each week, the two coding teams met separately to discuss the prevalent ideas and themes covered in the interviews. To ensure that all reported themes for the two age groups were verifiable and clearly supported by the data, the two team leaders revisited all interviews within their age group and copied and pasted primary data that had been directly linked with major themes. As a final check to increase rigor, two senior research assistants who had not participated in the open-coding process reviewed the data files (one file for each major theme) for accuracy and completeness. As a result, each of the major themes reported here had several pages of supporting data drawn from multiple interviews—consistent with Patton's (2002) recommendation of creating a data "audit trail" (p. 93).

For the major themes identified in this chapter, there was some overlap and similarity across the two age groups. There were, however, differences in the respective order of importance and salience across age groups—as well as some nuances that were captured during the process of team-based analysis. These themes are reported next along with more than 50 illustrative and supportive examples taken directly from the interviews.

Findings

In overview, we begin with *Materialism and True Colors Revealed: Despicable Deeds and Acts of Grace After the Storm* (Theme 1). In this theme, we focus on the polarizing effects of Katrina, where the best and the worst of humanity seemed evident after the storm. The next theme, *Helping Efforts Across Denominations* (Theme 2), overlaps substantially across the younger and older groups. Participants in both age groups revealed similar (sometimes strikingly similar) perceptions and reports in connection with this theme. However, our last theme, *Historical Ties that Bind: Old Roots Versus New Connections* (Theme 3), features noteworthy differences in responses between younger and older coastal fishers.

Theme 1: Materialism and True Colors Revealed: Despicable Deeds and Acts of Grace After the Storm

The first central theme voiced by our participants reflects a recurring, heightened awareness of the fleeting nature of material possessions. Many participants critically discussed some aspect of what might be broadly labeled *materialism*. With respect to money and the material possessions that money can buy, the catastrophic Hurricanes, Katrina and Rita, seemed to yield or "reveal" two diametrically opposed patterns of human response. One end of the spectrum involves the phenomena of looting and corruptly maximizing profits—the other end is an elevated sense of the worth of human life, often accompanied by generosity and unselfishness. In connection with Theme 1, we begin with a few brief references to the negative tendencies witnessed in Katrina's aftermath (see also Chap. 13, this volume).

One participant noted that several of the "kids" that lived around him started looting after the storm. He reportedly redirected their efforts:

> 361: They were coming back with TVs. They were stealing everything, you know. Radios, and TVs, and stuff like that…the kids [were]. I said, "But listen: Where you going to go with that? You can't eat it, and you can't drink it! You [are] going to starve to death with that! …Come back with food! ….You see anything floating [that we can eat], don't be stupid, pick it up, the canned goods, pick them up! Go gather food! And you all come right back here." So, boy, they go gather up [canned food] stuff and they come right back to me. And then I formed a posse, the kids got together, it was the kids that did everything [to keep us alive]. *(O)(57-year-old male)*

As looting of possessions reached its peak and began to spill from businesses to homes, the concerns of non-evacuated survivors spiked. One participant recalled:

> 334: "[At first] I left the gun out. [But then], I couldn't. I said, "What do I need a gun for? We don't need a gun, we just got hit with a hurricane." *(O)(58-year-old female)*

A few participants shared their view that the aftermath of the hurricane(s) revealed the "true identity" or "true colors" of people. The following excerpt is illustrative:

> 352: People were brought to their bare self. People…their *true identity* had become exposed. [You saw them] for what they really were…. You're at the mercy of whoever will show you any [mercy]…. But [some] people used and manipulated and lied and took advantage and abused [other people] on a scale that was—[well], it was despicable. And [some who did these things] showed no remorse, or respect for people because they felt [that others] owe them something, I guess. *(Y)(46-year-old male)*

Another woman (312) similarly concluded that the changes and financial upheaval surrounding the hurricanes created a context where "We got to see true colors of people." *(Y)(40-year-old female)*. While some storm survivors were eager to grab and acquire during the aftermath, first responders and other heroic citizens who had not evacuated before the storm were concerned with saving lives (for documentary evidence and specific description, see Buuck, 2007; Schaefer, 2007; Wells, 2008). A college-aged participant, who spoke of his mother (who was accustomed to providing for herself), provides a striking counter example to looting and stealing to improve one's own lot. He recalled:

> 314: We didn't have anything to eat, and the Red Cross would come around giving out lunches and my mom was crying because she didn't want to have to take food…. *(Y) (22-year-old male)*

The same young man, who was in high school at the time Katrina hit, also recalled:

> 314: [The] environment at Holy Cross [School] helped me be strong through times like that, and you see other kids at school and they're dealing with the same problems that you're dealing with. I know some kids that didn't have that strong family behind them like I did. I was…like I said, I was blessed to have that…. I know this one…guy I went to school with…he was working two jobs to help his mom rebuild their house [and he was still] in high school. I mean who should have to do that?

The crisis of Katrina placed new demands but also reportedly stimulated new opportunities and realizations in the lives of many of our participants.

As noted earlier, there were some reports and witnesses relating to persons who seemed to emphasize and cling to the monetary and material aspects of life through looting, dishonest manipulation, and other antisocial channels. Although this tendency to "grab" was mentioned, participants' reports far more frequently referenced changes *away* from a materialistic or acquisition orientation in their own lives (see Chap. 21, this volume). The remainder of this theme's discussion is devoted to conveying the participants' related experiences and differences in the outlook on life they reported. Some, for example, juxtaposed the fleeting value of possessions with the precious nature of life itself, as reflected in these five excerpts:

> 302: The one positive thing I could think of is that we're all living, we still, all my family made it through the storm; [our pets and] animals, and all my friends that I know made it

through the storm. And you know, *the possessions, you can always get back.... [But] life you can't.* ...I want to take every day...like it's the last day. *(O)(59-year-old male)*

346: [The initial shock] goes beyond just losing your home and pictures and your belongings. [What really makes you] emotionally distraught...[is] not knowing if your family members are okay and where you're going to end up next or what's going to happen [in] your future [life]. *(Y)(25-year-old female)*

339: [Y]ou got your babies, that's the main thing. *You can replace things, but you can't replace a life. (O)(63-year-old female)*

313: As long as it is not a human life and it is material things [that you lost], they can be replaced, and [things] are not really worth what you think they are anyway. *(Y)(47-year-old male)*

345: I hear...after Katrina, with [our] loss[es], "I'm so sorry" and I'm like, "Don't be. You know [what, our stuff might be gone but], we're still alive. *(Y)(51-year-old male)*

Several participants reportedly experienced a change in priorities following Katrina—a change away from an acquisition orientation or what finance scholars refer to as "conspicuous consumption" (Moore & Asay, 2008). The following excerpts are representative of a larger array of similar responses:

341: [I realized that] when I go out [of this life], I got to give [my stuff] to somebody else. But I done got that figured out. A lot of people are still trying to acquire things. I've done switched that off. I don't need to acquire no more things. And I find that's what makes living life a lot better, when you [see that you] only need so many things. When you get too overwhelmed with acquiring things, it messes your life up. *(O)(55-year-old male)*

Participant 341 mentioned that when this life is over, he will have to "give [his stuff] to somebody else." However, the next participant decided not to wait that long before passing along much of her wardrobe. She explained:

331: My biggest thing that I think everyone should know is not to take anything for granted. It's, because that's how I was before Katrina. I just figured that's how it was for everybody; and now I don't take anything for granted at all. ...That's the biggest thing that I learned from Katrina. And [I learned that] material possessions don't mean anything.... *I have so many clothes, I'm giving them all away...* [I was really down after Katrina but my friend], she told me one day that I had to get a grip and stop complaining and fix myself in my head. So, I just, I don't know, something just clicked. I just decided to go [and do things differently]... I kind of made "before-Katrina" life seem more like it was a different life, [that person was] not me. That was somebody else who lived that [way], that's kind of how I see it now.... *(Y)(21-year-old female)*

Two other shifts in perspective follow next:

330: The acts of kindness [from others], that is what was the silver lining. We really relearned what was really important. You know, before the storm we had a lot of material things and the kids were both in private schools. We were working really hard to supply the kids with a life that we thought was a good life for them. And after we went through everything, what we thought was good did not mean that much. And we had to go through [Katrina] to find [that] out.... And hopefully by us seeing it that way, the girls will live a life...[that is] more rewarding. *(Y)(43-year-old female)*

324: [An experience like Katrina] reminds us that...the material things in this life are really not that important because no matter how much you have, [no matter how many goods you] accumulate here, you're going to lose them sooner or later—whether you lose them in a disaster or…[well], if you don't lose them that way, you're going to lose them when you die anyway…. [Really remembering] that makes us realize [that] what's really important in life is your relationship with your friends and family and God. *(O)(55-year-old female)*

The latter reflection from participant 324 presents not only a reminder or remembrance that "the material things in this life are really not that important" but also an emphasis that what *is* "really important in life is your relationship with your friends and family and God." Several of the participants not only mentioned a personal or familial move away from materialism following Katrina—they also invoked the Divine in their discussion, as captured in the following two examples:

325: [God] helped me. The thing is that it is not about…material things, [material things] are not everything, you know. *(O)(60-year-old male)*

332: [Y]ou can show a young person that in spite of the devastation we had down here, we still had God. We still had family. We still had church. Despite losing everything [possession wise]…that [faith] was there, so we never really lost *everything*. *(Y)(52-year-old female)*

A final illustration of both a shift away from materialism and an invocation of God came from an individual who referenced significant financial resources and mentioned that they do not have "bills [they] can't pay." However, this participant framed the life-altering catastrophe of Katrina as something that reportedly awoke him and gave him "my soul back." He explained:

352: God took me out of my element because He knew that I had no chance of changing my life from what I was, in my surroundings. I had no chance of making it [spiritually, the way I was]…. There is a whole lot of worse things that could have happened to me. I feel quite blessed, very fortunate. I left. I saved not only my life, but gained a soul. I gained my soul back. I got my life. God gave me a new life…greater than any life I have ever had up to that point…. Who would you call upon to help you if not Him when you need it the most? People can only give you information or money. Maybe that is what you need sometimes, but it never seems to fill the void. You are always missing something…. I have lost everything behind me, and I have gained everything in front of me…. *(Y)(46-year-old male)*

For many of our participants, life after Katrina was never the same. However, in some cases, life was not only more challenging but also spiritually and relationally richer—sparked by a renewed emphasis on precious intangibles such as faith, true friendship, and family relationships. It is to these intangibles that we now turn.

Theme 2—Helping Efforts Across Denominations: "[God] was using His people to help His [other] people."

A discussion of religious denominational differences in Louisiana requires a brief note on social and religious historical context. Based on data from the US Census Bureau, the 2013 population of Louisiana was a little over 4.6 million. The largest denomination in the state is the Catholic Church with more than 1.2 million adherents followed by the Southern Baptist Convention with 709,650 members. No other faith exceeds 200,000 members (Louisiana Religion Traditions, 2010), making Louisiana a predominantly Catholic/Baptist state.

In terms of religious heritage, French Catholic settlers in Nova Scotia (called Acadians or "Cajuns") engaged in a series of battles with British troops during the early and middle eighteenth century that climaxed during the French and Indian War. Commencing in 1755, thousands of Acadians were expelled from Nova Scotia, and many of these refugees settled in regions that comprise present-day south Louisiana (Faragher, 2005). This "tragic…expulsion of the French [Catholic] Acadians" from Nova Scotia by the armed forces representing England and her Protestant faith laid a foundation for deep-seated tensions between Catholics and Protestants in Louisiana (Faragher, 2005). At least remnants of these tensions are apparent two and a half centuries later—indeed, the state remains divided into a northern, Baptist "Bible belt," and the heavily Catholic and Acadian ("Cajun") southern portion of the state that depends largely on the mouth of the Mississippi River and the waters of the Gulf of Mexico for economic and literal sustenance.

Consistent with this religious and demographic sketch, the Louisiana Gulf Coast fishing families interviewed during the present research project were predominantly Catholic (73.4 %). This context sets the table for our second emergent theme, which addresses significant reported and perceived differences in helping, rescuing, and assistance efforts made by churches and church members in the aftermath of both natural (Hurricanes Katrina and Rita) and man-made (Deepwater Horizon Oil Spill) disasters. As one participant summarized:

> 326: It just makes you realize that, you know, in times of trouble, you know, you will have somebody there to help you. *(Y)(52-year-old male)*

One young woman was sufficiently impressed by the "on-the-ground" disaster recovery efforts of diverse churches that she made an effort to attend and worship with some of them. After Katrina hit, she reported:

> 331: I would come home and read my Bible and pray. I think without all those different groups of churches [that helped out], I don't think I would've been able to cope as well as I did. Because I got something from each different church that I went to; I got a different little view on everything. *(Y)(21-year-old female)*

Another woman was also impressed by the array of engaged churches that she witnessed in action in the aftermath. She said of the churches,

> 318: They all wanted to help. And I think that in helping others, you feel like you have done something worthwhile. *(Y)(50-year-old female)*

A man reflected in his interview on his astonishment at diverse church involvement in the disaster aftermath. He admitted,

> 304: That was kind of surprising to me, I ain't going to lie. I was [blown away]. All of them people, [all of them] different religions, and they're all helping, you know? But they did. And like I said, it wasn't just one religion, it was all of them, you know? *(Y)(46-year-old male)*

From among the many denominations that helped, some participants singled out a specific group that impressed them. When talking about helpful faith community involvement, this woman told us:

> 332: Yes, [I remember] the Amish. And some of those men would just show up. We're not of the Amish faith and don't care to participate in the Amish faith, but it was another demonstration of the community of churches setting aside their philosophical differences to deal with the truly [incredible] physical devastation down here. Those men would come down here with hammers and shovels and whatever they needed…and help as much as they were able. And they didn't preach to you, but you got to see how they lived…. [T]he Amish guys were helping clean up around here, helping people hammer things back together or reconstruct from nothing. And the wives would be right behind them making sure that you had clean clothes, you had food. …[They] would take your children and just go play with your children so the grown-ups could do grown-up things without having to stress about the kids…. It reaffirms your faith in the compassion of man…. And they never forced their faith on you, but if you were willing to share God, they were willing to listen. So, I think that's pretty big. *(Y)(52-year-old female)*

Another man related his experience with a work group from a church whose name he did not mention and may not have even been aware of—although it was apparently not "their" church.

> 345: They were a church group [and they were] going to gut[1] this person's house out…[but] he changed his mind. So they had nothing to do so they all came down my way…. And I said, "Well, [I can sure use your help]." We knocked it out in an hour and a half. So that was a great blessing. And somebody happened to call and I said, "God sent me about twenty angels here. I'll be wrapped up this evening!" So that was really, really good. And they felt good about what they did. For a person who doesn't really like to ask for help, like myself, it was a real blessing…. God wrapped it up. *(Y)(51-year-old male)*

Even among our predominantly Catholic sample, several positive comments were made about the outreach efforts of the Baptist church, including the following report:

> 331: [One group that helped us was] the Baptist church, everything that they did for us. They showed me that we weren't alone. And that also helped me see that even though we had our house destroyed and everything destroyed, we weren't…God didn't abandon us completely. *(Y)(21-year-old female)*

Another Catholic participant recalled another kind "gesture" from members of the Baptist church that boosted her faith:

> 353: [A group that] was from a Baptist church, just came along and gave everybody ten dollars, and it was just so…it was a wonderful gesture. [M]y son said, "What's ten dollars?" I said, "It's not the ten dollars, it's the idea that these people came out to help." And I think that, that made you even have more faith in God, because *He was using His people to help His [other] people. (O)(71-year-old female)*

---

[1] When floods strike, a top priority in home cleanup is to remove soaked sheetrock and insulation to prevent the base of the lumber framing from rot. This urgent removal is referred to as "gutting." If gutting is done soon after the flooding, it can prevent rot from destroying the structural integrity of the home. If gutting is delayed and rot commences, the entire home must be razed. During hurricane aftermath, some church groups like the one referenced here go out in clean-up parties to do this urgently needed work without compensation.

The implicit use of language by this participant to indicate that both Baptists and Catholics are "His (God's) people" is representative of a post-disaster outreach of warmth and brotherhood that seemed to be present in several interviews. However, while goodwill for "His people" from Protestant denominations was apparent in several interviews with Catholic participants, another (not overpowering but discernible) theme was a recurring frustration with the Catholic Church's less than adequate outreach, as reported by some long-time Catholic parishioners (see Chap. 14, this volume). One man who had lost his home and business in Katrina went to Mass in a different state during his evacuation. He told us:

> 303: I just can't believe it either. I was standing there, I was shocked. I was standing there when [the priest at the church] says, "Well, if you're looking for a hand out, I can't help you. We lost the roof off our church and we need five thousand dollars to repair our roof." *(Y)(42-year-old male)*

Another participant reported a very similar experience with her sister when they visited a church during their evacuation shortly after Katrina. She reported the following interaction with a church representative:

> 312: [The] exact words to my sister—I turned around and walked away—[were], "We don't have anything for you." And my sister said, "I just want to go to Church services." He says, "Well, if you want to come to a service that's fine, but we don't have anything for you." *(Y)(40-year-old female)*

Our intent here is not to malign any church, including the Catholic Church.[2] Examples like the previous one recurred, but there were other Catholic participants who noted and applauded the efforts of specific Catholic churches in the area. For example, Participant 318 reported, "The Immaculate Heart of Mary is the church that my brother goes to.… They collected $25,000…in one weekend for Katrina [victims]." *(Y)(50-year-old male)*.

In Chap. 14 (this volume), we discuss the complexities and challenges of the Catholic Church's response in the Katrina aftermath in greater detail. However, the following excerpt fleshes out (and adds needed balance to) our brief discussion here: One of the cruelest consequences of the storms for our participants who were heavily invested in faith community was that those neighborhoods who suffered the most severe damage to homes were the same neighborhoods most likely to lose their (heavily damaged) neighborhood churches. Thus, those who arguably needed their *own* faith community, their *own* priest, (and) their *own* familiar sacred building most profoundly were least likely to have access to these spiritual and physical resources. As a 77-year-old female from our parallel study summarized:

> 215: When I came back here [after the flooding], everything was so disorganized…*the church was suffering the same way we all were*. The church lost everything too. Remember? The rectory, the church was flooded. Everything [was flooded]. The church was in dire

[2] The authors have published several previous articles or chapters containing largely or partly Catholic samples that present the faith from a constructive perspective, based on participants' reports. Indeed, one such article has focused solely on the strengths of Roman Catholic families (Batson & Marks, 2008).

> need of help itself. I mean as far as the community goes…basically, there was hardly any community. Everybody was in the same boat. Everybody…that came back was rebuilding their houses, rebuilding their lives. The church was trying to rebuild. The church lost everything [too]….

The recurring negative reports and perceptions regarding Catholic-based outreach (or lack of Catholic outreach) by the Catholic participants…and the recurring positive reports of the helping efforts of non-Catholic denominations are somewhat counterintuitive—based on documented trends in psychological research indicating that participants tend to rate the efforts and performance of groups to which one belongs *more* favorably (Roese & Olson, 2007).

In Theme 2 *(Helping Efforts Across Denominations)*, we have discussed the participant-lauded relief efforts of "outside" churches during the Katrina/Rita aftermath. These churches were often "outside" in two respects: (1) The faith-based groups were typically non-Catholic and (2) the groups were often from other cities, geographical areas, or even other states. Some groups stayed for days or even weeks—but eventually they had to return to their homes. As time progressed and infrastructure returned, the local or "insider" churches reportedly regained traction and influence. Indeed, support from "their" local faith communities was frequently referenced as participants learned how to live again during the long-term recovery.

As we conclude our discussions of Themes 1 and 2, we remind the reader that there were minimal age-related differences between the younger (<55 years) and older (55+years) groups with these themes. Indeed, the content of participants' responses was very similar. In the third and final theme, however, age group differences did emerge, and we saw discernible markers based on longevity and life experience, as discussed next.

Theme 3: Historical Ties that Bind: Old Roots Versus New Connections

Katrina's massive storm surge left no home or building standing; only tangled marsh grass and thick mud so deep that it was difficult to discern where one's property began. News media and press reports at the time document the destruction of coastal towns in St. Bernard and Plaquemines Parishes. In fact, the *Chicago Tribune* ran a story detailing the devastation of Reggio, Yscloskey, and Hopedale, noting that these small towns of eastern St. Bernard were seemingly wiped off of the map (see Fig. 18.1; Janega, 2005). Coastal residents without habitable dwellings or knowledge of whether services (electricity and gas) would be restored to these outlying areas were displaced for months—and up to 2 years or more for some.

Both younger and older fishers spoke of feeling unwelcomed and out of place in the communities to which they had evacuated (see also Chaps. 12 and 13, this volume). One younger participant (318) reported that after the mass evacuation and relocation, a woman in the community she had relocated to was lamenting on the influx and speaking in a derogatory way about the Chalmette evacuees in particular. This participant's loved one reportedly objected, spoke up, and said:

> "I am from Chalmette." [Then the woman], she says, "You and all the people from Chalmette, I wish all of you would go back."

Participant 318 went on to share her perception that:

> I guess it is the stress of having so many people move into your community. All of a sudden it is a population explosion [with so many people moving]…from one area to another. *(Y) (50-year-old female)*

Another participant (331), a high school student at the time, recalled that to the young people in the city where she and her family temporarily relocated, "I was the 'Katrina girl' from New Orleans who talked funny…" *(Y) (21-year-old female).*

Reports of "insider/outsider" perspective were not limited to fishers who temporarily resided in distant cities. In the eyes of some persons who went back to their coastal communities, the storms had a "cleansing" effect on the population, in that only those who deeply *wanted* to be there to rebuild returned. An older fisher related his views with blatant disdain for nefarious "opportunists" seeking to maximize personal gain at the expense of others, as follows:

> 341: [A]fter the storm, we had a lot of people in this parish that I would say that were undesirable…"trash." I hate to say that word. I try not to be a mean person. But they weren't born here, they just come [in] here… [Some of them were] opportunists and living and getting whatever they could get off of nothing. So the true people that wanted to stay here, that were born and raised here, *stood.* And the undesirables and the people that were just opportunists think they can just try and make hustles—well, they're gone. We got rid of them. So it basically cleaned, it cleansed the parish. *(O)(55-year-old male)*

In participant 341's remark, one can sense the depth of affinity and respect for his ancestral homeland, despite Katrina's devastation. Scholars use the term *place attachment* to describe the strong emotional bond that draws people to particular geographic areas that they consider "home." Affectionately known as "da parish," lifelong residents of eastern St. Bernard voiced concerns not only about the social environment but also about the insidious effects of coastal erosion, loss of marshland and barrier islands, and the long-term viability of the bayous and natural waterways of south Louisiana. Environmental concerns were both frequent and salient among the older fishers. Indeed, this was the sharpest point of contrast with the younger fishers who more often spoke of new social opportunities and forming lasting friendships with their displacement hosts in distant communities, as discussed more fully next.

Regarding new social ties, younger and older participants spoke with appreciation and gratitude toward those who had warmly welcomed them in host communities in neighboring states, including (but not limited to): Texas, Mississippi, Alabama, Georgia, Tennessee, and Florida. Organized relief efforts carried out by volunteers associated with faith-based groups made a tremendous difference, providing material goods and assistance with finding suitable housing for displaced fishers for the long months away from their ruined coastal homes. Many in the younger age group spoke of new connections and social relationships they had established with their displacement hosts. Some reportedly still keep in touch with their former hosts in other states. A counterpoint to the "insider/ outsider" mentality so many participants referenced, the kindness of strangers who warmly welcomed displaced fishers and provided for their material needs sometimes led to the formation of meaningful relationships that, in certain cases, continue today. The silver lining of new friendships and social ties was a frequent and salient trend coded in the primary data that was almost exclusively confined to those in the younger age group.

For those in the older age group, historical ties to multigenerational fishing communities and a deeply rooted cultural identity were frequent and salient in the primary data. A key factor was *fishing*—not only as a livelihood but also as a culture, an identity, a Gulf Coast-based society, and a "lifestyle" (see also, Wells, 2008). The following narratives capture and reflect a portion of the post-Katrina and post-Deepwater Horizon oil spill sense of the irretrievable loss of something more than boats, equipment, and fish—a loss disproportionately felt by the older group or participants. Commenting on what she missed most, one woman from the older group told us:

> 323: It was the *lifestyle*. It wasn't that my stuff was gone. I can deal with that. It was that you knew from this moment on, *your life is never going to be the same*. The people you've met, a lot of them you've been raised with…you might not ever see these people again in your life because they're gone from sight. You know?…And then, the [loss of the fishing] livelihood to people. Everything was disrupted…. That's what I was stressing over, not things. It was people. You see? And that was the hard part. *(O)(57-year-old female)*

The same participant (323) continued, "When I [re]-did the house, I thought of the possessions and stuff…[and I was able to] let it go, you know?" But for her, and many others, the fading out of a way of life—a fishing life—was a difficult and deeply painful prospect.

Another older fisher seemed to summarize in four brief sentences the essence of what many others struggled to convey, namely, that fishing was not just something they *did*—it was a large part of who they *were:*

> 341: Yeah, *I am a fisherman*. You can put me in my boat and if I got two bottles of water and cooking oil and a fire and a dozen oysters, [then] I am good for a week. The majority of people I was raised with, *that's how we are*. We just we don't need a lot. *(O)(55-year-old male)*

Like other folks in the fishing communities of south Louisiana, including the previous wife and mother (323) who was able to "let [her 'stuff'] go," participant 341 minimizes the importance of possessions ("We just don't need a lot"). However, the same centrality of fishing to life and identity seems to emanate from his brief, but clear statement.

Another participant, who was very young (22 years), showed a "stay and fight" persona reminiscent of many of the seasoned older fishers:

> 314: You know, people thought it was the end of the world, but I mean, if another Katrina came tomorrow, I would still be back here a couple of days later trying to rebuild. …Like my house. I worked hard to rebuild it, but like I said, if Katrina came tomorrow, I would be back fixing it. You just roll with the punches. Like I said last time, you can't cry over spilled milk. You [are] just going to have to deal with it and clean it up and get another glass…. It's not that big of a deal. It's just who I am. You just have to kind of roll with the punches; you

just learn to deal with stuff…. I kept my head up, and I didn't want people to feel sorry for me, I just did what I had to do. *(Y)(22-year-old male)*

If this young man's reflections convey some bravado, perhaps a high-held chin is well earned by one who absorbed several disastrous "punches" and still remained on his proverbial feet. This young man also showed a softer side. Discussing benefits of what he experienced, he said:

314: What matters is your family and, at least to me, I know one thing positive that came out of it for me was I learned how much my family really means to me.

Another participant from our younger group of fishers chose to frame Katrina in ways that emphasized two "good" outcomes of the tragedy. She said:

316: Well, for one, it [the storm] gave people a lot of knowledge that they can do it—that they do have the will power to do it. You just have to stick with it…. [T]here's no problems, there's only challenges…. [Another thing that was] good about the storm, it did umm… it didn't discriminate. It affected everybody, whether you were rich, poor, black, white… it just didn't matter. It didn't matter where you lived. Mm-hmm, yes, [it hurt us all] which united us all. We have a common…goal. [It] was to rebuild and to get back on with our life. *(Y)(51-year-old female)*

Importantly, "good" outcomes that came about after Katrina were not limited to younger fishers. New opportunities for cultural identity and growth in Plaquemines Parish, reflecting a deeply rooted Croatian heritage of hard work, perseverance, and love of family and friends (Ware, 2013), can be seen in this narrative from an older Croatian couple:

324: So…the positive outcome is that we do treasure our relationships with our, with our family and friends even more. And then, like last week, I thought about, some of our Croatian friends are closer now. They, some lived in Chalmette area, they lost their homes so they moved to Belle Chasse. Other people were like us in lower Plaquemines that ended up moving here so, the Croatian community has become a little more… *(O)(55-year-old wife)*

325: Close together *(O)(60-year-old husband)*.

324: [Yes] more clustered. And, we've been able to, we're starting our own Croatian [cultural center]. We've got a piece of property [two and a half acres in Jesuit Bend donated after the storm], we're building a center. We're redoing a little building into a [community] center and I think that would have been a lot harder…harder to come by if it wasn't for Katrina and Rita.

The older group seemed to report strong community ties and stronger ties to the "way of life" more often than their younger counterparts did, although overgeneralization should be avoided. As we see with participants 314 and 316, there were some younger fishers who were highly invested in literally and socially restoring hurricane-devastated communities. Further, there were some in the older group who seemed to have absorbed one blow too many and were preparing to try a life in a less perilous locale. One married couple with strong family ties to the oyster industry shared these sentiments just weeks after Hurricane Isaac swept through south Louisiana on the seventh Katrina anniversary (August 29, 2012):

359/360: No, we know we are not secure. And, you know, with [Hurricane] Isaac it just… reinforces that…. Yes, you do what you can and you fight and all, but then you realize this is not something that we have to endure. We do not have to live here, and we decided to live here by choice after the hurricane. We did not leave, but if you keep getting hit on the head, you know, I do not think we plan on staying here. I really do not. *(Y)*(359, *52-year-old female*; 360, *55-year old male*)

We conclude our discussion of Theme 3 with several excerpts from both younger and older fishers, which seemed to illustrate convergence of thinking—that the storms taught the lesson that historical ties with deep roots to one's cultural heritage and traditions, especially family relationships, are the "irreplaceable core" of life.

334/361: [The experience with the storms] brought people together. It made you realize just how close…your family is, and how much they mean to you. It brought a lot of families together…. It did. …My family's more important to me than anything. *(O)*(334, *58-year-old female*; 361, *57-year-old male*)

346: [One silver lining through all of this is] the quality time spent with family. *(Y)(25-year-old female)*

332: I know everybody in my family is only a phone call away, and if I say, "We've got to pray," then that's what we do. We stop right there. Don't even ask what's going on. Don't worry about what the problem is. Let's just pray, and God gives us the strength, and God gives us the…family camaraderie to get through it. *(Y)(52-year-old female)*

For many, the vital support of (and closeness with) family during "times of trouble" was a treasure pulled from the muck of the disasters. While the preceding three narratives specifically identify "family" as a coping support, other participants also referenced important assistance more generally—from "people" who were "there to help."

332: So many things had happened in a negative way since 9/11 [in 2001] that you begin to doubt, and you begin to be nervous about people's motives; and then post-Katrina, post-Rita, people's motives were simply to hold you up or lift you up or drag you up by your boot straps, depending on what you needed…as long as you weren't just sitting there with a hand out, these *people were there to give you a hand up.* ….I learned how truly loved we were and continue to be. *(Y)(52-year-old female)*

326: It just makes you realize that, you know, in times of trouble…you will have somebody there to help you. *(Y)(52-year-old male)*

Conclusions and Implications

Our focus in this chapter has been confined to lifelong residents of fishing communities in two south Louisiana coastal parishes where Katrina left a historically wide arc of destruction. Louisiana's Gulf Coast fishers and their families provide an authentic and generationally rich perspective on the experience of suffering related to natural disaster, having endured five major hurricanes in 7 years: Katrina and Rita in 2005, Gustav and Ike in 2008, and most recently, Isaac in 2012. Isaac, at first a tropical storm, then upgraded to a category 1 hurricane at landfall on August 29, 2012, was a haunting and cruel reminder of Katrina's legacy of loss, with destruction of property and homes lost once again in St. Bernard and Plaquemines Parishes.

The three core themes presented here were based on qualitative analyses of younger and older fishers' narratives at least 5 years after Katrina. Excerpts of primary data in connection with each core theme capture the diverse concerns, challenges, and coping resources utilized to counter traumatic stress associated with what has been described at the costliest natural disaster in US history (Kessler et al., 2009). Taken together, these themes bear witness to the horror of the first days after Katrina's landfall and unprecedented flooding following levee breaches (Theme 1). The tremendous outpouring of disaster relief assistance by faith-based communities and volunteers was illuminated next (Theme 2). Within this theme, an interesting counterpoint concerned numerous reports of assistance without regard to traditional denominational boundaries, where Baptists, Amish, and many others extended a helping hand to a predominantly Catholic community of fishers. The first two themes were based on remarkably similar responses across the two age groups compared in this study. On the contrary, the last theme provided evidence of age-related differences in responses, with salient trends for younger fishers on new connections and meaningful social relationships formed with their out-of-state displacement hosts, some of which continue today. In contrast, environmental concerns were voiced more frequently by the older fishers, bringing awareness to the problem of coastal erosion and the pervasive loss of land witnessed by generations of fishing families over the past century. For both younger and older participants, realization of the importance of family ties and a strong affinity to place were unifying and salient trends.

Interviews with fishers who have endured a decade of catastrophic disasters including the recent 2010 BP oil spill (see Chap. 4, this volume) are valuable in helping psychologists, and other social services professionals appreciate the core challenges that directly affected individuals and families must face. Evidence from the clinical and public health literatures indicates that previous trauma is one of several separate risk factors for PTSD (Brewin, Andrews, & Valentine, 2000; Tracy & Galea, 2006). Coastal fishers who have endured natural and technological disaster are at risk for adverse psychological reactions in the years after these events. In fact, over half of the fishers who participated in the present research had at least one symptom of clinical depression at the time of interview (51.6%; Cherry et al., 2015). On the contrary, individuals and families who have experienced recurring disasters and have recovered equilibrium are a valuable resource who may illuminate keys to successful coping after disaster.

Understanding the psychological and social factors that may lessen vulnerability and promote resilience is a timely challenge given the frequency of large-scale disasters in the world today (see Chaps. 5 and 15, this volume). Our participants' responses highlight resources that seem to be facilitative in assisting recovery, as well as how and why these resources were beneficial. We received a diverse array of reports regarding how the storms influenced the fishers' relationships with friends, family, and community. Based on many reports, the people who were "there to help" and to "give you a hand up" were often from faith communities. Our findings attest to the perceived benefits of organized disaster relief efforts carried out by faith-based communities, as well as humanitarian gestures and good will extended by beneficent strangers, some of whom have emerged as emotionally meaningful new friends. The individual and community-wide disaster relief efforts that displaced fishers described reflect social support, consistent with a voluminous literature on perceived social support, as key for positive outcomes after disaster (Boss, 2006; Silva Brown et al., 2010; Marks, Cherry, & Silva, 2009; Roberto, Kamo, & Henderson, 2009; see also Chap. 10, this volume).

Scholars have made the point that disaster outcomes depend critically on a combination of risk factors and resilience characteristics (Bonnano, Brewin, Kaniasty, & La Greca, 2010). In addition to perceived social support and reportedly closer family ties, findings from this study also highlight cultural identity as a potential resilience resource. The younger and older fishers of Isleño and Croatian descent provided novel insight into the roles cultural identity and tradition play in post-disaster recovery. The Los Isleños Museum and Village in southeastern St. Bernard and the annual fiesta to celebrate Isleños culture and heritage remind us of the longevity of commercial fishing and trapping for those whose forefathers immigrated to the Gulf Coast from the Canary Islands during the Spanish colonization of Louisiana. In Plaquemines Parish, religious observances and a special mass held in honor of St. Anthony, along with festivals and other celebrations throughout the calendar year strengthen Croatian cultural identity and ideals which include resilience and strong family ties (Ware, 1996, 2006, 2013). On a broader note, cultural identities and traditions passed down from generations of fishing families with deep roots to their coastal homes and lifestyles underscore the importance of place attachment for some, especially older fishers, and the potential for individual and community resilience despite hurricane devastation. Nonetheless, one must not forget the environmental realities of coastal erosion and the looming uncertainties associated with the BP oil spill (see Chap. 4, this volume), nor should one forget future hurricane risk in coastal communities.

In closing, our findings build on previous studies of commercial fishers and extend the literature by addressing long-term hurricane recovery in the context of exposure to an economically and environmentally devastating technological disaster (Lee & Blanchard, 2012; see also Chap. 4, this volume). The insights and practical information that disaster survivors can provide are keys to the development of evidence-based interventions to mitigate adversity. These data show that cultural ties affect younger and older adults' coping responses and adjustment in the years after a devastating natural disaster.

Acknowledgments We are grateful to George Barisich, President of the United Commercial Fishermen's Association, for his help with recruitment and Frank Campo of Campo's Marina in Yscloskey (southeastern St. Bernard) for providing space for interviews. We thank Pam Forest Nezat, Ashley Cacamo, Annie Crapanzano, and Benjamin Staab for assistance with data collection; Trevor Johnson, Savannah Ballard, Kyle Ryker, Priscilla Lebleu, Rachel Anderson, Katie Giordano, Mallori Seeger, and Caston Montgomery for help with qualitative analyses; and Sr. Mary Keefe, Robert Campo, Lauren Denley, Huey Gonzales, Charlie Robin, John Tesvich, and Eva Vujnovich for their contributions to the research effort.

This research was supported by grants from the Louisiana Board of Regents and the BP Gulf of Mexico Research Initiative, Office of Research and Economic Development, Louisiana State University. This support is gratefully acknowledged. Correspondence concerning this article should be addressed to Katie E. Cherry, Department of Psychology, Louisiana State University, Baton Rouge, LA 70803-5501 (e-mail: pskatie@lsu.edu).

References

Batson, M., & Marks, L. (2008). Making the connection between prayer, faith, and forgiveness in Roman Catholic families. *The Quantitative Report, 13*(3), 394–415.

Bonnano, G. A., Brewin, C. R., Kaniasty, K., & La Greca, A. M. (2010). Weighing the costs of disaster: Consequences, risks, and resilience in individuals, families, and communities. *Psychological Science in the Public Interest, 11,* 1–49.

Boss, P. (2006). *Loss, trauma, and resilience*. New York: Norton.

Brewin, C. R., Andrews, B., & Valentine, J. D. (2000). Meta-analysis of risk factors for posttraumatic stress disorder in trauma-exposed adults. *Journal of Consulting and Clinical Psychology, 68,* 748–766.

Buuck, M. M. (2007). *Firestorm: Hurricane Katrina and the St. Bernard Fire Department*. Xlibris Corporation.

Cataldie, L. (2007). *Coronor's journal: Forensics and the art of stalking death*. New York: The Penguin Group (USA).

Cherry, K. E. (Ed.). (2009). *Lifespan perspectives on natural disasters: Coping with Katrina, Rita and other storms*. New York: Springer

Cherry, K. E., Galea, S., & Silva, J. L. (2008). Successful aging and natural disasters: Role of adaptation and resiliency in late life. In M. Hersen & A. M. Gross (Eds.), *Handbook of clinical psychology: Volume 1* (pp. 810–833). NJ: Wiley.

Cherry, K. E., Sampson, L., Nezat, P. F., Cacamo, A., Marks, L. D., & Galea, S. (2015). Long-term psychological outcomes in older adults after disaster: Relationships to religiosity and social support. *Aging & Mental Health, 19*(5), 430–443.

Coles, F. (2012). Double identity: Isleños are Yats, too. *Southern Journal of Linguistics, 36,* 155–168.

Dunn, G. E., Davis, W. R., & Moore, P. L. (Dec, 1956). Hurricane season of 1956. *Monthly Weather Review,* pp. 436–443.

Faragher, J. M. (2005). *A great and noble scheme: The tragic story of the expulsion of the French Acadians from their American homeland*. New York: W.W. Norton.

Graumann, A., Houston, T., Lawrimore, J., Levinson, D., Lott, N., McCown, S., et al. (2005; updated 2006). *Hurricane Katrina a climatological perspective: Preliminary report*. Retrieved from the National Oceanic and Atmospheric Administration's National Climatic Data Center, from http://www.ncdc.noaa.gov/oa/reports/tech-report-200501z.pdf. Accessed 20 May 2013.

Janega, J. (11 Sept 2005). In some lost towns, Katrina went beyond destruction: Yscloskey, others wiped out entirely. *Chicago Tribune*. Retrieved from http://articles.chicagotribune.com/2005-09-11/news/0509110479_1_towns-parish-president-oil.

Kessler, R. C., Galea, S., Gruber, M. J., Sampson, N. A., Petukhova, M., & Wang, P. S. (2009). Hurricane Katrina. In Y. Neria, S. Galea & F. H. Norris (Eds.), *Mental health and disasters* (pp. 419–440). New York: Cambridge University Press.

Kilmer, R. P., Gil-Rivas, V., Tedeschi, R.G., & Calhoun, L.G. (2010). *Helping families and communities recover from disaster: Lessons learned from Hurricane Katrina and its aftermath*. Washington, D.C.: American Psychological Association.

Lee, M. R., & Blanchard, T. C. (2012). Community attachment and negative affective states in the context of the BP Deepwater Horizon disaster. *American Behavioral Scientist, 56*(1), 24–47.

Los Isleños Learn. (2014). In *Bienvenido Los Islenos.org*. http://www.losislenos.org/fiesta2014.html.

Louisiana Religion Traditions. (2010). http://www.thearda.com/rcms2010/r/s/22/rcms2010_22_state_adh_2010.asp. Accessed 5 Jan 2015.

Marks, L. D., Cherry, K., & Silva, J. (2009). Faith, crisis, coping, and meaning making after Katrina: A qualitative, cross-cohort examination. In K. Cherry (Ed.), *Lifespan perspectives on natural disasters: Coping with Katrina, Rita and other storms* (pp. 195–215). New York: Springer.
Moore, T. J., & Asay, S. M. (2008). *Family resource management*. Thousand Oaks: Sage.
National Hurricane Center. (23 Jan 2007). November 2005 Atlantic Tropical Weather Summary. NOAA. Retrieved August 2014, from http://www.nhc.noaa.gov/archive/2005/tws/MIATWSAT_nov_final.shtml.
National Hurricane Center. (2015). http://www.nhc.noaa.gov/. Accessed 5 Jan 2015.
Neria, Y., Galea, S. & Norris, F. H. (Eds.). (2009). *Mental health and disasters*. New York: Cambridge University Press.
Patton, M. Q. (2002). *Qualitative research & evaluation methods* (3rd ed.). Thousand Oaks: Sage.
Roberto, K. A., Kamo, Y., & Henderson, T. (2009). Encounters with Katrina: Dynamics of older adults' social support networks. In K. E. Cherry (Ed.), *Lifespan perspectives on natural disasters: Coping with Katrina, Rita and other storms* (pp. 133–152). New York: Springer.
Robin, C. J. (2000). *Remedies and lost secrets of St. Bernard's Islenos*. St. Bernard Village: Los Islenos Heritage and Cultural Society.
Roese, N. J., & Olson, J. M. (2007). Better, stronger, faster self-serving judgment, affect regulation, and the optimal vigilance hypothesis. *Perspectives on Psychological Science, 2,* 124–141.
Schaefer, M. (2007). *Lost in Katrina*. Gretna: Pelican Publishing Company.
Silva Brown, J., Cherry, K. E., Marks, L. D., Volaufova, J., Lefante, C., & Jazwinski, S. M. (2010). After Hurricanes Katrina and Rita: Gender differences in physical function and psychological well-being in middle-aged and older adults. Health Care for Women International, *31,* 997–1012.
Strauss, A., & Corbin, J. (1998). *Basics of qualitative research: Techniques and procedures for developing grounded theory*. Thousand Oaks: Sage.
Tracy, M., & Galea, S. (2006). Post-traumatic stress disorder and depression among older adults after a disaster: The role of ongoing trauma and stressors. *Public Policy & Aging Report, 16*(2), 16–19.
U. S. Census Bureau. (2013). *State and County Quick Facts from the U. S. Census Bureau*. http://quickfacts.census.gov/qfd/states/22000.html.
Vujnovich, M. (1974). *Yugoslavs in Louisiana*. Gretna: Pelican Publishing Company.
Ware, C. (1996). Croatians in southeast Louisiana: An overview. *Louisiana Folklore Miscellany, 11,* 67–85.
Ware, C. (2006). Croatians in Louisiana. In S. J. Bronner (Ed.), *Encyclopedia of American Folklife* (pp. 243–246). Armonk: M.E. Sharpe, Inc.
Ware, C. E. (2013). Louisiana's Croatian American society: A case study in adaptation and resilience. *Louisiana Folklore Miscellany, 23,* 97–128.
Weisler, R. H., Barbee, J. G., & Townsend, M. H. (2006). Mental health and recovery in the Gulf Coast after Hurricanes Katrina and Rita. *The Journal of the American Medical Association, 296,* 585–588.
Wells, K. (2008). *The good pirates of the forgotten bayous*. New Haven: Yale University Press.

Chapter 19
Trauma, Religion, and Spirituality: Pathways to Healing

Anna R. Harper and Kenneth I. Pargament

Introduction

When disaster strikes, religion and spirituality are commonly brought to the forefront of peoples' lives. Consider the following poignant examples:

- People talked about ghosts, especially in the beginning…or, people [could] smell the one they lost. Then, people go to the temple and give donations in [the victim's] name. It happened with me with my sister's "smell"—it only happened in the first few weeks, and I could smell her body decomposing. I would feel so badly, and it reminded me of her, but I was really busy. It still reminded me to go to the temple.
  Buddhist health-care provider in the Phang Nga Province of Thailand, after the 2004 Indonesian earthquake and tsunami (Varley, Isaranuwatchai, & Coyte, 2012, p. 665).
- Where is this peace and this evenness in my life coming from? Well, it is coming from God. It was coming from him ministering to me and helping me each day to cope with it [cancer] and live through it and heal, not just physically, but to heal spiritually as well.
  Cancer survivor (Denney, Aten, & Leavell, 2011, p. 379).
- "I really haven't found any meaning in my son's death. I don't understand it or accept it. I still get angry at times. I still cry frequently."
  Bereaved parent, 5 years after the tragic death of a child (Murphy, Johnson, & Lohan, 2003, p. 396).

A. R. Harper (✉) · K. I. Pargament
Department of Psychology and Counseling, Southern Nazarene University,
429 Don Beaver Science Building, Bethany, OK 73008, USA
e-mail: anharper@mail.snu.edu

K. I. Pargament
e-mail: kpargam@bgsu.edu

K. E. Cherry (ed.), *Traumatic Stress and Long-Term Recovery*,
DOI 10.1007/978-3-319-18866-9_19

As these quotations exemplify, traumatic experiences can have deeply spiritual consequences. The first statement illustrates one way in which a calamity may be interpreted through a religious or spiritual lens. The second statement describes the healing a cancer survivor achieved through the use of spiritual resources, while the third statement captures a bereaved parent's enduring spiritual struggles.

For better or worse, people often draw upon religion and spirituality in the wake of traumatic events. For example, a national survey about stress reactions to the September 11, 2011, terrorist attacks found that 90 % of American adults reportedly turned to "prayer, religion, or spiritual feelings" in order to cope during the week after the attacks (Schuster et al., 2001, p. 1510). In a qualitative study of older adults who had been displaced by Hurricane Katrina, interview responses revealed that approximately 37 % of the participants pursued active religious coping methods (i.e., praying, meditating, spiritual singing, scripture reading, exercising trust in God, participating in church-related activities), 29 % relied on maintaining attitudes of hopefulness, thankfulness, and/or gratitude (frequently directed toward God), and 13 % reappraised the situation in a positive existential light (i.e., focusing on being alive, seeking a posture of acceptance, holding a positive view about the event; Henderson, Roberto, & Kamo, 2010; see also Chap. 20, this volume). These findings are not particularly surprising, given that according to 2013 national surveys, 90 % of Americans endorsed belief in God or a universal spirit, while 39 % reported attending a church or synagogue at least once in the past 7 days (Gallup, 2014). Across the globe, tragic events often stimulate religious and spiritual expressions. Among the coastal and island people of Bangladesh who are frequently devastated by cyclones, for example, qualitative field data reveal an increase in diverse religious and spiritual activities (e.g., prayer, religious obedience, ritual sacrifices) in the Muslim and Buddhist communities during the days when a storm is imminent (Alam & Collins, 2010). The diversity of religious and spiritual responses to catastrophic events is striking; however, considerably more striking is the apparent ubiquity of religious and spiritual coping in the face of disaster.

In this chapter, we consider many ways in which religion and spirituality intersect with trauma. We focus on (a) the religious/spiritual facet of trauma, (b) religious and spiritual ways of coping with trauma, and (c) the outcomes of religious/spiritual coping with trauma. We end the chapter with a discussion of ways in which religion and spirituality can be integrated into the posttraumatic recovery process, with the goal of preventing enduring problems and enhancing lasting posttraumatic growth.

The Relationships Among Religion, Spirituality, and Trauma

As a prelude to this discussion, it is important to consider the meanings of religion and spirituality. *Religion* has been defined as "the search for significance that occurs within the context of established institutions that are designed to facilitate spirituality" (Pargament, Mahoney, Exline, Jones, & Shafranske, 2013b, p. 15). *Spirituality* has been defined as "the search for the sacred" (Pargament, 2007). These definitions rest on the assumption that people have a yearning to discover, pursue, sustain, and at times transform a relationship with something they perceive as sacred in their lives. While the *sacred* often directly references God or a higher power, any aspect of life may be deemed as sacred if it is perceived to have divine-like qualities, such as transcendence, boundlessness, ultimate meaning, and perfection (Pargament & Mahoney, 2005). In the words of Jones (2002), "The sacred is not, necessarily, a unique and special object or domain split off from the rest of life, but is rather the world of ordinary objects experienced in a particular way" (p. 61). The "particular way" in which we experience sacred things, according to Paden (1992), is the "immense role they play and the absolute priority they have in someone's world" (p. 73).

Indeed, people report making exceptional investments in the pursuit, maintenance, and transformation of special aspects of life they experience as sacred. For example, adults tend to invest more time, energy, and personal resources into work (Wrzesniewski, McCauley, Rozin, & Schwartz, 1997) and personal strivings (e.g., self-development, physical health, existential concerns; Mahoney et al., 2005b) when these domains of life are perceived to have sacred qualities. Likewise, the attribution of divine significance to aspects of the material world has been associated with greater personal investment, including greater care for one's body (Mahoney et al., 2005a) and the natural environment (Tarakeshwar, Swank, Pargament, & Mahoney, 2001). Furthermore, people who describe relational aspects of life as sacred exhibit similar patterns of increased personal investment in the domains of parenting (Dumas & Nissley-Tsiopinis, 2006; Murray-Swank, Mahoney, & Pargament, 2006; Volling, Mahoney, & Rauer, 2009), marriage (DeMaris, Mahoney, & Pargament, 2010; Lichter & Carmalt, 2009; Mahoney et al., 1999; Mahoney, Pargament, & DeMaris, 2009), and sexuality (Murray-Swank, Pargament, & Mahoney, 2005). The aforementioned list is certainly not exhaustive. As Durkheim (1915) stated, "By sacred things one must not understand simply those personal beings which are called gods or spirits; a rock, a tree, a pebble, a piece of wood, a house, in a word anything can be sacred" (p. 52).

Each person's search for the sacred is facilitated by a complex and dynamic system of beliefs, feelings, values, relationships, experiences, and practices that direct the person along spiritual pathways and toward spiritual destinations (Pargament, 2007). For many, religious institutions provide guidance regarding which spiritual pathways and destinations are of primary importance. While both religion and spirituality involve the sacred as a valued destination, religion can also be directed toward a variety of other goals, including psychological, physical, and social functions. Thus, religion and spirituality constitute overlapping yet distinct processes that are relevant to many peoples' experiences in times of crisis.

Traumatic events span multiple domains of life, including the interpersonal (e.g., violence, sexual assault, physical abuse, emotional maltreatment, neglect, death, separation), medical (e.g., physical injury, illness), ecological (e.g., natural disaster, man-made industrial accident), and political (e.g., war, terrorism, forced displacement). A holistic understanding of trauma must incorporate religion and spirituality because humans are complex beings with interrelated physical, psychological, social, and *spiritual* capacities. Traumatic events do not merely endanger a person's physical, psychological, and social well-being but can also have potent implications for spiritual well-being, to the extent that these upheavals threaten or damage aspects of life that have been deemed as sacred.

The spiritual impact of negative life events was illustrated when adults in a Midwestern community sample were asked to describe the most significant personal crisis that took place in the past 2 years (Pargament, Magyar, Benore, & Mahoney, 2005). These participants reported a variety of events, including the death or serious illness/injury of a loved one, parenting or family relationship difficulty, job loss, personal illness, and divorce/separation. Over 38 % of the sample appraised the event as a *sacred loss*, meaning that something once viewed as a manifestation of God or imbued with sacred qualities was perceived as lost. Nearly 25 % of the sample perceived the event as involving a *desecration*, or the violation of a sacred aspect of life by someone or something. Those who appraised the event more as a sacred loss reported greater intrusive thoughts and depression, while those who appraised the event more as a desecration reported greater intrusive thoughts and anger after the event.

In another study, college students living in the Midwest and New York City who reported greater desecration appraisals (e.g., "This event was both an offense against me and against God," endorsed by over 50 % of the sample) of the September 11, 2001, terrorist attacks reported higher levels of posttraumatic anxiety and depressive symptoms, as well as stronger approval of extreme forms of retaliation against the perpetrators (Mahoney et al., 2002). On the other hand, a qualitative study of Hurricane Katrina survivors found that many participants gained a greater appreciation for life and for the people in their lives, a greater sense of wholeness with family and community, and an enhanced sense of personal and spiritual strength (Tuason, Güss, & Carroll, 2012; see Chap. 21, this volume). These and other research findings have supported the notion that even seemingly secular aspects of life can be connected to the divine and that events that disrupt sacred aspects of life can have a significant impact on posttraumatic recovery, for better or worse.

Religious and Spiritual Coping with Trauma

Religion and spirituality do not only bear on peoples' perceptions of critical life events and their initial appraisals of traumatic incidents but also on the coping methods they select, the functions of coping methods, and the outcomes of coping. Efforts to measure posttraumatic coping often overlook religious and spiritual domains, and, when religion/spirituality is taken into account, it is often assessed by only a few items. A research study on the impact of the 2004 Indian Ocean tsunami found that religious affiliation alone did not predict Thai citizens' collective efficacy to cope with future natural catastrophes (Paton et al., 2008). This finding illustrates the importance of gaining a rich, fully dimensionalized picture of how religion and spirituality manifest during times of crisis. Because religion and spirituality are multifaceted and nuanced, it is important to go beyond broad measures of these constructs to gain specific information regarding *how* they are involved in coping, including *who* (e.g., clergy, congregation members, God) and *what* (e.g., prayer, reading sacred scriptures) is included in coping, *when* (e.g., acute stressors, chronic stressors), and *where* (e.g., privately, communally) coping occurs, and *why* (e.g., to find meaning, to gain control, to foster closeness and comfort) particular coping methods are pursued (Pargament, Falb, Ano, & Wachholtz, 2013a).

Theory and research arising from Lazarus and Folkman's (1984) influential account of stress and coping suggest that the outcomes of coping are not dependent solely on qualities of the traumatic event itself but also on personal reactions to the event (see Folkman & Moskowitz, 2004, for an overview of the history of coping theory and research). These personal reactions include primary cognitive appraisals (i.e., "What are the potential consequences of this event? Is it a challenge, a threat, or a loss?") and secondary cognitive appraisals (i.e., "Do I have the resources necessary to successfully handle this stressor?") of a stressful event, accompanied by an assortment of cognitive, behavioral, and relational coping strategies employed to deal with the stressor. Thus, religious and spiritual coping involves the use of cognitive appraisals and cognitive/behavioral/relational coping methods that promote the pursuit of the sacred. Pargament (1997) has described religious/spiritual coping as the intersection of the "search for significance in ways related to the sacred" (p. 32) with the "search for significance in times of stress" (p. 90). This search includes "the use of religious beliefs or behaviors to facilitate problem-solving to prevent or alleviate the negative emotional consequences of stressful life circumstances" (Koenig, Pargament, & Nielsen, 1998, p. 513). Religious and spiritual coping can take many forms. They may have a divine, intrapersonal, and/or interpersonal focus (Mahoney, Krumrei, & Pargament, 2008). In the divine realm, people may focus their coping efforts on countering threats to their thoughts, feelings, and general relationship with God or a Higher Power. In the intrapersonal realm, coping may center on resolving internal questions, doubts, and uncertainties about sacred aspects of life. In the interpersonal realm, coping may concentrate on relieving relational tensions and conflicts over spiritual matters. A relational, medical, ecological, or political disaster may conceivably trigger the need for religious/spiritual coping in all three of the aforementioned domains.

As with secular coping methods (Folkman & Lazarus, 1988), the effectiveness of a specific religious/spiritual coping strategy relies on how well the particular method fits the individual and his or her context. Across studies, however, two primary patterns of religious/spiritual coping have been identified: positive religious/spiritual coping and negative religious/spiritual coping (Pargament, Koenig, & Perez, 2000; Pargament, Smith, Koenig, & Perez, 1998). *Positive religious/spiritual coping methods* (also referred to as *positive religious/spiritual resources*) generally reflect a secure connection with the divine, oneself, and others, while *negative religious/spiritual coping methods* (also referred to as *religious/spiritual struggles*) are generally associated with conflicts with the divine, oneself, and others about sacred matters (Exline, 2013; Pargament, Falb, et al., 2013a).

Positive Patterns of Religious and Spiritual Coping

Positive patterns of religious and spiritual coping address five key coping functions: (1) finding meaning, (2) gaining mastery and control, (3) increasing comfort and closeness to God, (4) enhancing intimacy with others and closeness to God, and (5) achieving life transformation (Pargament et al., 2000). In the upcoming sections, we provide empirical examples to illustrate some of the ways in which these coping functions manifest in the lives of people healing from traumatic experiences.

Meaning In order to find meaning after a traumatic event, a person may attempt to redefine the stressor through a benevolent spiritual lens (Park, 2013). In a longitudinal qualitative study of 29 families in Louisiana who had survived Hurricane Katrina, 38 % of the respondents made sense of the storm by referencing "God" or "the Lord" (Garrison & Sasser, 2009). For example, one 25-year-old man explained, "I believe He (referring to God) has his reason and it is not for us to understand, it is for us to accept" (p. 120). Trauma is commonly perceived as serving a higher purpose or as evidence of God's perfect, mysterious will. This type of reappraisal is exemplified by the response of a person who experienced a paralyzing accident, "There must be some reason for it. Could be that He had a reason for it. Maybe somebody else needs my legs more than I do" (Bulman & Wortman, 1977, p. 358). Tragic events may also be reappraised as blessings in disguise or opportunities for spiritual growth and transformation. In a qualitative study of adults who had survived Hurricanes Katrina and Rita, one man stated:

> A lot of things are [not that important]…[the hurricane gets you] re-evaluating where you are in your life, what you're doing, what is important to you…. I am Christian…but I would think that even the atheist, after Hurricane Katrina, would have to sit down and…not suddenly believe in God, but they would have to sit back and re-evaluate where they are in life and realize how precious life is. (Marks, Cherry, & Silva, 2009, p. 201)

For some, disasters may be interpreted as spiritual challenges or tests of devotion to God. The following passage from the Hilali-Khan translation of the Qur'an provides an interpretation that believers will be rewarded for patience and devotion through trials and calamities:

> And certainly, We shall test you with something of fear, hunger, loss of wealth, lives and fruits, but give glad tidings to As-Sâbirin (the patient ones, etc.). Who, when afflicted with calamity, say: "Truly! To Allâh we belong and truly, to Him we shall return." They are those on whom are the Salawât (i.e. blessings, etc.) (i.e. who are blessed and will be forgiven) from their Lord, and (they are those who) receive His Mercy, and it is they who are the guided-ones. (Al-Baqarah 2: 155–157)

Mastery and Control To gain mastery and control in response to calamity, a person may pursue a collaborative problem-solving partnership with God. As one female breast cancer survivor stated, "God would help me but I had to do my part too, that was expected of me by the Providence to which I trusted my life" (Gall & Cornblat, 2002, p. 528). Others may cope by actively surrendering uncontrollable aspects of the situation. A Hindu, for example, may find encouragement from

Valmiki's Ramayana to accept unalterable circumstances: "Every man suffers the three pairs of opposites; hunger and thirst, pleasure and pain, life and death. Do not permit thyself to grieve for that which cannot be avoided" (2.77.23). A Christian may similarly find inspiration in the words of Jesus:

> Therefore I tell you, do not worry about your life, what you will eat or drink; or about your body, what you will wear. Is not life more than food, and the body more than clothes? Look at the birds of the air; they do not sow or reap or store away in barns, and yet your heavenly Father feeds them. Are you not much more valuable than they? Can any one of you by worrying add a single hour to your life? (Matthew 6:25–27 New International Version)

Comfort and Closeness to God To achieve comfort and closeness to God in the midst of grief, a person may seek connectedness with transcendent forces or pursue connection and support from God. As David recorded after he was delivered from the hand of his enemies in the Hebrew scriptures:

> I called to the Lord, who is worthy of praise,
> and have been saved from my enemies.
> The waves of death swirled about me;
> the torrents of destruction overwhelmed me.
> The cords of the grave coiled around me;
> the snares of death confronted me.
> In my distress I called to the Lord;
> I called out to my God.
> From his temple he heard my voice;
> my cry came to his ears. (2 Samuel 22: 4–7)

Sometimes people seek comfort and closeness to God by creating and adhering to helpful religious boundaries, engaging in spiritual cleansing rituals, seeking forgiveness for transgressions, or engaging in religious activities to shift the focus from the stressor. In another example from the Hebrew Scriptures, Job responds to a rapid series of calamities (i.e., raiding enemies, natural disasters) that strip him of his family and possessions with worship and a mourning ritual, saying, "Naked I came from my mother's womb, and naked I will depart. The Lord gave and the Lord has taken away; may the name of the Lord be praised" (Job 1: 21).

Intimacy with Others and Closeness to God In an effort to increase intimacy with others and closeness to God after disaster strikes, a person may seek support and reassurance from clergy, congregation members, and others in the community who share one's religious or spiritual faith. In a qualitative study of Hurricane Katrina survivors, participants who decided not to evacuate emphasized interdependence and connection with others in their community, strength, and faith in God as important factors in their decision to stay in the area (Tuason et al., 2012). Another way people may cope with disaster is to attempt to provide spiritual support and comfort to others. One Hurricane Katrina survivor recalled an encounter in which she had been emotionally and spiritually helped by others who had lost more in the storm than she had:

> I just vividly [remember] in my mind…a family from one of the hardest hit areas outside of Grand Isle…. They came…about a week or two after the hurricane and sang at our

> church.... [T]hey lost everything. I mean they lost every picture...everything.... Still to this day, [I remember thinking that day], "You are here and you lost everything and you are singing praises to the Lord." (Silva, Marks, & Cherry, 2009, p. 234)

For a breast cancer survivor, the power of spiritual intimacy with others was found within a support group: "I began to see that many had this same spiritual quest and experience, regardless of religion or no religion.... Here we support each other in our living and dying...[we created]...communities of spiritual seekers" (Gall & Cornblat, 2002, p. 529).

Life Transformation Sometimes people seek life transformation in the face of adversity. To achieve this, a person may offer forgiveness as a way to shift from a posture of anger and blame to one of peace, look to religion to find a new life direction, seek spiritual guidance, or pursue a radical religious or spiritual conversion. One individual who had suffered a paralyzing spinal cord injury explained that the event was a spiritual turning point:

> I see the accident as the best thing that could have happened 'cause I was forced to decide my faith, whereas there would have been the possibility that I would have lived and never made a decision—been lost the rest of my life. 'Cause an individual, they don't know how lost they are without faith.... (Bulman & Wortman, 1977, p. 359)

A Buddhist who turns to the following passage from Ṭhānissaro Bhikkhu's translation of the Dhammapada would find a different path toward spiritual transformation during times of crisis—to eschew mundane attachments:

> Abandon anger,
> be done with conceit,
> get beyond every fetter.
> When for name & form
> you have no attachment
> –Have nothing at all—
> no sufferings, no stresses, invade. (17: 221)

Taken together, these examples of positive religious/spiritual coping highlight the powerful capacity for religion and spirituality to facilitate the search for posttraumatic meaning, control, comfort, intimacy, and transformation. However, for some people, the search for the sacred also has a dark side. We now turn our attention to negative posttraumatic religious/spiritual coping.

Negative Patterns of Religious and Spiritual Coping

Negative patterns of religious and spiritual coping attempt to address the five coping functions described earlier, although these strategies typically exacerbate posttraumatic distress (Pargament et al., 2000). In the next sections, we share empirical examples to illustrate some of the ways in which these five coping functions manifest in the form of posttraumatic religious/spiritual struggles.

Meaning In the search for meaning after a traumatic event, a person may interpret the stressor as an act of evil forces, as a grandfather of two children killed in the Oklahoma City bombing exclaimed: "A year ago this week, Satan drove up Fifth Street in a Ryder truck. He blew my babies up. He may have looked like a normal man, but he was Satan" (Bragg, 1996). More often, people perceive traumatic events as punishment from God. A news report after the 2004 Indian Ocean earthquake and Indonesian tsunami described religious beliefs as coloring appraisals of the disaster; specifically, some Muslim survivors perceived the tsunami as punishment from Allah, some Israeli and Christian religious leaders interpreted it as God's wrath, some Buddhists believed the sea gods must have been angered, and some with beliefs rooted in Hinduism and Buddhism cited karma as the reason for the tragic deaths (Broadway, 2005). When calamity hits, the existential "problem of suffering" often arises: *How could a loving, all-powerful God allow terrible things to happen?* When faced with suffering, people often respond by (a) questioning God's love, or (b) questioning God's power (see Chap. 20, this volume, for related discussion). John Piper, an influential American evangelical Christian Protestant minister, has grappled with reconciling the concepts of God's power and love, as in his statement after the 2004 Indonesian earthquake and tsunami: "Destructive calamities in this world mingle judgment and mercy…. They are both punishment and purification. Suffering, and even death, can be both judgment and mercy at the same time" (Piper, 2004, section 3). However, for some, the problem of suffering is not as easily resolved. In a qualitative study of women who had battled breast cancer, one woman stated, "[I am] not sure if I will ever believe that God loves me again," while another woman fluctuated between attributing blame to God for her cancer and questioning the existence of God (Gall & Cornblat, 2002, p. 528).

Mastery and Control In the struggle to gain some semblance of mastery and control in the midst of crisis, a person may passively wait for God to control a stressor that calls for some degree of human agency, plead for divine intervention, or exclude God from one's coping attempts. The following college students' responses to their romantic breakups illustrate opposite sides of the control coin. One student explained, "I found myself begging God and making bargains with him to help us get back together," while another admitted, "I wasn't quite as close to God when I was dealing with my breakup. The breakup was something that I did not pray to God about" (Hawley, 2012, p. 140). Sometimes people struggle with both sides of the control coin. For example, a middle-aged woman seeking treatment for religious/spiritual struggles stemming from a history of sexual abuse described a pendulum of coping during childhood, in which she first tried pleading for divine intervention and then omitted God from her coping repertoire: "As a kid, I prayed for the incest to stop. He didn't answer my prayers. I became angry and disconnected" (Murray-Swank & Pargament, 2005, p. 199).

Comfort and Closeness to God Some people struggle to achieve comfort and closeness to God after a catastrophe. In a qualitative exploratory study of Hurricane Katrina survivors' images of God, some participants described God as distant, as illustrated in one man's response: "I don't feel like I heard Him [God] much lately"

(Aten et al., 2008, p. 252). Some may harbor resentment toward God or express confusion and dissatisfaction with God over the stressor (Exline et al., 2011). After hearing of her friend's pain from cancer and coping with the disappointment and confusion of her own unanswered prayers, one woman concluded, "It was then I decided that I wanted nothing to do with this cruel, unjust God" (Gall & Cornblat, 2002, p. 528). Another woman, who desired to work through her struggles with God, explained why she had decided to enter a spiritually–integrated intervention for survivors of childhood sexual abuse:

> I hope to gain a better understanding of abuse and God. Why He abandoned me and why I can't feel Him beside me now. I want a relationship with God back. I blame Him for what happened and I am very angry at Him. He wasn't listening to me when I prayed for it to stop. He betrayed me. (Murray-Swank & Pargament, 2005, p. 196)

Intimacy with Others and Closeness to God In the struggle to gain intimacy with others and closeness to God during times of upheaval, a person may harbor discontentment toward one's faith community or express confusion and dissatisfaction with clergy or others associated with the stressor. In a study examining the spirituality of patients diagnosed with HIV/AIDS, the most common religious/spiritual struggles expressed by participants were "disagreed with what the church wanted me to do or believe" (13 %) and "felt dissatisfaction with the clergy" (11 %; Cotton et al., 2006). Interpersonal religious/spiritual struggles are often particularly salient in matters that are perceived as within the sufferer's control. However, as one participant in a longitudinal study of coping with divorce explains, this attribution of personal responsibility for the trauma does not negate the sufferer's yearning for compassion and relational support:

> I felt that there was a lot of judgment on the part of the church towards my divorce and no support or grace…Friends from the church could not see past the scripture of divorce being a sin…If there's one message I would want to communicate, it's that those going through a divorce need compassion and grace, not judgment from the church. (Krumrei, 2008, p. 100)

Life Transformation In the struggle for life transformation following a tragedy, one's religious or spiritual faith may be severely hindered or abandoned completely. This brand of significant, life-altering struggle can be experienced in response to large- and small-scale stressors alike. In the words of a male college student who had experienced a difficult romantic breakup:

> The breakup totally changed my spirituality. I feel as though I no longer have a connection with God. I used to feel somewhat of a connection. I have stopped attending church almost entirely. Mostly my spiritual side of life has disappeared, or become focused on different things entirely. (Hawley & Mahoney, 2013, p. 245)

Outcomes of Religious and Spiritual Coping

It is important to note that positive and negative religious/spiritual coping methods are not mutually exclusive; they can occur simultaneously and in varying degrees over the course of the trauma recovery process. Moreover, each person's unique combination of positive and negative religious/spiritual coping patterns has significant implications for posttraumatic adjustment and growth. Positive religious/spiritual coping methods have been identified as primarily helpful and associated with greater positive posttraumatic outcomes (e.g., recent mental health, happiness, life satisfaction, optimism, hope, positive affect, self-esteem, social adjustment, posttraumatic growth, spiritual growth), while negative religious/spiritual coping methods have been associated with intensified problems and greater negative posttraumatic outcomes (e.g., global distress, depression, anxiety, posttraumatic stress symptoms, negative affect, anger/hostility, perceived stress, suicidality, social dysfunction, spiritual injury; Ano & Vasconcelles, 2005).

Focusing specifically on outcomes of positive religious/spiritual coping, a meta-analysis of coping with trauma indicated that positive religious/spiritual coping was a strong predictor of posttraumatic growth (e.g., enhanced personal strength, increased appreciation for life, more meaningful relationships with others, increased compassion), having a larger effect size than optimism, social support, and general spirituality (Prati & Pietrantoni, 2009). Likewise, positive religious/spiritual coping was associated with greater posttraumatic growth in a sample of university students, after taking into account secular coping styles (Gerber, Boals, & Schuettler, 2011). These findings illustrate the important point that religious/spiritual coping adds a unique dimension to the posttraumatic coping process that cannot be fully accounted for by secular forms of coping. In a longitudinal study of parental coping with the traumatic death of a child, participants who used positive religious/spiritual coping methods (e.g., seeking God's help, putting trust in God, finding comfort in one's religion, praying more frequently) found greater meaning during the 5 years after their child's death compared to parents who did not use such methods. Moreover, meaning–making was related to fewer symptoms of mental distress, greater marital satisfaction, and more favorable physical health status (Murphy et al., 2003).

On the other hand, negative religious/spiritual coping has been associated with more severe posttraumatic stress and mental health symptoms in female trauma survivors (Fallot & Heckman, 2005); greater posttraumatic symptoms and callousness toward others in people coping with the Oklahoma City bombing; greater emotional distress, more psychosomatic symptoms, and poorer physical heath in students who had experienced a negative life event within the past 3 years; and poorer health status and cognitive functioning, lower quality of life, and greater depression among hospital patients coping with medical illness (Pargament et al., 1998). Among medically ill elders, negative religious/spiritual coping has been linked to poorer cognitive and independent functioning, lower quality of life, more depressed mood, higher risk of mortality, and greater declines in mental and physical health status (Pargament, Koenig, Tarakeshwar, & Hahn, 2004b). Among university students who had experienced a variety of traumatic events, negative religious/spiritual coping was associated with greater symptoms of posttraumatic stress, after controlling for secular coping styles (Gerber et al., 2011).

It is important to note, however, that negative religious/spiritual coping is also sometimes associated with positive posttraumatic outcomes. For example, among members of churches that were close to the site of the Oklahoma City bombing, higher levels of spiritual struggle were linked with greater posttraumatic growth, while college students who encountered greater spiritual struggles with recent negative life events reported greater posttraumatic and spiritual growth (Pargament et al., 1998). Similarly, medically ill elders who described encountering more spiritual struggles also reported greater spiritual growth (Pargament et al., 2004b).

Findings from a study that was conducted six months after the 2010 earthquake in Haiti may help illustrate the complex relationships between positive religious/spiritual coping, negative religious/spiritual coping, and posttraumatic personal and spiritual growth (O'Grady, Rollison, Hanna, Schreiber-Pan, & Ruiz, 2012). Among 108 Haitian men and women, the majority experienced growth in their faith in God or a Higher Power (80 %) and an increase in religious practice (71 %) after the earthquake. In addition, 82 % agreed or strongly agreed that they "felt God's inspiration" to a greater extent during or following the earthquake. On the other hand, some reported feeling more distant from God or a Higher Power (23 %) and less spiritual (20 %) after the earthquake. Thus, it seems that a small percentage of the participants experienced *both* spiritual struggles and spiritual growth. Moreover, although those who suffered greater amounts of loss reported feeling greater disappointment, frustration, and betrayal in their relationship with God, these feelings did not directly impact posttraumatic and spiritual growth. Instead, perception of God's awareness and perceived interaction with God in daily life were linked to positive posttraumatic personal and spiritual outcomes. These and other research findings suggest that drawing upon one's religious and spiritual beliefs in the midst of adversity, including spiritual struggles, can promote long-term stress-related personal and spiritual growth. Because the results of cross-sectional studies reveal that symptoms of posttraumatic stress and posttraumatic growth often co-occur during the recovery process, longitudinal studies are needed in order to tease apart the long-term outcome trajectories of positive and negative religious/spiritual coping.

It should be noted that the majority of studies on religious/spiritual coping have been conducted with Christian samples. However, there have been recent efforts to investigate patterns of religious and spiritual coping among people of diverse religious traditions, including Jews (Rosmarin, Pargament, Krumrei, & Flannelly, 2009), Muslims (Ai, Peterson, & Huang, 2003; Raiya, Pargament, Mahoney, & Stein, 2008), Hindus (Tarakeshwar, Pargament, & Mahoney, 2003), and Buddhists (Phillips et al., 2009). Preliminary findings suggest that although specific religious/spiritual practices vary across religious identities, similar patterns of positive and negative religious/spiritual coping and posttraumatic outcomes are observed.

Integrating Religion and Spirituality into the Posttraumatic Recovery Process

We have explored so far the ways in which religion and spirituality can be deeply embedded in the process of appraising, coping with, and recovering from trauma. Moreover, because religious and spiritual coping can facilitate both recovery and growth and exacerbate distress during times of crisis (see Chap. 14, this volume), it is critical for helpers to be equipped with the therapeutic tools and skills necessary to effectively address the religious and spiritual dimension of trauma. For a more extensive discussion of how helping professionals can create a safe space for spiritual dialogue, initiate spiritual conversation, build clients' positive religious/spiritual coping resources, and address religious/spiritual struggles, see *Spiritually Integrated Psychotherapy: Understanding and Addressing the Sacred.* (Pargament, 2007)

Results of a meta-analysis by Smith, Bartz, and Richards (2007) indicate that religion and spirituality should be explored as potentially relevant topics in psychological treatment. They assessed treatment outcome studies featuring a variety of spiritually–integrated therapies in individual and group formats. These treatments featured an assortment of spiritually–oriented cognitive and behavioral techniques (e.g., teaching religious/spiritual principles, prayer, reading sacred texts, religious imagery, spiritual meditation) to help people cope with a variety of problems (e.g., posttraumatic stress, anxiety, depression, physical health symptoms). Results revealed a moderate effect size (0.56) for spiritually–integrated therapies across 31 studies, with a similar effect size (0.51) for studies comparing spiritually–oriented treatments with those lacking a religious/spiritual component. The helpful impact of spiritually–oriented therapy approaches seemed to be particularly strong in studies assessing positive functioning and well-being, compared to those only measuring mental health symptoms, which may speak to the unique capacity for religion and spirituality to facilitate growth and quality of life in the midst of ongoing stressors.

Outcome research on therapeutic meditation also illustrates the importance of investigating spiritually–integrated forms of mental health treatment. Although meditation is often presented by health-care professionals in secularized form, some evidence suggests that retaining the spiritual roots of meditation may enhance its effectiveness. For example, working with a sample of people who suffered from migraines, Wachholtz and Pargament (2008) compared the outcomes of meditating to spiritually–based phrases (e.g., "God is peace") with meditating to secular phrases (e.g., "I am content," "Sand is soft") and progressive relaxation. Results indicated that participants in the spiritual meditation group experienced relatively fewer migraine headaches, less negative mood and anxiety, greater pain tolerance and headache-related self-efficacy, increased daily spiritual experiences, and greater existential well-being. In a randomized controlled trial of the effects of meditation on coping with HIV, Bormann et al. (2006) found that participants who repeated spiritually–based mantras from a variety of religious traditions (i.e., Buddhism, Hinduism, Christianity, Judaism, Islam, Native American traditions) over 10 weeks reported significantly greater reductions in intrusive thoughts, trait anger, and depressive symptoms over time, as well as greater existential/spiritual well-being (e.g., faith, meaning/peace, spiritual connectedness) and perceived quality of life, compared to an attention control group.

Given the apparent helpfulness of accessing positive religious/spiritual coping resources and working through religious/spiritual struggles during times of stress, a number of spiritually–integrated psychotherapy treatments for coping with various forms of trauma have been designed and evaluated. For example, an eight-week psycho-spiritual intervention for women diagnosed with HIV has been developed to address existential concerns (e.g., healing, control and surrender, anger, guilt and shame, intimacy and isolation), facilitate positive religious/spiritual coping responses (e.g., meditation, prayer, ritual, spiritual support), and confront religious/spiritual struggles (e.g., feeling punished by God, anger toward God, stigmatization by religious communities; Pargament, McCarthy, et al., 2004a). A similar eight-week psycho-spiritual intervention was designed for adults diagnosed with HIV/AIDS to help them reflect upon the ways in which their spirituality helps and hinders their attempts to cope. Evaluation of this intervention revealed that participants experienced an increase in positive religious/spiritual coping methods (e.g., seeking strength from a Higher Power), a decrease in negative religious/spiritual coping methods (e.g., feeling punished by a Higher Power, anger toward a Higher Power), and a decrease in depressed mood (Tarakeshwar, Pearce, & Sikkema, 2005). A six-week psycho-spiritual intervention has also been developed for cancer patients suffering with severe medical conditions, in which participants draw upon their relationship with God for support while resolving spiritual struggles related to the search for control, identity, meaning, and relationships (Cole, 2005). A pilot outcome study revealed that participants maintained stability in mental and physical health, while nontreatment control group patients reported increased depression and pain severity. In a preliminary investigation of an eight-week psycho-spiritual intervention designed to address spiritual struggles in women who had experienced childhood sexual abuse, both participants experienced increases in positive religious/spiritual coping, spiritual well-being, and positive images of God (Murray-Swank & Pargament, 2005). Lastly, an evaluation of a nine-week group intervention for college students struggling with spiritual issues indicated that participants experienced significant improvements in the domains of psychological distress, spiritual struggles, emotion regulation, and congruence between their behaviors and spiritual values (Oemig Dworsky et al., 2012).

Large-scale natural disasters and man-made calamities often call for a two-pronged approach for spiritual and emotional support, including short-term triage interventions that focus on immediate physical, psychological, spiritual needs, as well as longer-term spiritually–integrated psychological interventions to ameliorate posttraumatic distress and facilitate long-term posttraumatic growth (Aten, 2012). Large-scale catastrophes also present an opportunity for helping professionals to offer spiritually–integrated psychological services through collaboration. Aten, Topping, Denney, and Hosey (2011) developed a three-tiered, faith-based model of disaster response in the Gulf Coast region of the USA, which features: (1) mental health professionals offering disaster response training and mental health education to the local clergy, (2) mental health professionals and religious leaders working together to educate congregation members, and (3) congregation members reaching out to others in their local communities with information about post-disaster mental health issues. Given that many mental health interventions tend to be individualistic in nature, this model has the strength of drawing upon communal resources and capitalizing on the relational facet of religion and spirituality. As one participant shared, “We all miraculously interacted with each other during Katrina. It was something like a great big family thing. All of the churches, all of the people came as one" (Aten, Topping, Denney, Hosey, 2011, p. 20).

Additionally, congregation-based psycho-spiritual interventions acknowledge the interrelatedness of psychological and spiritual well-being. Religious and spiritual coping resources (e.g., spiritual reappraisals, prayer, meditation, practicing forgiveness, seeking acceptance and hope, spiritual rituals and celebrations, participating in faith community services, congregational singing and artwork, renewed religious commitments, congregation-based activism) have been identified as serving a key role in family-based and community-based interventions addressing traumatic loss among people who have experienced many types of trauma, including community gang violence, Bosnian and Kosovar genocide and displacement, the 1995 Oklahoma City bombing, the 2005 Hurricane Katrina, and the 2001 World Trade Center terrorist attacks (Walsh, 2007). Further empirical research is needed, however, to test the effectiveness of spiritually–integrated, multisystemic disaster response interventions that are focused on ameliorating distress and facilitating growth in individuals, families, and communities.

Conclusion

In times of crisis, sacred dimensions of life become especially salient. Religion and spirituality are often embedded within multiple aspects of the posttraumatic recovery process, including the ways in which people understand crises, the methods they select to cope with adversity, and the short- and long-term outcomes of trauma. The relationships between religion, spirituality, and trauma are complex and dynamic. Religion and spirituality can be integrated into interventions designed to help people along in the coping process. Outcome data from spiritually–integrated interventions have been promising thus far (Bormann et al., 2006; Oemig Dworsky et al., 2012; Smith et al., 2007; Tarakeshwar et al., 2005; Wachholtz & Pargament, 2008). A dual approach to religious/spiritual coping that includes maximizing the use of positive religious/spiritual coping resources and resolving posttraumatic religious/spiritual struggles appears to be particularly effective. Researchers and helping professionals should continue to explore ways in which individuals' religious and spiritual experiences can play a key role in treatment. For many, religion and spirituality offer promising pathways to long-term posttraumatic adjustment and growth.

References

Ai, A. L., Peterson, C., & Huang, B. (2003). The effect of religious spiritual coping on positive attitudes of adult Muslim refugees from Kosovo and Bosnia. *The International Journal for the Psychology of Religion, 12,* 29–47. doi:10.1207/S15327582IJPR1301_04.

Alam, E., & Collins, A. E. (2010). Cyclone disaster vulnerability and response experiences in coastal Bangladesh. *Disasters, 34,* 931–954. doi:10.1111/j.03613666.2010.01176.x.

Ano, G. G., & Vasconcelles, E. B. (2005). Religious coping and psychological adjustment to stress: A meta-analysis. *Journal of Clinical Psychology, 61,* 461–480. doi:10.1002/jclp.20049.
Aten, J. D. (2012). Disaster spiritual and emotional care in professional psychology: A Christian integrative approach. *Journal of Psychology & Theology, 40,* 131–135.
Aten, J. D., Moore, M., Denney, R. M., Bayne, T., Stagg, A., Owens, S., et al. (2008). God images following hurricane Katrina in south Mississippi: An exploratory study. *Journal of Psychology and Theology, 36,* 249–257. http://journals.biola.edu/jpt/volumes/36/issues/4/articles/249. Accessed 5 May 2014.
Aten, J. D., Topping, S., Denney, R., & Hosey, J. (2011). Helping African American clergy and churches address minority disaster mental health disparities: Training needs, model, and example. *Psychology of Religion and Spirituality, 3,* 15–23. doi:10.1037/a0020497.
Bormann, J. E., Gifford, A. L., Shively, M., Smith, T. L., Redwine, L., Kelly, A., et al. (2006). Effects of spiritual mantram repetition on HIV outcomes: A randomized controlled trial. *Journal of Behavioral Medicine, 29,* 359–376. doi:10.1007/s10865-006-9063-6.
Bragg, R. (19 April 1996). A year of sorrow—A special report: Blast toll is no longer in deaths, but in shattered lives. *The New York Times*. http://www.nytimes.com. Accessed 24 May 2014.
Broadway, B. (8 Jan 2005). Divining a reason for devastation: Followers of various faiths differ on natural, supernatural explanations for tsunami. *Washington Post*. http://www.washingtonpost.com/wp-dyn/articles/A57758-2005Jan7.html. Accessed 19 May 2014.
Bulman, R. J., & Wortman, C. B. (1977). Attributions of blame and coping in the "real world": Severe accident victims react to their lot. *Journal of Personality and Social Psychology, 35,* 351–363. doi:10.1037/0022-3514.35.5.351.
Cole, B. S. (2005). Spiritually-focused psychotherapy for people diagnosed with cancer: A pilot outcome study. *Mental Health, Religion & Culture, 8,* 217–226. doi:10.1080/13694670500138916.
Cotton, S., Puchalski, C. M., Sherman, S. N., Mrus, J. M., Peterman, A. H., Feinberg, J., et al. (2006). Spirituality and religion in patients with HIV/AIDS. *Journal of General Internal Medicine, 21,* S5–S13. doi:10.1111/j.1525-1497.2006.00642.x.
DeMaris, A., Mahoney, A., & Pargament, K. I. (2010). Sanctification of marriage and general religiousness as buffers of the effects of marital inequity. *Journal of Family Issues, 31,* 1255–1278. doi:10.1177/0192513X10363888.
Denney, R. M., Aten, J. D., & Leavell, K. (2011). Posttraumatic spiritual growth: A phenomenological study of cancer survivors. *Mental Health, Religion, & Culture, 14,* 371–391. doi:10.1080/13674671003758667.
Dumas, J., & Nissley-Tsiopinis, J. (2006). Parental global religiousness, sanctification of parenting, and positive and negative religious coping as predictors of parental and child functioning. *International Journal for the Psychology of Religion, 16,* 289–310. doi:10.1207/s15327582ijpr1604_4.
Durkheim, E. (1915). *The elementary forms of the religious life*. New York: Free Press.
Exline, J. J. (2013). Religious and spiritual struggles. In K. I. Pargament, J. J. Exline, & J.W. Jones (Eds.), *APA handbook of psychology, religion, and spirituality (Vol. 1: Context, theory, and research)* (pp. 459–475). Washington, DC: American Psychological Association.
Exline, J. J., Park, C. L., Smyth, J. M., & Carey, M. P. (2011). Anger toward God: Five foundational studies emphasizing predictors, doubts about God's existence, and adjustment to bereavement and cancer. *Journal of Personality and Social Psychology, 100,* 129–148.
Fallot, R. D., & Heckman, J. P. (2005). Religious/spiritual coping among women trauma survivors with mental health and substance use disorders. *The Journal of Behavioral Health Services & Research, 32,* 215–226. doi:10.1007/BF02287268.
Folkman, S., & Lazarus, R. S. (1988). Coping as a mediator of emotion. *Journal of Personality and Social Psychology, 54,* 466–475. doi:10.1037/0022-3514.54.3.466.
Folkman, S., & Moskowitz, J. F. (2004). Coping: Pitsfalls and promise. *Annual Review of Psychology, 55,* 745–774. doi:10.1146/annurev.psych.55.090902.141456.
Gall, T. L., & Cornblat, M. W. (2002). Breast cancer survivors give voice: A qualitative analysis of spiritual factors in long-term adjustment. *Psycho-Oncology, 11,* 524–535. doi:10.1002/pon.613.

Gallup. (2 June 2014). Religion: Gallup historical trends. http://www.gallup.com/poll/1690/religion.aspx. Accessed 2 June 2014.

Garrison, M. E. B., & Sasser, D. D. (2009). Families and disasters: Making meaning out of adversity. In K. E. Cherry (Ed.), *Lifespan perspectives on natural disasters: Coping with Katrina, Rita, and other storms* (pp. 113–130). New York: Springer.

Gerber, M. M., Boals, A., & Schuettler, D. (2011). The unique contributions of positive and negative religious coping to posttraumatic growth and PTSD. *Psychology of Religion and Spirituality, 3,* 298–307. doi:10.1037/a0023016.

Hawley, A. R. (2012). *The roles of spirituality and sexuality in response to romantic breakup* (Master's thesis). https://etd.ohiolink.edu/ap/10?0::NO:10:P10_ACCESSION_NUM:bgsu1344123203. Accessed 5 May 2014.

Hawley, A. R., & Mahoney, A. (2013). Romantic breakup as a sacred loss and desecration among Christians at a state university. *Journal of Psychology and Christianity, 32,* 245–260. http://connection.ebscohost.com/c/articles/92531510/romantic-breakup-as-sacred-loss-desecration-among-christians-state-university. Accessed 14 May 2014.

Henderson, T. L., Roberto, K. A., & Kamo, Y. (2010). Older adults' responses to hurricane Katrina: Daily hassles and coping strategies. *Journal of Applied Gerontology, 29,* 48–69. doi:10.1177/0733464809334287.

Jones, J. W. (2002). *Terror and transformation: The ambiguity of religion in psychoanalytic perspective*. New York: Bruman-Routledge.

Koenig, H. G., Pargament, K. I., & Nielsen, J. (1998). Religious coping and health status in medically ill hospitalized older adults. *Journal of Nervous and Mental Disease, 186,* 513–521. doi:10.1097/00005053-199809000-00001.

Krumrei, E. J. (2008). *A longitudinal analysis of the role of religious appraisals and religious coping in adults' adjustment to divorce* (Doctoral dissertation). Available from ProQuest Dissertations and Theses database (UMI No. 3324024).

Lazarus, R. S., & Folkman, S. (1984). *Stress, appraisal, and coping*. New York: Springer.

Lichter, D. T., & Carmalt, J. H. (2009). Religion and marital quality in low-income couples. *Social Science Review, 38,* 168–187. doi:10.1016/j.ssresearch.2008.07.003.

Mahoney, A., Pargament, K. I., Jewell, T., Swank, A. B., Scott, E., Emery, E., et al. (1999). Marriage and the spiritual realm: The role of proximal and distal religious constructs in marital functioning. *Journal of Family Psychology, 13,* 1–18. doi:10.1037/0893-3200.13.3.321.

Mahoney, A., Pargament, K. I., Ano, G., Lynn, Q., Magyar, G., McCarthy, S., et al. (2002, August). The devil made them do it? Desecration & demonization in response to the 9/11 attacks. Paper presented at the Annual Meeting of the American Psychological Association, Chicago, IL.

Mahoney, A., Carels, R. A., Pargament, K. I., Wachholtz, A., Leeper, L. E., Kaplar, M., et al. (2005a). The sanctification of the body and behavioral health patterns of college students. *The International Journal of the Psychology of Religion, 15,* 221–238. doi:10.1207/s15327582ijpr1503_3.

Mahoney, A., Pargament, K. I., Cole, B., Jewell, T., Magyar, G. M., Tarakeshwar, N., et al. (2005b). A higher purpose: The sanctification of strivings in a community sample. *International Journal for the Psychology of Religion, 15,* 239–262. doi:10.1207/s15327582ijpr1503_4.

Mahoney, A., Krumrei, E. J., & Pargament, K. I. (2008). Broken vows: Divorce as a spiritual trauma and its implications for growth and decline. In S. Joseph & P. Alex Linley (Eds.), *Trauma, recovery, and growth: Positive psychological perspectives on posttraumatic stress* (pp. 105–124). New Jersey: Wiley.

Mahoney, A., Pargament, K. I., & DeMaris, A. (2009). Couples viewing marriage and pregnancy through the lens of the sacred: A descriptive study. *Research in the Social Scientific Study of Religion, 20,* 1–45. doi:10.1163/ej.9789004175624.i-334.7.

Marks, L. D., Cherry, K. E., & Silva, J. L (2009). Faith, crisis, coping, and meaning making after Katrina: A qualitative, cross-cohort examination. In K. E. Cherry (Ed.), *Lifespan perspectives on natural disasters: Coping with Katrina, Rita, and other storms* (pp. 195–215). New York: Springer.

Murphy, S. A., Johnson, C., & Lohan, J. (2003). Finding meaning in a child's violent death: A five-year prospective analysis of parents' personal narratives and empirical data. *Death Studies, 27,* 381–404. doi:10.1080/07481180390208621.

Murray-Swank, A., Mahoney, A., & Pargament, K. I. (2006). Sanctification of parenting: Links to corporal punishment and parental warmth among biblically conservative and liberal mothers. *The International Journal of the Psychology of Religion, 16,* 271–287. doi:10.1207/s15327582ijpr1604_3.

Murray-Swank, N. A., & Pargament, K. I. (2005). God, where are you? Evaluating a spiritually-integrated intervention for sexual abuse. *Mental Health, Religion & Culture, 8,* 191–203. doi:10.1080/13694670500138866.

Murray-Swank, N. A., Pargament, K. I., & Mahoney, A. (2005). At the crossroads of sexuality and spirituality: The sanctification of sex by college students. *The International Journal for the Psychology of Religion, 15,* 199–219. doi:10.1207/s15327582ijpr1503_2.

Oemig Dworsky, C. K., Pargament, K. I., Gibbel, M. R., Krumrei, E. J., Faigin, C. A., Haugen, M. R. G., et al. (2012). Winding road: Preliminary support for a spiritually integrated intervention addressing college students' spiritual struggles. *Research in the Social Scientific Study of Religion, 24,* 309–240. doi:10.1163/9789004252073_013.

O'Grady, K. A., Rollison, D. G., Hanna, T. S., Schreiber-Pan, H., & Ruiz, M. A. (2012). Earthquake in Haiti: Relationship with the sacred in times of trauma. *Journal of Psychology & Theology, 40,* 289–301. http://journals.biola.edu/jpt/volumes/40/issues/4/articles/289. Accessed 7 May 2014.

Paden, W. E. (1992). *Interpreting the sacred: Ways of viewing religion*. Boston: Beacon.

Pargament, K. I. (1997). *The psychology of religion and coping: Theory, research, practice*. New York: Guilford.

Pargament, K. I. (2007). *Spiritually integrated psychotherapy: Understanding and addressing the sacred*. New York: Guilford.

Pargament, K. I. & Mahoney, A. (2005). Sacred matters: Sanctification as vital topic for the psychology of religion. *International Journal for the Psychology of Religion, 15,* 179–198. doi:10.1207/s15327582ijpr1503_1.

Pargament, K. I., Smith, B. W., Koenig, H. G., & Perez, L. (1998). Patterns of positive and negative religious coping with major life stressors. *Journal of the Scientific Study of Religion, 37,* 711–725. doi:10.2307/1388152.

Pargament, K. I., Koenig, H. G. & Perez, L. M. (2000). The many methods of religious coping: Development and initial validation of the RCOPE. *Journal of Clinical Psychology, 56,* 519–543. doi:10.1002/(SICI)1097-4679(200004)56:4<519::AID-JCLP6>3.0.CO;2-1.

Pargament, K. I., McCarthy, S., Shah, P., Ano, G., Tarakeshwar, N., Wachholtz, A., et al. (2004a). Religion and HIV: A review of the literature and clinical implications. *Southern Medical Journal, 97,* 1201–1209. doi:10.1097/01.SMJ.0000146508.14898.E2.

Pargament, K. I., Koenig, H. G., Tarakeshwar, N., & Hahn, J. (2004b). Religious coping methods as predictors of psychological, physical and spiritual outcomes among medically ill elderly patients: A two-year longitudinal study. *Journal of Health Psychology, 9,* 713–730. doi:10.1177/1359105304045366.

Pargament, K. I., Magyar, G. M., Benore, E. & Mahoney, A. (2005). Sacrilege: A study of sacred loss and desecration and their implications for health and well-being in a community sample. *Journal for the Scientific Study of Religion, 44,* 59–78. doi:10.1111/j.1468-5906.2005.00265.x.

Pargament, K. I., Falb, M. D., Ano, G. G., & Wachholtz, A. B. (2013a). The religious dimension of coping: Advances in theory, research, and practice. In R. F. Paloutzian & C. L. Park (Eds.), *Handbook of the psychology of religion and spirituality* (2nd ed., pp. 560–79). New York: Guilford.

Pargament, K. I., Mahoney, A., Exline, J. J., Jones, J., & Shafranske, E. (2013b). Envisioning an integrative paradigm for the psychology of religion and spirituality: An introduction to the APA handbook of psychology, religion and spirituality. In K. I. Pargament, J. J. Exline, J. Jones, A. Mahoney, & E. Shafranske (Eds.), *APA handbook of psychology, religion, and spirituality*, (vol. 1, pp. 3–20).Washington, D.C.: American Psychological Association.

Park, C. L. (2013). Religion and meaning. In R. F. Paloutzian & C. L. Park (Eds.), *Handbook of the psychology of religion and spirituality* (pp. 357–379). New York, NY: Guilford Press.

Paton, D., Gregg, C. E., Houghton, B. F., Lachman, R., Lachman, J., Johnston, D. M., et al. (2008). The impact of the 2004 tsunami on coastal Thai communities: Assessing adaptive capacity. *Disasters, 32,* 106–119. doi:10.1111/j.0361-3666.2007.01029.x.

Phillips, R. E., III, Cheng, C. M., Pargament, K. I., Oemig, C., Colvin, S. D., Abarr, A. N., et al. (2009). Spiritual coping in American Buddhists: An exploratory study. *The International Journal for the Psychology of Religion, 19,* 231–243. doi:10.1080/10508610903143263.

Piper, J. (29 Dec 2004). Tsunami, sovereignty, and mercy. http://www.desiringgod.org/articles/tsunami-sovereignty-and-mercy. Accessed 20 May 2014.

Prati, G., & Pietrantoni, L. (2009). Optimism, social support, and coping strategies as factors contributing to posttraumatic growth: A meta-analysis. *Journal of Loss and Trauma, 14,* 364–388. doi:10.1080/15325020902724271.

Raiya, H. A., Pargament, K. I., Mahoney, A., & Stein, C. (2008). A psychological measure of Islamic religiousness: Development and evidence for reliability and validity. *The International Journal for the Psychology of Religion, 18,* 291–315. doi:10.1080/10508610802229270.

Rosmarin, D. H., Pargament, K. I., Krumrei, E. J., & Flannelly, K. J. (2009). Religious coping among Jews: Development and initial validation of the JCOPE. *Journal of Clinical Psychology, 65,* 670–683. doi:10.1002/jclp.20574.

Schuster, M. A., Stein, B. D., Jaycox, L. H., Collins, R. L., Marshall, G. N., Elliot, M. N., et al. (2001). A national survey of stress reactions after the September 11, 2001, terrorist attacks. *New England Journal of Medicine, 345,* 1507–1512. doi:10.1056/NEJM200111153452024.

Silva, J. L., Marks, L. D., & Cherry, K. E. (2009). The psychology behind helping and prosocial behaviors: An examination from intention to action. In K. E. Cherry (Ed.), *Lifespan perspectives on natural disasters: Coping with Katrina, Rita, and other storms* (pp. 219–240). New York: Springer.

Smith, T. B., Bartz, J., & Richards, P. S. (2007). Outcomes of religious and spiritual adaptations to psychotherapy: A meta-analytic review. *Psychotherapy Research, 17,* 643–655. doi:10.1080/10503300701250347.

Tarakeshwar, N., Swank, A. B., Pargament, K. I., & Mahoney, A. (2001). The sanctification of nature and theological conservatism: A study of opposing religious correlates of environmentalism. *Review of Religious Research, 42,* 387–404. doi:10.2307/3512131.

Tarakeshwar, N., Pargament, K. I., & Mahoney, A. (2003). Initial development of a measure of religious coping among Hindus. *Journal of Community Psychology, 31,* 607–628. doi:10.1002/jcop.10071.

Tarakeshwar, N., Pearce, M. J., & Sikkema, K. J. (2005). Development and implementation of a spiritual coping group intervention for adults living with HIV/AIDS: A pilot study. *Mental Health, Religion, & Culture, 8,* 179–190. doi:10.1080/13694670500138908.

Tuason, M. T. G., Güss, C. D., & Carroll, L. (2012). The disaster continues: A qualitative study on the experiences of displaced hurricane Katrina survivors. *Professional Psychology: Research and Practice, 43,* 288–297. doi:10.1037/a0028054.

Varley, E., Isaranuwatchai, W., & Coyte, P. C. (2012). Ocean waves and roadside spirits: Thai health service providers' post-tsunami psychosocial health. *Disasters, 36,* 656–675. doi:10.1111/j.1467-7717.2012.01274.x.

Volling, B. L., Mahoney, A., & Rauer, A. J. (2009). Sanctification of parenting, moral socialization, and young children's conscience development. *Psychology of Religion and Spirituality, 1,* 53–68. doi:10.1037/a0014958.

Wachholtz, A. B., & Pargament, K. I. (2008). Migraines and meditation: Does spirituality matter? *Journal of Behavioral Medicine, 31,* 351–366. doi:10.1007/s10865-008-9159-2.

Walsh, F. (2007). Traumatic loss and major disasters: Strengthening family and community resilience. *Family Process, 46,* 207–227. doi:10.1111/j.1545-5300.2007.00205.x.

Wrzesniewski, A., McCauley, C., Rozin, P., & Schwartz, B. (1997). Jobs, careers, and callings: People's relations to their work. *Journal of Research in Personality, 31,* 21–33. doi:10.1006/jrpe.1997.2162.

Chapter 20
Faith and Coping: Spiritual Beliefs and Religious Practices After Hurricanes Katrina and Rita

Loren D. Marks, Yaxin Lu, Katie E. Cherry and Trevan G. Hatch

Without God in my life, there's no hope. [And] when you lose hope, you have nothing.
(234; 59-year old male)

Introduction

In August and September of 2005, Hurricanes Katrina and Rita brought catastrophic destruction to the US Gulf Coast, including Texas, Louisiana, Mississippi, Alabama, and Florida. Nearly 2,000 people died and over a million Gulf Coast residents were displaced from their homes. Hurricane Katrina's devastating impact and the psychosocial consequences of this treacherous storm are described more fully elsewhere (see Cherry, 2009; Kessler et al., 2009). In this chapter, we focus on the role of faith as a coping resource hypothesized to promote resilience in the wake of the Katrina tragedy. In particular, we examine qualitative interview data that allowed deeper insights concerning not only *what* sacred beliefs and practices were helpful but also *why* they mattered to participants as they faced multiple stressors in the immediate aftermath and in the years following the 2005 storms.

K. E. Cherry (✉)
Department of Psychology, Louisiana State University, 236 Audubon Hall, Baton Rouge, LA 70803-5501, USA
e-mail: pskatie@lsu.edu

L. D. Marks
School of Family Life, Brigham Young University, 2092C Joseph F. Smith Building, Provo, Utah 84602, USA
e-mail: loren_marks@byu.edu

T. G. Hatch
School of Social Work, Louisiana State University, 335 Long Fieldhouse, Baton Rouge, LA 70803-5501, USA
e-mail: thatch8@lsu.edu

Y. Lu
Louisiana Department of Education, 1201 North Third Street, Baton Rouge, LA 70802, USA
e-mail: Yaxinlu3@gmail.com

K. E. Cherry (ed.), *Traumatic Stress and Long-Term Recovery*,
DOI 10.1007/978-3-319-18866-9_20

Overview of Coping and Resilience

A leading religious coping scholar, Ken Pargament, defines coping as a transactional process that involves maintaining and restoring multidimensional human functioning across cognitive, affective, behavioral, and physiological domains (Pargament, 1997; see also Chap. 19, this volume). Coping is further defined as the process through which resources are accessed and used to respond to stressor events within individuals and across people in various relationships and settings (Pargament, 1997). Although coping typically invokes a positive connotation, there are negative forms of "coping" as well (e.g., drinking, social withdrawal). A closely related concept, resilience, pertains to peoples' ability to "bounce back" and thrive after having experienced trauma, a potentially traumatic event (PTE), or other harsh circumstances (Cherry & Galea, 2015; see also Chaps. 1, 3, and 16, this volume).

With respect to religious coping, some religious practices, especially prayer, have been reportedly helpful for individuals in connection with both "acute" and "day-to-day stresses" of life in a variety of samples and contexts (Koenig, McCullough, & Larson, 2001, p. 94; Lambert, Fincham, Marks, & Stillman, 2010; Marks, 2008). Religious beliefs and practices have also been correlated with positive mental health outcomes including greater personal happiness and/or self-esteem and lower depression rates (Dollahite, Marks, & Goodman, 2004; Koenig, 1998; Mahoney, 2010)—but the science-based picture of religious coping is more complex than this, especially in a disaster context. For example, Cherry et al. (2015) found that non-organizational religiosity was associated with increased risk of posttraumatic stress disorder (PTSD), where people who were highest in non-organizational religiosity were nine times more likely to have PTSD symptoms than their low-scoring counterparts. Cherry et al. (2015) suggested that persons who suffer most severely from PTSD may seek solitary forms of religious coping to strengthen their sense of well-being, or perhaps they turn to non-organizational religiosity in response to emotional distress when former places of worship have been destroyed by natural disaster.

Religion is an important coping resource for many persons but, like other forms of coping, religious coping also has positive and negative manifestations (see Chap. 19, this volume). In connection with negative religious coping (i.e., "red flags"), Pargament et al. (1998b) have said: "Although religion is often a source of help and integration, *certain religious expressions appear to be part of the problem* in coping rather than part of the solution" (p. 88, emphasis added). Koenig, McCullough, and Larson's *Handbook of Religion and Health* (Oxford, 2001) and other volume-length reviews similarly identify religious belief as a beneficial psychological coping resource or as a correlate of better mental health with myriad samples—but also draw attention to harmful connections that sometimes surface (Koenig, 1998; Pargament, 1997; Pargament, Smith, Koenig, & Perez, 1998a; Paloutzian & Park, 2005). More recent article-length reviews continue to establish a generally positive connection between religion and psychological coping, but with greater sensitivity to positive *and* negative manifestations (Dollahite et al. 2004; Mahoney, 2010).

Regrettably, the influence of religious belief and practices on individual and family-level coping in response to major disasters has not been well researched. Much of what we do know is based on surface-level survey data, while many deeper and underlying questions regarding religious coping in the aftermath of both natural and man-made disasters are only beginning to be addressed (Cherry, 2009; Tausch et al., 2011). Closer examinations of underlying processes, like our attempt here, have been referred to as "mining the meanings" (Marks & Dollahite, 2011). Cherry, Galea, and Silva (2008) have made the point that natural disasters provide a context to study adaptation, resilience, and successful aging. The qualitative analyses reported here may shed new light on potential connections among religious coping and resilience outcomes in the years after Hurricanes Katrina and Rita's deadly impact on coastal communities along the US Gulf of Mexico.

To summarize, prior research has shown that positive religious coping may enhance posttraumatic resilience, while negative religious coping has been related to *higher* levels of depression (Abu-Raiya, Pargament, & Mahoney, 2010; Koenig et al., 2001). The "two-tailed" outcomes associated with religious coping beg more specific questions than "Is religion a factor?" Scholars must look deeper to examine the specific expressions of religious belief and practice that are facilitative and linked to successful adaptation and resilience without ignoring the potential for negative outcomes. The participants in the present study seem to be positioned to shed light on how spirituality and religious practice align with resilient outcomes and adaptation to stressful situations, as discussed next.

Method

Participants and Procedure

In all, 125 adults from the heavily affected parishes of St. Bernard and Plaquemines in south Louisiana participated in the study. All participants experienced significant property damage and storm-related displacement. Two groups were compared and contrasted: Group 1 was composed of 62 directly affected persons who ultimately *relocated* to new homes in non-coastal communities (M age = 58.4 years, SD = 17.1 years). Group 2 was composed of 63 directly affected persons who were displaced, and *returned to rebuild* and restore their lives in their home communities in the years following the 2005 storms of Katrina and Rita (M age = 60.7 years, SD = 15.0 years) (see Chap. 12, this volume).

Participants responded to open-ended questions regarding their experiences in coping with Hurricanes Katrina and Rita and were also encouraged to share illustrative personal stories and experiences, consistent with a narrative approach to qualitative methods (Josselson & Lieblich, 1993). All interviews were digitally recorded and transcribed verbatim. Transcribed interviews were then "audited" by additional research assistants who carefully checked the interview transcription with the digital audio interview, congruent with the spirit of careful data auditing promoted by leading qualitative researchers (Denzin & Lincoln, 1994).

Analyses

Qualitative grounded theory methods were employed to analyze the data. According to Strauss and Corbin (1998), open coding is an important initial analytic step in qualitative data analysis. In this study, we employed two coding teams of four members each (eight total coders) for the data analysis process. One team analyzed and open coded narratives from the 62 participants who relocated and identified recurring concepts in these interviews. The second coding team analyzed and open coded narratives from the 63 participants who returned and rebuilt their coastal parish homes.

Open coding and analysis were done on four different levels:

1. Each coder analyzed interviews independently.
2. The coders met (in pairs) with a coding partner on a weekly basis to compare and contrast their open-coding findings in a qualitative variation of inter-rater reliability.
3. Each team of four (i.e., two pairs per team) met to compare open-coding findings.
4. At the conclusion of the open-coding process, the two coding teams (team 1 representing the relocated participants and team 2 representing the returned/rebuilt participants) were reunited to compare and contrast central findings across the two groups.

During this process, we also conducted numeric content analysis (NCA) of the open coding in each interview. In NCA, high-frequency concepts and salient concepts are recorded and organized thematically. Major themes are identified and systematically documented (Chap. 12, this volume).

Findings

We have published work elsewhere based on quantitative analyses of survey responses from this sample which confirmed that participants lost their homes, property, and numerous personal possessions, including photo albums, journals, and family heirlooms (Cherry et al., 2015). Based on interview-by-interview qualitative analyses, we also found that many reported less tangible but equally profound losses including: their sense of "home," their sense of identity, and their lifelong affiliation with a particular faith community. By way of illustration, consider this woman who yearned for her friends and faith community "down the road" in eastern St. Bernard which sustained an estimated 30 feet of water and total destruction as a result of Hurricane Katrina's storm surge. Her church, San Pedro Pescador Catholic Church, named for St. Peter the Fisherman, as well as her entire community was lost in the storm (Janega, 2005):

235 (43-year old): Yes, church was a big, important thing [to me]. I wanted to go back, and I wanted to go back with the people down here [in Yscloskey]. I didn't want to [meet with a congregation somewhere else] because they didn't *suffer* like we did down here. I felt like I needed to be with [my] people down the road here, because the people that used to go to San Pedro [church] where I lived, they had nothing to go back to either. I think I needed to be around them…I wanted it back. I wanted my…I wanted to go to church on Sundays [in *my* church]…but they wouldn't allow us. They [the Archdiocese] said we could not touch this church. We couldn't do it.

San Pedro, among other churches in St. Bernard, was subsequently razed to the ground and never rebuilt. Where does one belong when his or her home, neighborhood, and faith community are suddenly destroyed? This is one profoundly painful and tragic question that many of our participants had to negotiate in the months and years after August 2005.

In addition, in most cases, the participants' close personal relationships were severely disrupted. Although the directly related death tolls of Katrina and Rita burst into four figures, for many participants it was *dispersion*, not death, that wreaked the greatest havoc on their relational ties. Some who were initially displaced, disconnected, and discouraged also reported frustrations and challenges in terms of their faith and faith community (Chap. 14, this volume). However, for most of the participants, religious belief and practices reportedly provided strength and encouragement.

Five themes related to faith and religious coping emerged from our participants' interviews. Three of these themes are connected to spiritual beliefs and two relate to religious practices. All five themes are presented with excerpts of original, primary data that illustrate and support the respective themes. Three themes related to spiritual beliefs are presented first.

Theme 1: "I Couldn't Have Done It Without My God's Help:" God as a Personal and Relational Being

Many participants reported that sacred beliefs played an important role in their coping during both the immediate aftermath and long-term adjustment that followed the hurricanes. The participants' discussions of their beliefs ranged from general reflection to discussions of specific beliefs and even specific scriptural verses. To illustrate, consider this man's response to our asking if religious beliefs helped him cope with the hurricanes:

216 (80-year old): If it wouldn't have been for believing in God and all, we never would have made it…. And after we got the [FEMA] trailer…*it* still helped us…. You never know what *it* is until you get into those predicaments…. If we wouldn't have believed in *it* or had faith in *it,* we never would have made it. That carried us through.

In his discussion of religious beliefs and coping, this participant repeatedly invoked the nebulous pronoun "it." Although referencing a belief "in God and all" in the opening line, four of the "it" references seem to denote faith or spiritual belief in a generalized way that leaves the reader wondering what, exactly, was helpful and why "it" was helpful.

In comparison, many others expressed their belief that it was not just "faith" or "belief" but very specifically *God* who "helped [them] through everything." Several identified God not only as their primary source of strength for coping during the hurricanes but also hastened to add that God had helped them through much more than the hurricanes of 2005—emphasizing that God had been both a fair-weather and foul-weather friend throughout their lives. Indeed, when many spoke about "God," they seemed to invoke a reverent, companionate, and deeply personal type of language. A 67-year-old woman provided an example of this personalized style of discourse:

207: I don't want to say [that it was] religion [that helped me] because it's not one religion, it's *God.* It's His son. It's Jesus. And it's my belief in [Him] that helps me get up every day. [He] helps me do everything I do every day. [He] helped me get through Katrina. [He] helped me with my husband passing….

This participant downplayed the importance of her specific denomination and centers her comments on her personal, relational belief in God and "His son." Note how God is described not in philosophical or theological terms but in a tangible and close-at-hand manner—almost as if the participant is describing a loving caregiver or family member. Many other participants discussed their beliefs about God and their "relationship" with "Him" in similarly intimate ways. Another woman discussed her belief in and connection with God in these personal terms:

208 (66-year old)**:** God's seen me through a lot of things. I go to Him for everything. Sometimes I feel a little guilty because I feel like I lay (so much) on Him. But He's there for me, and He helps me. Eventually I get together and try to handle things myself. He's seeing me through and getting me through everything.

One participant not only repeatedly referenced her "relationship" with God, she also referred to God's "touch" in a literal and tactile way that was unique and rather striking. She reported:

249 (51-year old)**:** Well, for me I have a very strong religious belief and *I am very, very close to God. [I have] a personal relationship with Him,* so even if no one is around… I had Him…. *You just have to have that close relationship with Him.* Because I believe [sometimes] you [may not] have anybody around you, and you may yearn, you know, for that human touch, but like one priest told me, he said he wished that Jesus had more skin. *[a good-natured chuckle].* Which I thought was so cute, because you do need that human touch, but you can…*I think you can pretty much survive if you're close to God.*

This same linkage between "survival" and "God" was drawn by others as well. For example, a 59-year-old woman also referenced how God carried her through both the immediate and residual challenges of Katrina. She emphasized:

259: *Without God in my life there's no way I would have gotten through something like this….* When I don't feel like I'm hanging on and I'm losing my faith in things and feeling so down and depressed, somewhere in the back of my head *I still know He's there carrying me* through these bad times…. For me personally, *[I] couldn't have done it without [Him],* because [Katrina] was very devastating to me personally. Katrina [was too much]…. So, no, *I couldn't have done it without my God's help.* There's no way I could've gotten through that [without Him].

In her brief excerpt, this participant referenced God directly or in pronoun form five different times. The mantra and theme that is continually reinforced seems to be: "I couldn't have done it without my God's help." The same core concept was reflected in several reports, as follows:

A 71-year-old female who lost an adult son in Katrina reflected:

> **241:** Well, I was always taught that there's only one person to turn over your troubles to, and that's Jesus…. He works in so many different ways. After Hurricane Katrina, I found that putting my trust in Him was the best thing that I could have ever done. [I needed His help to] not have a nervous breakdown, or try to, you know, try to do away with my life…. [He] helped me tremendously. If it wouldn't have been [for Him], if I had to do it on my own, I don't think I would have been able to handle [Katrina].

This participant specifically referenced "the Lord" directly or in pronoun form seven times in seven sentences. For participants like her, it was not optimism, positive psychology, or even "spirituality" in a general sense that reportedly helped them through—but a specific belief in (and reliance on) a personal and relational God who cared for them and "helped them through."

This sense of relationship with God was not necessarily a panacea. Several participants of apparent faith, including those cited in this section, referenced the longing for human touch. They contended with loneliness, "depression," "nervous breakdown," and even the temptation to "try to do away with my life." But even so, the recurring testimonial offered by those who found their faith most helpful was often an echo of (241), "[He] helped me tremendously."

Theme 2: "God is in Control:" Conceptualizations and Characteristics of God

As discussed in the previous section, a belief in a personal, relational God was a "tremendous help" to some participants. Other recurring beliefs addressed by those we interviewed dealt with the expansive power, scope, and involvement of God in the lives of those influenced and affected by Hurricanes Katrina and Rita. Again, the focus of the data was rarely on specific denominational doctrines, but instead on what might be called "attributes of God."

A small body of research has addressed individuals' "conceptualizations of God" (Dollahite, 1998; Hertel & Donahue, 1995; Vergote, 1980), although very little of the extant research examines ideas about God in the immediate or long-term aftermath of a disaster (for exceptions, see Aten et al., 2008; Marks, Cherry, & Silva, 2009). One spiritual belief or "conceptualization of God," voiced by some was that although God allows trials, trauma, and tragedy to touch human lives, "God doesn't give you more than you [can] handle." Examples of this sentiment included:

> **233** (49-year old female): Definitely my religious beliefs have helped me cope. I'm a firm believer that no matter how bad [your situation] is, *God doesn't give you more than you [can] handle.*

> **128** (49-year old female): [B]elieving in God helped me to remember that *He won't give us more than we can handle,* and He's here no matter what we're going through…. We can get through it.

From a capabilities-focused or positive psychology perspective, the conviction that God or life sometimes challenges you profoundly *but never beyond one's capacity* is a poignant belief because the inherent assumption promotes survival and success, even in the face of extreme difficulty. Covey (2004), among others, has discussed the elevating influence of the "Pygmalion effect" or self-fulfilling prophecy—namely, that when an individual *expects* a beneficial outcome, they are more likely to act in ways that will promote that outcome. In the immediate and long-term wake of Katrina and Rita, many of our participants were confronted by challenges that surpassed their previous life's experience, yet many reported that God "gave" them the additional strength, courage, and ability to bounce back and adapt to these challenges successfully. This belief seemed to be something of a supplement to the conviction that "God doesn't give you more that you handle"—in that if life *does* give you more than you are prepared to handle, God will provide additional strength and support to the individual and/or those surrounding them. From this vantage, whatever trials arose, God's "hand" was ready with a "plan." The reflection of this man captures a few of these interrelated ideas:

> **263** (73-year old male)**:** Yes. My spiritual beliefs helped me dearly because I knew that the Lord's hand was in everything that I done. He gave me the ability and the knowledge to do things that, like I said earlier, [I] had never done before in my life.

He went on to say, the experience "made me think of Psalms 23"—a portion of which reads:

> Yea, though I walk through the valley of the shadow of death, I will fear no evil: for thou art with me; thy rod and thy staff they comfort me (Psalm 23:4, KJV).

This man continued by directly quoting from another portion of the Old Testament. "Do not fear," he said, "For I know the plans I have for you." The verse this gentleman (263) cites reads in full:

> For I know the plans I have for you…plans to prosper you and not to harm you, plans to give you hope and a future (Jeremiah 29:11, NIV).

These latter three participants, like those directly cited earlier, seem to repeatedly return to a belief in a very personal and relational God "whose hand was in everything"—a God who has a "plan" with "hope and a future."

Consistent with our own previous research (Marks et al., 2009), a final representative reflection captures a recurring spiritual belief among the participants that God's involved hand "was in control." When asked if her spiritual beliefs helped her cope, one participant, the wife of 263 (the Bible-savvy gentleman mentioned earlier), responded:

> **262** (67-year old female): Oh, positively. Knowing that no matter what happened, in the past, in the present, or in the future, that *God was in control* [was a comfort]. No matter what emotions I was feeling, or when I would be depressed…. I knew that *He was in control.* And there was a purpose for everything. I may never know the answer [or the

purpose] but...I believe that with all my heart. There's no such thing as coincidence. [He's in control.]

Another participant similarly reflected:

124 (69-year old female): [Did my religious beliefs help me?]. Absolutely... [It was] comforting...knowing that there is...a God who...has taken care of me and who will continue [to]. And no matter what happens, He's going to make things right in the end, whether it is in this lifetime or in our next. You know, he never promised us a bed of roses. [laughs] And He did say we would have tribulation...[the Bible] says, "When things come, count it all joy," that's in James..."count it all joy," because *He's in control* and He'll make it better.

In this theme, participants have reported their belief in a God that "doesn't give you more than you [can] handle," a God whose "hand was in everything," a God with a "plan." A common theme through each of these conceptualizations of God, however, was a "God [that] was in control." We conclude our focus on the dimension of spiritual beliefs with the theme "The Katrina experience renewed your faith."

Theme 3: "The Katrina Experience Renewed Your Faith:" Spiritually Framing the Storm

We remind the reader that our data were obtained from in-depth interviews conducted 5–7 years after the storms. Revisionist history is always a threat in such interviews; however, this substantial length of time is likely to flatten some of the short-term trends (i.e., "spikes" in professed belief or church attendance for a couple of weeks or months). Our data provide a longer-term view of hurricane "effects" on spiritual belief. The data from a couple of our participants indicated little to no change on the faith-related front:

226 (81-year old male): God does...things for a reason, you know?.... Maybe people needed to be woke up. I don't know. But, far as waking up, I think a [small] percentage of people woke up after the hurricane [but] there's still a lot of people down here that [are] money hungry and they're doing things they're not supposed to be doing.

222 (66-year old male): [Were my religious beliefs helpful?] Not really. I'm not more religious than what I was before.... I am somewhat religious, and it did help (some). But I don't really depend on religion, you know. That's pretty much about it. And I'm not like a religious person. I'm not an atheist, but I kind of take [religion] with a grain of salt.

Reports such as these do not seem to indicate an epic post-Katrina revival of faith.

What lasting influence did the historic Hurricanes Katrina and Rita have on the participants' beliefs? Almost no dramatic changes in levels of religious faith were reported in our interviews. There were very few instances of atheists or agnostics experiencing a dramatic religious conversion[1], and seldom did strong believers report "losing their faith," although several had pronounced frustrations with perceived failures by their churches (see Chap. 14, this volume). Even so, the lack of dramatic increase or decrease of faith by persons at the poles of deeply avowed

[1] Two such incidents were directly reported (i.e., 352 and 361).

belief or disbelief should not be misinterpreted to mean that the Katrina/Rita experience had no faith-related influence on the participants' faith and beliefs. Some participants reported a "deepening," a "renewal," or a "return." One participant stated, "[The Katrina experience] just renewed your faith. That's all it did was, it renewed and confirmed…what you had grown up with as a child." A similar report was offered by a 20-year-old woman who explained:

> **261:** *[Katrina and Rita] definitely made me a more religious and faith filled person.* I do, I do…pray every night, I pray…. I try to thank God for what I have…because I mean, believe me, as bad as life can get sometimes, life can get one hundred percent worse.

Another participant spoke about a "turning" and a "realization" in more detail:

> **213** (64-year old male): [While coping with Katrina] most people turned back to God in their own ways…and you [do] turn to God. And you turn to religion. And you [plead], "Please God, help me. Please help us. We need help." That is a normal thing, I think, in a lot of cases…. Especially when you see dead people floating in the waters. [In most cases, those bodies were not recent deaths but] people that their bodies popped out of the tombs…. [But still, when you are confronted with death like that]…. You realize that, *You know, that's me twenty-five years from now in a tomb…maybe I ought to dog-gone get back to the way I was and start going to church or praying and all that.*

Some participants, like the individuals just mentioned, reported a sense of renewal of faith, a "turning," or a heightened realization of one's own mortality. Many others retrospectively captured their religion and coping experiences by using descriptive words such as "steady," "constant," and "peace." A 77-year-old woman was one of these. She reflected:

> **215:** *I could not have done anything without the help of God….* I think that's as simple as it gets. I can't think of anything else to say about that. *My religion was the one thing that remained steady in my life.* And it remained the same because in the Catholic Church, [well], no matter what church you go to, you feel at *home*. So I would have to say that was the most *constant* thing in my life right after Katrina…. *If I didn't have God in my life, I don't think I'd have a life.* That's the way I feel about my religion.

Earlier in this chapter, we emphasized the belief many participants manifested in a deeply personal and relational God. Although this woman specifically referenced her denomination, her emphasis is still on the personalized "help of God" she received—dramatically captured in the statement, "If I didn't have God in my life, I don't think I'd have a life." The next participant's language was, perhaps, not quite as dramatic as 215's, but this participant also conveyed a strong sense of relationship with and closeness to the Divine that is almost tangible:

> **136** (67-year old female): Before I left [to evacuate] I went through the house and blessed everything with holy water and just said "Lord you gave me this," [now] "I give it back to you."…I had done that…[when] we had evacuated the year before. And of course I came back [then] and everything was in perfect shape. This time, [with Katrina]…it wasn't in perfect shape but…God gave [it] to me to use, now I gave it back to Him…. *It was…God's will. So I think that helped me accept it.* He's here, better, faster than ever…. [T]here was a peace that came through all of this…. I would talk in my prayer to God [about]…what was going on and then I would just feel this peace. It was wonderful. *So it was an opportunity to get closer to God because you were dependent on Him….*

This section focused on participants' discussions of spiritual belief as a coping resource for those profoundly influenced by Katrina and Rita. As we have discussed and illustrated with nearly a score of interview excerpts, the reported influence of spiritual beliefs ranged widely from "none" to 215's personal synopsis that "If I didn't have God in my life, I don't think I'd have a life" and 136's report that "[I was] *dependent on Him*." Although the reports regarding the power of faith in coping with the hurricanes varied widely, the reports regarding the positive and negative influence of the hurricanes on faith were more modest and muted. Faith was rarely discovered or destroyed. Spiritual beliefs were, however, questioned, wrestled with, revisited, "renewed," and "strengthened."

The first three themes in this chapter dealt with sacred beliefs that reportedly helped many participants cope with the short- and long-term effects of the hurricanes. In the next section of the chapter, our lens is turned from beliefs to religious *practices* and their connection with storms, stress, and coping. Two themes related to religious practice is shared.

Theme 4: "Praying Helped Me Cope:" Prayer in the Immediate Katrina/Rita Aftermath

Based on our research team's open coding of the interviews, prayer was the most dominant and salient religious practice referenced, but the participants' narratives revealed that prayer was used for different purposes at different times. Even in interviews conducted at least 5 years after Katrina and Rita, several of the participants' prayer-related narratives referenced coping during the immediate aftermath, including the following four examples:

> **217** (80-year old female): [Do I believe my religious beliefs and practices helped me cope?] Of course I believe in that… I believe in miracles, I believe that if you pray and you believe, that [good] things will happen. Yes I believe strictly…I believe that *praying helped me cope*.

> **224** (51-year old female): [Do I believe my religious beliefs and practices helped me cope?] Definitely, for sure. I mean, *I prayed to God constantly*. You know, just to give us the strength to get through…. I wouldn't have gotten through all this without my faith.

> **245** (79-year old female): Well, I believe in my religion. And I prayed, and prayed. *That's all you could do was pray*…. Oh yes. I believe in God, and I prayed to God.

> **154** (57-year old male): "God grant me the serenity to accept the things I cannot change, courage to accept…courage to change the things I can, and wisdom to know the difference." I truly say that prayer at least once a week. And I don't know [for sure] who I'm praying to, *but I'm praying*…. I don't go to church, and I don't know if I see the value in that anymore, *but I pray*. So, does [prayer] help me cope with the stresses? When I'm in the highest stress, yes.

Some participants, like the four just reported, told us that they prayed. Others, however, explained *why* they prayed during the immediate aftermath and/or *why* they continue this religious practice. These explanations included various reported benefits and motivations. One woman reported:

> **223** (63-year old): *[When I pray], it just calms me down, and relax[es] me….* And I think since Hurricane Katrina, I say [prayers] more. I know I pray more since Hurricane Katrina.

Another man responded:

> **226** (81-year old male): In times of trouble…well…*I go to my religion before times of trouble…[I] pray a lot more when the storms come*, "[I] hope we don't get the storm" and [I] pray to God we don't get any severe damage, [and that] nobody loses their lives. Sure, I…definitely pray more.

For the former participant (223), prayer reportedly helped calm and relax her, while for the latter (226) prayer is a place to go in times of trouble and during the (literal) storms of life. Another participant provided this deeper glimpse:

> **208** (66-year old female)) I do pray constantly, and my beliefs have gotten me a long way, and they still do. *[My faith] has helped me to cope* because, I mean, a lot of times you sit down and you think about everything that you lost and all the friends that you lost and everything else, and all [of a sudden] you're [overwhelmed]…. *My big [prayer] is, "For God's sake, please take that out my mind for now*. I got something else I got to do. I mean please, take it out of my mind." But *[prayer] does help you to cope with everything….* I'm a great believer…God has brought me through a lot.

While many narratives portray prayer as a coping resource, this reflection is poignant because it captures a prayer for temporary relief from the emotional and psychological pain of loss—pain so severe that she wrestles with doing what she has "got to do."

Another participant offered multiple reasons why prayer was her path of choice before, during, and after the hurricanes. For this woman, prayer was the one thing she could do while struggling with multiple storm-related stressors that unfolded over time. For her, prayer was a comfort and pathway to healing. She reported:

> **203** (52-year old): [I remember] *praying for strength* to be able to get through this, and at the same time, *doing thankful prayers* that we didn't lose any more than we did. We lost stuff, but we only lost one person…. And so *[we said prayers of thanks] that we were all safe and that we were all together*. I think [that praying] was…you know, the best thing for me. *When I couldn't do anything else, or couldn't think, or couldn't write, or couldn't read [laughs], I could pray*. I could still do that. [I could still pray]. [I remember *praying] just to be able to bear it* and to have the strength to, even if it's a crawl, [praying to God] to let me go and *do something*. [Praying] was…*it was a big comfort and a big factor in my beginning to heal and recover….* Yes, *[I] prayed [for] the strength to go on,* but also prayed [with thanks] that we didn't lose more.

In this narrative, she (203) presents us with multiple "whys" behind her prayers: (a) praying for strength to get through; (b) offering prayers of gratitude that "we didn't lose more"; (c) prayers of thanks for the safety and unity of surviving family members; (d) praying because "I couldn't do anything else"; (e) praying for the ability to act, to contribute, and to "go and do something"; (f) praying for comfort, healing, and recovery; and (g) praying for the strength to go on.

We note that the extensive list of "whys" above begins with "(a) praying for strength to get through" and concludes with "(g) praying for the strength to go on."

"Praying for the strength to get through" seems to refer to weathering initial tragedy and trauma—the focal point of most of the interview excerpts in this theme. By contrast, "praying for strength to go on" is drawn from a marker later in the coping process, after the immediate and imminent danger has passed but when the foe of long-term recovery or adaptation must be faced. A fair metaphoric comparison might be that after absorbing the initial shock of the death of a beloved husband, the mourning wife must still confront the inevitable estate issues, insurance claims, funeral arrangements, and a home that is unalterably changed. The required actions, transitions, and decisions *increase* rather than mercifully subside. Even so, many of the hurricane survivors reported that prayer helped them not only with the initial shock but also with subsequent decisions. As we turn to Theme 5, the interview excerpts similarly turn from handling the initial shock to long-term coping and choices.

Theme 5: "I Prayed A Lot for Guidance:" God as a Guide in Post-Storm Decision Making

After the evacuation, after the storm surge, and after the breaching of the levees, our participants' lives would never be the same (see Chap. 13, this volume). As the floodwaters receded, the devastation of Katrina and Rita left two things, destruction and *decisions*. One participant explained that in the almost overwhelming aftermath of Katrina and Rita:

> **224** (51-year old female): *[I prayed to God] to just guide me*. What's the best way to handle things? [You know], I find myself never really asking for "things" anymore. [I find myself] just *asking [God] for guidance*….

Another participant similarly reflected:

> **161** (33-year old female): I was definitely praying a lot for *guidance*. And prior to that I've had a pretty strong relationship with God, so I knew, and I …reiterate[d] in my prayers that I understood this [disaster would work out] for my benefit. I will eventually see [God's purpose], but I needed *guidance* [in the meantime].

This participant (161) seems to be referencing and applying a Biblical verse that has surfaced in previous qualitative work on stress and coping (Marks, Nesteruk, Swanson, Garrison, & Davis, 2005). The verse reads:

> And we know that all things work together for good to them that love God, to them who are the called according to his purpose (Romans 8:28, KJV).

In spite of her conviction that the tragedies of the hurricanes would "work out for my benefit" she still "needed guidance"—guidance that was reportedly sought and found through prayer.

Another participant sought guidance, "steering," and "the right direction" through prayer:

211 (55-year old female): I think my religion and spiritual beliefs have always been with me, not just [during] Katrina and Rita.... And I think if you pray hard enough, *He'll steer you in the right direction.* He'll tell you what you have to do. [You have to] know where your strength is.

A third example of prayer as a source of guidance and decision making explained:

122 (69-year old female). *I prayed a lot for guidance and [for help in] making decisions,* and once *decisions* were made, [I prayed for help in] accepting them and just trying to lead a good life in the situation that I am placed in now. [I also tried] being of service to others because I think that..."Love God, love your neighbor," [those are the two great commandments].

For this participant, prayer was a resilience resource, not only in making decisions but also in accepting those decisions without unproductive second-guessing. Also note that for her, one of the steps in moving forward and "trying to lead a good life" was a concerted effort to "be of service to others." We have identified this effort in previous work and this giving of "service to others" is arguably a religious practice in its own right (Silva, Marks, & Cherry, 2009). In this narrative and others like it, prayer seems to provide the initial impetus that promotes "guidance," "making decisions," and "accepting" those decisions so that successful adaptation and a productive life can recommence. For participants like those whose voices we just heard, prayer was not "*the* solution," but it was an important catalyst that seemed to transform belief into facilitative action as they bounced back from Katrina's life-changing impact.

In the following narrative, we see a participant reference two religious practices that provided direction, consistent with the Theme 5 focus of "praying for guidance." Importantly, this participant's insights also seem to take us full circle as he, like the participants mentioned in theme 1, references a close, personal sense of relationship with a God who "speaks," guides, and "drew me closer." He recalled:

227 (54-year old male): Even though we went through Hurricane Katrina and Rita, *it drew me closer to the Lord.* I believe that [when you have a] prayer life, where you have an intimate *relationship,* where you pray, [then] you *spend time with the Lord.* [When you have that type of relationship], not only do you pray, but you listen [for His direction] and you read the Bible because the Bible is God's word. And I believe that the scripture's full of knowledge and not only is it full of knowledge, but it's actually God speaking to us [and guiding us].

This concluding example is rich—not because the participant tells us that prayer and faith were helpful, but because he explains the *processes* involved in almost clinical, step-by-step detail that seem to comprise the following pattern:

1. The storms hit, but the person had a previously established, close relationship with God (i.e., an active "prayer life") that yielded comfort.
2. (Even after the storms) the person continued to "spend time with the Lord" in (relational) prayer.
3. As part of this pattern of relational prayer, the person "listen[ed]" for God's direction.
4. The person read the Bible as a resource for receiving God's voice and direction.

5. God "speaks and guides."

As a result of these processes, the participant's sense of relationship was reportedly deepened: "Even though we went through Hurricane Katrina and Rita, *it drew me closer to the Lord.*"

We have endeavored to convey the participants' voices with fidelity—without muting their messages on the one hand or erring on the side of hyperbole on the other. While very few participants reportedly experienced a dramatic rise or fall from religious faith, a majority of our participants did tell us that they leaned on their religious beliefs or religious practices (or both) at some time during their Katrina and Rita coping experiences. The deeper point, however, is not that most "leaned on" their faith—but that many claimed to have experienced peace, comfort, direction, and guidance when they "leaned."

Conclusion

The richness of the participants' interviews and the recurring themes that emerged from them invite at least a few important points of discussion. We now revisit the themes and offer some additions, extensions, and counterpoints.

Based on our team-based analyses, the first three themes focusing on spiritual beliefs included: (a) "I couldn't have done it without my God's help" (Theme 1), (b) "God is in Control" (Theme 2), and (c) "The Katrina experience renewed your faith" (Theme 3).[2] Even so, a small minority of our participants explicitly wondered during their interviews how a loving God who cares about his children could allow such suffering and tragedy (see also Chap. 19, this volume). In our previous work, based on interviews conducted shortly after Katrina and Rita, we also found that a few participants openly wrestled with meaning making (Marks et al., 2009). One participant in our earlier study summarized:

> I heard somebody say that because New Orleans was a sin city, God cause[d] it (Katrina). I don't believe God causes things. I don't believe He causes cancer in children. I don't believe He causes these [hurricanes]. For one thing, Bourbon Street [in the heart of the French Quarter] was not really damaged and some churches *were* damaged. So, I mean I [don't think] that God would save…the "bad people" and ruin the churches. I mean God didn't have anything to do with it (Marks et al., 2009, p. 208).

[2] Although we presented data to support and illustrate each of these three themes, the discerning reader will note that (taken collectively) these beliefs represent but do not resolve the problem philosophers refer to as *theodicy* or "The Problem of Pain" (Lewis, 1940/2009). To outline this dilemma via our first three themes, if God is deeply concerned with helping humans on a personal level (Theme 1), and if God is truly "in control" (Theme 2), then why did God not prevent the hurricanes—or at least prevent the storms from wreaking cataclysmic damage? Although Theme 3 ("The Katrina experience renewed your faith") emerged from the data, this theme will (in light of the theodicy problem) be a *non sequitur* for some readers.

In our team-based qualitative analysis approach, we look for major, recurring, and well-documented themes. Even so, sometimes more subtle and less frequently referenced issues provide a colorful contextual backdrop that brings the foreground into sharper clarity. It is noteworthy that these participants' efforts to explain God "into" or "out of" the Katrina and Rita disasters were spontaneous—we did not ask any directly related questions. Apparently, however, meaning-making efforts were fundamental enough for a few that they continued to wrestle with these issues at least 5 years after the storm.

Given the chaos, looting, bedlam, and failure of systems in "The Storm after the Storm" documented elsewhere (Chap. 13, this volume; see also Cherry, Allen, & Galea, 2010), the collection of beliefs and themes from our participants extolling God's care and "control" in the face of historic carnage will strike some readers as oddly incongruent at best and hopelessly naïve at worst—perhaps calling to mind variations on Voltaire's definition from *Candide:* "[Optimism is] a mania for insisting that everything is all right when everything is going wrong" (1759/1959, Blair trans., p. 73). Conversely, other readers may instead perceive a flame of authentic faith in many of these participants that could not be extinguished, not even by tragic back-to-back hurricanes, as exemplified by this participant who told us how she got through the Katrina tragedy:

> **228** (52-year old female): [How did I cope?] Through my faith. If it were not strong-based and [if I did not have] a strong sense of humor, there is no way that…we could have gotten over all the hurdles, obstacles and stuff. You know, I just, I have a flame of faith that my Grandmother passed along [to me]. She tended to the church, and she went to Mass everyday until she died and so did my Father. Everyday, everyday, until he got to where he couldn't, and so that strong flame of faith was just passed along….

Let us now turn from the featured spiritual beliefs to some discussion of the central religious practice that emerged in the data, *prayer*. In previous work, we have raised the concern that "certain forms of prayer that abdicate personal action may lead *away* from [healthy] objectives and toward a type of passive fatalism" (Marks, 2008, p. 682). The data from the current project provided little to no support for this position. The two major recurring reports from our participants were that: "Praying helped me cope" and that "I prayed a lot for guidance." These themes seem to capture *motivations* for and *benefits* of prayer (e.g., assurance, peace, strength, and the need of comfort and guidance in post-storm decision making).

The efficacy of prayer as both a coping resource in the immediate aftermath and as guide in making post-Katrina/Rita decisions is especially vital to note. Pauline Boss (1999, 2002), a leading researcher on the topics of stress, coping, trauma, and ambiguous loss (see Chap. 15, this volume) has indicated that trauma and loss seem to have a freezing effect on some individuals and families—to the degree that some persons stall and fail to progress and make essential decisions. Several participants in our study specifically discussed prayer as a core source of "guidance" that helped them to move through the grief and loss, enabling them to make vital decisions, thereby avoiding the trap of posttraumatic freezing.

For some in our sample, prayer seemed to be important, but not necessarily central. By comparison, prayer (as a coping resource) seemed to be most potent and dynamic for those who spoke about God in personal and relational ways. It was this collection of deeply faithful participants who identified various expressions of prayer, explained why prayer was helpful to them, and even outlined the processes involved in their own active "prayer life." From these persons who were most centered on their faith and "prayer life," we learned that it was possible to emerge from tragedy with faith not only intact but also strengthened. Again, in the words of this gentleman (227), "Even though we went through Hurricane Katrina and Rita, *it drew me closer to the Lord*." The deeper understanding provided by these faithful hurricane survivors called to mind the words of perhaps the greatest of American psychologists, William James:

> We may learn most about a thing when we view it…in its most exaggerated form. This is as true of religious phenomena as of any other kind of fact. The only cases likely to be profitable enough to repay our attention will therefore be cases where the religious spirit is unmistakable…. Its fainter manifestations may tranquilly pass by (James 1902/1997, p. 48).

As we consider what our participants conveyed and taught us about the influence of their spiritual beliefs and religious practices, their shared experiences and insights, and their coping with both the immediate and long-term aftermath of two catastrophic hurricanes, we are convinced that these real-life cases have been "profitable enough to repay our attention." Perhaps the most profitable and profound finding is that the participants who reportedly received the deepest measure of support from their spiritual beliefs and religious practices were those who tended to speak of God in the closest and most personal terms. These men and women conceptualized and discussed God in ways that captured and reflected not only a belief but also a being, not only religion but also a relationship, and not only faith but also a friend.

Acknowledgments We are grateful to Sr. Mary Keefe and Fr. John Arnone of Our Lady of Lourdes Catholic Church in Violet, LA, and Gayle Buckley, Judy Chiappetta, and Catherine Serpas for their assistance with recruitment. We thank Susan McNeil of the St. Bernard Council on Aging and Sean Warner of the Gulf Coast Trust Bank in Chalmette, LA, for providing space for interviews. We thank Susan Brigman, Kelli Broome, Ashley Cacamo, Pamela Forest Nezat, and Mary Beth Tamor for their assistance with data collection. We also thank Emily Allen, Savannah Ballard, Timothy Benedetto, Trevor Johnson, Keri Kytola, and Bethany Pinkston for their assistance with data coding and qualitative analyses. This research was supported by grants from the Louisiana Board of Regents and the LSU Office of Research and Economic Development. This support is gratefully acknowledged.

References

Abu-Raiya, H., Pargament, K. I., & Mahoney, A. (2010). Examining coping methods with stressful interpersonal events experienced by Muslims living in the United States following the 9/11 attacks. *Psychology of Religion and Spirituality, 3,* 1–14.

Aten, J. D., Moore, M., Denney, R. M., Bayne, T., Stagg, A., Owens, S., et al. (2008). God images following hurricane Katrina in South Mississippi: An exploratory study. *Journal of Psychology and Theology, 36,* 249–257.

Boss, P. (1999). *Ambiguous loss: Learning to live with unresolved grief.* Cambridge: Harvard University Press.
Boss, P. (2002). *Family stress management.* Thousand Oaks: Sage.
Cherry, K. E. (Ed.) (2009). *Lifespan perspectives on natural disasters: Coping with Katrina, Rita and other storms.* New York: Springer.
Cherry, K. E., & Galea, S. (2015). Resilience after trauma. In D. Ajdukovic, S. Kimhi & M. Lahad (Eds.), *Resiliency: Enhancing coping with crisis and terrorism* (pp. 35–40). NATO Science for Peace and Security Series. The Netherlands: IOS Press.
Cherry, K. E., Galea, S., & Silva, J. L. (2008). Successful aging and natural disasters: Role of adaptation and resiliency in late life. In M. Hersen & A. M. Gross (Eds.), *Handbook of clinical psychology* (Vol. 1, pp 810–833). NJ: Wiley.
Cherry, K. E., Allen, P. D., & Galea, S. (2010). Older adults and natural disasters: Lessons learned from hurricanes Katrina and Rita. In P. Dass-Brailsford (Ed.), *Crisis and disaster counseling: Lessons learned from hurricane Katrina and other disasters* (pp. 115–130). Thousand Oaks: Sage.
Cherry, K. E., Sampson, L., Nezat, P. F., Cacamo, A., Marks, L. D., & Galea, S. (2015). Long-term psychological outcomes in older adults after disaster: Relationships to religiosity and social support. *Aging & Mental Health, 19*(5), 430–443.
Covey, S. (2004). *The 7 habits of highly effective people.* New York: Free Press.
Denzin, N. K., & Lincoln, Y. S. (Eds.) (1994). *Handbook of qualitative research.* Thousand Oaks: Sage.
Dollahite, D. C. (1998). Fathering, faith, and spirituality. *The Journal of Men's Studies, 7,* 3–16.
Dollahite, D. C., Marks, L. D., & Goodman, M. (2004). Religiosity and families. In M. J. Coleman & L. H. Ganong (Eds.), *The handbook of contemporary families: Considering the past, contemplating the future.* Thousand Oaks: Sage.
Hertel, B. R., & Donahue, M. J. (1995). Parental influences on God images among children. *The Journal for the Scientific Study of Religion, 34,* 186–199.
James, W. (1902/1997). *The varieties of religious experience.* New York: Touchstone.
Janega, J. (2005, Sep 11). In some lost towns, Katrina went beyond destruction: Yscloskey, others wiped out entirely. *Chicago Tribune.* Retrieved from http://articles.chicagotribune.com/2005-09-11/news/0509110479_1_towns-parish-president-oil. Accessed 1 Oct 2014.
Josselson, R., & Lieblich, A. (1993). *The narrative study of lives.* Newbury Park: Sage.
Kessler, R. C., Galea, S., Gruber, M. J., Sampson, N. A., Petukhova, M., & Wang, P. S. (2009). Hurricane Katrina. In Y. Neria, S. Galea, & F. H. Norris (Eds.), *Mental health and disasters* (pp. 419–440). New York: Cambridge University Press.
Koenig, H. G. (1998). *Handbook of religion and mental health.* San Diego: Academic.
Koenig, H. G., McCullough, M. E., & Larson, D. B. (Eds.). (2001). *Handbook of religion and health.* New York: Oxford University Press.
Lambert, N. M., Fincham, F. D., Marks, L. D., & Stillman, T. F. (2010). Invocations and intoxication. *Psychology of Addictive Behaviors, 24,* 209–219.
Lewis, C. S. (1940/2009). *The problem of pain.* New York: HarperOne.
Mahoney, A. (2010). Religion in families, 1999–2009: A relational spiritual framework. *Journal of Marriage and Family, 72,* 805–827.
Marks, L. D. (2008). Prayer and marital intervention: Asking for divine help…or professional trouble? *Journal of Social and Clinical Psychology, 27,* 678–685.
Marks, L. D., & Dollahite, D. M. (2011). Mining the meanings from psychology of religion's correlation mountain. *Journal of Psychology of Religion and Spirituality, 3,* 181–193.
Marks, L. D., Nesteruk, O., Swanson, M., Garrison, M. E. B., & Davis, T. (2005). Religion and health among African Americans. *Research on Aging, 27,* 447–474.
Marks, L. D., Cherry, K. E., & Silva, J. L. (2009). Faith, crisis, coping and meaning making after Katrina. In K. E. Cherry (Ed.), *Lifespan perspectives on natural disasters: Coping with Katrina, Rita and other storms* (pp. 195–215). New York: Springer.
Paloutzian, R. F., & Park, C. L. (2005). *Handbook of the psychology of religion and spirituality.* New York: Guilford.

Pargament, K. I. (1997). *The psychology of religion and coping*. New York: Guilford.
Pargament, K. I., Smith, B., Koenig, H., & Perez, L. (1998a). Patterns of positive and negative religious coping with major life stressors. *Journal for the Scientific Study of Religion, 37,* 711–725.
Pargament, K. I., Zinnbauer, B. J., Scott, A. B., Butter, E. M., Zerowin, J., & Stanik, P. (1998b). Red flags and religious coping: Identifying some religious warning signs among people in crisis. *Journal of Clinical Psychology, 54,* 77–89.
Silva, J. L., Marks, L. D., & Cherry, K. E. (2009). The psychology behind helping and prosocial behaviors: An examination from intention to action. In K. E. Cherry (Ed.), *Lifespan perspectives on natural disasters: Coping with Katrina, Rita and other storms* (pp. 219–240). New York: Springer.
Strauss, A., & Corbin, J. (1998). *Basics of qualitative research: Grounded theory procedures and techniques*. Newbury Park: Sage.
Tausch, C., Marks, L. D., Silve Brown, J., Cherry, K. E., Frias, T., McWilliams, Z., et al. (2011). Religion and coping in the aftermath of hurricanes Katrina and Rita: Qualitative themes from the Louisiana healthy aging study. *Journal of Religion, Spirituality, and Aging, 23,* 236–253.
Vergote, A. (1980). Religion after the critique of psychoanalysis. *The Annual Review of the Social Sciences of Religion, 4,* 1–29.
Voltaire. (1759/1959). *Candide* (L. Blair translation). New York: Bantam.

Chapter 21
Seeing Silver Linings After Catastrophic Loss: Personal Growth, Positive Adaption, and Relationships that Matter

Trevan G. Hatch, Katie E. Cherry, Yaxin Lu and Loren D. Marks

> *I don't believe God does bad things to people. I think he may allow things to happen in your life and then give you things for you to make your own choices, where you go with it, and how do you learn from it? And...even though Katrina's been several years, we're still learning, we're still processing the losses and the blessings.*
> (308; 52-year-old female)

Introduction

In 2005, Hurricanes Katrina and Rita brought catastrophic destruction to the US Gulf Coast. Nearly 2,000 people died, and hundreds of thousands were displaced as a result of what has been described as the worst natural disaster in US history (see Chaps. 12 and 13, this volume). There is a sizeable literature on the psychosocial and mental health consequences of Hurricane Katrina (Chan & Rhodes, 2013; Cherry, 2009; Galea, Tracy, Norris, & Coffey, 2008). In this chapter, we focus on a counterintuitive topic, namely, the reported benefits and blessings that some people perceive after disaster. Drawing on verbatim quotes from participants at least 5 years after sustaining catastrophic losses associated with the 2005 storms, the

T. G. Hatch (✉)
School of Social Work, Louisiana State University, 335 Long Fieldhouse,
Baton Rouge, LA 70803-5501, USA
e-mail: thatch8@lsu.edu

L. D. Marks
e-mail: loren_marks@byu.edu

K. E. Cherry
Department of Psychology, Louisiana State University, 236 Audubon Hall,
Baton Rouge, LA 70803-5501, USA
e-mail: pskatie@lsu.edu

Y. Lu
Louisiana Department of Education, 1201 North Third Street,
Baton Rouge, LA 70802, USA
e-mail: Yaxinlu3@gmail.com

K. E. Cherry (ed.), *Traumatic Stress and Long-Term Recovery*,
DOI 10.1007/978-3-319-18866-9_21

concept of silver linings is revealed. In the paragraphs that follow, an overview of the silver lining concept and a theoretical model from the literature on family stress are given to contextualize our findings.

A Brief Overview and Explanation of "Silver Linings"

The dictum, *every cloud has a silver lining,* refers to "some basis for hope or comfort in the midst of despair" (Webster, 1996, p. 577). Several qualitative researchers have found that reports of *silver linings* frequently surface in connection with challenges and temporal and/or existential crises including immigration, loss of employment, the death of a loved one, and parenting a child with special needs (Dollahite, Marks, & Olson, 1998; Dollahite et al. 2002; Marks, Swanson, Nesteruk, & Hopkins-Williams, 2006; Nesteruk, Marks, & Garrison, 2009). In addition to qualitative research, a meta-analytic review of 87 cross-sectional studies between 1985 and 2005 (Helgeson, Reynolds, & Tomich, 2006) revealed the following about posttraumatic reports of silver linings—also referred to in the literature as "benefit finding," "posttraumatic growth," or "stress-related growth":

a. Benefit finding was related to better mental health outcomes (i.e., "depression" and "positive well-being"), but also related to more intrusive and avoidant thoughts about the stressor.
b. Benefit finding was more strongly related to less depression and greater positive affect when the time since the traumatic event was more than 2 years, and it was related to greater global distress only when the time since the traumatic event was 2 years or less.
c. Women and non-White individuals engaged in benefit finding more than did men and White individuals, respectively (Helgeson et al., 2006).

Helgeson and colleagues' findings are consistent with Tamres, Janicki, and Helgeson's (2002) previous meta-analytic review, where these authors found that women engage in more benefit-finding and optimistic self-talk than do men following traumatic events. Age and gender, among other sociodemographic variables, are widely recognized as important to coping behaviors which in turn may affect psychological outcomes. Further discussion is beyond the scope of the present chapter, so interested readers are referred to other scholarly reviews (for disaster, see Bonnano, Brewin, Kaniasty, & La Greca, 2010; for stress and coping; see Carver & Connor-Smith, 2010; Folkman & Moscowitz, 2004; for benefit finding, Tennen & Affleck, 1999, 2002).

In the years following World War II, family sociologist, Reuben Hill propounded the seminal empirical and theoretical work capturing the range of outcomes that can result from stressors and crises. In particular, Hill (1949, 1958) developed an ABC-X model of family stress which remains useful in assessment and family studies today (Boss, 2002; Ingoldsby, Smith, & Miller, 2004). Figure 21.1 presents a graphic version of Hill's (1958) ABC-X conceptual model, adapted from prior

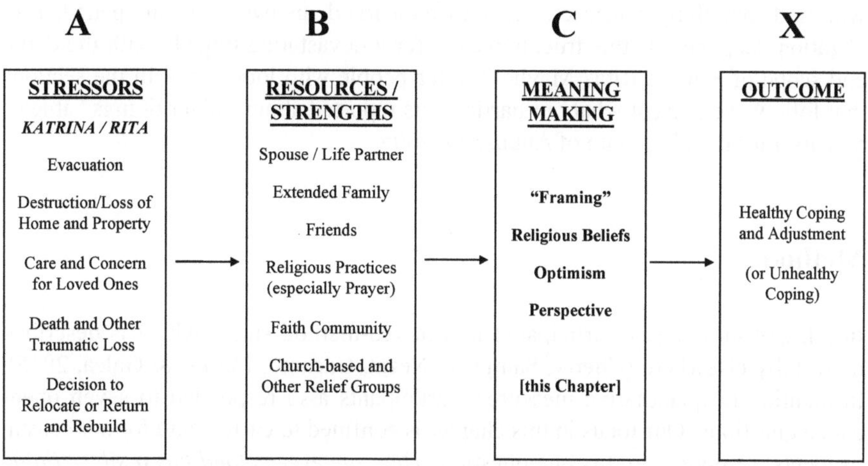

Fig. 21.1 Model for understanding post-disaster family stress adapted from prior work (Marks et al., 2012) based on Hill's ABC-X Model (1958). ***A*** Several of these stressors are discussed in Chaps. 12 and 13 (this volume). ***B*** Several resources/strengths are discussed in Chaps. 14 and 20 (this volume). ***C*** This chapter ("On Seeing Silver Linings after Disaster"). ***X*** Processes and outcomes (see Part 3, this volume)

work (cf. Marks, Hopkins, Nesteruk, Chaney, & Baumgartner, 2012) to portray the present study sample and their collective experience of living through Hurricanes Katrina and Rita (see Chaps. 12 and 13, this volume). Several key "A" factors *(stressors)* for our sample are listed in the model (see Chaps. 12 and 13, this volume); along with several key "B" factors *(strengths/resources)* that are addressed in Chaps. 14 and 20. This chapter centers on "C," the *meaning making* implied as hurricane survivors in our sample coped (and continue to cope) with the Katrina/Rita experience. By identifying silver linings from Hurricanes Katrina and Rita, our participants engaged in meaning making, which helps individuals cope with stressful or traumatic events by highlighting positive aspects of life (e.g., family relationships and personal growth; see Chap. 15, this volume, for related discussion).

Hill's ideas, as we have adapted them in Fig. 21.1, have been further developed by several scholars over the years with a wide range of applications (see Lavee, McCubbin, & Patterson, 1985). One of these scholars—Pauline Boss, a leading researcher and clinician of psychological stress, crisis, and trauma (see Chap. 15, this volume)—has observed that the Chinese character representing stress/crisis also means *opportunity* (Boss, 2002). Similarly, "a crisis, according to the psychological theorist, Erik Erikson, is not a disaster but a choice point…an opportunity for growth" (Marks, Cherry, & Silva, 2009). From these theoretical viewpoints, profound challenges can potentially yield benefits for at least some of those involved. This statement should not be overextended or misinterpreted to mean that disasters and crises are "positive" in a net sense (e.g., that more good than bad ultimately emerges). It means that in the wake of challenge, trauma, and crisis there are some who find something constructive…a lesson learned, an awareness sharpened, a realization deepened. Is this true, however, for a devastating tragedy with the depth and scope of Katrina/Rita? Maybe it is for people who look for it. In the sections that follow, we present what our participants reported about "silver linings" at least 5 years after the nightmare of August 29, 2005.

Method

In all, 219 individuals participated in a mixed-method study, which is described more fully elsewhere (Cherry, Sampson, Nezat, Cacamo, Marks, & Galea, 2015). In addition to quantitative measures, participants also responded to seven open-ended questions. Our focus in this chapter is confined to current and former coastal residents' responses to this one question: *They say every cloud has a silver lining and even the most awful events can have positive outcomes. Do you think there are any positive outcomes that can come from Hurricanes Katrina and Rita? If so, what are they?*

Data were coded using the same team-based qualitative analysis techniques described at length in Chap. 12 (this volume). Using this methodology, three central, emergent themes related to "silver linings" were identified and documented. These themes are presented in the next section. We also provide illustrative (verbatim) excerpts and narratives from former and current residents (see Chaps. 12 and 13, this volume) and where relevant, supplementary quotes from commercial fishers (also current coastal residents) from this research program are provided (see Chaps. 4 and 18, this volume).

Findings

Participants' responses to the silver linings question yielded several insights regarding the processes involved in coping with disasters. Although many lost friends, employment, and their personal possessions (Cherry et al., 2015), most participants *did* identify positive outcomes of Hurricanes Katrina and Rita. Our multiple-team content analysis yielded the following themes from the silver linings question:

Theme 1: Personal Growth and Change in Perspective
Theme 2: Appreciation for a New Positive Social Environment
Theme 3: Relationships with Friends and Family are What Matter Most

These three themes are presented and discussed in turn next.

Theme 1: Personal Growth and Change in Perspective

In Theme 1, we present excerpts from individuals who mentioned "silver linings" related to individual development. This theme is divided into two subthemes: (1) A Change in Attitude: "[Katrina] helped me to become a better person;" and (2) Material Possessions Do Not Ultimately Matter: "I don't need all of that anymore."

Subtheme 1: A Change in Attitude: "[Katrina] helped me to become a better person"

The interview question relating to positive outcomes of the storms elicited responses of an introspective nature from several participants like the following:

> **132** (22-year old male): I felt…before the storm, I was…a pretty selfish person. Everything was there that I needed. You know, it was…everything was convenient. I have or had everything that I ever wanted and needed, you know? Without a question. And I didn't really think much beyond myself. But then Katrina happens and your life is turned upside down. And, all of a sudden, I've got to make sacrifices that I wasn't used to making. And, *that really helped me to become a better person*, a more giving person. I feel as though I've become a lot more selfless and understanding from Katrina.

Participant 132 recognized that a life-altering event, like a severe natural disaster, can be a catalyst for personal growth and humility. He specifically mentioned that being forced to sacrifice in the wake of the storms helped him to become "a more giving person" and also "more selfless and understanding." By having many of their personal possessions and their previous way of life snatched away, many of our participants were motivated or even compelled to combine resources and serve other people in an unprecedented way.

Other participants reported that they felt immense gratitude for life and family after the storms. Participant 125, for example, was grateful just for being alive as she was aware of several people who died in the community:

> **125** (20-year old female): The majority of how you deal with stuff is attitude. You know, my mother is one of those who she'll say about all the stuff she lost. She lost her clothes, but it's like, *but you're alive*. You have people who didn't make it out, [like the people] at that nursing home [where] thirty-something people died…. So, when you look back…our family was all together, our family was all alive. To me, it's just,…[there] was much more positive [that] came out of it.

> **352** (53-year old female): "So you know, as far as you know the positive outcomes of this, every day is a positive outcome. That God allows me to wakeup. That's as positive as it gets. I woke up on the right side of the dirt."

Becoming a better person—a more selfless and grateful person—includes recognizing what ultimately matters most in life. This process of self-evaluation for several of our participants included the identification of the "more important" things that will occupy their minds, focus, and emotional energy as they continue forward. For several participants, a change in perspective meant that material goods do not matter as much as personal serenity or warm and close relationships. Notice that participant 125 was not only happy to be alive but she also recognized that the "stuff" that her mother lost meant nothing compared to family and physical safety. A similar idea is expounded in the next subtheme to which we now turn.

Subtheme 2: Material Possessions Do Not Ultimately Matter: "I don't need all of that anymore"

Several participants seemed to experience a shift away from materialism in the wake of the storms, as articulated by the following excerpts:

> **313** (47-year old male): …as long as it is not a human life and it is material things, they can be replaced, and they are not really worth what you think they are anyway.

> **151** (62-year old female): We just don't worry about things and all anymore. When I say "things," what I mean is possessions. That's not—it's not a big deal to us anymore. We like the things that we have that we've bought in place of the things that we lost, but none of it takes up a whole lot of time with us anymore as far as, "Oh we need to get this. Oh, we need to get that." Now, we kind of let go of the materialism. It's very humbling. It's very humbling. It's—you just think to yourself. I have got to the point where I realize I had too much anyway, as far as material things. I had way too much. *I don't need all of that anymore*. What I want is peace of mind. I want—just peace.

Even though participant 151, for example, replaced many of her material possessions after the storm, her family is reportedly no longer investing much emotional energy on acquiring and displaying them; instead, they sought "peace of mind." Many participants similarly acknowledged, like the woman just quoted (151), that they "had too much anyway as far as material things" and did not "need all of that anymore." It is important to note, however, that this perspective may be related to the 5 years that had passed since Katrina and Rita. This tempered and reflective state of mind may not have been evident in the immediate aftermath. To illustrate, consider participant 137 who recalled the following observations among people in her neighborhood immediately after the storms:

> **137** (71-year old female): It's surely interesting. This was a clinical observation of mine. When we first came back and we would talk to people about their problems, about what you lost, it was all *loss:* "I lost this. I lost that." The ladies that lost the pictures like of their babies and of their weddings, they were off the wall. They were nuts. And I'm thinking… [all this fuss over] a piece of paper? I mean, I don't know…a picture only makes you recall a memory; [but] the memories are [still] there.

Based on some reports, like the previous quote, as well as our own observations of changes in participants across time, shifts in perspective are not typically immediate and may require months or even years.

Participant 203, although having lost much (like all of our participants) reflected that for her, "The silver lining is realizing how important your relationships are in your life, not your new sofa" (52-year-old female). Another woman (124) provides an additional and final example of a change in perspective regarding material possessions:

124 (69-year old female): Things are tangible. Home…it's a tangible thing. It's not…it's a touchable thing, but it's not the most important thing. Things are not important. I look back, I can see my grandmother's little lavatory that was so beautiful that was [broken] in pieces. And I looked at my children's grandmother's rocker that was beautiful, and it's…all that's gone. So we can't put so much of our minds and bodies and souls into these material things. It…that's not where it's at. It's in…people and most of all it's in the knowing that God is there. That is, to me, the most important part, that He's in control. [Whatever] things that have occurred, whether I like them or not…He's going to make it work. He's going to make things okay. And as I said, I have seen beauty [rise] from the ashes. And that's it. I don't think I can advise people on how to cope with all this. Just got to keep on trucking. That's it.

Like many other participants, this woman (124) emphasized that "things are not important," and also recognized that investing "so much of our minds and bodies and souls into these material things" is pointless. The shift away from material possessions to relationships, including a relationship with God, is another major theme discussed by the participants (see Chap. 20, this volume). Notice that 124 believed that "knowing that God is there" is more important than knowing that your material possessions are there. We now shift our focus from the "personal growth" and antimaterialist foci of Theme 1 to a "silver linings" discussion of positive new environments in Theme 2.

Theme 2: Appreciation for a New, Positive Social Environment

In addition to a new perspective on life and a rejection of materialism as a means to happiness and increased feelings of self-worth, several individuals we interviewed expressed deep appreciation for their new (post-evacuation) neighbors and new social environment. Some mentioned that, in some ways, the hurricanes seemed to have an elevating effect on their neighborhoods in that only those who were most committed to St. Bernard as a *community* seemed to be willing to invest the time, effort, money, and risk required to rebuild the devastated area. In other words, the people who moved back into the area to rebuild were *happy* to be there, even at high personal cost. For many of these, their local community was reportedly like an extended family. One participant (254) described the new social ambiance of his neighborhood after he returned, which was reminiscent of the 1960s when many people seemed happier to him:

254 (59-year old male): The people that live here are better people. The only people that you see in Chalmette [now] are the people that want to be here. So, every neighbor you talk to is glad to see you. Just, it's almost like it was in the '60s when we moved here. You know, semi-rural and everybody's…just happy to be here. The one third of the population that said, "You know what? I don't think real estate is disposable stuff, and I'm going to rebuild my house and my life where I used to live." That one third that you see on the street are just happier, easier to get along with. You know, it's just a better environment. When I see the kids in religion class [at church], it's like night and day. Before the storm, we had a lot of behavior problems…kids that just, you know, come from obviously poor parental environments. [Things have improved].

From a different perspective, another participant (153) did *not* want to return to New Orleans and was unhappy with the area. Despite considering her family to be among the "founding fathers" of the area, she was grateful that the storms gave them a ticket out of the old neighborhood. She explained that from her vantage:

> **153** (52-year old female)**:** I think there's positive outcomes. We moved to Baton Rouge which has a much better attitude on life.... It's positive. It's a happy place. I found St. Bernard to be sort of depressing in that it was oppressed. You know it was the Lower Ninth Ward and then sort of brought bad feelings. You're down at the bottom of New Orleans and like you said, no one knew anything about us. [The public] still doesn't know.
> We were a family, a foundation, a family that came from St. Bernard, you know. The founding fathers of it. But it too was starting to change in that different people were just coming in. And I'm not saying Black, White, or anything, just different...it wasn't the old neighborhood, you know. ...You hear about the killings on the street. And you ride over there and you can see the blood, on the street. One time that happened to me.
> Yes, and then you also had the bridge problem. You had...the railroad problems...It just... It didn't seem like it wanted to grow. [But in] Baton Rouge...you've got lovely homes, lovely places. Ninety percent of the people here are educated, even if it's just high school, it's a good education.

For many participants, resettling in another community was their silver lining. Participant 153 expressed her gratitude to be out of her original and (from her perspective) declining area. For her, living in a community where "ninety percent" of the population was "educated" and where everyone seemed "happy" was new and refreshing.

To summarize briefly, in the present theme two narratives from two different participants present us with two different variations of neighborhood and environment-related "silver linings." The "return and rebuild" group (represented by participant 254) appreciated his perceived reality that only those who were most attached to and invested in his beloved Chalmette community returned to start again from scratch—and that this selection effect seemed to have an elevating influence on the quality of life in his local community and faith community. By contrast, for participant 152, the silver lining of the Katrina/Rita thundercloud was a fresh start in a new city and environment that better fit her ideals of the good life. These two perspectives exemplify the reports of other participants and remind us that a strength of qualitative reports can be the opportunity to not only receive a participant's report but also hear the explanations and rationale behind the response. Both 152 and 254 are reportedly pleased with their post-Katrina environments but for different reasons and in different locations. We now turn from the silver lining of improved environment to a focus on close personal relationships in our final theme.

Theme 3: Relationships with Friends and Family are What Matter Most

Theme 3 is divided into two subthemes. The first concerns close friendships and the second concerns family relationships.

Subtheme 1: The Formation of Lasting Friendships: "I have met some new, wonderful people…"

Although personal growth, change in perspective, and appreciation for a more positive social environment were all recurring themes among those we interviewed, participants collectively identified *relationships* as the most salient silver lining of the hurricane aftermath. Notably, relationships with family and friends were emphasized even more than God and religious faith. Numerous participants did discuss their reliance on God and/or their religious faith in subsequent questions (see Chaps. 14 and 20, this volume); however, the silver lining question seemed to foster an emphasis on social, relational, and practical (positive) outcomes of the storms, like the importance of close friendships and family ties. Several participants, for instance, talked in glowing terms about the friends they had made after the storms as they mingled with new neighbors and volunteers. Participants 157 and 203 offered the following examples that illustrate this relationship-centered theme:

> **157** (44-year old female)**:** Oh man. One of the things that I enjoyed about it was getting to meet so many different people. You know, the amount of people, the volunteers that came in, the different groups we gave disaster tours to. Heck, I wouldn't have met *you* [*referring to the interviewer herself*]. I mean…just moving into a new neighborhood, having to make new friends, new friends at school, there's just so many people that I would have never gotten to meet if it hadn't happened.
>
> **203** (52-year old female): One of the things that's been the best thing that's happened to me through this whole course of Katrina is [that] I have met some new, wonderful people that I would never have been able to meet prior to Katrina…I've met one of my closest friends now, [and] would never have had the opportunity because she did something else before the storm and now our jobs have intermingled because she had to switch jobs…. I would have never…become friends with her or her husband and their kids…and it's turned out to be a wonderful friendship….
> We had a lot of people come into St. Bernard Parish, teachers, counselors, that were willing to go back to work, and they have just been splendid to work with. I've become friends with some of them and have a wonderful working relationship with most of them…. So what's been created down here as far as friendships and…working relationships…has been absolutely incredible. So that's been a big silver lining for me. My original set of friends, I'm still friends with. They don't live here anymore, but life has gone on and I still see them, but there's been an opportunity to go ahead and…meet new people, and have them become a wonderful part of life… for me.

While some participants, like 157, seemed to emphasize meeting "new friends" in a general sense, participant 203 also spoke passionately about specific friends she had made after the storms and seemed to place paramount value on a relationship with one particular new friend and her family. She implied that her new friendship was more than just nice or even "wonderful"—she identified it as foundational in her post-Katrina adjustment and coping. She identified this particular friendship as "one of the best things that's happened" to her in the wake of Katrina. Another participant similarly explained to us that a new friendship was the "only positive outcome" of the storms. This new friendship developed after participant 141 was hired as a nanny following Katrina. She reflected:

141 (55-year old female): The only positive outcome I can see is this little girl, right here, I take care of because…it seems like she just been a blessing. She doesn't know it because she's a child, a baby, but I just feel like God put her there for me for a reason; to help me get over, or try to get over, [Katrina]. And I started when she was three months and now she, next month, she will be four years old. So I will, in June, [have been] with them for four years. She really helped me cope. Like days when I was feeling bogged down or whatever and I'd come here and she'd just run up to me and want me to hug her or just kiss me on the cheek. She's a very, very affectionate child. [She's got me through].

The bond between this participant (141) and the small child in her care was powerful enough to be framed by her as a great "blessing." Indeed, she believed that God had intervened by placing the child in her life to help her cope. Narratives like this illustrate the major role that deep bonds of new friendship played in the coping process after the storms for some participants. In the next subtheme, we turn from the bonds of friendship to familial relationships.

Subtheme 2: The Fundamental Importance of Family Relationships: "My son…became more family-oriented"

As much as new friendships were viewed as a silver lining, the most pronounced and most frequently identified "silver lining" was a heightened awareness and deeper appreciation of the fundamental importance of family relationships. Many participants described at length how members of their families supported each other by splitting up tasks, combining resources, or serving one another in various ways. Special efforts were occasionally reported in behalf of those who seemed least able to cope—and persons who were clearly not faring as well as the rest.

Some participants explained that their familial relationships were strengthened by the storms, as illustrated by the following comment:

334 (58-year old female): [The hurricane] brought people together. It made you realize just how close your family is, and how much they mean to you. It brought a lot of families together." […] "It did… I'll never stay for another hurricane, because my family's more important to me than anything. I can always buy a new house or new sofa…

Another participant offered a more specific example of the storm's role in strengthening family relationships. Participant 229 had become distant from his brothers in the years preceding the storms; however, after the storms hit the relationships reportedly changed. He said:

229 (56-year old man): This tragedy [of Katrina/Rita] was shared among you and your friends and your family. It kind of brought you all closer together…. You kind of depend on each other, you reached out to each other more. Family you ain't talked to for a while, you realize how much they really love you when something like this happens, I think. Like all my brothers, they all thought I was dead, and then they all cried.

Participant 142 lost his house and job, yet he identified that as a silver lining because he was able to relocate. The relocation meant that he could move in with and care for his terminally ill father during the last year of his life. In his own words, he tells us:

142 (59-year old man): So [after Katrina] I was going to have to work someplace else, I knew that. And my first prospect was in Jefferson. So that would be a nice commute each day I'd be making. Then my father became sick. So if Katrina never would have happened, I'd be working in Jefferson Parish, my father would've got ill, and I could have only possibly seen him on weekends. [However, with] Katrina happening, ex-ing out where I worked, and my chance of working, and then putting all of us together, [that] was a silver lining.... Katrina gave me a possibility of being with [Dad] for his last year on Earth. Being with him every day, doing different things that I wouldn't have done, because he would've been in his house [and I would have been somewhere else].

As previously highlighted in Theme 1, devastating and traumatic events like a severe hurricane apparently present opportunities that enrich the lives of some and invite others to assess what matters most and to change for the better. We found that many participants reportedly became more compassionate and selfless; others became more grateful for what they had. As discussed previously, many participants felt that their attitudes changed regarding materialism—and some even reported shifts in overall perspective on life. The final example we will share again demonstrates that not only do people have the capacity to change for the better and become more responsible individuals and citizens, but that traumatic events have the potential to help heal families and bring people together:

262 (67-year old female): My son used to stay out nights at a time...drinking. Well, after Katrina, he became more family-oriented. Very family oriented. So, that was an absolute positive...and he tells me all the time..."Momma, if Katrina wasn't for anybody else, it was for me." .... Even though he still has the anger issues.... [Now], he is involved with his son and his family and they do things together now and it never used to be like that.

Without seeking to minimize the related horrors of Hurricanes Katrina and Rita, it is apparent that there were perceived benefits and silver linings for many of the participants who weathered these storms and coped with the long-term, psychological, and emotional storm surge that took years to relent. Even so, there were at least some, like the son just mentioned, who felt, "If Katrina wasn't for anybody else, it was for me." Can anything good come out of a hurricane? Many of our participants give us reason to hope that the answer can be yes...and in some cases, a profound yes.

Conclusion

As the years passed and life returned to a new version of "normal" (with the old "normal" gone forever; see Chap. 12, this volume)—many participants had progressed from a wrestle for survival to a point where they could reflect on the Hurricane Katrina/Rita experience with new perspective. Accordingly, when we began our project of interviewing individuals with long-term resilience and recovery in mind, we decided to include an open-ended question on optimistic appraisals of the storms. We sought to determine if our participants could identify "silver linings" (i.e., benefits and blessings) in the wake of Katrina and Rita, and if so, what these benefits were or how they were explained.

From Theme 1, we learned that many of our participants acknowledged that the traumatic experience was a catalyst for personal growth. Participants specifically mentioned that they enjoyed a new attitude on life, and many remarked that the situation forced them to sacrifice more of themselves and to become more aware of the needs of others. Many of our participants served in their communities by volunteering at food stations and handing out water. Others expressed their increased gratitude for life and family. In addition to describing a more altruistic and optimistic attitude, many participants articulated a fresh perspective on materialism. They reportedly shifted away from investing a lot of time and energy acquiring and maintaining "things" towards a different emphasis of developing and enjoying more meaningful (and less tangible) aspects of life, like spirituality, improved relationships, peace of mind, and a clear conscience.

Theme 2, "Appreciation for a New Positive Social Environment," revealed that many of our participants were deeply appreciative of their new environment, whether they returned to their coastal neighborhood to rebuild or relocated elsewhere permanently. Some commented that they were glad to escape their former communities and resettle in different communities with greater opportunities for entertainment and educational advancement. Comparatively, others expressed gratitude that they were lucky enough to return with many of their lifelong friends to rebuild the old neighborhood together.

Theme 3 was arguably the most salient silver lining among our participants, which concerned the importance of relationships. Many participants described a heightened awareness of the importance of family and friends in the immediate aftermath of the storm. The reality that their personal relationships are what mattered most to them was intensified and clarified. Data from our interviews, regarding the nurturing of relationships with friends and family, are congruous with findings of Dolińska (2008), who compared data gathered 9 months after the 1997 flood in Poland and 3 years later (conceptual replication). Her analysis of benefit finding after severe flooding revealed that participants who were directly affected and those who were threatened but did not lose homes and property in the flood reported various positive outcomes and frequently emphasized improved interpersonal relationships more often than did the non-affected comparison groups.

Participants in our study mentioned, more than anything else, that the formation of lasting friendships (e.g., new neighbors and volunteers) and the nurturing of family relationships are what matter most to them. Many participants commented that while the storms scattered their friends, neighbors, and fellow church parishioners all over the USA, the storms also brought new people into their social circles, many of whom have become close friends. Most of our participants articulated that familial relationships were strengthened by the storms because each member of the family had to sacrifice for everyone else. Some reported that every family member had a role to play after the storms. Older children, for example, assisted with the care of their younger siblings so that the parents could deal with the Federal Emergency Management Agency (FEMA) and insurance companies. Some worked tirelessly on "gutting" the flooded house while others resolved concerns with food, clothes, and school arrangements. The necessity of sacrifice and of combining resources to survive in the immediate aftermath of the storms strengthened relationships in ways that were vividly remembered at least 5 years after the storms. The potential role of natural disasters in unifying communities and families, even for several years afterword, is congruous with Dolińska (2008), underscoring the need for and importance of further research on this topic.

In conclusion, a growing body of research has examined post-disaster threats to individual and familial well-being during the immediate impact period (Cherry, 2009). Other studies have examined the phenomenon of benefit finding after traumatic events (Helgeson et al., 2006). Fewer studies, however, have addressed long-term (5 or more years) disaster resilience and recovery, especially in relation to benefit finding—and in-depth qualitative studies are almost nonexistent. The present research adds to the small but growing literature on long-term recovery after exposure to a natural disaster. Our findings suggest that traumatic, life-changing experiences like a natural disaster, may elicit not only the worst (e.g., looting and predatory behaviors, see Chaps. 13 and 18, this volume) but such disasters may also call forth the best from many individuals and families involved, as illustrated by the comments and reflections of our participants.

Acknowledgments We are grateful to Sr. Mary Keefe and Fr. John Arnone of Our Lady of Lourdes Catholic Church in Violet, LA for their assistance with recruitment. We thank Susan McNeil and Janet Hood of the St. Bernard Council on Aging and Sean Warner of the Gulf Coast Trust Bank in St. Bernard for their assistance and providing space for testing. We thank Susan Brigman, Kelli Broome, Ashley Cacamo, Pamela F. Nezat, and Mary Beth Tamor for assistance with data collection and Dina Anbinder, Kayla Holland, Beth Lyon, Kyle Ryker, and for help with data scoring. We thank George Barisich, Gayle Buckley, Judy Chiappetta, and Catherine Serpas for their contribution to the research effort.

This research was supported by grants from the Louisiana Board of Regents and the BP Gulf of Mexico Research Initiative, Office of Research, and Economic Development, Louisiana State University. This support is gratefully acknowledged.

References

Bonnano, G. A., Brewin, C. R., Kaniasty, K., & La Greca, A. M. (2010). Weighing the costs of disaster: Consequences, risks, and resilience in individuals, families, and communities. *Psychological Science in the Public Interest, 11,* 1–49.

Boss, P. (2002). *Family stress management* (2nd ed.). Thousand Oaks: Sage.

Carver, C. S., & Connor-Smith, J. (2010). Personality and coping. *Annual Review of Psychology, 61,* 679–704.

Chan, C. S., & Rhodes, J. E. (2013). Religious coping, posttraumatic stress, psychological distress, and posttraumatic growth among female survivors four years after Hurricane Katrina. *Journal of Traumatic Stress, 26,* 257–265.

Cherry, K. E. (Ed.). (2009). *Lifespan perspectives on natural disasters: Coping with Katrina, Rita and other storms*. New York: Springer.

Cherry, K. E., Sampson, L., Nezat, P. F., Cacamo, A., Marks, L. D., & Galea, S. (2015). Long-term psychological outcomes in older adults after disaster: Relationships to religiosity and social support. *Aging & Mental Health, 19*(5), 430–443.

Dolińska, B. (2008). Positive consequences of the experience of disaster. *Polish Psychological Bulletin, 39*(3), 165–170.

Dollahite, D. C., Marks, L. D., & Olson, M. M. (1998). Faithful fathering in trying times: Religious beliefs and practices of latter-day Saint fathers of children with special needs. *The Journal of Men's Studies, 7,* 71–93.
Dollahite, D. C., Marks, L. D., & Olson, M. M. (2002). Fathering, faith, and family therapy: Generative narrative therapy with religious fathers. *Journal of Family Psychotherapy, 13,* 263–294. [Published simultaneously in T. D. Carlson & M. J. Erickson (Eds.), *Spirituality and family therapy* (pp. 259–290). New York: Haworth.]
Folkman, S., & Moskowitz, J. F. (2004). Coping: Pitsfalls and promise. *Annual Review of Psychology, 55,* 745–774.
Galea, S., Tracy, M., Norris, F., & Coffey, S. E. (2008). Financial and social circumstances and the incidence and course of PTSD in Mississippi during the first two years after Hurricane Katrina. *Journal of Traumatic Stress, 21,* 357–368.
Helgeson, V. S., Reynolds, K. A., & Tomich, P. L. (2006). A meta-analytic review of benefit finding and growth. *Journal of Consulting and Clinical Psychology, 74*(5), 797–816.
Hill, R. (1949). *Families under stress: Adjustment to the crisis of war separation and reunion.* New York: Harper and Brothers.
Hill, R. (1958). Generic features of families under stress. *Social Casework, 49,* 139–150.
Ingoldsby, B., Smith, S., & Miller, J. E. (2004). *Exploring family theories.* New York: Roxbury.
Lavee, Y., McCubbin, H. I., & Patterson, J. M. (1985). The double ABCX model of family stress and adaptation: An empirical test by analysis of structural equations with latent variables. *Journal of Marriage and the Family, 47,* 811–825.
Marks, L. D., Swanson, M., Nesteruk, O., & Hopkins-Williams, K. (2006). Stressors in African American marriages and families: A qualitative study. *Stress, Trauma, and Crisis: An International Journal, 9,* 203–225.
Marks, L. D., Cherry, K. E., & Silva, J. (2009). Faith, crisis, coping, and meaning making after Katrina: A qualitative, cross-cohort examination. In K. Cherry (Ed.), *Lifespan perspectives on natural disasters: Coping with Katrina, Rita and other storms* (pp. 195–215). New York: Springer.
Marks, L. D., Hopkins, K., Nesteruk, O., Chaney, C., & Baumgartner, J. (2012). A qualitative exploration of why faith matters in African-American marriages and families. *Journal of Comparative Family Studies, 43,* 695–714.
Nesteruk, O., Marks, L. D., & Garrison, M. E. (2009). Immigrant parents' concerns regarding their children's education in the U.S. *Family and Consumer Sciences Research Journal, 37,* 422–441.
Tamres, L. K., Janicki, D., & Helgeson, V. S. (2002). Sex differences in coping behavior: A meta-analytic review and an examination of relative coping. *Personality and Social Psychology Bulletin, 6,* 2–30.
Tennen, H., & Affleck, G., (1999). Finding benefits in adversity. In C. R. Snyder (Ed.), *Coping: The psychology of what works.* New York: Oxford University Press.
Tennen, H., & Affleck, G. (2002). Benefit-finding and benefit-reminding. In C. R. Snyder & S. J. Lopez (Eds.), *Handbook of positive psychology* (pp. 279–304). London: Oxford University Press.
Webster. (1996). *Webster's New World Dictionary and Thesaurus.* New York: Wiley.

Chapter 22
On Bereavement and Grief: A Therapeutic Approach to Healing

M. Katherine Shear and Susan Delaney

Introduction

Case Study: An Illustration of Complicated Grief

Mary is a widow who sought treatment 18 months after her husband David's sudden unexpected death of a heart attack. She was referred by her family doctor who was concerned about her physical and emotional health. Mary blamed herself for David's death because though she had been encouraging him to see his doctor and take some exercise, she had left it up to him to make the appointment. After he died, she was full of self-recrimination. Further, she frequently reminded herself about how terrible it was that she had not been present when David died alone in their bedroom. She became reclusive, took time off work, and began smoking again. Mary had started on a course of antidepressants but after nearly 6 months showed little improvement.

When Mary presented for treatment, her therapist administered a screening questionnaire, the 19-item Inventory of Complicated Grief (ICG) and Mary's total score of 56 out of a possible 76 was well above the threshold of 30 considered a positive screen for complicated grief (CG). She also completed the Grief-Related Avoidance Questionnaire (GRAQ) and endorsed a total score of 33, a moderately high level of avoidance. She completed the Typical Beliefs Questionnaire (TBQ) that rates problematic grief-related thoughts and beliefs that again indicated symptoms with a total of 56, also a high score.

M. K. Shear (✉)
School of Social Work, Columbia University, 1255 Amsterdam Avenue,
New York, NY 10027, USA
e-mail: ks2394@columbia.edu

S. Delaney
Irish Hospice Foundation, 32 Nassau St.,
Dublin 2, Ireland
e-mail: susan.delaney@hospicefoundation.ie

K. E. Cherry (ed.), *Traumatic Stress and Long-Term Recovery*,
DOI 10.1007/978-3-319-18866-9_22

Mary arrived at her first clinic appointment in a somewhat disheveled state, and she cried copiously during the session. She described a rewarding and very loving relationship with David and their two daughters and stated that life held no interest for her now that he was gone. She hoped to die soon, but would not hurt their daughters by taking her own life. The therapist confirmed that Mary was experiencing prolonged acute grief with strong feelings of yearning, longing, and sadness as well as anxiety about a future without David. She had frequent insistent thoughts of him that were both deeply sorrowful and also warm and comforting. She still could not believe he had died in this way. In addition, Mary showed evidence of grief complications, including ruminative counterfactual thoughts (e.g., “If only I had insisted on his going to the doctor his heart condition would have been diagnosed and he would still be alive”), catastrophic misinterpretation of a future without him (e.g., “My life is over if David is not here.” “If I am not very careful I will forget him.”), and extensive avoidance of reminders of the loss. She could not understand how other family members were “getting on with things.” She was annoyed at people who seemed to be suggesting that she was not trying hard enough, yet she also felt they might somehow be right. Since his death, Mary had not slept in the bedroom she shared with David. She was unable to look at photos of her husband and would not discuss him with their daughters other than to tell them that her heart was broken. She was not attending to self-regulation as evidenced by low levels of self-compassion; by returning to smoking; and by paying little attention to getting good nourishment, enough sleep, adequate exercise, or engaging in pleasurable activities. After completing the rest of her standard assessment, the therapist diagnosed Mary with CG.

The therapist asked Mary to begin using a daily diary to record her grief levels. During the first week, her levels were consistently very high, 9 and 10 on a scale of 0–10. However, during week 2 Mary recorded an 8 and said she was noticing that while her grief was really hard “it was not terrible all of the time.” In the second session, the therapist asked Mary to try to imagine that her grief was at a manageable level and to think about what she would want for herself if that happened. Surprisingly, given her catastrophic thinking about the future, it took little prodding for Mary to explain that she had a wish to complete her education. She also said she had long wanted to take a trip to Italy. She agreed to begin getting information on both aspirational goals, although she said it was unlikely that she would be able to do either without David’s help.

The therapist urged Mary to invite someone to the third session. Initially, she was quite reluctant to do so, but finally agreed to bring her sister, Pauline. As frequently happens in these sessions, Pauline validated the report that Mary and David had enjoyed a very loving and enviable relationship. She also explained that she loved her sister very much, and she was so sad that David had passed in this way, but she felt stymied in trying to support Mary as her calls mostly went unanswered. Pauline said she would help in any way—in fact, it would be a great relief to her if there was anything at all she could do to relieve her sister’s pain. The therapist explained the syndrome of CG and briefly described the planned treatment procedures and their rationale. Pauline offered to be available to meet Mary for coffee after her appointments or to phone her after Mary listened to the recording of the story of the death that she would make as a part of the treatment. Mary was moved by her sister's offers of support and said she appreciated this very much. She added tearfully that she was not very good at asking for help, but she was very lonely without David.

The fourth session began a sequence of the treatment in which Mary was asked to revisit the story of the death. She found it very difficult to comply when she was asked to close her eyes and imagine herself back at the time when she learned that David had died. However, she completed the exercise as best she could. The story she told was audiotaped, and she took the tape home with a plan to listen daily. However, when the therapist phoned as planned, she said she had not been able to listen to the tape as she feared her grief would be out of control. With gentle encouragement, she tried again and gradually began to engage with the story of receiving a phone call from her daughter who had gone over to the house and found her father. Mary's grief was hard to witness, and she struggled with the "shoulda, woulda, couldas". The revisiting sequence continued for 5 weeks; Mary managed to listen to the tape four or five times per week. Her willingness to engage and reflect on the story slowly led to the realization that she was not responsible for David's death. As she put it, "Sure if his heart was going to give out it made no difference if I was there or not—his time was up." She was sad that she was not with him and that he was alone when he died, but, on reflection, she came to realize that this, too, was likely not as devastating as she had been imagining. She said she was confident that he knew how much she loved him, and that he might not have even realized that he was dying and if that was so, he would not have missed her. Moreover, even if he had been aware, he would have known that she would have been by his side in the blink of an eye had she known he needed her. These thoughts gave her considerable relief. She began to think that it was up to her to live a full rich life for them both.

The therapist also asked her to begin revisiting things that she was avoiding. They first worked to develop a hierarchy of such situations and then began planning how she could start to go places and do things she was avoiding. This would help her continue to process the loss and allow her to move around more freely in the world. A goal of the planned revisiting exercises was to feel more comfortable being in the bedroom she shared with David. This was very challenging for her to even consider at first, and she admitted sheepishly that a "mad part of me believes he isn't really dead if I don't go in." However, after thinking about this for a number of weeks while revisiting less challenging situations she was also avoiding, she made the decision around week 10 to move back into the bedroom. She told the therapist "I know he's not there but I feel close to him in here and I remember the happy times we had cuddling up at night."

Mary and the therapist began working with memories. Mary brought photos of David to the sessions and looked at them for the first time since he died. She said they still made her very sad, but it also felt really good to be able to see him and remember the good times they had together. She shared memories of David with considerable pleasure, struggling to find something negative. She finally settled on his annoying habit of folding the newspaper the wrong way around and reading her out snippets when she preferred to read them herself. She commented that while she found those things irritating at the time, she missed them now. She also noted that he was stubborn and quickly became irritated if he perceived she was nagging. When she talked about this she suddenly remembered that she had, in fact, nagged him about going to the doctor, and he got annoyed with her so she stopped. The final exercise was the imaginal conversation. The therapist invited Mary to imagine that she was with David right after he died, and that even though he truly was gone, she should imagine that she could talk, and he could listen and respond. The therapist suggested that Mary could say anything or ask anything she wished. This was a poignant, bittersweet experience for Mary. She apologized for not being there when he died and beautifully answered for David with: "Mary, my love, you were always there for me." She said she wished she had made him go to the doctor and allowed herself to hear him reply: "Now Mary, who could ever make me do something I didn't want to?".

After completing the 16-session program, Mary had returned to sleeping in her own bedroom, had given up smoking, and had joined a choir, something she was interested in but never pursued because David did not care for singing. She had gone on a short trip to Italy with her daughters and enjoyed it ("but not as much as I would have with David"). She had collected all the documentation for returning to school but did not yet feel ready to apply to a program. Mary thought about what had been most helpful in opening the way for these positive changes. She said the imaginal revisiting ("I never thought I would be able to think about his dying without going crazy") and the conversation with David where he had imaginally acknowledged that she had been there for him throughout their marriage, and he was too stubborn to go to the doctor. She still missed him and reckoned she always would, but was now engaging in life again, accepting some social invitations and enjoying time with her newest grandson, who had been named after David and was stubborn just like him. At the last session, she produced a note that someone had written saying: "you can grieve that he is gone or rejoice that he was" and declared that was what she was going to try to do from now on. Mary continues to miss her husband, but her grief is back on track to find its rightful place in her life. She can remember and think about him with warmth and pleasure, though always with a tinge of sorrow. Her memories contain her love and with it her yearning and sorrow. She has come to understand that grief is the form love takes when someone we love dies.

Mary's story illustrates the syndrome of CG, a condition that is gradually becoming better recognized and for which targeted treatments have now been devised. The remainder of this chapter describes the syndrome of CG and an innovative efficacy-tested treatment called complicated grief treatment (CGT). We outline the principles and procedures used to develop this treatment and briefly describe building blocks upon which it rests.

The Syndrome of CG

The term CG is used to describe a syndrome consisting of acute grief symptoms that persist beyond the time frame that is considered adaptive or culturally appropriate in the bereaved person's social network accompanied by complicating thoughts, feelings, and behaviors. Acute grief is the result of a destabilized attachment system (acute attachment insecurity) in which the attachment behavioral system is activated while caregiving and exploratory systems are inhibited. The configuration and course of grief is different for each person and each loss. Nevertheless, we can still identify generic symptoms of acute grief based on the instinctive response to attachment loss.

Typical symptoms of bereavement-induced acute attachment insecurity include separation distress with intense yearning, longing or searching, preoccupation with thoughts and memories of the lost person that frequently include hallucinatory experiences, pronounced feelings of emotional loneliness, feelings of emptiness and anxiety about a future without that person, feelings of mistrust and detachment from others, and feelings of anger at being abandoned. Caregiver inhibition in the setting of loss is often associated with a sense of caregiver failure. Feelings of guilt or remorse are common, and there is sometimes shame. Self-blaming thoughts may accompany feelings of caregiver ineffectiveness. Exploratory system inhibition in adults produces feelings of incompetence and disinterest in learning and performing in the world. By definition, bereavement entails confrontation with death which may trigger a trauma response with feelings of shock and disbelief and a sense of confusion and disorientation.

Acute grief is variable with respect to the specific symptoms it entails and the time course over which it is transformed and integrated. However, for most people, acute grief does not last indefinitely. Like physical wound healing that takes differing amounts of time and has varying residual impairment based upon the nature of the wound, the health of the person who suffers that wound, and the availability of support and care, healing after loss is variable in its course based on similar considerations. Wound healing can be complicated by an infection or a compromised immune or cardiovascular system. Healing after loss can be complicated by thoughts, feelings, or behaviors that derail the natural process of adaptation. People we love are deeply interwoven in our lives. Essentially, they become a part of us, and when they die, we must make many adjustments in order to adapt to their loss. These adjustments can be generally grouped as loss-related and restoration-related. For most of our lives, we inhabit the present feeling connected to the past and ready for the future. We move through time bringing supplies from the past and inventing our future in ways that seem so natural that we do not notice that we are doing this. Bereavement disrupts this reassuring sense of continuity making the past seem lost and invention of the future challenging or even impossible. It is as though an earthquake has struck, and we are suddenly stranded on a path with the way back blocked and the way forward across a seemingly impassable chasm. The adaptation process requires us to reclaim supply lines from the past and find a way to bridge the chasm so we can move forward.

In order to reconnect to the past, we first need to learn what the finality and consequences of the death means to us. We must reconfigure our internalized relationship with the person who died and reenvision our lives going forward in a way that has purpose and meaning and possibilities for joy and satisfaction. We need to live in a world without the deceased person, observing and reflecting upon what that is like. We need to begin to imagine ways we can feel enthusiastic about the future. Adapting to bereavement is fundamentally a learning process that takes place in a setting of intense emotional activation and takes place best when emotions are adequately regulated. Adaptation can get derailed. Rumination and/or avoidance can complicate grief and hinder the learning process. So too can an inability to regulate intensely painful emotions.

When complications derail the progress of grief, the result is a repetitive loop where feelings of intense yearning, longing, and sorrow persist along with frequent insistent thoughts of the deceased often accompanied by frustration of endless pain; bitterness about the loss, anger, or disappointment with oneself, with others, or with the unfairness of the world; or a belief that it is wrong to now enjoy life. Concurrently, the bereaved person eschews a myriad of reminders that the person is gone. They may stay away from the final resting place, shun activities once shared with the deceased, refrain from disposing of possessions, or avoid countless other reminders. Counterfactual rumination and avoidance prevent the bereaved person from coming to terms with the finality and consequences of the loss. Instead of finding a way to integrate the painful information, they remain caught in a cycle in which the death seems to have been wrong, unfair, or even preventable. The mental representation of the deceased is not revised, and life goals are not reviewed or redefined.

The number of people who develop CG ranges from an overall population estimate of 2.4–4.8 to 10–20% for spousal bereavement (Prigerson, 2004) to even higher rates for loss of a child (Meert et al 2011). Neimeyer and Burke (2013) points out that in considering risk of CG, clinicians need to "consider both fixed and relatively enduring characteristics of the survivor and shifting or circumstantial factors that bear on his/her ability to adapt to the death of a loved one." Their review of prospective risk factors for developing CG include background factors (close kinship, female gender, insecure attachment style), death-related factors (bereavement overload, violent death, low acceptance of pending death), and treatment-related factors (caregiver burden, aggressive medical intervention, family conflict regarding treatment). It is important to remember in any risk assessment that the presence of risk factors does not always predict CG, and the absence of risk factors does not preclude the development of CG. CG can be identified using a standardized tool such as the ICG (Prigerson et al., 1995) along with a detailed clinical interview (Shear, 2015).

A systematic review of the literature on CG (Kristjanson, Lobb, Aoun, & Monterosso, 2006) further suggests that a small percentage of the population experience complications in their grief, and that these individuals appear to be at greatest risk for adverse health effects. CG is a syndrome that causes distress and impairment for a minority of people bereaved of a significant person in their life. People with CG have prolonged, impairing grief symptoms that affect both mental and physical health, including increased risk of suicide. Researchers in CG have over the past 20 years been developing tools for diagnosing and treating this condition. Our work entails developing and testing a treatment approach underpinned by rigorous research that integrates current knowledge on trauma processing with current models of emotion regulation, coping, and self-determination needs. CGT has been studied in two National Institute of Mental Health (NIMH)-funded randomized controlled trials and found to be significantly (Shear, Frank, Houck, & Reynolds, 2005; Shear et al., 2014) better than interpersonal psychotherapy (IPT) at relieving symptoms of CG. As a result, this work equips practitioners with innovative ways to help clients resolve grief complications, reconfigure their relationship to the deceased loved one, and find bridges to a new normal and a future with possibilities for joy and satisfaction.

Typical Grief

The experience of grief is universal, and the majority of bereaved people find their own path through the grief process using a combination of their own intrinsic adaptive capacity and the help of a supportive network. Human beings are hardwired to adapt to threatening events and have a natural adaptive process that is triggered by the loss. Bowlby (1980) defined mourning as the set of psychological processes set in motion by the loss and described successful mourning as acknowledging the finality of the loss and its consequences, revision of the internal representation of the deceased person, and redefinition of life goals. In early or acute grief, most people will experience periods of intense distress with yearning, sadness, anxiety, and preoccupation with thoughts and memories of the person who died. These acute reactions usually subside over time as natural resilience is activated; painful feelings lessen and interest and engagement in daily life is rekindled. As grief decreases in intensity and recedes into the background, it no longer dominates the emotional landscape and no longer interferes with the day-to-day functioning of the bereaved person. Acute grief is transformed and integrated (Shear, 2010).

Death is a part of all life and loss is virtually universal. Yet acute grief is one of life's most dreaded experiences, and perhaps with good reason. Can grief kill you? Can you actually die from a broken heart? An article by Anna Hodgekiss published in the *Daily Mail* in November 2013 entitled; "You really CAN die of a broken heart" drew comments such as (Hodgekiss, 2013):

> I had an aunt who collapsed and died in her garden on the first anniversary of my uncle's death. She really couldn't live without him and the doctor said it was a broken heart that killed her." And; "My stepfather died late Friday evening, my mother also in the same hospital on the Saturday saying that she had nothing left to live for and died that day.

Ms. Hodgekiss was referencing a study by Mostofsky et al. (2012) in Harvard which reported an increased risk of heart attack within the first week after the loss of a significant person and a 66 % higher risk of dying in the 3 months after a partner's death. The authors specifically acknowledged that psychological stress such as that caused by intense grief can increase heart rate, blood pressure, and blood clotting and Mostofsky, lead researcher, noted that neglecting to take medications, poor sleep, loss of appetite, and higher cortisol levels can all increase the risk of heart attack. Commentators on the article also pointed to the possibility that the cardiac event might have been something called stress cardiomyopathy. Regardless of the exact mechanism, what is clear is that bereavement can be a severe stressor, and that acute grief is associated with physiological changes that increase the risk for negative health outcomes. Additionally, the media "hook" of unbearable grief easily resonates with the public. This raises the question of why is it that losing a loved one creates such havoc in our lives?

The answer to why acute grief is so intensely painful lies in understanding what it is that our loved ones provide. It is because of what they do for us that their loss rocks our world so profoundly. It is useful to define what we mean by a loved one and, in our work, we use the definition employed by attachment researchers. An attachment figure is someone who is rewarding to be with; who we do not want to be separated from; and who is a person we turn to when we are upset, threatened, or stressed. This person provides support that is often instrumental as well as emotional. Our attachment figures also serve as a secure base from which we explore the world and function autonomously. They encourage us to take risks, express confidence in our abilities, and share in happiness for our successes. Losing someone who provides these functions is difficult enough. But there is more. It turns out that people we love influence our lives in a range of ways that are out of our awareness, and that loss affects our caregiving and exploratory motivational systems as well as attachment.

Theoretical Underpinnings of CGT

Attachment theory, first developed by Bowlby in the 1950s, underpins the current understanding of the impact of the disruption of affectional bonds. The theory emphasizes the critical role that close relationships play in our lives and posits that motivation is inborn to seek, form, maintain, and respond to the loss of these relationships (see Chap. 7, for related discussion). Rupturing of a security-enhancing attachment bond provokes a reaction of separation distress with symptoms that typically emerge following the death of a significant person. According to Bowlby (1980), the attachment system has important implications for personality and interpersonal behavior. The system is activated by perceived physical and psychological threat, including the threat of meaningful separation from a loved one. Activation of the attachment behavioral system causes the threatened individual to seek proximity to protective others who provide a safe haven. The attainment of proximity and protection results in feelings of relief and security as well as positive mental representations of relationship partners and the self. Bowlby (1988) viewed the optimal functioning of this behavioral system as important for the maintenance of emotional stability and mental health, the development of a positive self-image, and the formation of positive attitudes toward close relationships. Attachment theory posits individuals come into the world equipped with interrelated behavioral systems including:

Attachment: the propensity to form strong emotional bonds with particular individuals to whom we seek proximity when distressed and who serve as a secure base for exploration. *Exploration:* the desire to engage the world to work, play, discover, and create. *Caregiving:* motivation to provide a relationship partner's attachment and exploration needs.

John Bowlby (1980) posited that individuals thrive when they have attachment figures that enable them both to seek comfort when needed and to explore the world in a confident way. Researchers have begun to identify brain circuitry that might be involved in the attachment system. For example, Bartels and Zeki (2004) used functional MRI (fMRI) to explore areas of the brain activated when mothers viewed pictures of their infants and compared it to individuals experiencing romantic love. Both types of attachment activated regions specific to each type of relationship, as well as overlapping regions in the brain's reward system that coincide with areas rich in oxytocin and vasopressin receptors. They suggested that human attachment employs a push–pull mechanism that overcomes social distance by deactivating networks used for critical social assessment and negative emotions, while it bonds individuals through the involvement of the reward circuitry. However, as James Coan, another researcher interested in attachment has noted (Coan 2008), the entire brain is a social brain and so far it has not been possible to find specific circuitry associated with attachment functioning.

Nevertheless, we make the assumption that such brain circuitry exists and entails implicit and explicit memory, positive and negative emotion centers, and cognitive centers for self-monitoring, attention, appraisal, goal setting, and planning. These brain mechanisms work to enable attachment relationships that are rewarding; provide a foundation of security, support, and shared competence; and play a central role in emotional and physiological regulatory processes. With bereavement, these functions are temporarily disabled and adaptation requires that the brain's internalized representations of the deceased person be updated to reflect the reality of the death. We hypothesize that failure to do so is one consequence of CG.

Our minds naturally resist accepting finality of loss, creating a sense of ambivalence about conceding the reality of a death. Thankfully, most of the time, bereavement sets in motion an adaptive process by which information about the death is gradually acknowledged and incorporated into our internal representations of the deceased, and our relationship with them and goal orientation are correspondingly amended to foster the potential for renewal of rewarding activities and relationships. CGT aims to address the complicating factors in grief and to facilitate and reinvigorate the interrupted instinctive healing process. This is accomplished using a highly structured treatment approach that uses seven core procedural modules administered in a way that is personalized to the individual client.

CGT is also informed by some aspects of the dual process model (DPM) of coping with bereavement (Stroebe & Schut, 1999). This model organizes the stresses entailed in bereavement as loss or restoration orientated. The loss orientation is defined as the processing of the grief experience and attending to what has been lost, and the restoration orientation focuses on coping with the various stressors entailed in living without the deceased loved one. Both kinds of coping are challenging but are thought to be required for grief resolution. The DPM posits a dynamic coping process in which there is oscillation between loss-related and restoration-related coping. They consider this similar to Bowlby's idea that oscillation promotes adaptive coping through alternating confrontation and avoidance ("defensive exclusion") of emotional pain. CGT incorporates the idea that a bereaved person needs to address both loss- and restoration-related issues but differs from DPM in positing that emotional pain exists in both arenas as does the potential for positive emotions. Oscillation toward and away from emotional pain is seen as one of several emotion regulation strategies that are supported by the therapist. CGT incorporates a focus on both loss and restoration in each of the 16 treatment sessions.

Most bereaved people have some ambivalence about accepting the reality of the loss, and people with CG often feel ambivalent about the evolution of grief because they believe that the intensity of their grief is a sign of the intensity of their love. To address ambivalence, CGT incorporates aspects of motivational interviewing (MI). MI techniques can be used to encourage a client to think differently about her behavior and to consider what can be changed and the possibility of envisioning a brighter future. MI contributes to the collaborative aspect of the work and to an acknowledgement that change is difficult, and an inspiration of hope (Miller & Rollnick, 2002)

CGT also draws on three other bodies of theoretical work, one entailing study of self-determination needs, another on the role of self-compassion as a response to suffering (Neff, 2011; Gilbert, 2009), and a third related to the adaptive unconscious (Gilbert, Pinel, Wilson, Blumberg, & Wheatley, 1998). CGT posits that bereavement undermines the ability to fulfill basic human needs of autonomy, competence, and relatedness (Deci & Ryan, 2000) and seeks to help clients find new ways to meet these needs. CGT also encourages clients to practice kindness to themselves rather than self-criticism in the face of their continued suffering and to remember that suffering and acting imperfectly are one of the most important universalities of human life. Suffering often makes us feel estranged from others, and we encourage our clients to see it instead as connecting us to others. We further encourage clients to practice mindfulness when confronting painful emotions. CGT is based on the principle that there is a natural adaptive process that can help us make needed adjustments to loss. This process operates out of awareness, in the implicit system and is especially strongly activated when we face a threat to our psychological well-being that is severe and out of our control.

CG Principles and Procedures

CGT is a short-term approach that contains seven core content modules: psychoeducation, self-regulation, rebuilding connection, aspirational goals, revisiting the story of the death, revisiting the world, and memories past and future. The treatment is usually administered in four phases (getting started, core revisiting sequence, midcourse review and closing sequence) comprising a total of 16 sessions.

Throughout the treatment, the therapist encourages oscillation between confronting pain and setting it aside, mirroring the process described by Bowlby (1980).

Each session entails some work on loss (past focus) and some on restoration (future focus), following the idea put forward by Stroebe and Schut (1999) that loss and restoration are best addressed in tandem. Throughout the treatment, the therapist works to facilitate the three main processes of acknowledging the death and its consequences, revising the mental representation of the deceased, and redefining life goals.

The introductory sessions (getting started) focus on information gathering, introducing the treatment, and alliance building. Grief symptoms and maladaptive behaviors are assessed via clinical interview and the administration of several monitoring instruments which are repeated throughout the treatment. This allows both practitioner and patient to note where changes have occurred and where additional focus needs to be brought. Psychoeducation is provided regarding the model of CG, and an overview of the rationale and procedures of the treatment is presented. The idea that grief is a form of love and is not pathological is discussed with its important implication that a successful outcome of treatment is that grief can now find its rightful place in the life of the client. We expect that emotional activation will recede, and its quality will be predominantly bittersweet as the bereaved person continues to feel connected to the person who died, remembering them in ways that honor their love and their life together. The therapist might use a metaphor of grief such as a train journey and CG as a "what happens if the train is derailed"? Treatment can then be understood as attending to the derailing factors (the "debris on the track") and facilitating a return to the natural adaptive process that results in integrated grief.

Session 1 includes introductions and a brief personal and social history, attending to both prior mental health problems and also to interests and achievements. The therapist takes a history of the relationship with the deceased, the story of the death, and the experience of grief, including who has been in the person's life and the quality of current relationships. At the end of session 1, the therapist introduces the grief-monitoring diary and invites the client to bring someone to the third session. The grief-monitoring diary is a simple tool that is used throughout the treatment. It simply asks the client to pay attention to grief intensity during the day and to take a few minutes at the end of each day to rate on a scale of 1–10 the highest level for that day, the lowest level, and the average level for the whole day. The therapist also makes a brief note about what was happening when the grief was highest and when it was lowest that day (Turret & Shear, 2012). Clients may find this difficult at first, but if they are encouraged to try and to stick with it, the diary becomes a very useful way of following grief intensity and of discussing and working with ways to support the natural oscillation between confronting the pain and setting it aside.

In the second session, the therapist provides information about how grief can be understood using research findings about close relationships. The therapist explains the concept of grief as the form love takes when someone we love dies and outlines and clarifies that grief is not one thing—that it is different for each person, and that it usually evolves over time. The therapist then explains CG and outlines the plan for the remaining sessions. During the last 10 min of session 2, the therapist asks to shift gears to do a different kind of exercise. The therapist says that if she could wave a magic wand and the client's grief was at a comfortable level, what would the client want for himself/herself? This question is aimed at eliciting a long-term aspirational life goal. The exercise is continued during the last 10 min of each session thereafter and included as an assignment between the sessions each week. When an aspirational goal has been identified, clients are asked to think about what they would be doing that would tell them they are on their way to accomplishing the goal, how committed they are to the goal, what might stand in the way of their achieving it, and who could help them achieve it. Then, at each session, a specific activity related to one of these topics is planned for the interval until the next session.

The third session is generally held with a significant other. The therapist invites the client and his/her guest to explain briefly the history of their relationship and what it has been like since the death that the client is grieving. Often the friend or family member is feeling helpless and frustrated. The therapist explains the CGT model of loss, grief, and CG and outlines the treatment procedures, explaining what we do and why. They then discuss whether and how this person might be helpful in some aspect of the program. Most importantly, the therapist helps the client see their friend or family member's love and concern and helps the guest see the client's grief in a different way and instills hope that things can be better for the client.

Sessions 4–9 make up the core revisiting sequence. These sessions contain most of the imaginal revisiting exercises and begin the situational revisiting sequence. Aspirational goals work is continued throughout these sessions during which the therapist and client develop and plan strategies to work toward a major life goal. Imaginal revisiting is an exercise in which the client is asked to close his/her eyes and visualize herself at the time when he/she first learned of the death and tell the story of what happened from that point forward. Similar to the procedure of prolonged exposure for post-traumatic stress disorder (PTSD), the therapist asks for distress level ratings and provides simple encouragement during the story but does not intervene in any other way. The client's story is audio recorded, and she is encouraged to listen to it once each day until the next session. After about 10 min, the client opens her eyes, and the therapist invites him/her to reflect on the experience of telling this story. This is done by simply asking the client what it was like to tell the story and then asking if he or she noticed anything while telling the story. The therapist and client discuss these observations as needed and the client's distress level is tracked. At the end of another 10 min, the client is encouraged to put the story away and think about a rewarding activity he or she might do after the session is concluded. A visualization exercise can be done if there is difficulty setting this story aside. The story is retold in the next session, recorded, and listened to over the ensuing weeks. This procedure is repeated for about three to five sessions.

Situational revisiting is begun in session 5. This exercise focuses on daily life activities that the patient is avoiding. It is helpful to begin with situations that have been pleasurable or satisfying in the past and that have the potential to be so again. The idea is twofold: to foster acknowledgement of the death and emotion processing and to remove restrictions to the person's ongoing life. During both imaginal and situational revisiting, the patient is asked to report levels of distress in "subjective units of distress" (SUDS) rated on a scale of 0–100.

The core revisiting sequence uses a toolbox approach drawing upon strategies and techniques in other efficacious treatments. Among the tools are IPT strategies and techniques including exploratory techniques, both directive and nondirective, encouragement and acceptance of painful as well as positive emotions, and examining and coaching interpersonal interactions. Each session has a similar format, beginning with review of the prior week, moving to an exercise and/or discussion focused on the story of the death and its consequences, to activities and discussion of aspirational goals, and ending with plans for the upcoming week. Session 10 is the midcourse review, devoted to reassessment of symptoms and progress and plans for the remaining six sessions.

Structured memories work and imaginal conversation are used in the closing sequence to reinforce a deep sense of connection to the deceased that the client can draw comfort from beyond the therapeutic sessions as he or she moves forward in life. Following successful completion of two revisiting exercises, the client is given a memories work sheet for each of the next 5 weeks. These guide exploration of positive and negative memories of the deceased. The patient is encouraged to bring in pictures of the deceased. Following successful completion of core revisiting sequence work, the client is invited to have an imaginal conversation with the deceased in which he or she imagines being with the loved one shortly after death. A two-way conversation is facilitated by the therapist, in which the client is invited to say, ask, or clarify anything that feels unfinished and then to take the role of the deceased loved one and respond. The conversation goes back and forth in this manner.

The closing sequence also contains work on treatment termination. The patient is encouraged to talk about his or her feelings about ending the treatment. Treatment gains are reviewed, and plans are made for the future, including plans for difficult times (calendar days that are emotionally activating, e.g., birthdays and other anniversaries or holidays). A decision is made regarding possible need for further treatment, for either grief or other conditions. For CG, the therapist makes a global judgment of improvement. People who are much or very much improved can be discharged without further treatment as follow-up data show maintenance of gains. This improvement is usually associated with a decrease in ICG score below 30 and a clear increase in the client's enthusiasm for a future without the deceased, a sense of reconnection with significant others, and a sense of comfort in moving through the world without deceased loved one.

CGT Outcomes

CGT was evaluated in a pilot study and tested in two prospective randomized controlled trials comparing it to standard grief-focused IPT. In addition, several other groups have now tested similar approaches (Shear, 2015). In our studies (Shear et al., 2005; Shear et al. 2014), participants who received CGT showed significantly better response to treatment than those treated with IPT. Among study completers, 66% of those receiving CGT were rated as either much improved or very much improved, compared with only 32% of those receiving IPT. Correspondingly, reductions on ICG total score was almost twice as great (−20.6 vs. 12.8 in study 1 and −21 vs. −16 in study 2) for the targeted CG treatment compared with standard IPT. Overall, CGT has been tested in samples diverse with respect to age, race, and relationship to the deceased, and there were no significant differences in response based on these variables. Secondary analysis of data from our randomized, controlled study indicated that participants on stable doses of antidepressant medication had significantly greater adherence to CGT than those not on medication (91 vs. 58 %) and marginally better outcome. Medication doubled the response to IPT without affecting treatment adherence.

Learning CGT

The competent delivery of the CGT protocol assumes strong therapeutic skills with an ability to foster hope and develop a therapeutic alliance and a willingness to work in a new way with clients. Therapists need a basic understanding of attachment theory and a knowledge of grief theory. Some therapists find it difficult to move away from a traditional, client-centred, and client-led approach to more structured, focused work. This can challenge our beliefs, our training, and our assumptions about what is efficacious in therapy. Therapists may erroneously believe that CGT does not privilege the therapeutic relationship or may think it does not allow clients time to "tell their story." It is worth remembering that CGT targets a very specific segment of bereaved people. When clients present with CG, they usually have already seen several kind and caring therapists who validated their grief and listened to these stories, but this was not sufficient to get their grief back on track. Validating the pain of grief, while gently avoiding repetition of stories about the deceased, is a delicate task that requires a light and practiced touch. The grief story is of great interest in CGT because it provides the clinician with a hypothesis for why a person's grief has become stuck, locked in place, or derailed, borrowing from the prior train metaphor of CG. The clinician is then tasked with gently structuring exercises and the inquiry that follows them, to allow new perspectives to emerge which challenge the current thoughts, feelings, and behaviours. This demands a deep presence, and an ability to attend to content and process simultaneously on the part of the clinician.

CGT sessions differ from a more traditional therapy session in several ways including use of set focus and structure. Therapists need to review the session outline and prepare the required materials prior to each session. Adherence to time is of greater importance than usual as activating exercises must be accomplished early in the hour to allow time for a shift to self-care, self-compassion, and future orientation before the close of a therapeutic session. In learning the treatment, we encourage taping of the sessions (with the client's permission) and reflecting on what went well and what could be improved, ideally also having the tapes listened to by a more advanced CGT practitioner who can provide constructive feedback. This is a humbling but worthwhile exercise. In doing so, it becomes clear that there is a flow to the protocol, and one exercise naturally leads to the next piece of work. However, one should recognize that initially learning CGT often requires therapists to move out of a familiar comfort zone into a new and possibly anxiety-provoking learning zone.

In all treatments, the clients are our best teachers. Through them, the value of learning to lean into grief becomes clear. Our clients demonstrate the natural healing process at work. Observing the indomitable spirit that can be reawakened affirms this way of working with loss. People with CG have to learn new ways of being in the world, they have to give up on or let go of assumptions they held dear, be willing to try new things, and keep hope alive. Perhaps learning CGT is a little like that. Our ability to stay open and curious to new ways of working can serve us and those who seek our help.

Conclusion

CG is a syndrome that causes distress and impairment for an important minority of people who have lost a close attachment. People with CG have prolonged, impairing grief symptoms that can affect both mental and physical health, including increased risk of suicide. The development of valid, reliable assessment instruments, and a therapeutic intervention tested in rigorously designed and carefully implemented clinical trials represent major advances in the field of grief treatment. While more research in this area is clearly needed, we now have sufficient information to inform clinicians. Unfortunately, the majority of cases of CG currently remain undiagnosed and untreated. Greater awareness of the syndrome, as well as understanding of its underpinnings and principles of effective intervention, is needed. It is our hope that growing awareness of CG within the mental health community will result in increased recognition and treatment. Far from an assumed wisdom that there is no point in life when a loved one dies—these new treatment protocols are helping people to process painful experiences, to find a way to accept an unwanted reality, and to regain their interest in life and experience joy again.

References

Bartels, A., & Zeki, S. (2004). The neural correlates of maternal and romantic love. *Neuroimage, 21*(3), 1155–1166.

Bowlby, J. (1980). *Loss: Sadness and depression (attachment and loss)* (Vol. 3). New York: Basic Books.

Bowlby, J. (1988). *A secure base: Clinical applications of attachment theory*. London: Routledge.

Coan, J. A. (2008). Toward a neuroscience of attachment. In J. Cassidy & P. R. Shaver (Eds.), *Handbook of attachment: Theory, research, and clinical applications* (2nd edn., pp. 241–265). New York: Guilford.

Deci, E. L., & Ryan, R. M. (2000). The "what" and "why" of goal pursuits: Human needs and the self-determination of behavior. *Psychological Inquiry, 11*, 227–268.

Gilbert, D. T., Pinel, E. C., Wilson, T. D., Blumberg, S. J., & Wheatley, T. P. (1998). Immune neglect: A source of durability bias in affective forecasting. *Journal of Personality and Social Psychology, 75*(3), 617–638.

Gilbert, P. (2009). *The compassionate mind: A new approach to life's challenges*. London: Constable & Robinson, Ltd.
Hodgekiss, A. (2013). You really CAN die of a broken heart: Surviving spouses have a 66 % higher risk of dying in the three months after their partner's death. http://www.dailymail.co.uk/health/article-2507829/You-really-CAN-die-broken-heart-Surviving-spouses-66-higher-risk-dying-months-partners-death.html#ixzz2uuTqeKNI. Accessed 27 Jan 2015.
Kristjanson, L., Lobb, E., Aoun, S., & Monterosso, L. (2006). A systematic review of the literature on complicated grief. *Department of health and ageing, Australian Government*.
Meert, K. L., Shear, K., Newth, C. J., et al. (2011). Follow-up study of complicated grief among parents eighteen months after a child's death in the pediatric intensive care unit. *Journal of Palliative Medicine, 14,* 207–214.
Miller W., & Rollnick, S. (2002). *Motivational interviewing*. New York: Guilford.
Mostofsky, E., Maclure, M., Sherwood, J. B., Tofler, G. H., Muller, J. E., & Mittleman, M. A. (2012). Risk of acute myocardial infarction after the death of a significant person in one's life: The determinants of myocardial infarction onset study. *Circulation, 125*(3), 491–496.
Neff, K. D. (2011). *Self-compassion: The proven power of being kind to yourself*. New York: William.
Neimeyer, R. A., & Burke, L. A. (2013). Complicated grief and the end-of-life: Risk factors and treatment considerations. In J. L. Werth (Ed.), *Counseling clients near the end-of-life* (pp. 205–224). New York: Springer.
Prigerson, H. (2004). Complicated grief. *Bereavement Care, 23*(3), 38–40.
Prigerson, H. G., Maciejewski, P. K., Reynolds III, C. F., Bierhals, A. J., Newsom, J. T., Fasiczka, A., et al. (1995). Inventory of complicated grief: A scale to measure maladaptive symptoms of loss. *Psychiatry Research, 59*(1), 65–79.
Shear, K., Frank, E., Houck, P. R., & Reynolds, C. F. (2005). Treatment of complicated grief: a randomized controlled trial. *JAMA, 293*(21), 2601–2608.
Shear, K. M. (2010). Exploring the role of experiential avoidance from the perspective of attachment theory and the dual process model. *Omega, 61*(4), 357–369.
Shear, K. M. (2015). Complicated grief. *New England Journal of Medicine, 372,* 153–160.
Shear, M. K., Wang, Y., Skritskaya, N., Duan, N., Mauro, C., & Ghesquiere, A. (2014).Treatment of complicated grief in elderly persons: A randomized clinical trial. *JAMA Psychiatry, 71*(11), 1287–1295.
Stroebe, M. S., & Schut, H. (1999). The dual process model of coping with bereavement: Rationale and description. *Death Studies, 23,* 197–224.
Turret, N., & Shear, M. K. (2012). Grief monitoring diary. In R. A. Neimeyer (Ed.), *Techniques of grief therapy: Creative practices for counseling the bereaved*. New York: Routledge/Taylor & Francis Group.

Chapter 23
Triumph Over Tragedy: The Healing Power of Forgiveness

Eva Mozes Kor

Introduction

It was the last week of May 1944, and my family and I had been shoved into a train cattle car along with many other people, so tightly packed like sardines that we could not sit. The car only stopped to refuel, and we were given no food, water, nor rest. The inside of the train was stifling hot. When we stopped to refuel the train, the adults asked the Nazi guards for water. The guards responded that they would provide water to us if five gold watches were given to them. After collecting the watches, the Nazis threw a bucket of water through the window. I held my small cup above my head, but I did not receive more than a few drops. At the time, I wondered why we had to resort to such measures, but I did not dare ask. In retrospect, I believe that people who are scared to death do not verbalize their thoughts. On the third day, when the train had once again stopped to refill, we asked a guard for water. Although we knew that receiving a substantial amount of water was hopeless, this was our only method of receiving information. If we asked and the answer was in a different language, we knew we had crossed into another country. The guard responded in German. Although I was only 10 years old, I instantly realized what had happened, and I believed the end of my life was near. During the previous 4 years, there were rumors around our village that Jews were being sent to Germany to be killed. We did not know when nor how, but our one hope for survival had vanished.

Many people were crying over the next 8 hours. We had stopped once more, and when we asked for water but did not receive a response, I had concluded that we were at our final destination. I was correct. Finally, after 4 days of exhaustion, the doors to the car slammed open. The German Schutzstaffel (SS) guards screamed out "*Schnell! Schnell!*" [Fast! Fast!] and, in a frenzy, we and hundreds of others poured

E. M. Kor (✉)
CANDLES Holocaust Museum and Education Center, 1532 South 3rd Street, Terre Haute, IN 47802, USA
e-mail: evakor@abcs.com

K. E. Cherry (ed.), *Traumatic Stress and Long-Term Recovery*,
DOI 10.1007/978-3-319-18866-9_23

out of the car as they had ordered. Inside the cattle car, my mother, father, and two older sisters had all stayed together. Miriam, my twin sister, and I were holding onto my mother's hands as we stepped down onto the selection platform. There was a lot of noise and confusion, with people crying, orders being shouted, and even dogs barking. I think my mother believed, as long as she held onto our hands, she could protect us. We had been on the platform for 10 minutes when childhood curiosity led me to try and comprehend where we were. As I looked around, I realized that my father and two older sisters had vanished into the crowd. We had not even passed selection yet, but, in the midst of the chaos, we had lost them. I never saw my father and two old sisters again.

Miriam and I gripped even tighter onto our mother's hands, petrified of losing her like we had the rest of our family. Nazi guards began bellowing out for twins. At first, we did not volunteer because we did not know what to expect. A guard saw Miriam and me in our matching burgundy dresses that our mother loved and demanded to know if we were twins. Before answering, my mother asked, "Is that good?" The guard responded affirmatively. As quickly as "yes" was out of her mouth, we were torn away from my mother, with one guard dragging Miriam and me away, while our mother was pulled in the opposite direction. The last memory I have of her is her reaching out her arms in despair, sobbing for her children, as we went separate ways. Miriam and I were very upset. I never got to say goodbye, but, at the time, I did not understand that I would never see my mother again. Within that 30 minute span, Miriam and I were now orphans. We had lost our family forever, our only crime being our Jewish heritage.

Bewildered and all alone, Miriam and I were marched to the other end of the selection platform. We became part of a group of 13 other sets of twins, ages 2 to 16 years. In our group was Mrs. Csengeri and her twin daughters who were close to our age. Mrs. Csengeri owned a shop in a nearby city called Şimleu Silvaniei, Transylvania, and my mother liked to shop there and compare notes with her about raising twin girls. She convinced the Nazi guards that she would be able to provide valuable information about her daughters, so they allowed her to stay with them. We were taken to a huge building where we were immediately forced to remove our clothing. We sat on long benches, naked and afraid, for most of the day. All of the twins were given short haircuts, and Mrs. Csengeri's head was shaved as were the heads of all adult prisoners. When we received our clothes back, a huge, red, oil-painted cross was on the back. We were then lined up for registration and tattooing. When my turn came to be tattooed, I decided I would give the women inmates and guards as much trouble as a 10-year-old could. It took four people, two women prisoners, and two Nazis, to restrain me as they heated a gadget that looked like a ballpoint pen with a needle. Then they pressed into my left arm, dot by dot; they tattooed A-7063. Miriam became A-7064. Auschwitz was the only concentration camp to tattoo its prisoners.

Once our group of twins was processed and tattooed, we were led to our barracks, a modular, wooden horse barn, filthy and crude. I have never encountered a filthier place. The barrack was divided in the middle by a brick bench that ran from the beginning to end of the building. The bench was made of two rows of brick and would prove very useful in the winter. Because the Nazis did not provide any source of heat for us, we would "organize" coal from the Nazis and make a fire in one of the ovens in the barrack, sitting on the brick benches for warmth. We used the term "organizing" because we did not believe a person taking items in order to survive should be classified as a thief.

On each side of the brick bench was a walkway and then three-story high bunk beds. They were covered in a thin straw mattress, and the only linen we received was a soiled blanket. Miriam and I were assigned a bunk bed together on the bottom. After 4 days of not being able to stretch my body, unable to rest, and the sudden separation from my family, I thought I would fall asleep as soon as I shut my eyes. But in my experience, a person who has experienced such a traumatic event cannot function normally. I tossed and turned throughout the night, desperately trying to fall asleep. As I squirmed about, I noticed something large moving in the dark alongside my bed. I slowly counted five figures before jumping out of bed screaming. "Mice! Mice!" I was very scared because I was always scared of mice.

A voice spoke from above me. "Silly kid," another twin answered. "Those are not mice. Those are rats, and you better get used to them, because they are everywhere."

Earlier that night, we had received our first "meal" at Auschwitz. This had consisted of a black liquid in a cup which they called "coffee," and a slice of brown bread. Although Miriam and I had not eaten nor drank for 4 days, we were very religious little girls. We could not eat the bread because it was not kosher, bread that is prepared according to very strict Jewish laws. Miriam and I gave our portions to two girls who were showing us around the barrack. We wanted to remain our father's perfect religious daughters, and we would not violate the strict religious laws.

We were so upset we could not sleep so we went to the latrine. As I entered the latrine, the scattered corpses of three children stared back at me. I had never seen a dead body before. In that latrine, I realized in order to survive Auschwitz, I would have to do everything to stay alive. I made a silent pledge that I would do everything in my power to make sure that Miriam and I would not end up on the filthy latrine floor, and that we would survive and walk out of this camp alive.

Life at Auschwitz

Our daily routine at Auschwitz: Every morning at 5 a.m., we were woken. We helped the toddlers and youngest children put on and lace up their shoes. We never had to worry about helping with clothing because we never took off our clothes. The only possessions any of us had were literally the clothes on our back. By 6 a.m., we were outside for roll call, regardless of season or temperature. In the winter, we were forced to stand throughout multiple blizzards, only wearing the clothes we had arrived in Auschwitz with. After we were counted, we would file back inside the barrack and stand by our bunk bed for Dr. Josef Mengele's daily inspection. Mengele would perform his inspection 6 days a week. He never came on Sundays and that allowed us to know what day of the week it was. Even though we had already been counted outside, Mengele and his entourage of eight people would come in and recount us. At every moment, Mengele wanted to know how many of his guinea pigs were still alive. The first day that Miriam and I were there, Mengele became enraged at the sight of a dead child's body in a bunk bed. I would soon learn that this would become a normal routine: Mengele walks in, sees a dead child and becomes very angry. But I was puzzled as to why. We and the other twins had inferred that Mengele had probably killed our parents, so why was it so important that the children stay alive? Today, I understand. If a child died in the barracks, it was a result of improper conditions, thus eliminating another guinea pig for Mengele's procedures. Mengele did not care if we lived or died in the name of science, but, if arbitrary conditions led to death, he would become very vehement.

Once Mengele would leave, we received our breakfast. Breakfast was nothing more than the brown "coffee" liquid, boiled so it would be safe to drink, but lacking any calories. If we were in the barrack for lunch, we had a substance that is similar to cream of wheat. However, I could not spoon this gooey mush nor could I swallow it. I am convinced that we were only served this as a form of torture because it was impossible to swallow. At night, we would receive our brown bread, and even though it was only about 2.5 inches long, it filled my stomach. After a few days at Auschwitz, I began to learn the routine. I realized that I could sleep at night on an empty stomach, but going the whole day without food was agonizing. I had a tough decision to make. If I saved my bread for the morning, the terrifying rats may steal it, and I would have no bread. Although Mengele supposedly wanted his twins to survive until they were in his hands, we twins were not given our bread for breakfast like workers in the camp were.

After breakfast on Mondays, Wednesdays, and Fridays, we were marched to the two-story buildings that were Auschwitz I. Every time, we were placed naked in one of the barracks alongside approximately 50 other sets of twins. For 8 hours a day, we were forced to stand or sit naked. Every part of my body was measured and then compared to my twin sister, noting how we were alike and different, and how close we were to the Aryan race that Hitler so desired. These "experiments" were not dangerous, but they were incredibly demeaning. Even in Auschwitz, I could not cope with the fact that I had been reduced to the lowest form of human existence—just a mass of breathing, living cells.

On Tuesdays, Thursdays, and Saturdays, we were taken to another building which I called "the blood lab." There, they would draw blood from my left arm while I received a minimum of five injections in my right arm—concurrently. The contents of the injections were unknown to us at the time and are still unknown to this day. They were rumored to be drugs, germs, and diseases, and I believe this to be true. The Kaiser Wilhelm Institute for Human Genetics, and Eugenics, a prestigious German research institution, had been conducting a study on twins since 1920. Before the war, volunteers had been recruited through the newspaper, and noninvasive, observational notes were taken. If a volunteer decided to not participate, they simply stopped. In 1937, Mengele, who held both an MD as well as a Ph.D. in anthropology joined the staff of the institute, very excited to work with twins. However, in 1939, all German men were drafted, and Mengele was sent to the Russian front lines where he was injured in 1942 and sent back to Berlin to recover.

In 1943, he was declared unfit for battle; he visited his former advisor, Dr. Otmar von Verschuer, an expert in eugenics, the science of selective breeding. While von Verscheur wanted to eliminate mental diseases like schizophrenia, Hitler wanted to utilize eugenics to create a pure Aryan race. When Mengele returned to von Verscheur, his advisor lamented that since the war began, no twins were volunteering for the study. So the two doctors thought that there were many twins on the incoming cattle cars. As soon as the major German pharmaceutical companies heard about Mengele's plans, money began to pour in for Mengele to run experiments.

Surviving and Defeating Mengele

One day, in August, after receiving an injection, I became very ill with an incredibly high fever I desperately tried to hide. There were rumors that twins who were taken to the hospital never made it back to the barrack, and I myself had seen some twins disappearing. If one twin went to the hospital, the other twin vanished as well. This meant that they had been murdered. Instead of receiving injections that day, my temperature was taken, and I knew I was in serious trouble. In the blazing August sun, my body trembled and shook. My arms and legs were extremely swollen and painful, and red spots covered my body. I was taken to the hospital, another barrack filled with people who looked more dead than alive. The next morning, Mengele came up to my bed with four other doctors. He looked at my fever chart, laughed sarcastically, and declared, "Too bad she's so young. She only has two weeks to live." I was conscious enough to realize he was right, but I would not give up. I made my second silent pledge to survive my illness and return back to the barrack to be reunited with Miriam. For the next 2 weeks, I only have one recollection. In the hospital barrack, food and water were not given out, as the Nazis did not want to waste on people who would die. All I could do was to crawl to the other end of the barrack where a faucet with water was located. On my hands and knees I trudged through the filthy floors, fading in and out of consciousness. Delirious, malnourished, and very ill, I had but one thought in my mind: I must survive. I must survive. *I must survive.*

After 2 weeks, my fever broke, and I knew I had defeated Mengele. Me, a 10-year-old girl, had the power and will to defeat the Angel of Death himself. When I was finally allowed to return to my old barrack and to my sister, I was concerned. Miriam looked very sick. I asked her what had happened to her, and she responded, "I cannot talk about it, and I will not talk about it." It would not be until 1985 that Miriam and I finally discussed our experiences at Auschwitz with one another.

The next day, I volunteered to be a food carrier from the kitchen to our barrack. I volunteered because I knew I would have an opportunity to organize raw potatoes. At Auschwitz, raw potatoes became our medicine for every illness. When I walked into the kitchen, I saw the potatoes sitting there. I knew people had been hanged for being caught stealing, but if I did not organize these potatoes, Miriam would die. I decided to conquer my fear and take two potatoes. As I bent down, somebody grabbed the back of my dress and hair and began yelling into my face, "It's not nice to steal." I nearly burst out laughing. Here, I thought I would be killed for my crime, but instead I received a slap on the wrist. I learned an important lesson in Auschwitz that day. As long as Mengele wanted us alive, no one dared harm us. I left my fear of organizing behind and became the happy owner of three raw potatoes. We would fill cups with water, place a potato inside, and boil them in our barrack ovens. I became a very good organizer, allowing us to have potatoes three to four times a week. The steady diet of potatoes gave Miriam the strength to continue to survive.

Miriam's Hardships

In 1985, as Miriam and I began to finally talk about Auschwitz, my sister revealed what had happened to her when I was in the infirmary. She told me that she was kept in isolation for 2 weeks under 24 hour supervision. They were waiting for something to happen, but I spoiled the experiment. I survived. Later on, I found out that if I were to die, Miriam would have been instantly killed via an injection to the heart, and Mengele would have performed comparative autopsies on my diseased organs versus Miriam's "healthy" ones. Miriam went on to explain that after the 2 weeks, she was taken back to the blood lab and injected with many different substances that made her quite ill. After the war ended, we would find out that Miriam was much weaker than me. In 1960, while expecting her first child, Miriam had a severe kidney infection that would not respond to antibiotics. In 1963, she had a second child, with her kidney infection becoming worse. After examining Miriam, the doctors concluded that her kidneys were malfunctioning because they had never grown larger than an average 10-year old's kidneys. For the sake of her health, I begged her not to have a third child, but she did, and her kidneys started to rapidly deteriorate. By 1987, her only options were either a lifetime of dialysis or a kidney transplant. Being her twin sister with two functioning kidneys, the choice was easy. On November 16, 1987, I donated my left kidney to my sister. Unfortunately, Miriam was the only individual out of 2000 successful transplants to develop cancerous polyps in the bladder a year after the transplant. The doctors were very puzzled and stated that if we could find the files of what we were injected with at Auschwitz, an antidote might be possible. I do not know to this day what we were injected with. Mengele's files have never been found. On June 6, 1993, my twin sister, Miriam, passed away. Out of the 1500 sets of twins who were in the experiments, only around 200 individuals survived (a 6% survival rate).

A Child Coping in Auschwitz

Many people have asked me how, as a 10-year-old child, I could survive and cope in a place like Auschwitz. First, I must explain that children cope differently than teenagers and adults. When I was in Auschwitz, I thought the whole world was a concentration camp, with everybody in the world living like we were—miserable, orphaned, and malnourished, surrounded by Nazi guards day and night. Children lose their point of reference very quickly. In order for a child to survive, they have to exert more energy than an adult because they cannot project hope forwards nor can they project backwards. A child functions only in the moment.

In August 1944, I heard a lot of planes flying above us, but very low. One of the planes had an American flag, and that provided me with the hope and determination to survive one more day, suffer through one more experiment. Hope in Auschwitz was in very limited supply, so I grasped onto that picture of the American flag and kept on fighting. By the end of September, we were experiencing two air raids a day. In my childlike innocence, I thought that the good guys must be winning, and the bad guys, the Nazis, were losing. My childhood intuition proved me right. Suddenly, the experiments dropped from 6 days a week to 5 days a week. By October, the air raids increased to three a day, and our experiments once again were reduced to 4 days a week. In November, we were receiving up to four air raids a day, and our experiments completely stopped. Our camp was like a continuous battlefield, with explosions and gunshots happening more often than not. Once again, I found hope in this. Although I was only a child, I truly believed the war could not go on much longer like this. Someday soon, we would be free, and we would go home.

In early January of 1945, the Nazis told us after the evening meal to evacuate the barracks to go deep into Germany to "protect us from the fighting." My childhood logic led me to believe that if the Nazis were winning the war and they were mean, I certainly did not want to go on a march with them when they were losing. Besides, it was bitterly cold weather, and the only clothes I possessed were the ragged and torn ones I brought to Auschwitz 8 months before. We decided in our barrack that it would be safer to stay inside. Later on, this march would be described as "the death march." I have asked survivors why they left the camp to go on the march when they could have stayed behind and not suffered. I was surprised to find out that Nazi guards had come into the barrack, held a gun to their head, and forced an evacuation. Due to what can only be described as a guardian angel, no Nazis ever came into our barrack. The next morning when we woke up, I opened our barrack door and cautiously peeked outside. There were no guards to be found in the towers. All the Nazis were gone. It was just us prisoners left. The adults who had stayed behind cut through the barbed fence so we could go in between camps, trying to organize blankets, water, and bread.

One day when I was in the kitchen trying to organize loaves of bread, I heard the strange noise of a car. Puzzled, because no one had cars except the Nazis, I stepped outside to investigate. A Nazi jeep pulled up and four Nazi guards jumped out, immediately spraying the area and the people around with their machine gun bullets. The last thing I remembered was seeing the barrel of the gun pointed at my head. I soon collapsed. When I woke up some time later, I tried to feel my arms and my legs. Looking around, I could see piles of bodies surrounding me. I touched a girl next to me and was surprised to find she was ice cold. I understood then that I had not died. Somehow, I had fainted before any of the bullets were able to hit me. Hurrying back to Miriam, I told her what happened. We wondered why the

Nazis had come back. That night, the Nazis tried to destroy all evidence of their war crimes. The gas chambers were blown up and our barracks set on fire. As we escaped from the barrack, the same four Nazi guards who had almost taken my life earlier caught us. They ordered us to march, and if anyone did not march fast enough, they were immediately shot and killed.

We were forced to march to Auschwitz I, where the two-story buildings were located. Miriam and I ran to the buildings as soon as we saw them for our safety. The Nazis could not take us any further into Germany because the Allies were outside the city limits. For the next 9 days, we hid in the buildings, listening to the very heavy fighting outside. We needed water desperately. We were on our own. The Nazis no longer controlled the camp. I went to the nearby river, broke the ice, and lowered a container tied to a string. When I looked across the river, I saw a girl about Miriam's age and my age. She was not in torn rags like we were. She wore a beautiful dress like the kind our mother used to have made for us. She had long braids with ribbons. What really shocked me the most; she was carrying a school bag. In my 10-year-old mind, I had believed everyone in the world was in a concentration camp under Nazi rule. This naivety was shattered. This was my first realization that beyond the camp, there were children who looked like children, who had parents, clothes, food, and went to school. The only school I had attended for the past 8 to 9 months was the school of survival.

Liberation

A few days later, when we awoke, an eerie silence had fallen over the camp. It was Saturday, January 27, 1945. We knew deep down that something was going to happen, but we had no idea how or where it would occur. In the late afternoon, a woman came running into our barracks yelling, "We are free! We are free!" While this was very exciting to hear, as I peered down from the second-story building, I could see nothing. Miriam and I walked outside to get a closer look. Snow was falling heavily and made it challenging to see. I stood in that spot for 30 minutes when in the distance I could make out lots of people, all wrapped in white camouflage raincoats. As they came closer, I could see very big smiles on their faces, and the most important part: These were not Nazis. Miriam and I ran up to the Soviet soldiers, and they gave us cookies, chocolate, and hugs. This was my first taste of freedom. The silent pledges I had made to myself became a reality: Miriam and I had survived Auschwitz, and we would walk out hand in hand as planned.[1]

[1] For the next few days, the Soviets surveyed the camp and brought in huge cameras in order to film us. They wanted to have photographs and films of the Soviets liberating us. An iconic picture of Miriam and I marching in the front was taken, albeit posed. Any time a photo was taken, it was a staged event: We were already free. I have a hard time believing that any liberation photos taken by the Allies were not staged events. We, the victims, hid until we absolutely knew who was coming from the other side.

Life Lessons

I have told my story of my experience at Auschwitz to many people. Every time I share my story, it is because I want the people I am sharing with to learn my "life lessons." I call them that because I have learned them throughout my life.

1. **Never Give Up on Yourself or Your Dreams**
   As I lecture to many young people, I can sympathize with their struggle to find their place in the world, regardless of where or how they grew up. When I was a teenager, you would have never convinced me that I could someday lecture and write to an audience of thousands of people. I encourage everyone who is reading this to persevere through their troubles and make a serious effort to accomplish their goals and dreams. If I had not actively fought to live through Auschwitz, I would not be alive today. You can accomplish anything if you truly try hard enough.

2. **Do Not Judge a Person Based on Prejudice**
   Hitler's rise to power was based on prejudicial judgments. Bad economies cause genocides, and, before World War II, Germany's unemployment rate was at 33 %. Thus, Hitler found a scapegoat—the Jews. However, taking a minority and attributing them to the cause of the economic slump does not solve the actual problem.
   I encourage every American to exercise their human responsibility and vote. Inform yourself before voting, and find a candidate who will have both solutions for the economy and strict policies that advocate and practice human rights.

3. **Forgive Your Worst Enemy and Everyone Who Has Hurt You: It Will Heal You and Set Your Soul Free**
   After liberation, I was a good victim. I was angry at the world, I hated everyone, and I yelled a lot. As I mentioned earlier, Miriam had passed away on June 6, 1993. I founded the organization, CANDLES, an acronym for Children of Auschwitz Nazi Deadly Lab Experiments Survivors in March of 1984 to locate surviving Mengele twins. I founded the CANDLES Holocaust Museum and Education Center in April of 1995, 2 years after Miriam's death. While still mourning, I was invited by Dr. Mihalchick to speak at a conference at Boston College about Nazi medicine. He had one request though: to bring a Nazi doctor along with me! I asked him incredulously, "And where do you think I'll find a Nazi doctor? Last I checked, they were not advertising in the Yellow Pages." He laughed but encouraged me to use my resources to find somebody. I remembered a documentary I worked on together with Miriam where they included footage from a Dr. Hans Münch, a Nazi doctor who was still living in Germany. Through the production company, I asked for Dr. Münch's telephone number. Would he meet with me in the memory of my late sister, Miriam? He agreed and I was heading to Germany to meet a Nazi doctor.

An array of emotions filled me as I prepped for the trip. What if that man treated me like the other Nazis had treated me? Although it had been nearly 50 years since liberation, I felt a fear deep inside I had not felt for many years. What if reliving the experience was too traumatizing? I tried to put these worries aside. To my surprise, Dr. Münch was nothing but gracious towards me. We talked for many hours. Right away, I asked about Mengele's experiments. Dr. Münch responded that he did not know much, unfortunately. Mengele had declared the information "top secret" and not many Nazi associates viewed the files. Suddenly, I found myself asking him if he knew of the details of the gas chambers. He looked at me and said solemnly, "That is the nightmare I have to live with every day." I learned that while Dr. Münch was not a part of the selection process (he refused to do so), his job was to look in the peephole of the gas chamber, verify that the bodies were perished, and sign the mass death certificates. I was taken aback. Since 1978, I had been actively involved in Holocaust research, and I had never read anything like he told me. The words came out of my mouth without hesitation: "Dr. Münch, will you accompany me to Auschwitz?" I explained how I was going back for the 50th anniversary of the liberation of the camp. I wanted Dr. Münch to sign a statement at the gas chambers in the company of witnesses so no Holocaust denier could say that he did not sign the form. He eagerly agreed.

Beginning of the Healing

When Dr. Münch agreed to accompany me to Auschwitz, I felt an overwhelming sense of gratitude. But how does one go about thanking a Nazi doctor? I thought and struggled for 10 months in trying to find a meaningful gift for Dr. Münch, then it popped in my mind that I could give him a letter of forgiveness. With the help of my former English professor, I carefully crafted a letter of amnesty, forgiving Dr. Münch for his part in the Holocaust. During one revision, my professor stated, "Eva, you need to think about forgiving Dr. Mengele, too." Forgiving Mengele? This was not in my plans. Did I have the power within myself to forgive the person who nearly killed me and my sister?

On January 27, 1995, I walked hand in hand with Dr. Münch through the gates of Auschwitz. With our families by our sides, I read my declaration of amnesty, and Dr. Münch signed his statement by the ruins of gas chambers. Almost instantly, I could feel the emotional wounds starting to lift and heal. I had the power to forgive, and no one could take that from me. In that moment, I realized that I could forgive *everyone* who had hurt me, for there was no reason to hold unnecessary pain. In my declaration of amnesty, I forgave all of the Nazis for their war crimes. In my heart, I was finally able to forgive my parents for not saving us from Auschwitz.

Not all survivors were happy with my declaration. Some questioned how I could possibly forgive the Nazis when so many people had perished at their hands. I explained to them that my forgiveness was coming from me—no one else. If I were to forgive on behalf of all survivors and victims, there would be no benefit to them. When it comes to forgiveness, you, the individual, have the power. Unlike the traditional sense of forgiveness, my forgiveness does not involve contact with the perpetrator. They could be alive or dead, but it does not matter because this healing experience is for me the victim. You are not hurting the perpetrator; rather, you are reclaiming the power that they had taken away from you. Everyone has the human right to live free from the pain of the past.

How to Forgive

I receive many letters and e-mails from people inquiring how to go about forgiving someone. I tell everyone the same thing. First, you must remove yourself from the situation in which you are a victim. Now, I know that this is not easy for every person, such as children who are being abused by their parents. But in order to truly forgive and accept your past, it cannot be in the present. You cannot subject yourself to constant torment and forgive at the same time.

Second, take your feelings and emotions and put them on paper. Writing a letter to the person(s) you are trying to forgive can be difficult and time-consuming, but that is okay. When you write your letter, you want to be completely honest with the person who hurt you. If you are angry and mad, write *why* you are feeling these emotions. Remember, the other person never has to see this letter. This is for you.

Lastly, you must realize that you, and you only, have the power to forgive. As I said before, this interaction is not two-way. The person(s) who hurt you do not need to know that you are forgiving them, nor do they need to accept the forgiveness. By declaring forgiveness, you are rising above the other person and stating that they are no longer in control or influence of your life. You are the only person who will lead your life, and no one will ever take that power away from you again.

Benefits to Forgiveness

I believe that society could greatly benefit from my form of forgiveness. Rather than always seeking vengeance and justice, why not try forgiveness? After the war ended, our country was so focused on prosecuting the Nazis that little information was gleaned from them. If Mengele had testified, perhaps we would know what Miriam had been injected with, along with other twins who had developed illnesses as a result of their time at Auschwitz. We also could have information on the studies Mengele was supposedly conducting as well. But as of today, we do not have that information because of our thirst for retribution.

Many survivors of traumatic events carry their pain with them because they have not been given a chance to speak. I believe this is true of many Holocaust survivors. By not telling your story, you are keeping others uninformed and unenlightened. By lecturing to others, I have given thousands of people an insight to a terrible thing that they never want to happen again. That is another misconception people have with forgiveness—you do not forget what happened to you. How can anyone forget an event that changed your life forever? Best of all, forgiveness is free! You do not have to pay a single thing to start the healing process. And if you do not like how you feel after you forgive someone, you can always take your pain back. However, in my many years of telling people this philosophy and having them enact it in their own lives, I have never had a single person tell me they wanted to take back their pain.

In conclusion, I think forgiveness helps break the cycle of victims creating victims. You see, when people do not forgive, they keep their pain and trauma with them, and they pass it down through generations. By forgiving, the line of hurt stops. I would like to look at the world someday and see what I see in myself now—an empowered individual who took control over the events in her life. I desire to see a world with a lot fewer victims. Forgiveness gives us power over our life. We are in control over our feelings today and tomorrow. It removes the power and hold the perpetrator had over the victim. Therefore, forgiveness is the best revenge. It is a gift I give myself. Anger is a seed for war. Forgiveness is a seed for peace.

Acknowledgments This chapter was prepared based on a transcript of public lecture sponsored by the Louisiana State University (LSU) Life Course and Aging Center and LSU School of Social Work on March 20, 2014, in Baton Rouge, Louisiana, USA. I wish to thank Katie E. Stanko for her assistance in preparing this chapter.

Sources

CANDLES Holocaust Museum and Education Center. (n.d.). http://www.candlesholocaustmuseum.org/. 1 October 2014.

Eva Kor—The Triumph of the Human Spirit [Video file]. (2014, March 20). Retrieved from https://www.youtube.com/watch?v=ijsKCSr5U5o. 1 October 2014.

Hercules, B., & Media Process Educational Films. (2005). *Forgiving Dr. Mengele*. Brooklyn: First Run/Icarus Films.

Kor, E. M. (2013, August 31). Interview by K. E. Cherry. [Transcript].

Kor, E. M. (2014, September 26). Interview by K. E. Stanko. [Transcript].

Rojany-Buccieri, L., & Kor, E. M. (2012). *Surviving the angel of death: The true story of a Mengele twin in Auschwitz*. Terre Haute: Tanglewood.

Index

K. E. Cherry (ed.), *Traumatic Stress and Long-Term Recovery*,
DOI 10.1007/978-3-319-18866-9

I

J

T

MIX
Papier aus verantwortungsvollen Quellen
Paper from responsible sources
FSC® C105338

If you have any concerns about our products,
you can contact us on
ProductSafety@springernature.com

In case Publisher is established outside the EU,
the EU authorized representative is:
Springer Nature Customer Service Center GmbH
Europaplatz 3, 69115 Heidelberg, Germany

Printed by Libri Plureos GmbH
in Hamburg, Germany